MACLEOD'S

CLINICAL EXAMINATION

The Editors

John F Munro OBE FRCPE FRCP(Glasg) FRCP

Formerly Consultant Physician,
Eastern General Hospital, Edinburgh;
Honorary Fellow, Faculty of Medicine,
University of Edinburgh

Ian W Campbell MB ChB FRCPE FRCP(Glasg)

Consultant Physician,
Victoria Hospital,
Kirkcaldy, Fife;
Honorary Professor,
Department of Biological and Medical Sciences,
University of St Andrews, Fife

CHURCHILL LIVINGSTONE

EDINBURGH LONDON NEW YORK OXFORD PHILADELPHIA ST LOUIS SYDNEY TORONTO 2000

TENTH EDITION

MACLEOD'S CLINICAL EXAMINATION

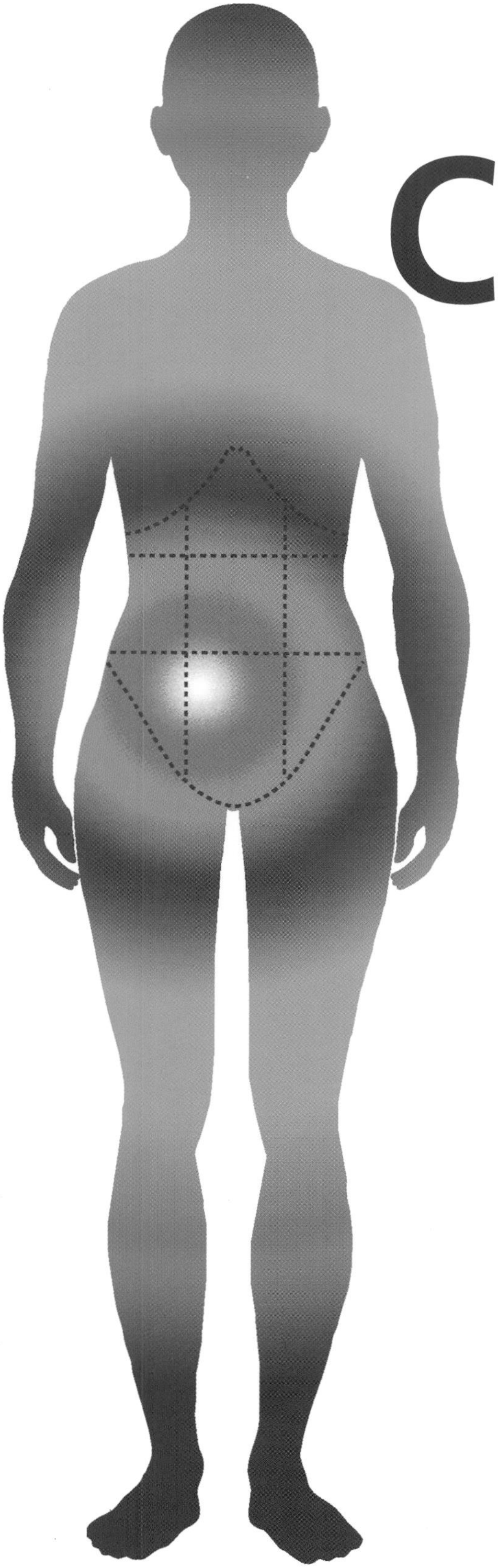

CHURCHILL LIVINGSTONE
An imprint of Elsevier Limited

First edition	1964	Sixth edition	1983
Second edition	1967	Seventh edition	1986
Third edition	1973	Eighth edition	1990
Fourth edition	1976	Ninth edition	1995
Fifth edition	1979	Tenth edition	2000

ISBN 0 443 061726
Reprinted 2001, 2002, 2003 (twice)
International Student Edition 0 443 061866
Reprinted 2000, 2001, 2002, 2003 (twice)

British Library of Cataloguing in Publication Data
A catalogue record for this book is available from the British Library

Library of Congress Cataloging in Publication Data
A catalog record for this book is available from the Library of Congress

Medical knowledge is constantly changing. As information becomes available, changes in treatment, procedures, equipment and the use of drugs become necessary. The author and publishers have, as far as it is possible, taken care to ensure that the information given in this text is accurate and up to date. However, readers are strongly advised to confirm that the information, especially with regard to drug usage, complies with current legislation and standards of practice.

Printed in China
C/05/06

Commissioning editor: Laurence Hunter
Project development manager: Barbara Simmons
Project manager: Nancy Arnott
Designer: Erik Bigland
Illustrations by: Robert Britton and Hardlines

Preface

The practice of medicine is constantly changing. Some diseases are controlled, or even eradicated, while others increase in frequency and significance. New diagnostic techniques are developed and therapeutic regimens introduced. There is an increasing awareness of the importance of preventative medicine within the community, and also of the special needs of patients, relatives and carers. The tenth edition of this textbook is designed to keep abreast with changes in medical practice and to maintain the impetus for change in medical education.

This new edition has provided a further opportunity to alter the previous text extensively. Nine new contributors have joined the balanced team of specialists in medicine and surgery. Professor I.W. Campbell has replaced Professor C.R. Edwards as an editor.

The book has been extensively rewritten and numerous new sections have been added, for example the use of case histories to illustrate important aspects of clinical examination. There is an additional chapter on case history recording. The introduction of colour throughout the book has provided the opportunity to add new tables and figures as well as making increased use of clinical photographs.

The basic aim of the book remains unchanged, namely to describe the various skills involved in taking a history, performing a physical examination and providing the patient with an explanation. These are attributes that every clinician requires in order to form satisfactory relationships with patients and to manage them appropriately. The book is intended to complement the information available in standard surgical and medical textbooks.

Throughout the book emphasis is placed on the method of obtaining an accurate history and of performing a physical examination appropriate to the clinical problem. The main chapters conform to a basic pattern. Each starts by describing the relevant symptoms and by discussing their significance. The normal findings in physical examination are detailed and related to important aspects of applied anatomy and physiology. The examination sequence is then described in detail. Thereafter, the relevance of abnormal signs is discussed. Investigations are described only to illustrate the approach to the diagnostic process. Throughout the text 'key points' are highlighted.

The book is intended primarily for undergraduates in their clinical years. It has also proved to be of value to general practitioners and postgraduates, particularly for those working for a higher clinical examination or returning to clinical medicine after a period of research or working in a highly specialised field.

The tenth edition of *Macleod's Clinical Examination* is closely integrated with *Davidson's Principles and Practice of Medicine*, both at an editorial level and with shared contributors, and both titles have established a wide international appeal

Edinburgh — J.F.M.
2000 — I.W.C.

Acknowledgements

The editors are very grateful to all the past contributors and editors of the previous editions and in particular acknowledge their continuing debt to Dr John Macleod. The editors have received generous help from many sources and are grateful to those students and doctors from all over the world who have provided constructive suggestions towards the development of the book.

The editors wish to thank Ian Ramsden for taking the examination photographs in this edition. They are also indebted to Jamie Ramsden, Lyndsay MacMillan and Janice Urquhart for acting as the clinical models, and to Dr Caroline Providence, Dr Catriona Duncan and Dr Elizabeth Arnold and various others for their assistance with the photographic sessions. We also thank Robert Britton and Hardlines for producing the line drawings.

Acknowledgements are made in the text to the source of the original photographs which have been kindly provided.

Finally, the editors wish to thank Laurence Hunter, commissioning editor, and Barbara Simmons, project development manager, at Harcourt. Their cheerful support and encouragement was greatly appreciated.

Contributors

Peter J Abernethy MB ChB FRCSE
Formerly Consultant Orthopaedic Surgeon, Royal Infirmary and Princess Margaret Rose Orthopaedic Hospital, Edinburgh

Elaine D C Anderson MB ChB BSc (Hons) FRCSE MD
Consultant Surgeon, Breast Unit, Western General Hospital, Edinburgh

Andrew W Bradbury BSc MD FRCSE
Professor of Vascular Surgery, University of Birmingham, Birmingham

Nicki R Colledge BSc MB ChB FRCPE
Consultant Geriatrician, Liberton Hospital and Royal Infirmary, Edinburgh; Honorary Senior Lecturer, Department of Medicine, University of Edinburgh, Edinburgh

Graham K Crompton MB ChB FRCPE
Formerly Consultant Physician, Respiratory Diseases Unit, Western General Hospital, Edinburgh; Formerly Part-time Senior Lecturer, University Departments of Medicine, Western General Hospital and Royal Infirmary, Edinburgh

Roger E Cull BSc (Hons) PhD MB ChB FRCPE
Consultant Clinical Neurophysiologist, Western General Hospital; Honorary Senior Lecturer in Clinical Neurosciences, University of Edinburgh, Edinburgh

Allan Cumming MB ChB MD FRCP
Senior Lecturer and Honorary Consultant Physician, Department of Medicine; Associate Dean (Teaching), Faculty of Medicine, University of Edinburgh, Edinburgh

Michael J Ford MB ChB (Hons) MD FRCPE
Consultant Physician, Western General Hospital, Edinburgh; Clinical Sub-Dean and Part-time Senior Lecturer, Faculty of Medicine, University of Edinburgh, Edinburgh

John A A Hunter OBE BA MD FRCPE
Formerly Professor of Dermatology, University of Edinburgh, Edinburgh

Nigel Peter Hurst MB BS PhD(Edin) FRCPE
Consultant Rheumatologist, Lothian University Hospitals NHS Trust, Edinburgh

Margaret J MacDonald FRCSE FRCOphth
Consultant Ophthalmologist, Queen Margaret Hospital, Dunfermline, Fife and Victoria Hospital, Kirkcaldy, Fife

George Masterton BSc MD FRCPsych
Consultant Psychiatrist and Honorary Senior Lecturer, Royal Infirmary, Edinburgh

John J V McMurray BSc (Hons) MB ChB(Hons) MD FRCPE FESC FACC
Professor of Cardiology, University of Glasgow; Consultant Cardiologist, Western Infirmary, Glasgow

David Northridge MB FRCP
Consultant Cardiologist and Honorary Senior Lecturer, Western General Hospital, Edinburgh

Anthony Toft BSc MD FRCPE FRCP(Glasg) FRCP
Consultant Physician, Royal Infirmary, Edinburgh

Ian R Whittle MD PhD FRACS FRCSE
Forbes Professor of Surgical Neurology and Honorary Consultant Neurosurgeon, University of Edinburgh and Department of Clinical Neurosciences, Western General Hospital, Edinbugh

Contents

MACLEOD'S
CLINICAL
EXAMINATION

The principles of a clinical examination

1

G. MASTERTON • A.D. TOFT

CLINICAL EXAMINATION

The public is fascinated by developments in Medicine, whether these comprise better understanding of disease, sophicated investigations or new drugs. What is probably more directly relevant to patients is the less dramatic evolution in the manner in which doctors examine and communicate with patients. These changes have occurred partly in response to increasing knowledge about the consultation process and partly because of patients' expectations. These shifts in emphasis in the training of doctors for the 21st century go to the heart of the consultation process.

Phases of a clinical examination

A clinical examination has three phases (Table 1.1). The relative weighting given to each element varies, depending on the nature of the problem and the time available, but this structure is basic to all clinical consultations. However, the skilled clinician is forming an impression of the patient and seeking clinical clues from the moment of first meeting the patient. For example, a 55-year-old man, visiting his daughter and her children, attended the daughter's general practitioner to obtain a repeat prescription for his wife's hormone-replacement therapy. The doctor noticed unduly prominent arterial pulsations in his neck. He wondered if the man might have significant incompetence of the aortic valve and that his occupation and life-style were sedentary. The visitor insisted that he was well. However, the clinician persuaded him to take off his shirt. On auscultation the doctor confirmed his initial assessment. With a little knowledge of cultural habits and disease patterns it is possible to paint an accurate picture, simply by observation, and such an approach makes the practice of medicine even more interesting and more stimulating.

Importance of good interview technique

The ability to elicit an accurate history from the patient is crucial. It is the history which provides the basis for priorities in the clinical examination and subsequent investigation, and management. The style of obtaining a history leads to the therapeutic alliance between doctor and patient – so essential for establishing trust and satisfaction (Fig. 1.1).

TABLE 1.1 The phases of a clinical examination

	Title	Purpose
Phase 1	History-taking	Information gathering
Phase 2	Examination: physical and mental	Objective findings
Phase 3	Explanation	Information giving, decision making

Some people are naturally better communicators than others. Useful assets are listed in Table 1.2. From the patient's perspective the most important component of the clinical examination is the explanation. Clinicians who are courteous and patient, appear interested, encourage patients and relatives to ask questions and who spend time explaining the situation in a way which is understood, are judged to be 'good doctors' irrespective of their other attributes. Most patients and relatives will respect a clinician who tells them that a mistake has occurred much more than one who tries to conceal an error. Indeed most complaints about doctors are attributable, at least in part, to poor communication. All clinicians can improve their communication skills by practice and experience, especially if they make a positive effort to learn from their own mistakes and those of their colleagues. Support and encouragement will assist those with weaknesses in their inter-personal skills, supplemented as necessary by counselling, the use of role play and simulated interviews. With help and effort, an effective clinical technique can be established which will not only advantage patients, but also enhance professional fulfilment.

Role of the student

Medical students are expected to learn and to practise history-taking and examination techniques. They should take every opportunity to observe, when appropriate, the phase of explanation. However, this element is best conducted by qualified doctors who are responsible for the patient's care. If students are asked by a patient to give a medical opinion, they should remind the patient of their status and either suggest that the inquiry is redirected to the doctor or offer to raise that concern with the doctor.

PREPARATION

The setting

Patients attending the general practitioner will either be seen at home or in the surgery. In hospital, although teaching may be ward-based, most examinations take place in consulting rooms. Privacy is a key requirement for all clinical examinations, which can be difficult in a ward setting. If the patient can get up then it is preferable to conduct the examination in an office or a single room. If a bed-bound patient has to be interviewed there may be no alternative to pulling the curtains at the beginning of the interview. This will obscure vision but not sound. Other patients may unavoidably be eavesdropping, so it is important to proceed by talking in as quiet a voice as possible to enable understanding and by avoiding discussing sensitive topics unnecessarily.

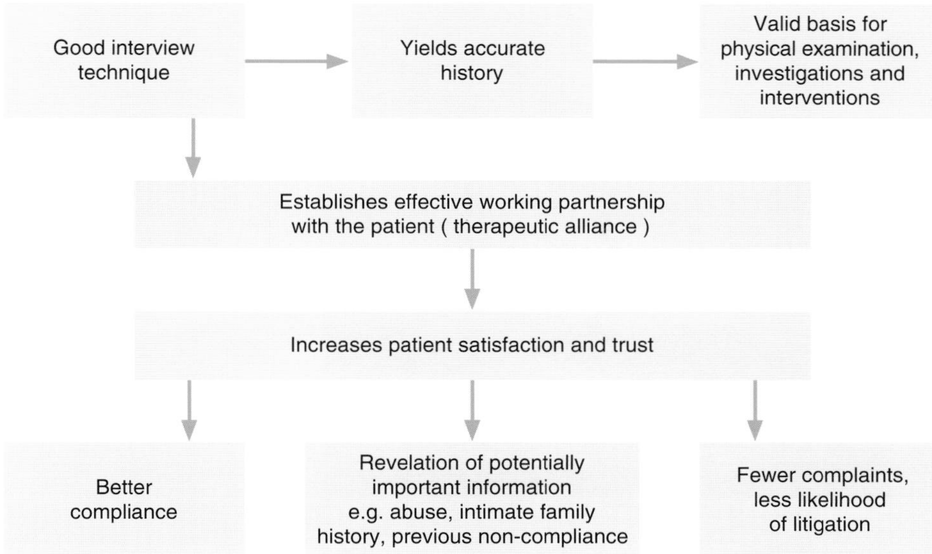

Fig. 1.1 Benefits of good interview technique.

TABLE 1.2 Assets valuable for obtaining a good clinical history

- *Being empathic* – having the capacity to put yourself in somebody else's shoes, to understand and share the patient's thoughts and feelings
- *Being an attentive listener* – the quality that patients rate as the most important attribute in a doctor from their perspective
- *Being articulate* – recognising when to speak, what to say and how to express it
- *Being a good nonverbal communicator* – using body language appropriately and responding to nonverbal cues from the patient
- *Being friendly* – rather than businesslike
- *Being interested in other people* – and enthusiastic if a student

The ambience, arrangement of furniture and relative positions of patient and doctor all matter in facilitating communication. The aim is to establish a comfortable, relaxed, quiet and friendly environment which enables rapport to develop and the patient to talk.

Ideally doctor and patient should be seated about 1 metre apart on similar chairs which are positioned in such a way that the doctor can observe the patient but the patient can look away without awkwardness (Figs 1.2, 1.3 and 1.4).

The arrangements should allow the clinician to write during the interview. Doctors develop a style of interviewing which suits them best. Some record detailed notes during the consultation, others take rough notes as aides-mémoire, whilst some write little or nothing at the time but record the content as soon as the patient has left. There are advantages and disadvantages with any technique. During training it is useful to take detailed notes while the patient is being seen. This enables the record to be more complete and accurate. However, it is necessary to learn how to do this without damaging rapport, and it is important to recognise that the consultation demands that full concentration is paid to the patient. Writing should temporarily cease, for instance, with the revelation of sensitive information or signs of distress or irritation.

Time

In General Practice a consultation of 5–10 minutes is usually adequate because the family doctor will have seen the patient on previous occasions. The doctor will not only be familiar with the past and social history, but may also have cared for other members of the family and household. In hospital the appointment time of new outpatients will depend upon the nature of the speciality and the patient's problem. It may be as much as 2–3 hours in child psychiatry.

It is important to plan the consultation to the time available. To fail to do so may result in other patients being kept waiting, thereby diminishing the value of their consultations. When a problem arises that clearly requires much more than the allocated time, it may be advisable to arrange a further consultation.

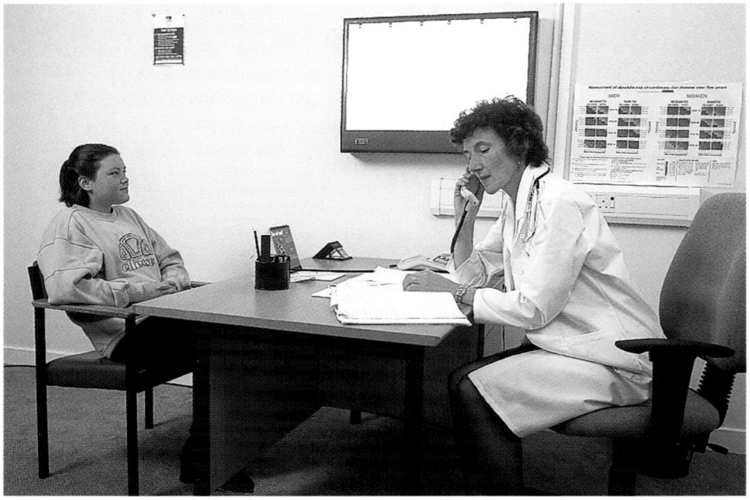

Fig. 1.2 The desk as a defence mechanism. Note also the failure to give the patient full attention, the stethoscope and white coat and the illuminated viewing box.

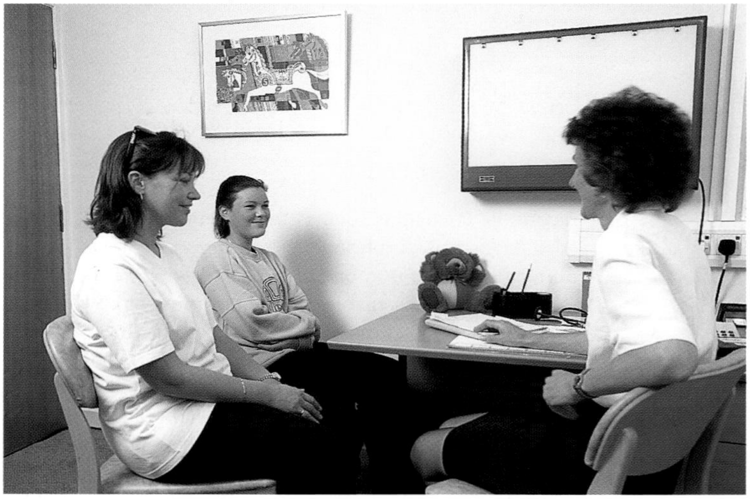

Fig. 1.3 A more appropriate arrangement of doctor and patient designed to put the patient at ease. Note the eye contact, the presence of the patient's mother, the picture and the 'cuddly toy'.

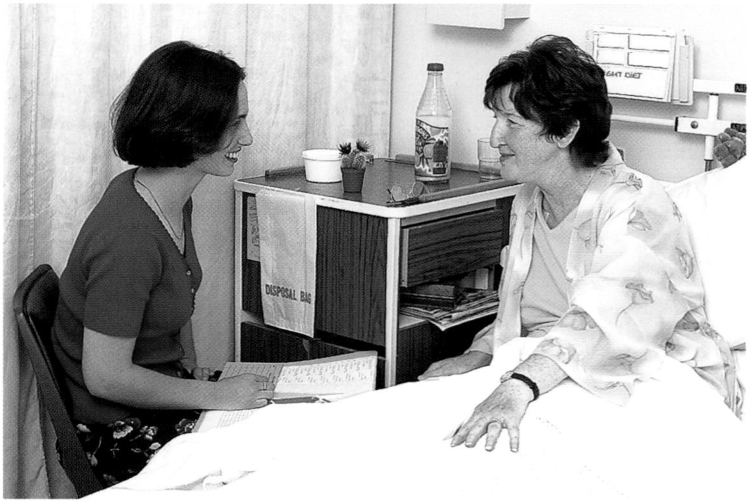

Fig. 1.4 Appropriate arrangement of doctor and patient for a bedside interview.

Appearance and demeanour

Many patients are influenced by how doctors and students present themselves. The medical profession retains a respected status in society. People may be put off if their doctor does not conform to their expectations. Invariably different people have different preconceptions of how they expect clinicians to behave and to dress. In hospital, patients and relatives appreciate doctors, and other hospital staff, who wear a badge which provides their name and clinical status. Many would like to meet doctors who dress smartly, whether or not they wear a white coat, and to be addressed by their title and surname. Others may prefer a more informal approach, especially in primary care. Informality may be a sign of a close and friendly relationship, but, if misplaced, runs the risk of losing respect. Informality can be a positive therapeutic force, particularly in the long-term management of patients with chronic disease, in the case of the dying and the support of the bereaved. The development of the doctor–patient relationship should be in response to the patient's needs. Doctors who behave and dress naturally are often successful at establishing good professional relationships.

Transference/countertransference

A clinical interview involves the establishment or renewal of a relationship between two people, who happen to be in specific roles of a doctor and a patient. While it is a professional encounter, the doctor needs to be aware that both parties bring other feelings, attitudes and expectations to the consultation.

Doctors continue to be held in higher esteem by the public than any other profession. Doctors are often seen like parents, powerful figures who are due respect and who can be trusted. This may be used to facilitate treatment by fostering compliance and enhancing confidence. *Transference* is the term applied to this unconsciously driven process by which patients develop feelings and attitudes to their doctor which are transferred from important figures in their past: this is normal, and is usually helpful, and occurs without the awareness of either the doctor or the patient.

However, if the patient's early life was unhappy, particularly in relationships with parents, this may adversely influence the relationship with the doctor. Most often this involves either unmet dependency or mistrust. With the former the impetus is to attempt to break down normal professional boundaries, while with the latter rapport cannot be established and hostility and suspiciousness may permeate the consultation. The doctor requires to recognise when abnormal transferences develop and then to stick to the reality of the relationship; occasionally it may be necessary to bring the development of abnormal transference to the patient's conscious awareness so that the feelings can be re-attributed appropriately or, if necessary, to arrange alternative medical help.

Countertransference refers to those feelings that the patient stirs up in the doctor, which can originate in the doctor's own past. Countertransference is important to recognise and resolve if it repeatedly affects the doctor-patient relationship, or causes personal difficulties for the doctor.

KEY POINTS

- The clinical examination has three phases – history-taking, examination (physical and mental) and explanation. Of these, the last is the most important to the patient.
- Good interview skills enhance the therapeutic alliance with the patient. This may benefit the diagnostic process and the clinical management.
- Some people are naturally better at communicating than others, but training will remedy deficiencies in the motivated.
- Personal appearance and demeanour may also influence the patient–doctor relationship

HISTORY

Introduction

Unless the patient is well known, clinicians should introduce themselves by name and explain their position and who they work for. If appropriate, the patient's identity should be confirmed along with that of any accompanying person. The patient may wish to be accompanied during the interview. This can help allay anxiety, and may be necessary in some situations, such as memory impairment and language difficulties. At other times it may be counterproductive. The most advantageous time to involve a third party is during the discussion after the clinical examination, as this may improve the patient's subsequent understanding of the information given by the doctor.

Interview technique

What to ask about

History-taking involves inquiries into a series of topics (Table 1.3). It is helpful to think in terms of nests or clusters of questions which are multilayered. Hence a negative response to a stem inquiry moves the clinician on to the next topic, whereas a positive response leads to further questioning (Fig. 1.5).

How to ask

The patient needs to understand what is being said. Generally speaking, technical terms are best avoided. The

TABLE 1.3 Elements in a clinical history

Presenting complaint
Past medical history
Drug history
Family history
Social history
Systemic or general symptom inquiry
Further information from a third party
Alternative order
Past medical history
Presenting complaint
Systemic inquiry
Drug history
Family history
Social history
Further information from a third party

TABLE 1.4 Examples of inquiry techniques

Open inquiries
Tell me about your pain
What effects has this illness had on your life?
What happened next?
How did you react to that tragedy?
Closed inquiries
When did your headache begin?
Have you had chest pain?
Has anyone in your family had a similar problem?
Do you smoke? If so, how many cigarettes per day?
Remember – phrasing inquiries as open questions extracts more information and is to be preferred, e.g. 'what effect did painkillers have?' is a better question than 'did painkillers ease the headache?'

public is becoming increasingly informed on medical matters through the Internet and mass media, but their use of medical jargon does not necessarily mean they understand the terms. Similarly there are terms such as 'shock', 'stress', 'nervous breakdown' and 'gastric flu' which need to be clarified, if used by the patient.

There are two main types of inquiry – *open* and *closed* (Table 1.4).

- *Open inquiries* are generally 'how', 'what', 'why' questions: 'tell me about' inquiries. Such questions give patients the opportunity to say what they want to say, and to tell the doctor the history as they perceive it.
- *Closed enquiries* are generally 'who', 'when', 'where' questions: 'is it or is it not' inquiries. They are mainly used to expand the patient's story and to clarify specific points.

History-taking normally begins with open questions to establish the nature of the presenting problem or problems. Only then is it appropriate to introduce more closed inquiries as the doctor focuses on the problem to establish facts and details. As the information is collected some

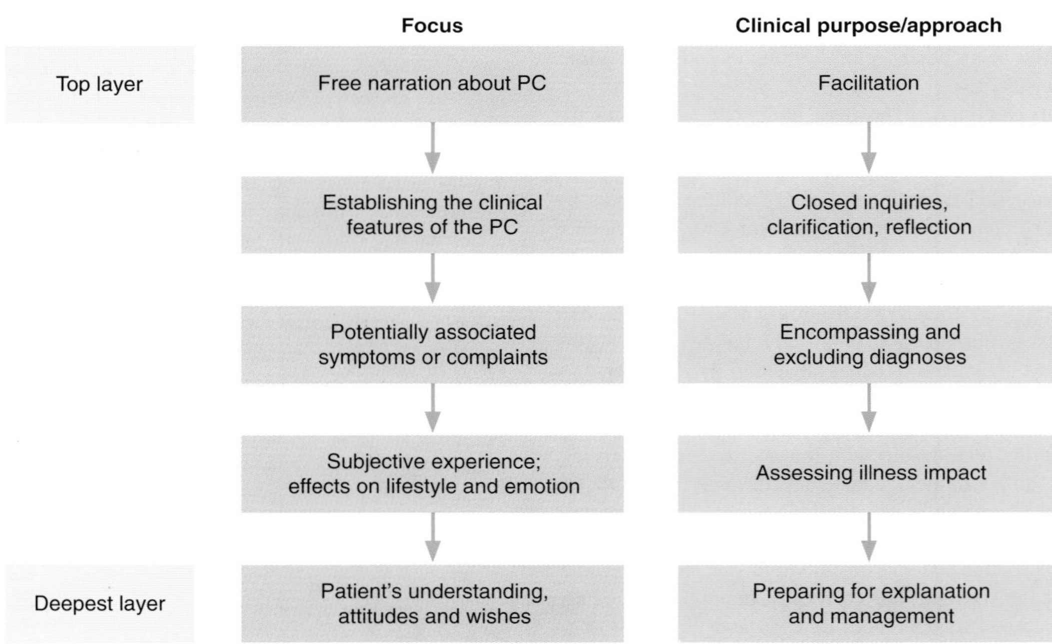

Fig. 1.5 Example of nests and layers in history-taking.

diagnostic possibilities are discounted while others are raised. This processing leads to inquiries which involve *clarification*, *reflection* and *summary*, all techniques to be used selectively.

- *Clarification* enables the clinician and the patient to resolve apparent contradictions, ambiguities and uncertainties in the history.

  Sometimes these issues arise because clinicians' questions have been confusing. On other occasions, apparent contradictions occur because the patient is acutely ill or in severe pain. Sometimes contradictions in the history should alert the clinician to the possibility that the patient is either confused or dementing.

  As a principle, the clinician should seek to clarify the history as tactfully as possible. For example, not infrequently patients may say that they do not have a cough but then describe their sputum. Rather than confront them with this paradox, the clinician should resolve the uncertainty by asking further specific questions regarding the nature of the sputum. Rarely it may be appropriate to challenge the patient's story: 'You mention that you only drink fifteen pints of beer in a week, but tell me that you spend between £60–£80 on alcohol every week. How does this add up?'
- *Reflection* involves putting back to the patient a symptom or remark the patient has provided either for confirmation or development. This also emphasises a matter of importance.

  'You said that you developed a tingling sensation in your arms after you became light-headed. Can you tell me anything more about these symptoms?'
- *Summary* is an expansion of reflection, in which chunks of history are condensed and reiterated for the patient to confirm and correct.

  'Let's see if I've got this right – and please correct me if I'm wrong. You were fine until 8 o'clock this morning when you suddenly developed severe, crushing pain in the centre of your chest while you were in the toilet. You felt sick but didn't vomit, you felt cold and sweaty and became breathless. You thought you were about to die; your wife dialled 999.'

KEY POINTS

- History-taking involves knowing what to ask and how to ask it.
- How inquiries are framed largely determines the information elicited. Open-ended questions are better than closed questions in establishing the framework of the history. Closed questions provide detail and sharpen the account.
- Avoid using technical terms which the patient may not understand.
- Techniques such as clarification, reflection and summary should be used when and where appropriate.

These techniques can be used to facilitate rapport, building up the doctor–patient relationship through the demonstration of attentive listening.

Presenting complaint (PC)

After the initial introduction, many clinicians obtain basic details of the patient's background such as age, date of birth, marital status, previous or present occupation and the number of dependants. Thereafter it is important to establish the patient's presenting complaint or complaints. Sometimes questions such as 'what are you complaining of?' may be misinterpreted. While recommending a flexible approach to different situations, one format is to ask the patient 'what is your main problem' and then 'when were you last in your usual state of health?' This leads to the request 'please tell me what has happened to you since then'. This approach is also useful in documenting the nature of the presenting complaint, or complaints if several (Table 1.5). Case recording is dealt with at length in Chapter 9.

TABLE 1.5 Examples of the presenting complaint(s)

PC	'Headache at the back of my head'	Duration 2 hours
PCs	1. 'Crushing chest tightness with breathlessness'	Duration 40 minutes
	2. Increasing tiredness	Duration 2 weeks

Note the wording. Use the patient's language and not technically correct terms like occipital headache, retrosternal pain and dyspnoea.

The presenting complaint, as described by the patient, is the body of the history. Patients should be encouraged to give their history right up to the time of the interview with a minimum of interruption. The clinician's aims at outset are threefold: first, to keep the history flowing, e.g. 'so what happened then?'; second, to identify those aspects of the history which are incomplete and require further closed questions, and finally to observe the patient, picking up clues about the patient's emotional state, intelligence and understanding that may also influence subsequent inquiries, the physical (or mental) examination and the explanation.

The history of the presenting complaint can be viewed as a series of layers, not all of which need to be explored in each case (Fig. 1.6). Patients vary in how they react to the same pathology. The clinician has to take account of this when assessing the significance of the disease to this individual, and when deciding how best to handle the problem.

Pain: a common presenting complaint

Pain is the commonest presenting problem, accounting for about half of all consultations. Specific presentations of pain that arise in each system are described in the chapters

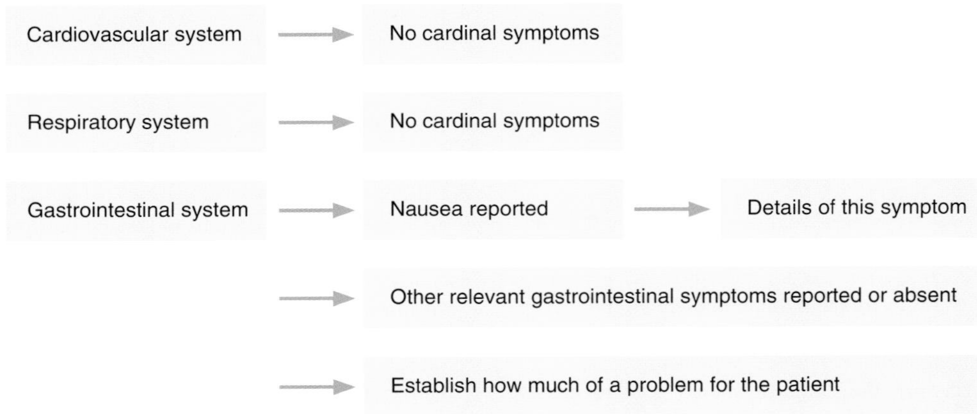

Fig. 1.6 The layers of the HPC. In the absence of cardinal cardiorespiratory symptoms, the clinician rapidly proceeded to eliciting gastro-intestinal symptoms which were described in detail before continuing to the next system.

that follow: here the approach to all presentations of pain is described as an example of the multilayered history.

Characteristics of the pain. Although Table 1.6 may seem complex, with practice, information can be gathered within a few minutes and accurately and briefly summarised as in the case of a patient presenting with a myocardial infarction.

> A 58-year-old man with a history of infrequent angina of effort for the previous 6 years developed retrosternal chest pain radiating to his left arm. The pain appeared suddenly while he was watching television, was crushing in nature and associated with nausea and sweating. It was not relieved by sublingual glyceryl trinitrate used to control his angina but settled spontaneously on his arrival in hospital 2 hours later.

Associated symptoms. Symptoms that develop along with the pain often help towards making the diagnosis. However, part of the body's response to pain or stress is autonomic arousal. As a result, the patient may experience symptoms, such as faintness, sweating, nausea, vomiting, diarrhoea and increased frequency of micturition. The effects of pain on sleep and appetite should be noted. The persistent disturbance of sleep by pain suggests a physical as opposed to a psychological cause.

Effects on lifestyle. 'How has the pain affected your life?' Areas to be considered are presented in Table 1.7, and reflect the normal psychosocial adaptation to disease or disability. Plainly, these issues are irrelevant in the acutely ill.

Attitudes to illness. This is a difficult area to evaluate. In most chronic conditions insight into patients' response to illness may be obtained by considering their overall attitude toward their illness. This is subject to numerous influences; that two people may behave quite differently and yet suffer from the same disease.

TABLE 1.6 Characteristics of the pain

Main site	Somatic pain often well localised, e.g. sprained ankle; visceral pain more diffuse, e.g. angina pectoris
Radiation	Through local extension, or referred by a shared neuronal pathway to a distant, unaffected site, e.g. in diaphragmatic pain at the shoulder tip via the phrenic nerve (C_3, C_4)
Character	Described by adjectives, e.g. sharp/dull, burning/tingling, boring/stabbing, crushing/tugging, perferably using the patient's own description rather than offering suggestions
Severity	Difficult to assess as so subjective. Sometimes helpful to compare with other common pains, e.g. toothache
Onset	Speed of onset and any associated circumstances
Duration	Since onset
Course	Episodic or continuous. If episodic, duration and frequency of attacks; if continuous any changes in the severity
Pattern	Variation by day or night, during the week or month (e.g. relating to menstrual cycle)
Aggravating factors	Circumstances in which pain is provoked or exacerbated (e.g. food). Specific activities or postures, and any avoidance measures that have been taken to prevent its onset
Relieving factors	Effects of specific activities or postures. Includes effects of medication – painkillers in particular and alternative medical approaches

TABLE 1.7 The social effects of chronic pain

Employment	Ability to maintain work If so, any changes to duties If not, duration off work and reasons for not working Attitude to work
Money	Changes in income Benefits Compensation claim Deprivations
Relationships	Effects on key relationships Changes in physical and emotional aspects of marriage Changes in role, decision-making, etc. within the family Changes in contact with family or friends
Leisure	Effects on social activities, holidays, hobbies and interests Changes in habits such as smoking and drinking Increased interest in illness, e.g. joining a patients' group

- The *pain threshold* can be increased considerably by factors like physical activity and analgesic drugs, a positive emotional state and suggestion. Autohypnosis is an example of this.
- Patients vary in their *tolerance of pain* and their *willingness to communicate* this to others; anxious patients tend to request more pain relief.
- *Past experiences*, both personal and family, influence how patients respond to symptoms. For instance a family history of death from heart disease can affect how a patient interprets and reacts to chest pain.
- *Somatisation* is the development of physical symptoms as an expression of emotional distress or illness. It is sometimes easier and more acceptable for patients to present a physical complaint to the doctor rather than a worry. For example, they will concentrate on the headache rather than the source of the stress responsible for the tension headache.
- *Gains from remaining sick*; where these exist they are not always obvious or fully appreciated and frequently are not disclosed by the patient. Benefits may include financial advantages, avoiding unenjoyable or stressful work, or obtaining opiate medication. Alternatively there may be emotionally based needs, such as trying to stabilise an insecure marriage. In such circumstances patients may be poorly motivated to get well but may continue to attend their doctor.

Failure by the clinician to recognise anxiety, somatisation and abnormal illness behaviour may lead to unnecessary investigation and inappropriate treatment.

Past medical history (PMH)

Some clinicians obtain the past medical history after the presenting complaint because it is often highly relevant. Indeed, others take the past history first. Certainly it is not uncommon to discover a direct relationship between the previous history and the presentation which may be inapparent to the patient. For instance, a patient with a past history of rheumatic heart disease, who presents with recurrent fever and malaise, may have developed infective endocarditis.

It is useful to begin with an open inquiry such as 'what significant illnesses have you had?' Patients who report all episodes of ill health may be anxious, obsessional or hypochondriacal: what matters are illnesses that are clinically significant or potentially relevant to the presenting complaint. For example, if a patient complains of haemoptysis, it is relevant to ask if the patient has ever been treated for tuberculosis or has been in contact with that disease. Any positive response establishes a nest which should be explored by further questions.

The past psychiatric history should be incorporated into the PMH as this helps to establish the sequence of events and any interactions among medical and psychiatric episodes.

Drug history (DH)

It is important to obtain full details of the prescribed drugs and any other medications the patient may be taking. These include over-the-counter remedies and alternative medicine treatments, particularly herbal remedies, laxatives, analgesics and vitamin/mineral supplements. The name of each drug, the dose, dosage regime and duration of treatment should be noted, along with significant side-effects. In hospital, not uncommonly, the patient may not know the name of a drug and may have omitted to bring the medication. In such circumstances the patient's general practice should be contacted to obtain the details. This is also advisable when doubt arises about the accuracy of the information – for instance when the account seems unlikely or potentially hazardous. A drug addict may be intentionally misleading the doctor about his or her regular supply.

Compliance

Prescribing drugs is one matter, taking them is another. About 50% of patients are non-compliant. However, many doctors assume compliance unless the contrary is obvious. Sometimes non-compliance can be established by absent plasma concentrations of drugs or suspected by the lack of common adverse effects such as a dry mouth with tricyclic antidepressants. Inquiring about compliance requires tact

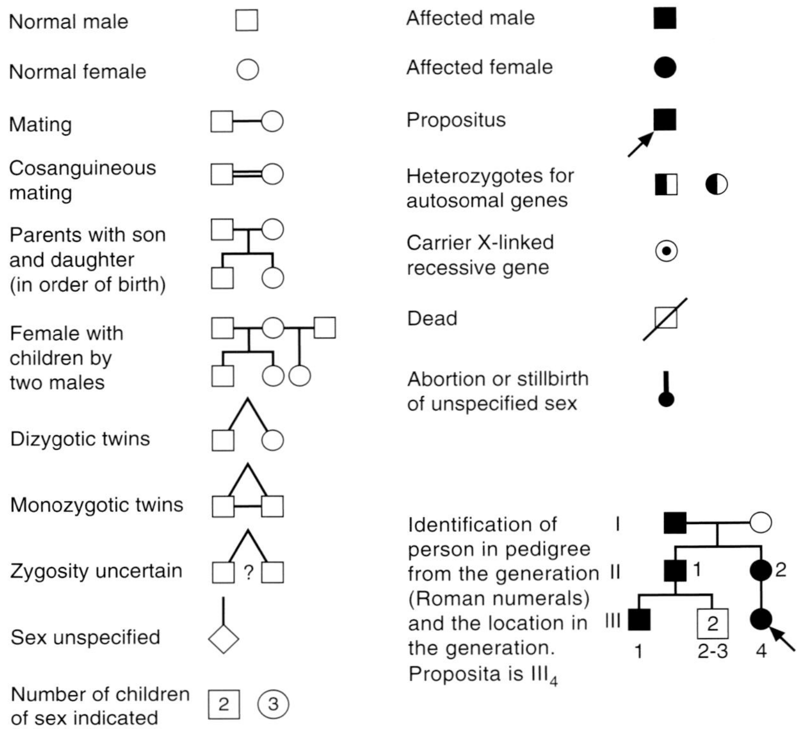

Fig. 1.7 Symbols used in pedigree charts. Drawing up a family tree begins with the affected person first found to have the trait (propositus if male, proposita if female). Thereafter, relevant information regarding siblings and all material and paternal relatives is included. (Reproduced with permission from Emery A E H, Mueller R F 1992 Elements of medical genetics, 8th edn. Churchill Livingstone, Edinburgh.)

and rapport. Poor compliance may not be wilful and many patients may be unaware of the extent of their non-compliance and embarrassed when questioned.

Drug allergies/reactions

It is important to determine whether the patient has ever experienced an adverse reaction to a drug and, if so, to record the information prominently so that it is immediately obvious at any future presentation. Failure to obtain and record an adverse reaction may lead to serious illness or even death.

Family history (FH)

As with other aspects of history-taking, it is preferable to begin with an open inquiry – 'tell me about any illnesses that run in your family'. The nature of the reply may provide grounds for asking further questions. Often closed questions should be asked regarding particular diseases or specific relatives.

The extent of enquiry will probably be constrained by time, and the clinician has to judge the relevance of determining how detailed a family history is required. Plainly this element is most important with potentially inherited disorders.

The symbols used in the construction of a family tree (pedigree chart) are illustrated in Figure 1.7.

The genetic basis is most striking in disorders which are autosomal dominant, e.g. Huntington's disease, or sex-linked, e.g. haemophilia. The pattern of inheritance in autosomal recessive conditions is less apparent as siblings only have a 1 in 4 chance of developing the disorder.

In many common disorders such as coronary artery disease the mode of inheritance is more complex and variable, and there may be additional environmental influences such as diet and smoking. Apparently unrelated illness may be associated through a common pathological process, such as atheroma, with one relative presenting with a heart attack and another with a stroke or with intermittent claudication. Environmental factors may emerge through family proximity; for instance a lifelong non-smoking woman with a bronchogenic carcinoma may have had a husband who smoked heavily before he died of a smoking-related illness. It is necessary also to consider the implications of diseases; for instance a patient presenting with a depressive illness may (truthfully) say that no member of the family has had a similar illness yet further inquiry may reveal that several relatives committed suicide.

Finally, it may be important to establish if the patient or a close relative has been adopted.

Social history (SH) (Table 1.8)

Unlike the general practitioner, hospital doctors usually have little or no awareness of the patient's personal and social background. This information can prove useful in identifying the patient's problem and how best to manage the situation. For instance the management of a patient who has to care for a disabled spouse may differ from that of a patient with the same disease and a healthy supportive partner.

The same principles of nests and layers in the selection of the appropriate questions to ask apply. For example, if an elderly patient presents with dementia or a fractured hip, the sexual orientation will be irrelevant and illicit drug misuse (although not alcohol abuse) so unlikely that any inquiries may cause upset and antagonism. However, inquiries about with whom the patient lives, whether there is additional help at home, and whether the house is on the ground floor or at the top of a tenement building may be crucial.

A social history should not only include basic information about current domestic arrangements and occupation, and the usage of alcohol and tobacco, but also whether any major previous, recent or imminent life changes have occurred.

TABLE 1.8 The social history: areas of potential relevance

Upbringing
Birth injury or complications
Early parental attachments and disruptions
Schooling, academic achievements – difficulties
Behavioural problems
Home life:
emotional, physical or sexual abuse*
experiences of death and illness
interest and attitudes of parents
Further education/occupation
Higher education and further training
Occupation:
current and previous
exposure to hazard, e.g. chemicals, foreign travel, accidents and compensation claims
Unemployment – duration and reason
Attitudes to job or unemployment
Finance
Financial circumstances including loss of income and debts
Relationships/domestic circumstances
Marital status:
quality of relationship and any problems
spouse's occupation, and attitudes to the patient's illness
Sexual identity – any problems
Other occupants of the house – any problems, e.g. violence, health and bereavement
House:
type of home – size, owned or rented
problems with the house
neighbours
Supporting friends or family
Community support:
social and health services involvement
pastoral support and church involvement and other voluntary groups
Attitudes to help being provided or offered
Leisure activities
Habits
Tobacco
Alcohol
Caffeine
Illicit drugs
Dietary restrictions/eating habits

**Note*: Inquiring about sexual abuse requires training and experience, and should be conducted, when indicated, by an appropriately trained clinician.

Habits

Because of the extent to which smoking cigarettes, drinking alcohol and abusing drugs contribute to disease, inquiries into these habits is often necessary. Patients tend to be defensive and are quite likely to deny or minimise their substance use. If there are clinical grounds for suspecting misuse, questioning has to be tactful but firm and persistent. It may be important to seek collateral information from a relative or the general practitioner.

Tobacco

It is important to determine whether the patient is a smoker, an ex-smoker or a lifelong non-smoker. If the patient smokes, the following information is required: form (cigarettes, cigars or pipe); quantity (number of cigarettes/cigars or amount of pipe tobacco per day); duration. If the patient is an ex-smoker, the length of time since the practice ceased should be noted. Staining on the fingers or teeth should raise strong suspicion that the patient is or until recently was a heavy smoker. In smokers, the possibility of tobacco-related disease should be considered (Fig. 1.8).

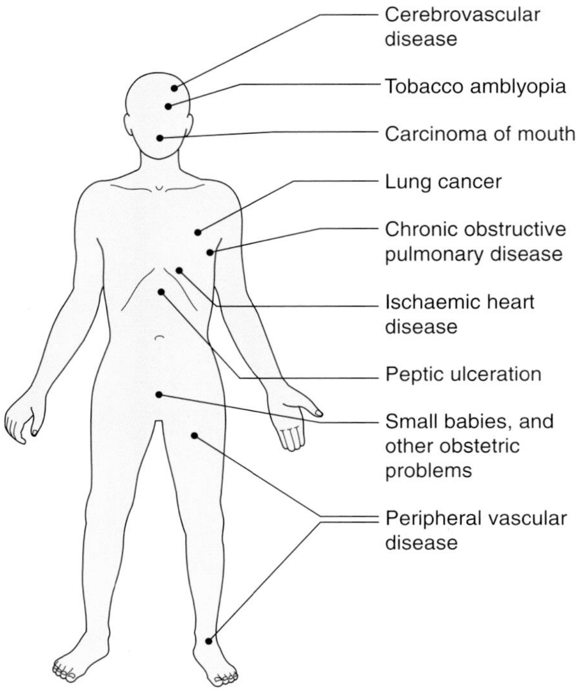

Fig. 1.8 Tobacco-related disorders.

TABLE 1.9 Calculating units of alcohol

Method one
Standard measure = one glass of wine, one half pint of beer, one 'short' of spirits
= 1 unit of alcohol

Method two
Assumptions:
1 unit = 10 ml of pure alcohol
x% proof = x units of alcohol per litre

Examples:
40% proof spirits contains 400 ml pure alcohol or 40 units per litre, so one standard 750 ml bottle contains 30 units of alcohol
4% beer contains 40 ml of pure alcohol or 4 units per litre, so one large (500 ml) can contains 2 units of alcohol

TABLE 1.10 The content of a detailed alcohol history

Drinking habits
Quantity and type of drink
Amount of money spent on alcohol
Daily/weekly pattern (especially binge drinking and morning drinking)
Usual place of drinking
Alone or accompanied
Purpose
Attitudes to alcohol

Alcohol

It is often necessary to ask whether the patient is teetotal or drinks alcohol, with the approximate weekly quantity in units. A past or current history of an alcohol problem should be noted. Comments like 'social drinker' are meaningless and should be clarified.

The approximate quantity of alcohol consumed in an average week should be calculated in units. This is usually obtained by asking the patient to go through a typical week's drinking day by day and then calculating the total alcohol consumed.

There are two ways of calculating units. The first, which is less accurate and may underestimate intake is in terms of standard measures. The second method is based on direct calculation of the alcohol content of drinks. This is more accurate given the range of alcohol strengths in beers, cider and wine in particular (Table 1.9).

Comparing the methods. A patient says she drinks two glasses of wine every evening. By method one this equates to 2 units per night. By method two, if the wine is a standard bottle (750 ml) with an alcohol content of 12%, one bottle contains 9 units so each glass is 1.5 units and the patient is drinking 3 units per night – 50% greater than by method one.

The recommended limits for 'safe' drinking are 21 units per week for men and 14 units per week for women. Such guidelines should be interpreted with caution. A man who drinks 21 units per week in a single binge could develop alcohol-induced problems. On the other hand, drinking above these levels does not necessarily imply an alcohol problem – it is simply that complications become increasingly more likely. Certainly, average weekly intakes above 50 units in men and 40 units in women imply hazardous drinking. If excessive drinking is suspected, either currently or in the recent past, the clinician requires to take a more detailed history of drinking habits (Table 1.10).

In taking a history from a defensive or evasive patient it may be necessary to concentrate on closed questions requiring direct yes or no replies. It is also useful to cross-check the history through its internal consistency, for instance whether the quantity the patient admits to drinking tallies with the stated amount of money being spent on alcohol. Similarly patients who evade questions that evaluate the extent of their drinking through direct inquiry may reveal useful information when asked about the duration and circumstances of periods of abstinence.

Additional questioning may be indicated to assess if the patient has developed an alcohol dependence syndrome, exhibiting withdrawal symptoms such as 'the shakes'. A

Ask about:
- Problems at work (e.g. dismissal)
- Problems with personal relationships (e.g. domestic violence; separation)
- Problems with the law (e.g. drink driving)
- Psychological problems (e.g. depression, attempted suicide)

Consider:

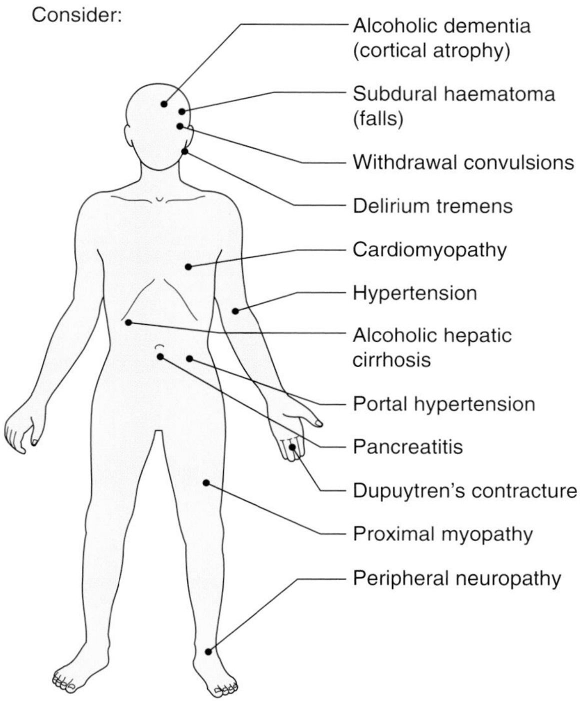

Fig. 1.9 Alcohol-related disorders.

further layer of questions relate to assessing the presence of the different aspects of alcohol-related problems (Fig. 1.9).

Illicit drug use

Clinical common sense is required in deciding whether or not to ask about the use of illicit drugs. In many situations, questioning is unnecessary and could damage the patient–doctor relationship. However, illicit drug consumption is rising rapidly and if there is any doubt, it is advisable to approach the subject with tact and firmness. If illicit drugs are being used or have been used, the following should be noted: the type(s) of drug involved; the frequency and duration of use; intravenous use and whether needle-sharing occurred; whether drug dependence occurred; any physical, mental or social problems arising from drug misuse (as for alcohol history); any treatment interventions.

Inquiries concerning illicit drug use are fraught with even greater difficulty if the patient has been indulging in other illegal activities such as theft to fund the purchase of drugs. How far questioning should be pursued depends upon the urgency of the clinical problem. Information about drug-taking by a young person brought into casualty having collapsed may prove crucial. The past medical history may also include disorders which could be due to intravenous drug misuse while the social history may include interests like attending 'raves' where the use of stimulants is common. The patient may be more forthcoming if there is an established dependence on drugs which are being medically prescribed to control dependence and to reduce harm.

When asking about substance misuse it is necessary to advise the patient that medical confidentiality affords protection but that affirmative responses would need to be recorded in the casenotes. This information need not be conveyed in correspondence if it is not clinically relevant. If a patient refuses to disclose details of drug-taking, this should be noted.

General symptom (systemic) inquiry

It is inconceivable that any patient will require to be asked all the questions that may be important on some occasions. For example, enquiry about contact with birds may be critical in a patient with atypical pneumonia but is a waste of time in many situations. It follows that the choice of questions selected to ensure that the history, as obtained, is sufficiently comprehensive is a matter of clinical judgement. As a general principle, it is important for the clinician to pay particular attention to those diagnostic options which require specific treatment.

During training experience can be obtained from undertaking a thorough general symptom inquiry, asking the patient the 'cardinal' symptoms relevant to each system (see Table 1.11). Otherwise, it is useful to start with an open inquiry such as 'what other symptoms have you noticed?' or 'tell me about your health in general' (i.e. not 'have you any other symptoms?'). A positive response precipitates an examination of the system cluster – and its layers – as undertaken for the presenting complaint, but usually in less detail.

There are other cues to checking cardinal symptoms in one or more systems:

- when the putative diagnosis for the presenting complaint raises possibilities of disease or disorder in other systems, e.g. a patient presenting with palpitations due to atrial fibrillation may have hyperthyroidism

TABLE 1.11 The general symptom inquiry: 'cardinal' symptoms

General health
General well-being
Sleep
Appetite
Weight change
Energy

Cardiovascular system
Ankle swelling
Palpitations
Breathlessness when lying flat (orthopnoea)
Attacks of nocturnal breathlessness (paroxysmal nocturnal dyspnoea)
Chest pain on exertion
Pain in legs on exertion

Respiratory system
Shortness of breath: exercise tolerance
Wheezing
Cough
Sputum production (colour, amount)
Chest pain related to respiration or coughing
Blood in sputum (haemoptysis)

Alimentary
Condition of mouth
Difficulty with swallowing (dysphagia)
Nausea and vomiting
Indigestion
Heartburn
Abdominal pain
Weight loss
Change in bowel habit
Colour of motion (e.g. pale, dark, black, fresh blood)

Urogenital
Pain on passing urine (dysuria)
Frequency of passing urine by day or night (nocturia)
Abnormal colour of urine (e.g. blood)
Number of sexual partners
Males
- If appropriate age, prostatic symptoms such as difficulty in starting to pass urine, poor stream, terminal dribbling
- If appropriate, mental attitude to sex (libido), morning erections, frequency of intercourse, ability to maintain erections, ejaculation, urethral discharge

Females
- If premenopausal, age of onset of periods (menarche), regularity of periods (e.g. 28-day cycle), length of period, blood loss (e.g. clots, flooding), date of last period, contraception if relevant, presence of vaginal discharge
- If post-menopausal, bleeding
- Stress and/or urge incontinence
- If appropriate, libido, pain during intercourse (dyspareunia)

Central nervous system
Headaches
Fits
Faints and blackouts
Tingling (paraesthesiae)
Numbness
Muscle weakness
Hearing symptoms (e.g. deafness, tinnitus)

Visual
Appearance of eyes
Pain
Disturbance of vision, including dyplopia

Locomotor
Joint pain or stiffness
Muscle pain or weakness

Endocrine
Heat intolerance
Cold intolerance
Change in sweating
Prominence of eyes
Swelling in neck
Excessive thirst

- when further information raises possibilities of disease or disorder affecting other systems, e.g. family history of a particular disease, past medical history, patient's medication, admission of alcohol abuse
- when observation of the patient raises possibilities of disease or disorder in other systems, e.g. smelling of alcohol, being breathless, having exophthalmos
- a more general, speculative 'trawl' in a patient who may be at greater risk of unrecognised disease, e.g. the homeless, the elderly, or patients who are not registered with a general practice.

It is better to incorporate any positive or important negative information gained during the systemic enquiry into the main history, rather than considering this part as a separate entity.

Completing the history-taking

It is helpful to both the patient and the doctor to signal the end of the taking of the history as a preliminary to the physical (or mental) examination. There are two elements to closure – an opportunity to acquire further information which has been forgotten or undisclosed, then a review of the history.

The opportunity to provide further information should be given to the patient. As the history is being taken, anxiety and embarrassment may diminish, and rapport and trust develop. This may enable the patient to divulge information to the doctor that the patient had not disclosed earlier. This is not always relevant, but from the patient's perspective it may need to be shared. The fact that this has happened should signal to the doctor that an effective interview has taken place.

History-taking also acts as a prompt, directing the patient's attention, and this may result in retrieval of memory.

The summary should be presented by the clinician and pick out what the clinician considers to be the main points. Anything incorporated from the background history should have an obvious relevance. This summary should be put to the patient for confirmation, correction, expansion or alteration of emphasis. The aim is to agree a distillation of the problem for which the patient seeks help.

KEY POINTS

- A clinical history has a basic structure consisting of a series of elements or 'nests' which vary in relevance and importance from case to case.
- The history of the presenting complaint is the first and most important nest. It should be considered in layers, beginning with the patient's free account, then refining the clinical features, then reviewing the subjective effects of the illness and finally evaluating the patient's standpoint (attitudes, understanding and wishes).
- The essence of history-taking is to place emphasis on those diagnostic possibilities which require to be urgently excluded or for which there is specific treatment. The specific questions which should be asked will depend upon the nature of the problem.
- Drug allergies/reactions require specific inquiry.
- The social history should be slanted appropriately for the patient's age, background and presentation. Inappropriate inquiries may antagonise patients. Sensitive areas of inquiry need to be recognised and managed as such.
- The use of tobacco and alcohol should be determined with an estimate of consumption.
- Closed questions and cross-checking of inquiries may be necessary when assessing the use of tobacco, alcohol and illicit drugs, and compliance with treatment.
- The completion of history-taking should be signalled with a summary of the presentation which the patient can correct or amplify.

PATIENTS WHO PRESENT DIFFICULTY IN HISTORY-TAKING

Taking a history from a patient may pose problems for a variety of reasons. This is rarely the patient's fault: it is necessary to bear this firmly in mind and remain objective and professional throughout what may be a protracted and less than productive interview.

Patient too unwell (triage, severe pain, profuse bleeding, vomiting, severe breathlessness, agitation or distress)

Principles:
- Rapidly assess the situation.
- Treat the patient.
- Obtain history from third party.
- Review in detail when the patient is fit enough.

Mental incapacity (coma, confusion, acute psychosis, severe learning disability)

Principles:
- Ascertain what, if any, history can be obtained from the patient.
- Seek history from a third party or third parties – relatives, neighbours, friends or professionals. Establish the basis of their knowledge of the patient through how long, how often and how recently they have had contact.

Communication difficulties

No English language (foreign visitors, members of an ethnic minority).

Principles:
- Establish competence to understand and express English – it is not uncommon for people to understand considerably more than they can express.
- If accompanied, ask whether the friend or relative could and would act as interpreter. Proceed if the patient agrees to this.
- If alone, or involving a friend or relative is unacceptable or inappropriate, seek an interpreter (most clinicians have access to a translator service. Occasionally an Embassy has to be approached).

Sensory deficit (deafness, mutism).

Principles:
- Check the hearing aid is working.
- Establish a means of communication. This may involve:
  - obtaining a history through written questions
  - lip reading
  - involving a relative who is acceptable and can communicate with the patient
  - involving someone who is proficient in sign language (may be a staff member, or volunteer).

Expressive problem (dysphasia, dysarthria, stammering).

Principles:
- Establish the nature of the problem.
- If the patient understands, then agree with the patient how best to proceed, e.g. could involve the patient communicating in writing, or via a relative.
- If the patient cannot understand, then proceed as for mentally incapacitated.

Emotionally disordered (angry or abusive/threatening).

Principles:
- Ascertain the nature of the problem and try to establish

the basis for the patient's reaction: 'I get the impression that you are angry. Can you tell me why?'

- Encourage patients to talk through the problem from their perspective, even at the expense of interrupting the history-taking. The problem may involve a previous unsatisfactory medical consultation or a misunderstanding arising during the current one.
- Try to correct any misunderstanding, apologising if appropriate.
- Set limits. Abuse, threats or violence may be understandable but are unacceptable reactions which are counterproductive. If the problem remains unresolved, consider terminating the interview and offering an alternative appointment.

During, or before a hospital consultation, it is frequently useful to contact the patient's family practitioner, not just to obtain or verify the medical history, but to establish how the communication problem has been managed in the primary care setting. Ideally this information should be obtained before the patient and family are interviewed.

Consultations that involve a third person present special problems in terms of maintaining patient confidentiality. This is why, whenever possible, the clinician should establish the patient's agreement with this arrangement. Potentially sensitive areas of the history should not be broached unless it is clinically imperative, the third party is acceptable and the patient is given warning and choice before proceeding.

Rapport is often impaired when an intermediary is required to establish a communication link between clinician and patient. The doctor can improve matters, however, by increasing the emphasis on nonverbal communication – greater eye contact, more smiles and encouraging nods – and making a point of directing inquiries to the patient rather than to the intermediary.

THIRD PARTY INFORMATION

Speaking to a third party to obtain important information about the patient's presenting problem or background is often useful and sometimes vital. This may prove crucial in arriving at the correct diagnosis, for instance if the patient is withholding information about an alcohol problem, or in establishing the best management, for instance the capacity of a frail elderly patient to maintain independent living.

It is ideal if the patient suggests that the doctor speaks to the friend or relative but the stimulus for third party involvement may have to come from the clinician. Sometimes it is not practical for the interview to take place in the patient's presence, but this is generally preferable. It may be necessary to gain urgent information by telephone, again with the patient present, and the third party aware of that presence. The purpose of the third party interview should be made clear to the patient.

Rarely, a patient may refuse to agree to a relative being approached. This decision should be respected. If the patient is ambivalent, the problem may be resolved by agreeing on a different person from that suggested first.

In addition to those special situations in which it is necessary to obtain the history from a third party, sometimes the clinician is approached by a third party who is anxious to provide information without the patient's knowledge. In this situation, the doctor should first establish who the person is, the relationship with the patient and, crucially, the reason for the unwillingness to let the patient know about the approach. Depending on the responses, the doctor may wish to proceed with the conversation. In these circumstances the informant should be invited to continue on the clear understanding that this is to be a one-way exchange.

The topics involved are often highly sensitive, for instance sexual abuse, offending behaviour, drug misuse, eating disorder or domestic violence, and the informant may be genuinely concerned for the patient and apprehensive about the outcome should the patient discover the intervention. In these circumstances, clinically relevant information obtained from a third party should be written on a separate sheet of paper, clearly identified as such and, located separately in the clinical records, preferably behind a casenote divider headed 'Third Party Information'. This ensures that the patient would not have access to this part of the clinical record (under the Health Records Act 1990), and this assurance should be given to the informant.

KEY POINTS

- When the acquisition of a good history proves difficult it is rarely the patient's fault, and the clinician should not react as if it is.
- Problems may vary, e.g. deafness, expressive dysphasia following a stroke. Most problems can be surmounted.
- Third party information is sometimes vital, often helpful, and rarely motivated by considerations other than the patient's welfare. The doctor needs to be aware of potential confidentiality problems and how to avoid or handle these.

THE PHYSICAL EXAMINATION

There is no correct sequence of performing a physical examination. It is important for all doctors to develop their own approach. By so doing the clinician will reduce the risk of making mistakes. The time-honoured sequence of physical examination is:

1. inspection
2. palpation
3. percussion
4. auscultation.

These have to be integrated into the examination and can be altered as deemed necessary. For example, it may be advisable to listen to bowel sounds before palpating the abdomen.

Although the tendency is to teach the techniques of physical examination system by system, in practice these require to be integrated because this approach is less tiring to the patient.

Environment and equipment

Whenever possible the physical examination should be performed in privacy and with optimal conditions of lighting and heating. Privacy may be readily obtained in a patient's home. It may be more difficult to achieve in a hospital ward.

The examination couch should be of an adjustable height or a stool provided to facilitate access. It is useful if the couch has an adjustable back-rest. This is particularly valuable is the patient is unable to lie flat without becoming breathless.

The part of the body being examined needs to be properly exposed and illuminated. The rest of the patient should be covered with a blanket or sheet, and care should be taken to prevent the patient becoming cold or unnecessarily embarrassed.

Not uncommonly a patient's relatives attend a consultation en masse. They should be tactfully asked to leave prior to the physical examination. However, sometimes it is helpful for one to remain behind, especially if the patient is a child or if there is a language problem. If a rectal or vaginal examination is to be performed then the presence of a nurse or relative is essential.

The equipment that is required will depend upon the nature of the examination. The clinician will usually have a stethoscope, pen-torch and measuring tape. Other equipment such as an ophthalmoscope, auroscope, sphygmomanometer, tendon hammer, tuning fork, cotton wool, pins, disposable wooden spatula to use as a tongue depressor, disposable gloves, lubricant jelly and proctoscope, and facilities for obtaining blood samples and for testing urine should be readily available. An accurate weighing machine and height scales (preferably a Harpenden stadiometer) should be standard equipment on a ward, outpatient department and a General Practice surgery. When visiting the patient's home the doctor will require a fairly wide range of similar equipment.

THE MENTAL STATE EXAMINATION (MSE)

A mental state examination is an intrinsic component of the clinical examination because:

- mental disorders frequently present with physical complaints
- some physical disorders may present as mental illnesses
- physical and mental disorders coexist much more often than can be explained by chance.

Some aspects of the mental state examination, such as appearance, demeanour and speech form part of the general assessment of every patient. A more formal mental state examination should be undertaken when indicated by:

- symptoms and signs suggestive of a mental disorder
- a past history of mental disorder
- evidence in the history-taking of mental abnormalities, e.g. memory impairment
- evidence on observation of behavioural disturbance.

The clinician should bear in mind particular diagnostic possibilities. Three types of mental disorder are especially common, namely, *organic mental disorders* (especially delirium and dementia), *illnesses of mood* (especially anxiety and related conditions, and depressive disorders), and *substance abuse* (especially harmful effects of alcohol).

The procedures

The mental state examination is systematic and is slanted towards the presenting complaint and the diagnostic possibilities especially those requiring specific treatment. It is usually performed with the patient seated and dressed. There are several components.

Appearance and demeanour. This involves assessing what the patient looks like and how the patient behaves. Abnormalities include:

- evidence of self-neglect or emaciation
- lack of cooperation and difficulty in establishing rapport
- drowsiness, evasiveness, lack of eye contact or marked suspiciousness.

Motor activity. This includes facial expression, posture and gait. The main abnormalities are:

- too much activity such as tremor or restlessness
- too little activity such as retardation
- involuntary activity such as tics or dystonia.

Speech. Again, abnormalities divide into:

- too much talk such as pressure of speech (a feature of mania or stimulant misuse)
- too little talk such as retardation or poverty (features of depression)
- talk abnormalities such as elective mutism or stuttering.

Mood. Mood is traditionally divided into subjective and objective mood state, but there is considerable overlap with thought content and sometimes behaviour or autonomic activity.

TABLE 1.12 Questions to ask to determine the possibility of suicidal thoughts in a patient

How have you been feeling recently?
Do you feel brighter in the morning or in the evening?
Have you any difficulties with sleeping/night waking?
Do you feel worried, irritable or depressed?
Has life seemed less worthwhile?
Have you ever seriously considered taking your own life?

Subjective mood is assessed by an introductory open inquiry such as 'how have you been feeling recently?' As with history-taking the aim is first to establish whether a nest exists and then to explore the layers through a series of inquiries, moving from the general to the specific to determine the possibility, for example, that the patient is suicidal (see Table 1.12).

Objective mood is assessed by observation of the patient – facial expression, behaviour and emotional state, resonance and responsiveness – and by picking up the general demeanour of the patient and ambience of the interview. Assessing mood objectively takes experience and awareness.

The difficulty is compounded by many patients who suffer from depression or anxiety denying or failing to recognise their abnormal mood state. Conversely, the strain of the interview itself can provoke emotional reactions such as weepiness, irritability or emotional lability in some patients, and there exists a danger that the unwary clinician can misinterpret these responses as signs of mood illness.

Sometimes features like the loss of normal resonance in mood or the persistence of anxiousness long after the patient should have settled provide useful clues – but often the diagnosis of mood illness has to rely on other sections of the history, notably thought content.

A rapid, reliable way of assessing a suspected mood disorder is presented in Table 1.13.

Thought. Thought is traditionally divided into form and content.

Form refers to how thought processes are constructed and the relationships between ideas.

Content is often more important. It should be considered in terms of preoccupations and abnormal beliefs (delusions), the former being more often relevant. Preoccupations are the thoughts that recurrently run through the patient's mind, or particularly trouble the patient. These are usually understandable and appropriate to the circumstances, but they can come to dominate the patient and so become a problem in their own right (Table 1.14).

Delusions are rare. A delusion is a mistaken belief which is held with conviction; not shared by others with the same cultural or social background, or intellectual level; and cannot be shaken by persuasion or evidence to the contrary.

TABLE 1.13 Two short mood scales

A. *Anxiety*
- Have you felt keyed up, and on edge?
- Have you been worrying a lot?
- Have you been irritable?
- Have you had difficulty relaxing?

If YES to any ONE of above, go on to:
- Have you been sleeping poorly?
- Have you had headaches or neck aches or tightness in head?
- Dizzy; trembly; sweating, diarrhoea; frequency; tingling etc. (autonomic anxiety)?
- Been worried about health?
- Difficulty falling asleep?

D. *Depression*
- Low energy?
- Loss of interest?
- Lost confidence in yourself?
- Felt hopeless?

If YES to any ONE of above, go on to:
- Unable to concentrate?
- Lost weight (owing to poor appetite)?
- Early waking?
- Felt slowed up?
- Felt worse in mornings?

1 point for each answer
Add A-score; add D-score
Anxiety states usually score > 3 on A and depressive illness > 3 on D

TABLE 1.14 Typical preoccupations associated with mood disorder

Anxiety state	Anxiousness, worry, fear, apprehension, doubt, uncertainty
Depressive disorder	Loss of self-worth, confidence, ability Guilt, burden, failure, catastrophe, hopelessness Death, suicide Unlovable, unlikeable, self-denigration

Delusions are always erroneous but not always absurd; they are evidence of serious mental illness and require to be distinguished from overvalued ideas which arise from eccentricity or cultural factors.

Disorders of perception. The most important abnormalities are *hallucinations* which are defined as apparently normal perceptions occurring in the absence of the appropriate stimulus. *Illusions* differ in that these are misinterpretations of external stimuli. Hence a coat hanging behind a door which the patient misperceives as a person amounts to an illusion, but if there is no person or coat and the patient perceives somebody, then this is a visual hallucination.

Hallucinations and illusions can occur in any sensory modality, but the commonest forms are visual and auditory, and common causes are delirium and drug intoxication. Auditory hallucinations also occur in schizophrenia, but

TABLE 1.15 Abbreviated mental test

1. Time (nearest hour)?
2. Day of week?
3. Month?
4. Year?
5. Age?
6. Place?
7. Names of three objects at 2 minutes, e.g. apple, table, coin (score 1 if one item, or more, is remembered)
8. Dates of Second World War?
9. Name of Prime Minister?
10. Count backwards from 20 to 1 (0 for any uncorrected error)

Each item scores 1 point
Normal scores 8–10
Mild–moderate dementia 4–7
Moderate–severe dementia 0–3

may be a feature of other mental illnesses including organic brain disorders.

Attention/concentration. An inability to concentrate on a task, increased distractibility and occasionally an inability to attract the patient's attention, are important mental state abnormalities often cued by the history. For example patients may volunteer that they have difficulty in following the thread of a book or TV programme. Deficits occur in most mental disorders but particularly organic brain states and mood illnesses.

Simple tests of concentration include repeating the months in reverse or performing serial sevens (starting at 100 and continuously subtracting 7). In some patients, serial threes from 40 is preferable. It takes experience to establish what amounts to an abnormal response given the patient's educational attainment, but in general, patients should be able to complete serial sevens in less than 1 minute with no more than two errors.

Orientation. Disorientation is the cardinal feature of organic brain disorder, occurring in delirium, when it is frequently accompanied by clouding of consciousness, and in dementia. Orientation is considered in terms of time, date, place and person, and this forms the basis of most of the brief tests of organic brain impairment (Table 1.15).

Memory. Memory abnormalities take a variety of forms, but the important practical division is between recent/short-term memory (STM) and remote/long-term memory (LTM). Various ways of testing registration of memory, STM and LTM exist.

- *Registration* can be assessed by digit span. The patient simply repeats back immediately a set of randomly chosen numbers that the clinician announces. It is usual to start at three digits and work up to seven if possible. Most unimpaired adults of average intelligence can manage seven. Five or fewer indicates impairment.
- *STM* can be tested by asking the patient to recall a six-item name and address. After explanation, the patient is given a fictitious name and full address which consists of six key facts to remember, e.g. Mrs Margaret Brown, 32 Blackford Crescent, Edinburgh EH12. This is checked immediately to ensure accurate registration, any errors are corrected, and the name and address are repeated until the patient scores 6/6. The errors and number of trials are noted. After 5 minutes during which other matters are discussed the patient is asked to repeat the name and address. Unimpaired adults usually score 5 or 6, while 3 or fewer strongly suggests a significant deficit.
- *LTM* is tested by the clinician asking about some past well-known events. Deficits in LTM are often evident in the history-taking when, characteristically, details such as names, places and sequence of events are lost. It is important to ask verifiable questions, and it is also necessary to bear in mind that remote memory overlaps with intellect, educational attainment and interests, so for example, an elderly lady's failure to remember the year of Scotland's last rugby Grand Slam is more likely to reflect a lack of interest in rugby!

It is a characteristic feature of dementia that patients may have remarkable preservation of LTM, compared with gross impairment of STM, and that LTM for the distant past is better than for the previous few years.

Intelligence. Assessing a patient's intelligence in the clinical interview is based on factors evident when taking the history, such as the use of vocabulary, complexity of concepts, understanding of and reactions to the illness, and the level of educational and occupational attainment.

If the patient has a learning disability this may affect the ability to understand the explanation at the end of the interview and comply with treatment.

Formal tests of intelligence can be employed, such as simple sums or factual knowledge. It may also be appropriate

KEY POINTS

- Because of the close association between physical and mental disorders, mental state examination is an intrinsic component of clinical examination.
- Three categories of mental disorder are especially common in general medical practice – organic mental disorders, mood illnesses and substance abuse.
- A mental state examination should be slanted towards the diagnostic possibilities raised by the history or the physical examination.
- Assessing aspects of the mental state involves a combination of observation, good interview technique and standard clinical tests. Brief scales can be useful in evaluating specific areas such as intellectual impairment.

to check for literacy. Plainly this requires to be handled sensitively and only when circumstances necessitate.

Insight. It may be important to explore the patient's awareness of the nature of the illness, particularly with disorders in which insight may be partially or totally lost, e.g. multiple sclerosis. The same consideration applies to somatised presentations of mental illness – can the patient recognise the basis may be mental rather than physical? Lack of insight sometimes has diagnostic significance and frequently has crucial implications for the management.

THE EXPLANATION

The third and final stage of the clinical interview is the most important element from the patient's perspective. It is the area to which relatively little attention has been paid when training doctors. Skilful communication develops with experience from a foundation of personal attributes and training. The need to acquire these skills, which will be put into use every time a patient is interviewed, cannot be overemphasised.

Preparation

Whilst examining the patient, the clinician should be developing not only a view of the problem, but also the way to most effectively explain the situation to the patient.

If it is, or may be, bad news, it may be useful to give the patient warning before a word is spoken – by the use of nonverbal cues, particularly facial expression. It is preferable to have any accompanying relative present, with the patient's agreement, as a common, automatic reaction to unwelcome news is dissociation, which prevents the patient taking in anything else.

The way in which the doctor presents the information is as important as the substance of the information; compassion is as important as factual accuracy. This is also important when conveying 'good' news. Otherwise patients may get the impression that they have been accused of wasting a clinician's time. Although all patients should have the opportunity of having their condition fully discussed, some patients, especially the elderly, do not wish a detailed explanation. Denial is a coping strategy. Such patients' wishes should be respected. The key to success is the ability to be natural and flexible and to recognise that each patient presents a unique situation. The principles of communicating the content include the following.

Content

Speak clearly and audibly, providing cues to the patient about the significance of the illness through the tone of voice. Go at a slow but steady pace which should be flexible in response to the patient.

Avoid jargon. Use words appropriate for the patient's educational background and intelligence.

Avoid emotive words. Phrases like 'cancer', 'failure' or 'multiple sclerosis' may so distress patients that they stop paying attention. Such words may have to be used, but it may be advisable to discuss the management and prognosis in general terms first.

Give the most important information first. This is usually an explanation for the presenting symptoms – it may be a diagnosis, or if there is doubt, what the main possibilities are. Patients are more prepared to relate to doctors who are uncertain and open about their doubts, than doctors who appear overconfident.

Packet the information. Categorise the information. In general, move through diagnosis, to investigations or referrals, then to immediate treatment and possible treatments, and end with prognosis. Identify areas of doubt, and qualify what is or is not likely, bearing in mind widely held myths such as cancer invariably kills.

Monitor the patient's reactions and encourage dialogue. Observe the patient's reactions and respond to facial cues such as puzzlement or distress. Check that patients understand what is being conveyed by asking them to summarise. Then tactfully correct any misunderstandings. Try to ensure that the patient is neither unduly positive or negative. Answer any immediate questions as truthfully and completely as possible. Break off if the patient is plainly too anxious or distressed to continue.

Provide the patient with as much choice as possible. Patients have differing views on what is appropriate for them, and it is important to take this into account when determining the management plan. For example, women who have breast cancer are more satisfied with their treatment and less likely to suffer from mood illness if their wishes are taken into account about the type of surgical operation when choice is feasible. Choice is not always possible, but issues where choice is available should be highlighted.

Repeat and reinforce the key points. Repetition should be used selectively to be effective. The same points can be repeated using other techniques, for example a surgeon may usefully explain an operation using a diagram or model – if the patient shows an interest in this (for some patients this might prove upsetting). Other ways of providing information which have been shown to be effective include audiotaping the interview, providing written information immediately or even a version of the medical assessment letter (which has the advantage of permitting errors of fact to be corrected). Such elaborate reinforcement is unnecessary in most clinical interviews; these techniques are adjuncts to be used selectively, usually when serious disease is established or likely and compliance with sometimes arduous investigations and distressing treatment is vital.

Encourage questions at the end of the main information-giving. Patients vary in their concerns, and it is important to allow airing of such worries – even if they are inappropriate. Patients may hold elaborate and sophisticated theories about their illness sometimes commonly understanding it in terms of some event in their life, either recent or remote, which may be relevant or not. Patients also vary in what and how much they want to know. Many want to know the answers to three basic questions – Why me? Why now? Why this particular illness?

Prognosis. 'How long have I got doctor?' This is a common question. Sometimes the best initial response is to ask why the patient wishes to know. This may then provide the opportunity to discuss particular fears and anxieties before dealing with the prognosis. It may also alert the patient to the nature of the problem. It is important to emphasise that nobody can predict life-expectancy accurately. It is best not to mention any specific time or range, and to maintain and share the uncertainty with the patient – 'neither of us knows'. The focus can then be switched to something practical and relevant, such as whether the patient would want to know the signs or symptoms that might herald deterioration or what steps the patient ought to consider taking now, given the current status of the disease.

However, giving patients an approximate life-expectancy enables them to make important decisions about how they intend to use their remaining life and to prepare for death. The advice given to each patient should be influenced by the disease process, the patient's personality and circumstances and especially by their wishes.

Follow-up appointments/arrangements. One session may not suffice. If further information needs to be conveyed or it is essential that the patient's understanding is adequate or the patient needs time to come to terms with the news, then follow-up will be required. This is often best undertaken by the same clinician, but sometimes it may be more appropriate for the general practitioner or a trained counsellor to take over. In such circumstances the person who is to take over should be personally briefed by the clinician about the original session but it is far better if this can be anticipated; for instance, the attendance of the breast nurse counsellor at the first consultation of a woman with breast cancer with the surgeon is crucial in facilitating effective communication as much of the dialogue and information-giving will be taken over by the counsellor, who is usually better trained in this aspect and more approachable from the patient's perspective.

TABLE 1.16 The health gains of effective communication

Better understanding of the disease
Reduced immediate psychological distress
Reduced long-term mood disorder
Fewer stress-induced physical symptoms
Better compliance with treatment
Greater likelihood of favourable behavioural change
Better disease outcome

Reassurance. Reassurance is a potent therapeutic tool which, like all treatments, has to be used appropriately and carries potential risks. Inappropriate reassurance is counterproductive. Reassurance given in response to specific anxieties is both necessary and usually beneficial. It is of special value in helping to allay specific fears such as the control of pain and the fear of dying alone.

Table 1.16 summarises the main health gains that arise from effective communication with patients. Beneficial clinical communication does not unduly prolong an interview, provided the clinician has acquired the relevant skills.

Communicating with other health professionals

Much of the effort involved in the explanation may be wasted if the clinician fails to inform colleagues of the substance of the discussion. This is particularly the case if the patient has been seen by a hospital-based doctor and the continuing care is the responsibility of the family practitioner. Nurses and other health care professionals should also be appropriately informed, always respecting the overriding wishes of the patient. Very occasionally a patient may insist that the family doctor is not contacted. A doctor can overrule this refusal if clinical necessity demands but this should be documented and the general practitioner informed of the situation.

Conclusion

The explanation is a critical component of any consultation. In patients with chronic illness or disability and in those with terminal disease, it also forms the foundation for the development of the patient–doctor relationship. This will be required to provide continuing support and comfort to patients and to their relatives, especially for those coming to terms with a bereavement.

KEY POINTS

- The explanation is the most important phase of the interview from the patient's perspective.
- Skilful communicating by doctors is vital. Effectiveness stems from a combination of personal attributes and training.

General examination and the external features of disease

2

E. D. C. ANDERSON • I. W. CAMPBELL • J. A. A. HUNTER

There is no one correct way or correct sequence of performing the physical examination. Some clinicians may start by examining that system which appears to be most affected; others may first examine the hands and others examine the patient from the feet upwards. It is best to develop one's own sequence and 'style' of examination rather than to follow a rigid regime uncritically. This book does not attempt to describe the method of physical examination but rather to provide a satisfactory and effective method of examination. The purpose of this chapter is to describe the following:

- the significance of those general observations that can be made before formally examining the patient
- an assessment of height, weight, temperature and state of hydration
- the examination of the hair and skin
- the examination of the hands and head (which can be performed before asking the patient to undress)
- those other components of the examination which cannot be assigned to any single system. This includes examination of the lymphatic system and the breasts and an assessment of the endocrine system.

Physical signs may be easily missed during a routine examination unless the clinician looks specifically for them. The very concept of performing a complete physical examination is misleading and should be avoided except as an exercise in practising examination techniques. It is time-consuming and inappropriate to test every patient's sense of smell and colour vision and to always examine the abdomen for shifting dullness. But it is essential to perform these tests in certain circumstances. It follows that, once the history has been obtained, the clinician should consider what physical features may be present and then to examine the patient accordingly. A useful maxim is 'You only find what you look for'.

GENERAL OBSERVATIONS

The physical examination starts as soon as the clinician meets the patient and begins to assess the general appearance, which includes demeanour, personal hygiene and the nature and state of clothing.

Examination sequence

- ☐ Greet the patient with a handshake and note its characteristics.
- ☐ Observe and define any abnormality of gait or posture.
- ☐ Note any features beside the bedside.
- ☐ Assess the facial expression and the state of the clothing.
- ☐ Identify any abnormalities in complexion, movement, sounds or odours.

Common abnormalities

Many conditions can be identified at first glance. Some are very obvious, such as gross obesity; others less so, such as the increased arterial neck pulsation in aortic incompetence or the blue sclera of osteogenesis imperfecta (Fig. 2.1A). Other examples of 'spot diagnoses' are shown in Figure 2.1B–D. Skills of making these observations can be tested on the general public! First impressions are often invaluable. For example, hypothyroidism may be identified on first sight but overlooked by somebody in regular contact with the patient who has failed to appreciate the insidious onset of the changes in voice and facial appearance.

The handshake

A friendly handshake at the onset will offer reassurance and provide an opportunity for the clinician to make contact with the patient as a useful prelude to the more intimate aspects of examination. The handshake may provide an index of the patient's personality and may also give diagnostic clues.

It is abnormal in many neurological or locomotor disorders, such as spastic hemiparesis or severe Dupuytren's contracture (Fig. 2.2). Indeed, it is advisable to check surreptitiously that the patient's right hand is present and reasonably functional. If this is not the case, it is best to avoid shaking hands or to offer the left hand. Much information may be available from a 'normal' handshake (see Table 2.1).

Posture and gait

Useful information can be obtained by observing a normal gait, which ranges from the brisk and erect to the slouched and shuffling. Abnormalities in gait should be carefully analysed as they may indicate a neurological (p. 194) or a locomotor disturbance (p. 265). Similar observations should be made about the posture of the patient sitting or lying in bed. Much information may also be available by observing the bed itself and the surrounds, for example:

- Is the bed level or tilted?
- Has the bed got 'cot sides'?
- Is there a bed cage, monkey rail, ripple mattress or other apparatus?
- How many pillows are in use?
- Is there a sputum mug?
- Is oxygen in use or available for use?
- Has the patient been catheterised?

Facial expression

Facial expression, including the presence or lack of eye-to-eye contact, is a useful index of physical and psychological well-being (see Table 2.2).

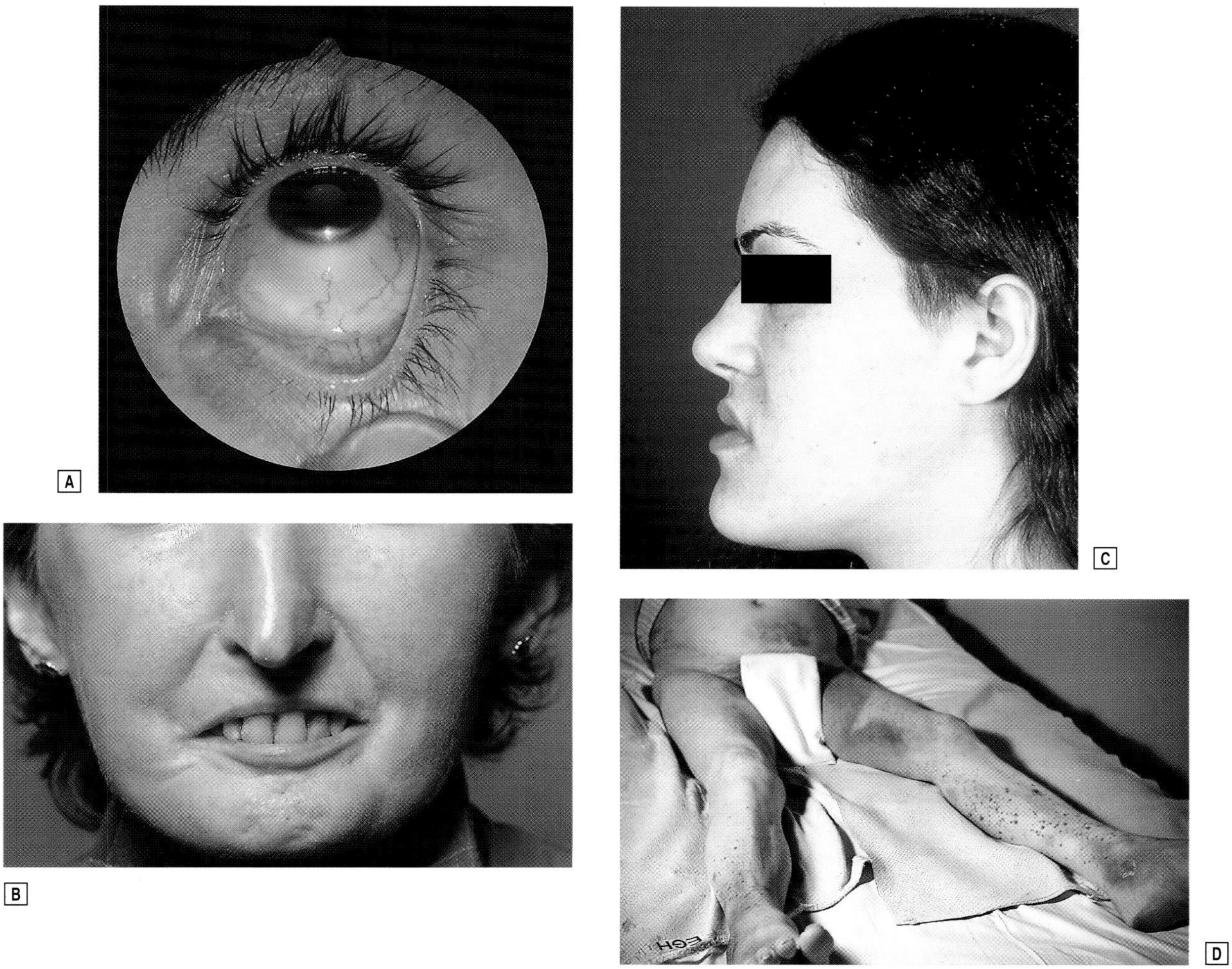

Fig. 2.1 Examples of the value of 'spot diagnoses'. [A] Blue sclera in a patient with osteogenesis imperfecta. [B] Scleroderma facies with 'beaking' of nose and taut skin around mouth. [C] The facies in acromegaly. [D] Leg of elderly male with scurvy showing large ecchymosis in thigh ('woody leg') with perifollicular haemorrhages in calf.

The recognition of the looks of pain, fear, anxiety, anger or grief does not require medical training but should alert the clinician to explore the underlying emotional issues. Some patients may manage to conceal their apprehension or cloak their feelings in an air of feigned cheerfulness. The doctor should avoid adopting, or being misled by, such an apparently lighthearted attitude. The experienced clinician behaves naturally and thereby reduces risks of misunderstanding.

Clothing

Useful information about the patient's personality, state of mind and social circumstances can be obtained from a surreptitious inspection of the clothing. Examples include faecal soiling of underwear in patients with learning difficulties or dementia and the inappropriately juvenile dress of some patients with anorexia nervosa.

COMPLEXION

Abnormalities of complexion may be first noticed by patients or by their friends or relations. The colour of the face depends upon variations in oxyhaemoglobin, reduced haemoglobin, melanin and, to a lesser extent, carotene. Unusual skin colours, excluding those which have been applied externally, are due to abnormal pigments such as the sallow brownish tinge seen in uraemia. The bluish tinge

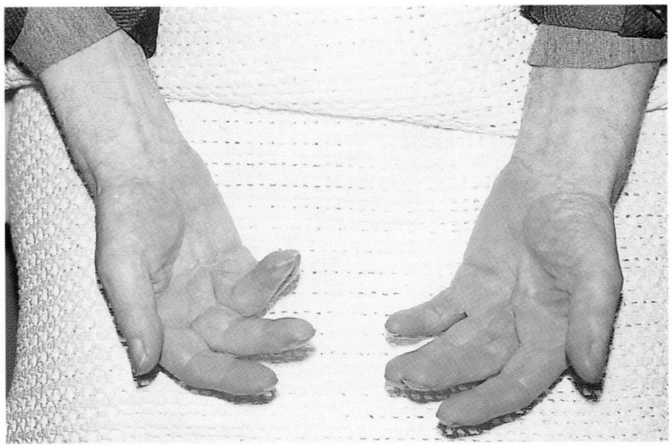

Fig. 2.2 Bilateral Dupuytren's contracture with thickening and shortening of palmar fascia resulting in flexion deformities.

TABLE 2.1 Some information available from a normal handshake

Features	Diagnosis
Large hands with excessive sweating	Acromegaly
Hot and sweaty hands	Thyrotoxicosis
Cold and sweaty hands	Anxious
Dry and coarse skin	Hypothyroidism
Delayed relaxation of grip	Dystrophia myotonica

TABLE 2.2 Examples of abnormal facial expressions

Features	Diagnosis
Poverty of expression	Parkinsonism
Startled	Hyperthyroidism
Apathy and poverty of expression	Depression
Agitation	Hypomania
Peering	Myopia
Apparent indifference	Dissociative (conversion) disorder

of 'enterogenous' cyanosis, produced by abnormal haemoglobins such as sulphaemoglobin and methaemoglobin, may be caused by drugs such as dapsone and some sulphonamides.

The pink colour characteristic of carbon monoxide poisoning from coal gas is due to excessive carboxyhaemoglobin in the blood. Metabolites of some drugs cause striking abnormal coloration of the skin, for example mepacrine (yellow), clofazamine (red) and phenothiazines (slate grey on exposed areas) (Fig. 2.3A). The appearance of skin complexion may be influenced by artificial lighting.

Haemoglobin

Untanned Caucasoid skin is pink owing to the red pigment oxyhaemoglobin in the capillary-venous plexuses of the superficial dermia. The contribution of haemoglobin to the complexion is influenced by the proportion which is oxygenated or reduced.

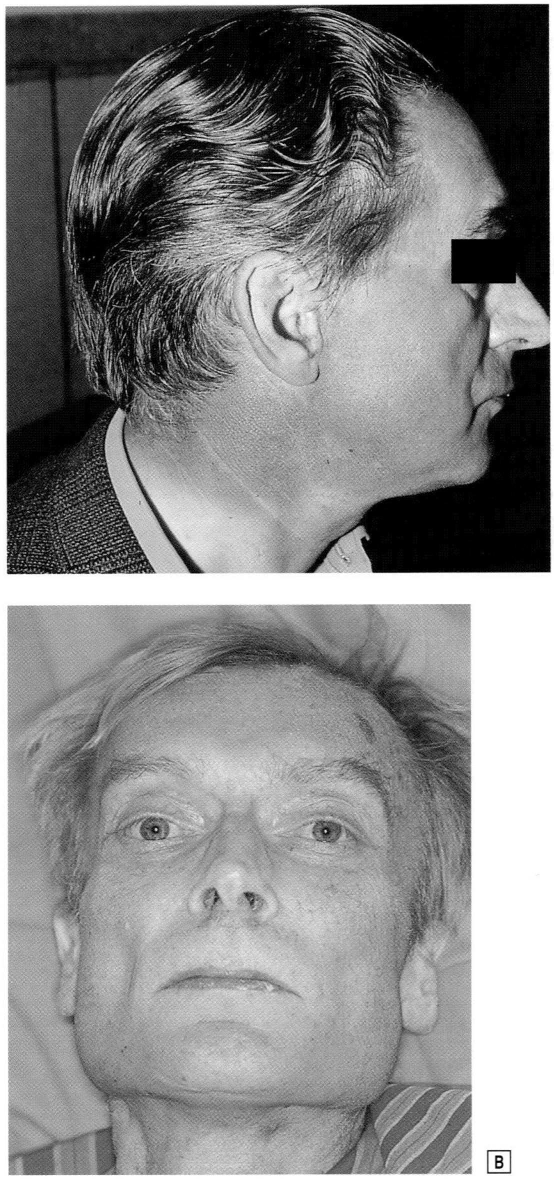

A

B

Fig. 2.3 Abnormal coloration of the skin. A Phenothiazine-induced pigmentation. B Jaundice (by permission of M. Eastwood).

Pallor may be due to anaemia or to vasoconstriction, which may occur when subjects faint or are frightened. The observation by relatives or friends of increasing pallor may be an early feature of progressive anaemia. Examination of the mucous membranes may help to distinguish the pallor of anaemia from that of other causes.

Vasodilatation may produce a deceptive pink complexion even in the presence of anaemia. An unduly plethoric complexion may be seen in polycythaemia, some alcohol abusers with a pseudo-Cushing's syndrome and in Cushing's syndrome itself (see Fig. 2.8A, p. 32). The plethora of Cushing's syndrome is due to thinning of the skin with enhanced visibility of superficial blood vessels.

Cyanosis

This is discussed on page 126.

Melanin

The amount and distribution of melanin is modified in a number of situations (see Table 2.3).

Vitiligo and albinism may affect any race, whereas the characteristic pallor of hypopituitarism is only apparent in white races.

The overproduction of melanin in adrenal insufficiency results in the development of brown pigmentation of the skin, particularly in creases, in scars, overlying bony prominences and on areas exposed to pressure from belts, braces and tight clothing. Melanin may also be deposited in the mucous membranes of the lips and of the mouth, where it results in patches of slatey grey-brown pigmentation (Fig. 2.38, p. 55). Pregnancy is commonly associated with a blotchy pigmentation of the face, 'melasma' or 'chloasma', and increased pigmentation of the areolae, the linea alba and around the genitalia.

In both Addison's disease and hypopituitarism vasoconstriction occurs in the skin, so that pigmentation and pallor respectively are accentuated.

TABLE 2.3 Local and generalised causes of abnormal melanin production

Underproduction	
Patchy (vitiligo)	Autoimmune loss of melanocytes
Total absence (albinism)	Genetic failure to form tyrosinase
Partial absence (hypopituitarism)	Diminished pituitary formation of melanotrophic peptides
Overproduction	
Adrenal insufficiency (Addison's disease)	Excessive pituitary formation of melanotrophic peptides
Pregnancy	Owing to oestrogen, progesterone and pituitary melanotrophic peptides
Heavy metals including iron	As in haemochromatosis
Freckles, lentigines and pigmented naevi	Local overproduction

Carotene

Hypercarotenaemia occasionally occurs in subjects who eat a lot of raw carrots and tomatoes. The orange-yellow pigment carotene is unevenly distributed in the subcutaneous fat and epidermis. It is seen particularly on the face, palms and soles but not in the sclerae. A yellowish discoloration of the face may appear in hypothyroidism because of impaired hepatic metabolism of carotene.

Bilirubin

In jaundice, the sclerae, mucous membranes and skin are lemon-yellow in colour (Fig. 2.3B). A useful site to look for jaundice is the sublingual mucosa. Jaundice that may be obvious in daylight may be undetected in artificial light.

In haemolytic jaundice there is an increase in circulating unconjugated bilirubin, which is not excreted in the urine. The stools are dark and the urine looks normal but contains an excess of urobilinogen.

In hepatocellular and obstructive jaundice, bilirubin has been dissociated from plasma albumin and conjugated with glucuronic acid by the liver. Conjugated bilirubin is water soluble and readily passes through the renal glomeruli. The urine is brown like beer and the stools tend to be pale in colour like putty, because of the reduction in the amount of bile in the faeces.

If jaundice is deep and long-standing, a distinct greenish colour develops in the sclerae and in the skin owing to the presence of biliverdin. Scratch marks may be prominent in obstructive jaundice; the precise cause of the associated pruritus is unknown but may be attributed to the retention of bile acids. The causes of hepatocellular and obstructive jaundice are discussed on page 154.

Haemosiderin

This is another haemoglobin breakdown product. It may be difficult to distinguish from melanin though it has a more gingery hue. It occurs frequently in the wake of purpura (Fig. 2.1D, p. 25) and is seen most commonly on the lower legs, like a sprinkling of pepper, where blood under the influence of gravity is most likely to leak from small capillaries.

MOVEMENTS

Involuntary movements may be due to organic disease of the central nervous system, particularly when the extrapyramidal system is involved (see p. 216). Disorders of movement may also result from primary disease elsewhere (see Table 2.4).

The 'flapping tremor' of encephalopathy due to hepatic failure may only be apparent when the patient's arms are

TABLE 2.4 Some abnormal movements

Nature	Condition
Increase in physiological tremor	Anxiety Thyrotoxicosis Beta agonists (e.g. salbutamol)
Twitching and myoclonic jerks while falling asleep	Chronic renal failure with uraemia Respiratory failure with carbon monoxide retention
Flapping tremor	Hepatic encephalopathy

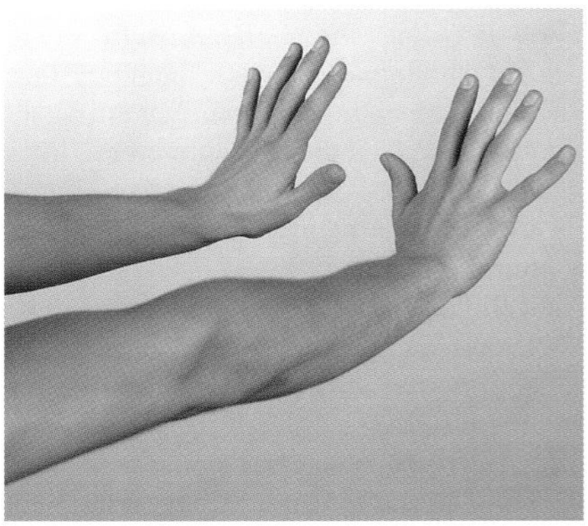

Fig. 2.4 Hand and arm position for observing the 'flapping tremor' of hepatic encephalopathy.

outstretched with the hands dorsiflexed (see Fig. 2.4). The sign consists of irregular jerky movements of the hands due to flexion and extension of the wrists and fingers.

SOUNDS

Normal speech depends upon the tongue, lips, palate and nose, the integrity of the mucosa, muscles and nerve supply of the larynx and the ability to expel sufficient air from the lungs.

The neurological abnormalities which cause disturbances of voice and speech are described on page 194. Many of the other causes can be recognised by inspection, for example a cleft palate, nasal obstruction, loose dentures or a dry mouth. Hoarseness of the voice may be neurological in origin, due to laryngitis or the result of excessive smoking. The voice in myxoedema may be so characteristic that the diagnosis can be made over the telephone without seeing the patient. The normal inflections of tone disappear, speech is low-pitched, slow and deliberate, and seems to require more effort than normal; it sounds 'thick'. Many of these changes are due to myxoedematous infiltration of the tissues concerned in voice production.

Several other types of abnormal sound may be heard. Wheezing, rattling or stridor (p. 123) may help in the differentiation of dyspnoea. The character of a cough may be revealing (p. 189). Witnesses may give an account of a whoop suggestive of pertussis or the cry of an epileptic fit. Audible noises of cardiovascular and alimentary origin are described in the appropriate chapters.

ODOURS

The body normally produces an odour. This largely arises from apocrine sweat contaminated by diphtheroid bacteria and may be reduced by deodorants or concealed with perfume. Excessive sweating causes an increase in body odour, which becomes pungent. Poor personal hygiene results in an exaggeration of this smell, which may be compounded by the odour of dirty and soiled clothing and the smell of dried-out urine. Where washing and toilet facilities are available, malodour usually occurs only in:

- the very elderly and infirm
- those with a physical disability that prevents normal toileting
- subjects with severe learning difficulties or personality disorders
- those with dementia and other causes of progressive brain disorders.

Some odours are sufficiently characteristic to be diagnostic:

- the sickly 'fetor hepaticus' of liver failure
- the sweetness of the breath in diabetic or starvation ketoacidosis, obvious to some observers but not appreciated by others
- the smell of wounds or ulcers infected by *Pseudomonas aeruginosa*
- the characteristic smell of wet gangrene, chronic suppuration, necrotic tumours or some skin disorders.

Halitosis or malodorous breath is often unrecognised by the patient but offensive to others. Sometimes, halitosis occurs without any obvious explanation. It may be caused by decomposing food wedged between the teeth, gingivitis, stomatitis, atrophic rhinitis and tumours of the nasal passages, as well as pulmonary suppuration. Bronchiectasis may be associated with offensive breath and, in some cases, the patient may notice that expectorated sputum tastes foul. In patients with gastric outlet obstruction from scarring or carcinoma of the stomach, foul-smelling eructations may occur, but probably the most offensive odour of this type is associated with a gastrocolic fistula caused by the faecal contents of the stomach.

Tobacco has a characteristic lingering smell which pervades clothing. Marijuana can also be identified by smell. Its presence and that of alcohol should prompt the doctor to ask appropriate questions from the patient and, if necessary, from others about the subject's habits. If alcohol can be detected in the breath before midday, there is a high probability that the patient has a significant drink problem.

MEASUREMENT OF HEIGHT, WEIGHT AND TEMPERATURE

A clinical examination should include the measurement of weight and height, both for their immediate value and for future reference. Measurements such as span, sitting height and pubis to ground height are made only where a more precise evaluation of growth and development is required, especially in infants and young children.

In an adult 70-kg male, total body water (42 kg) accounts for 60% of body weight and fat accounts for about 10 kg. In females, there is a greater percentage of total body water and, in the premenopausal, there are often marked fluctuations in weight owing to premenstrual fluid retention. Body weight may fluctuate by several kilograms from year to year.

In adults, nutritional status is best assessed in terms of body mass index (BMI), which is derived from the formula Wt/Ht^2, measured in kg/m^2. BMI can be readily calculated from this formula or derived from the nomogram (Fig. 2.5), which also indicates the relationship between BMI and nutritional status as follows.

	BMI
Underweight	<18
Normal	18–25
Overweight	26–29
Obese	30–39
Morbid obesity	≥ 40

The normal oral temperature is 37°C. Circadian variations of 0.5°C occur, the lowest temperature being in the early morning. Rectal temperature is usually about 0.5°C higher than that in the mouth, which in turn is 0.5°C higher than in the axilla. Body temperature is best recorded either beneath the tongue, which is convenient, or in the rectum, which is reliable. Alternative sites, the axilla, groin or natal cleft, should be avoided as much as possible. Digital thermometers are becoming increasingly available.

Examination sequence

- ☐ Assess any abnormalities in stature.
- ☐ Measure height on a vertical scale with a rigid, adjustable arm-piece with the patient standing erect and without shoes.
- ☐ Determine the weight of outpatients in indoor clothing without shoes, and of inpatients with pyjamas and dressing gown.
- ☐ Where necessary determine the BMI.
- ☐ Determine waist–hip ratio in the erect patient by measuring the girth at the level equidistant between costal margin and iliac crest and at the level of the greater trochanters.

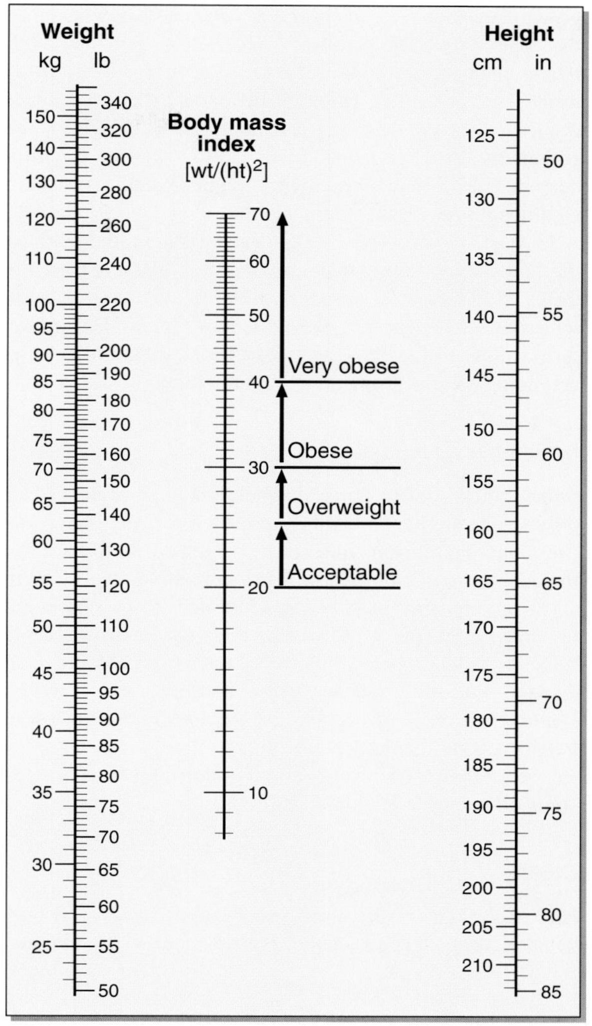

Fig. 2.5 Desirable weights of adults according to body mass index.

- ☐ Look for any evidence of malnutrition or abnormal fat distribution.
- ☐ Take the temperature either by using a digital thermometer inserted into the external auditory meatus, or with a mercury thermometer beneath the tongue or in the rectum. Use a low-reading thermometer if there is a possibility of hypothermia.

Common abnormalities

Increase in height

Gigantism is very uncommon as a feature of hyperpituitarism because of increased levels of prepubertal growth hormone. The sex hormones normally serve to close the epiphyses after puberty. In some patients with hypogonadism, the limbs continue to grow for longer than usual. Thus the sitting height of the patient (head, neck and trunk) will be considerably less than half the height of the patient measured standing. Likewise the span of the fully extended arms will exceed the height standing or, more significantly, twice the sitting height.

In Marfan's syndrome, the appearances are rather similar, the limbs being longer than appropriate to the length of the trunk. Additional features in Marfan's syndrome include long slender fingers and narrow feet, a high arched palate, dislocation of the lens and sometimes dilatation of the ascending aorta, causing aortic regurgitation.

Decrease in height

Short stature is often familial. Adult height is influenced by polygenic inheritance and has a normal distribution. However, any significant illness in childhood will have an impact on the rate of growth. Most conditions that result in short stature can usually be identified from coexistent features (see Table 2.5). Possible exceptions include selective failure of growth hormone secretion, chronic renal disease, intestinal malabsorption and, in girls, Turner's syndrome if the neck webbing is overlooked. Reduction in height is a normal process of ageing. It is accentuated by severe kyphosis, multiple compression fractures of the spine or extensive lumbar disc disease.

Obesity

Life expectancy is shortened by obesity. Obesity will only develop when dietary intake exceeds energy expenditure. The causes are probably multifactorial, but in some subjects, a vicious circle situation may develop whereby weight gain results in 'comfort eating' and further weight gain. Obesity is associated with hypertension, hyperlipidaemia and diabetes mellitus. Its presence should alert the clinician to consider these possibilities and various other complications (see Fig. 2.6).

Regional distribution of fat is of greater prognostic significance than the absolute degree of obesity. Waist–hip ratio provides a simple assessment of visceral adipose fat. Subjects with a 'pear-shaped' configuration and a waist-hip ratio of 0.8 or less in females or < 0.9 in males have a good prognosis; 'apple-shaped' subjects with a greater waist–hip ratio have an increased risk of developing cardiovascular disease.

TABLE 2.5 Some causes of short stature

Hereditary	Constitutionally small
Genetic	Down's syndrome Turner's syndrome Achondroplasia
Nutritional	Intrauterine growth retardation Protein and energy deprivation Rickets
Systemic disease	Chronic wasting diseases including renal failure and biliary disease
Endocrine	Juvenile hypothyroidism (cretinism) Hypopituitarism, craniopharyngioma
Alimentary	Malabsorption including gluten enteropathy, Crohn's disease, cystic fibrosis
Cardiorespiratory	Congenital heart disease Suppurative lung disease
Locomotor	Severe scoliosis

Ask about:

- Family history
- Obstetric history
- Psychological stress
- Anxiety and depression
- Binge eating
- Alcohol and other fluid intake
- Symptoms of diabetes

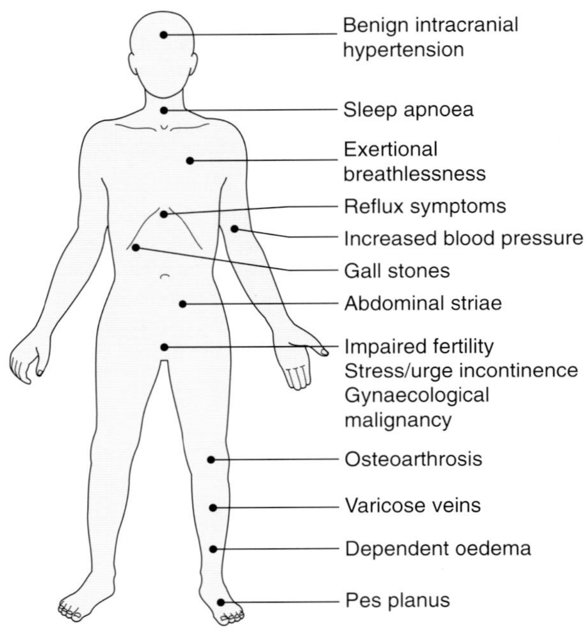

Fig. 2.6 Complications of obesity.

Subnutrition

Malnutrition and starvation remain major problems in many parts of the world. In developed countries, malnutrition due to poverty is rare. Malnutrition occurs in the psychological disorder anorexia nervosa. It may be associated with chronic abuse of alcohol and other addictive drugs and is a feature of HIV infection.

Scurvy affecting elderly people living alone is almost the only vitamin deficiency disease of dietetic origin seen in British adults (Fig. 2.1D). In its most florid form it may present with extensive ecchymosis. In Asian immigrants, vitamin D deficiency used to be quite common and probably resulted from differences in dietary intake and absorption of the vitamin and from its decreased formation in the skin.

Specific abnormalities of fat distribution

- *Localised deposits*. Lipomas are commonly found around the trunk and are soft, circumscribed, lobulated swellings.
- *Progressive lipodystrophy* is a rare condition in which subcutaneous fat is reduced in the face, neck, arms, chest and trunk but may be deposited in excess on the lower trunk and thighs, the line of demarcation varying from patient to patient. Diabetes mellitus is common and mesangiocapillary glomerulonephritis may also occur.
- *Localised atrophy of subcutaneous fat* occasionally may develop in diabetics at the site of injection of some insulin preparations (Fig. 2.7).
- *In Cushing's syndrome* the distribution of fat is abnormal. This syndrome can result from excessive endogenous secretion of cortisol or much more commonly as a result of administration of supraphysiological amounts of glucocorticoids or from injections of adrenocorticotrophic hormone (ACTH). Fat deposition tends to be restricted to the trunk, neck and face, when it causes mooning (Fig. 2.8A and B), together with an increase of the normal pad of fat over the lower cervical and upper thoracic vertebrae. The limbs remain relatively thin or are actually wasted, the whole impression giving rise to the term 'buffalo obesity'. Other features that may alert the clinician to the possibility of Cushing's syndrome are shown in Table 2.6.

Temperature

The warmth of the skin to the touch usually provides a good indication of fever, but the skin of a patient with a normal temperature may feel cold, and an apparently normal skin temperature does not exclude hypothermia.

Fever is usually due to organic disease. An otherwise inexplicable transient rise may be due to a recent hot drink or a hot bath. Individuals sometimes falsify their temperatures by a variety of tricks, including the use of hot-water bottles, in order to feign illness.

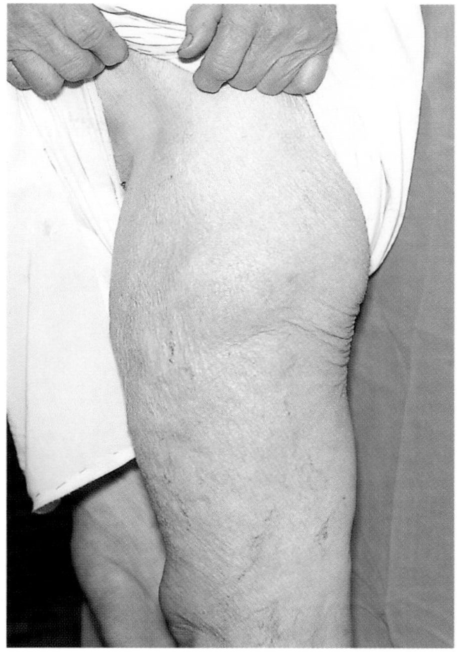

Fig. 2.7 Insulin-induced lipodystrophy.

Hypothermia may be overlooked, particularly if the ordinary clinical thermometer, which reads from 35°C, is not shaken down below this level before use.

Low-reading clinical thermometers are readily available and should be used when hypothermia is suspected. Temperatures as low as 27°C are not uncommon and core body temperatures below 20°C have been recorded in patients who subsequently survived.

Hypothermia is associated with various situations:

- elderly patients living alone who have lain overnight after falling
- near-drowning
- prolonged unconsciousness in low environmental temperatures, especially as a result of alcohol intoxication (which causes peripheral vasodilation), other drug overdosage or head injury
- severe hypopituitarism and hypothyroidism.

Because many of the features of severe hypothyroidism and near-drowning mimic death, such subjects may require to be fully resuscitated and rewarmed before assessing viability.

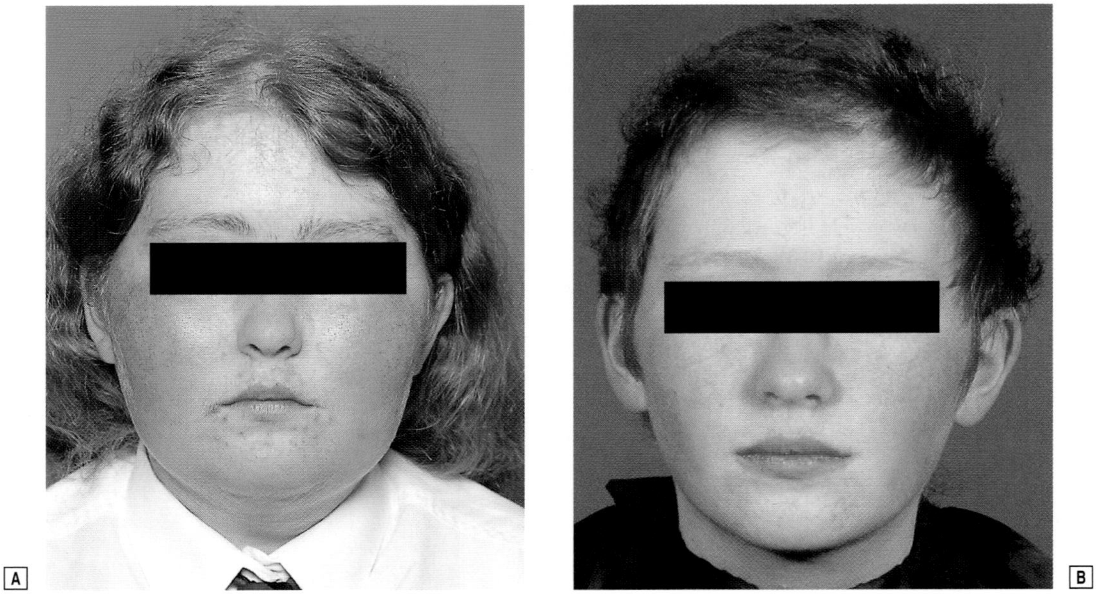

Fig. 2.8 Patient with Cushing's syndrome showing [A] mooned face and [B] facial appearance 6 months after removal of ectopic ACTH-producing tumour.

TABLE 2.6 Other features of Cushing's syndrome	
Features	**Comment**
Facial mooning	Face round and plethoric (see Fig. 2.8)
Plethoric appearance	Caused by thinning of dermis
Purple striae	Noticeable on trunk and limbs
Bruising	Increased capillary fragility
Diabetes	Glucocorticoid effect
Hypertension	Mineralocorticoid effect
Vertebral collapse	Osteoporosis may lead to shortening of stature
Personality change	May progress to psychosis

KEY POINTS

- First impressions are often invaluable.
- The concept of performing a complete physical examination is inappropriate. As a general rule 'you only find what you look for'.
- Check to make sure that the patient's right hand is functional before shaking hands.
- Skin complexion is influenced by artificial lighting.
- A liver 'flap' may only become apparent when the outstretched hand is dorsiflexed.
- Regional fat distribution can be roughly assessed from the waist–hip ratio and is probably as useful a prognostic index as overall degree of obesity.
- Hypothermia may be missed if a clinical thermometer is not shaken down to below 35°C.

STATE OF HYDRATION

In an adult, body water comprises 60–65% of the body mass. It follows that a subject weighing somewhat more than 70 kg has about 45 litres of body fluid. Two-thirds of this is intracellular (30 litres); of the remainder, two-thirds comprises interstitial fluid (10 litres) and roughly 5 litres is included in the circulating blood volume.

Examination sequence

- ☐ Assess the state of hydration by testing skin elasticity and intraocular pressure, recording the blood pressure and looking for a postural drop.
- ☐ Check for dependent oedema by firm pressure at the ankle behind the medial malleolus and, when present, assess its extent elsewhere by pressing over the tibia, in the medial thigh and in the sacral area.
- ☐ Examine the jugular venous pulse (JVP, p. 88).

Common abnormalities

Dehydration

The state of hydration should be assessed in all cases of fluid loss, including vomiting, diarrhoea, sweating and polyuria. Unless the possibility of dehydration is considered, its existence may be overlooked or its severity underestimated. A detailed history of the nature and the quantity of fluid loss is important but, if the patient's usual weight is known, the most satisfactory assessment is obtained by weighing. A dry tongue is apt to be deceptive as it may be due to mouth breathing. In an adult, a total of 4–6 litres has to be lost before the skin becomes dry, loose and wrinkled. Loss of skin elasticity is a poor index, relating more to collagen damage than to water loss. It can be demonstrated by pinching up a fold, which then remains as a ridge and subsides abnormally slowly. The eyeballs are soft, due to lowering of the intraocular tension but this is difficult to assess manually. The blood pressure may be low and the presence of a postural drop in blood pressure may be a useful index of intravascular volume depletion. Elevation in the haemoglobin concentration, packed cell volume and plasma osmolality provide evidence of the severity of dehydration, and serial readings will indicate when treatment has been adequate.

Oedema

Oedema means swelling of the tissues due to an increase in interstitial fluid.

Generalised oedema may be due to a disorder of the heart, kidneys, liver or gut or may be nutritional in origin. Occasionally the cause is idiopathic.

Localised oedema may arise from venous or lymphatic obstruction, allergy or inflammation.

Postural oedema is relatively common but unimportant.

Clinical manifestations of oedema

When oedema is due to generalised fluid retention, its distribution is determined by gravity. It is usually observed in the legs, back of the thighs and the lumbosacral area in the semirecumbent patient. If the patient lies flat, it may involve the face and hands, as in children with acute glomerulonephritis. Regional rises in venous pressure also influence the distribution of oedema as exemplified by pulmonary oedema in left heart failure and by ascites in portal hypertension.

The cardinal sign of subcutaneous oedema is the pitting of the skin, made by applying firm pressure with the examiner's finger or thumb for a few seconds. The pitting may persist for several minutes until it is obliterated by the slow redistribution of the displaced fluid. However, pitting on pressure may not be demonstrable until body weight has increased by as much as 10–15%. Day-to-day alterations in weight usually provide the most reliable index of progress or response to treatment.

Myxoedema is due to infiltration of the tissues by a firm mucinous material. In contrast to oedema, it does not pit on pressure. Chronic lymphoedema may also fail to pit.

Genesis of oedema

Increase in interstitial fluid will occur if fluid intake exceeds fluid loss from the urine, skin, breath and other sources. The renal excretory capacity may be reduced by disease of the kidneys or by extrarenal factors. For example, in the early stages of cardiac failure, a fall in renal blood flow leads to a reduction in glomerular filtration rate and an increase in obligatory water absorption by the proximal tubule. Renal tubular reabsorption of water may be enhanced when a rise in circulating aldosterone increases the reabsorption of sodium and chloride, as occurs in some patients with hepatic cirrhosis, the nephrotic syndrome or cardiac failure (secondary hyperaldosteronism).

The traditional concept that the accumulation of interstitial fluid is caused by a change in the balance between hydrostatic pressure within the vessels and the osmotic pressure of the proteins in the interstitial fluid fails to take into consideration the importance of the pulsatile nature of the capillary flow. Although the mean capillary pressure is equal and opposite to the osmotic gradient, it is the capillary pulsation which is responsible for fluid exchange between plasma and interstitial space.

The mean capillary pressure varies widely at different sites. For example, in the pulmonary capillaries during recumbency, it is less than 10 mmHg, while in the glomerular capillaries it is about 75 mmHg. The theoretical mean capillary pressure in the feet of a person of average height during quiet standing is at least 110 mmHg. It is not surprising that some swelling of the feet may occur by the end of the day.

The types and causes of oedema

Oedema may be generalised or localised and it results from factors disturbing the physiological control of body fluid.

Generalised oedema (Fig. 2.9). There are two principal causes of generalised oedema, *hypoproteinaemia* and *fluid overload*. Clinically, these two causes can be distinguished because fluid overload usually results in a rise in JVP (p. 89), whereas the JVP is not elevated in hypoproteinaemia.

Hypoproteinaemia. The osmotic pressure is mostly due to the serum albumin so that a fall in the concentration of this protein predisposes to oedema. Hypoproteinaemia may arise for a variety of reasons:

- Kwashiorkor may develop when there is a selective inadequate intake of protein. This, and true famine, are the most important nutritional disorders in the world. Self-imposed dietary restrictions or pyloric obstruction with vomiting may also impair protein intake.
- Failure of digestion of dietary protein results from impairment of the exocrine secretion of the pancreas, as in chronic pancreatitis.
- Failure of absorption of the products of digestion may occur in conditions such as Crohn's disease or gluten enteropathy, or after extensive small bowel resection.

Ask about:

Cardiac causes (e.g. past history of rheumatic fever, breathlessness, palpitations)
Malabsorption (e.g. stool odour, bulk and colour)
Malnutrition
Liver disease
Renal disease (e.g. diabetes, sore throat, colour of urine, frothing of urine)

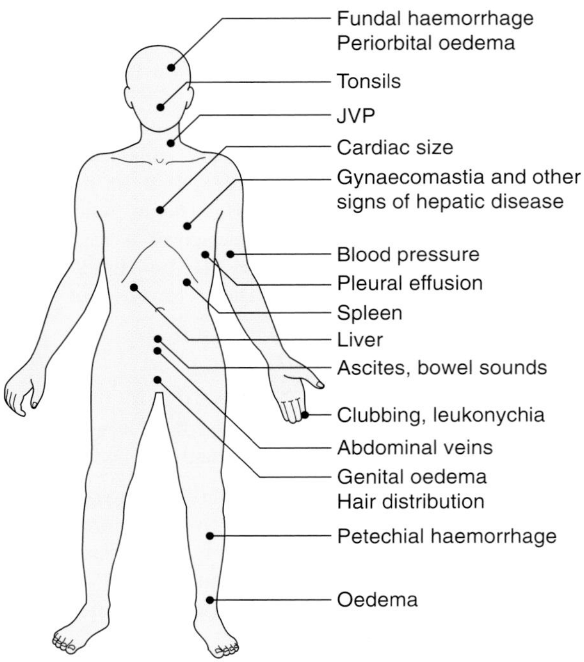

Fig. 2.9 Generalised oedema checklist.

- Reduced synthesis of albumin is found in hepatocellular disease, including cirrhosis. When the portal venous pressure is high, ascites is a more prominent feature than dependent oedema.
- Excessive loss of protein may occur in the urine in the nephrotic syndrome. The repeated removal of body fluids, especially ascites, will also aggravate depletion of protein. Uncommonly protein may be lost into the gut in protein-losing enteropathy, which occurs in a variety of gastrointestinal disorders.

In one patient several of these reasons may coexist. In addition, a low intravascular volume may cause secondary hyperaldosteronism via the renin–angiotensin system, promoting sodium retention and an increase in the oedema.

The cause of hypoproteinaemia can usually be identified from the history. The nephrotic syndrome can be excluded in the absence of heavy proteinuria and most patients with a hepatic cause will show the features either of hepatocellular failure (Fig. 5.14, p. 167) and/or of cirrhosis, which is associated with venous changes, splenomegaly and ascites (p. 169).

Fluid overload. This may have a number of causes:

1. *Cardiac causes.* The causes of oedema in cardiac failure are multiple and are not fully understood.
   Significant factors are:
   - *Impairment of renal blood flow.* The reduction in renal blood flow, alteration in the pulsatile pattern of renal perfusion, and possibly alteration in the distribution of blood flow within the kidney promote excessive reabsorption of salt and water – this is the main cause of 'cardiac' oedema.
   - *Increased venous pressure.* There is a rise in venous pressure proximal to the failing chamber. In right-sided failure this can be detected by inspection of the neck (p. 88). In left-sided failure, pulmonary venous congestion may produce dyspnoea and cough and the auscultatory finding of crepitations in the lungs. However, the heights of the rises in venous pressure do not correlate with the degrees of oedema and the hydrostatic effect alone does not account for the fluid retention.
   - *The effect of aldosterone.* In some cases secondary hyperaldosteronism occurs and contributes to the oedema.
   - *Antidiuretic hormone.* There is evidence of increase in antidiuretic substances in the urine of some patients.
   - *Lymphatic factors.* Lymphangiectasis, incompetent valves and poor lymph drainage have been demonstrated.
   - *Osmotic pressures.* A combination of chronic passive congestion of the liver reducing albumin synthesis, a poor appetite and loss of protein into the oedema fluid and the urine may sometimes account for a significant drop in the concentration of the serum albumin. The protein content of the interstitial fluid may rise to as much as 1 g/dl compared with 0.02 g/dl in normal interstitial fluid. This change has sometimes been interpreted as evidence for an increase in capillary permeability supposedly due to ischaemia, but it is unlikely to be mainly due to lymphatic failure.
2. *Renal causes.* In acute glomerulonephritis, the cause of

the fluid retention is not fully understood. There is an expansion of the circulating fluid volume as well as the extracellular space, due at least in part to increased tubular reabsorption of sodium and consequent reduction in urine volume. Should normal fluid intake be maintained, oedema results.

3. *Iatrogenic.* Excessive fluid replacement, especially if given intravenously, will result in fluid overload. The danger is greatest in infants and young children. The same mechanism can operate if oral intake is unrestricted when urine production is diminished or absent in renal failure.

Localised oedema. This may be due to venous, lymphatic, inflammatory or allergic causes.

Venous causes. External pressure upon a vein, venous thrombosis or incompetence of the valves due to previous thrombosis may each contribute to a rise in capillary pressure. A common example is deep thrombosis in the leg veins. Venous return will also be impaired if the normal pumping action of the muscles is diminished or absent. Accordingly oedema may occur in an immobile bedridden patient, in a paralysed limb or even in a normal person sitting for long periods, as, for example, during air travel.

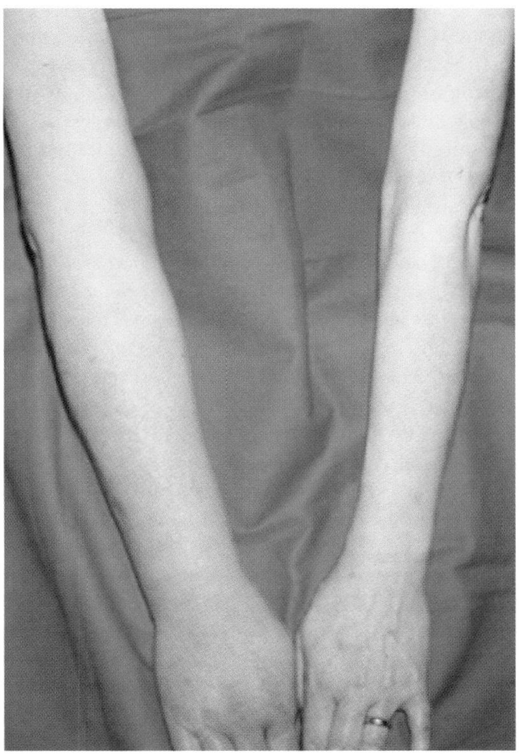

Fig. 2.10 Lymphoedema of the right arm. This patient had been treated with a simple mastectomy of the left breast and a radical mastectomy with radiotherapy on the right side.

Lymphatic causes. The small quantity of albumin filtered at the capillary is normally removed through the lymphatics. In the presence of lymphatic obstruction, the water and solutes are reabsorbed into the capillaries as the tissue pressure rises, but the protein remains until its concentration approaches that in the blood. Ultimately, fibrous

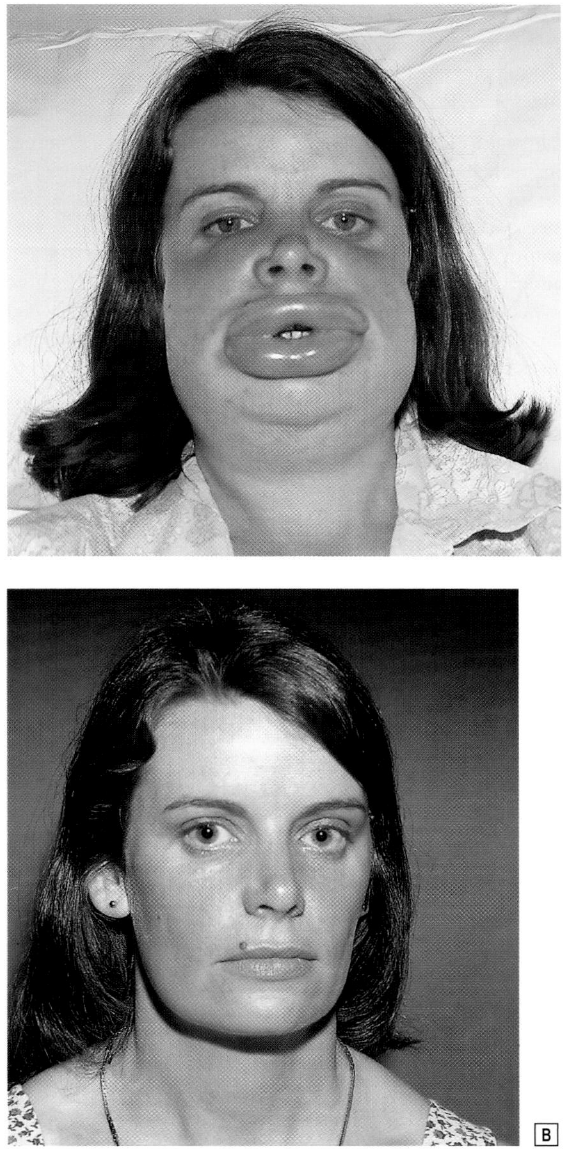

A

B

Fig. 2.11 Angio-oedema [A] following wasp sting and [B] after treatment.

tissues proliferate in the interstitial spaces and the whole part becomes hard and no longer pits on pressure. Lymphatic oedema (lymphoedema) is common in some tropical countries owing to lymphatic obstruction by filarial worms. One or both legs, the female breast, or the external genitalia in either sex, are the parts most frequently involved. The skin of the affected area may eventually become very thick and rough – elephantiasis. Lymphoedema is comparatively rare in Britain. It may be due to congenital lymphangiectasis or hypoplasia of the lymph vessels of the legs (Milroy's disease), recurrent lymphangitis (resulting in fibrosis of lymphatics) or may affect an arm after radical mastectomy and/or irradiation for carcinoma of the breast (Fig. 2.10).

Inflammatory causes. Damage to tissues by injury, infection, ischaemia or chemicals such as uric acid results in liberation of histamine, bradykinin and other factors which cause vasodilatation and an increase in capillary permeability. The inflammatory exudate has a high protein content. The resulting oedema is accompanied by the classical signs of inflammation, namely redness, heat and pain. Testing for pitting on pressure in inflammatory oedema causes pain and should be avoided.

Allergic causes. Increased capillary permeability occurs in allergic conditions, but in contrast to inflammation, there is no pain, there is less redness and the exudate, which has a high protein content, contains eosinophil cells rather than polymorphs and red cells. Angio-oedema is a specific example of allergic oedema; it is particularly prone to affect the face and lips. The swelling develops rapidly, and it is pale or faintly pink in colour. The condition may be life-threatening if the tongue and glottis are affected (Fig. 2.11A and B).

CASE HISTORY

A 27-year-old female was admitted to casualty with sudden severe swelling of the lips and periorbital region immediately following a wasp sting (Fig. 2.11A). The patient had been stung by a wasp some 10 years previously with marked swelling on her arm at the site of the sting.

On this present occasion, she had increasing difficulty with breathing with evidence of stridor. Puffiness was also present around her eyes. 1 ml (1 mg) of 1:1000 adrenaline was given subcutaneously. 4 mg chlorpheniramine orally and 100 mg hydrocortisone intravenously were also given. Her breathlessness improved rapidly and the facial features settled to normal within 6 hours (Fig. 2.11B).

Learning points

- An anaphylactic reaction may occur following initial sensitisation by an antigen.
- Early treatment is the safest way of aborting a life-threatening reaction; this patient has been taught how to give self-medication should she be stung again.

KEY POINTS

- Dehydration in an adult only becomes clinically apparent after substantial fluid loss.
- The JVP is useful in distinguishing between the oedema of fluid overload and that of hypoproteinaemia.

THE PHYSICAL ASSESSMENT

THE HAIR

Anatomy

The hair follicle is the sac-like housing of the hair shaft. The germinative part of the hair shaft is the hair matrix (see p. 39, Fig. 2.15). Melanocytes migrate into the matrix and the melanins that they produce are responsible for the different colours of hair. Each follicle passes, independently of its neighbours, through regular cycles of growth (anagen) and resting/shedding (telogen), the duration of these stages varying in different regions of the body. The anagen phase of scalp hair may last for up to 5 years, accounting for its length. This phase is shorter and the telogen phase longer in eyebrow and sexually determined hair. Moulting does not normally occur in humans unless the hair cycles in neighbouring follicles become synchronised, as sometimes occurs after childbirth and various pyrexic illnesses (telogen effluvium).

There are three different types of hair. Fine long *lanugo* hairs cover the fetus but are shed about 1 month before full-term. They are replaced by fine short *vellus* hairs, which cover much of the body surface. *Terminal* hairs then replace vellus hairs on the scalp. At puberty, the vellus hair of the pubic region is replaced by darker, coarser and curlier hair. This begins earlier in girls (average age 11.5 years) than in boys (average age 13.5 years). The development of pubic hair is related to adrenal androgen production (adrenarche). This occurs in the absence of gonadotrophin secretion. Thus patients with isolated gonadotrophin deficiency may have pubic hair but no other signs of pubertal development.

Axillary hair appears about 2 years after the start of pubic hair growth and, in boys, coincides with the development of facial hair. Last of all, body hair develops, and its extent increases throughout the years of sexual maturity though there is a wide variation in its pattern.

The amount of hair varies considerably in normal subjects and is influenced by familial and racial factors. Asians tend to have straight hair, Negroids to have curly hair and Europeans to have wavy hair. Mongoloids have sparse facial and body hair. Mediterranean people have more hair than northern Europeans.

Examination sequence

- ☐ Inspect the scalp hair for its lustre, calibre, structure, tensile strength and density.
- ☐ If alopecia is present, determine if the abnormality affects the hair shaft or the scalp itself.
- ☐ Inspect for evidence of fungal infection, nits and lice.
- ☐ Examine the body and secondary sexual hair for its nature and distribution.

Common abnormalities

Scalp hair

Certain follicles of the scalp regress with age to produce fine vellus instead of coarse terminal hairs. This patterned baldness often starts as temporal recession, progressing to thinning of hair over the crown. It is common in males and is androgen dependent, prevented by prepubertal castration but not reversed by castration in maturity. Temporal recession is less common in women and may suggest virilisation. Loss or thinning of hair over the frontal region is an almost constant finding in the rare condition myotonic dystrophy, and is also seen in systemic lupus erythematosus.

Alopecia is the term used to describe hair loss. It has many causes and patterns. Complete hair loss may occur following the administration of some cytotoxic drugs. The most common local disease of the hair of the scalp is alopecia areata, in which the hair falls out in patches. In active spreading alopecia areata, hairs shaped like exclamation marks (Fig. 2.12) are found at the periphery of the bald area, which is clean and smooth. Alopecia areata may rarely cause total scalp baldness (alopecia totalis) or loss of all body hair (alopecia universalis), both distressing conditions. Alopecia may also be caused by a fungal infection. In this condition, the affected area contains hairs broken off close to the skin. In assessing alopecia it is helpful to distinguish if the hair loss is due to an abnormality of the hair shaft (as in some inherited disorders of sparse hair) or of the scalp and, if the latter, whether or not there is evidence of scarring. A search for nits and lice is essential in patients with an itchy scalp and posterior cervical lymphadenopathy. Nits (the ova of lice) are firmly adherent to the hair shaft, whereas dandruff (desquamating scalp scales) is easily shed.

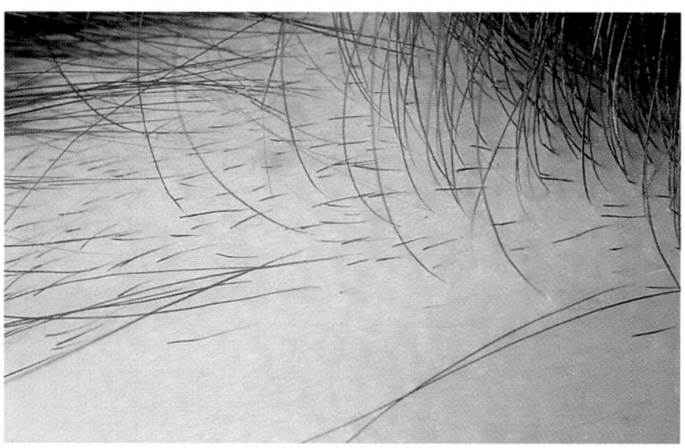

Fig. 2.12 Alopecia areata.

Facial and body hair

Hirsutism is an excessive growth of coarse hair in the female on the face, trunk and limbs in the pattern normally seen in males. The pubic hair spreads from its normal flat-topped distribution up towards the umbilicus, this being described as a male escutcheon. Mild hirsutism is a common condition, often associated with higher than average levels of testosterone. In some subjects it may be a cause of considerable psychological distress. Some increase in facial hair is common after the menopause.

Hirsutism associated with other signs of virilisation (the development of masculine physical features in a female), including enlargement of the clitoris and menstrual irregularity or cessation, may be a sign of an androgen-secreting or pituitary tumour (Fig. 2.13).

Hypertrichosis is an excessive growth of coarse hair which does not follow an androgen-induced pattern. It may be due to many different causes including drugs

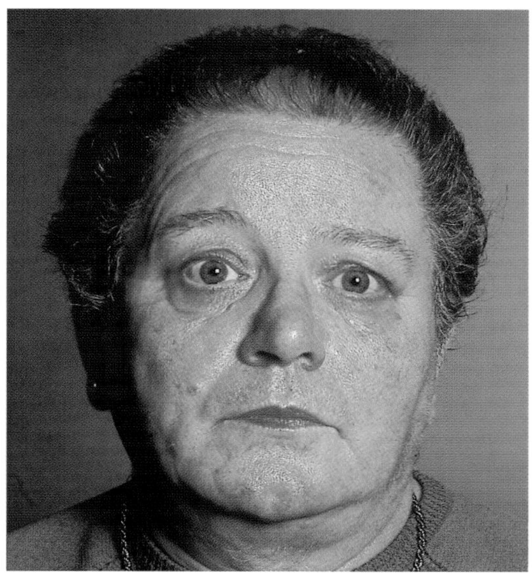

Fig. 2.13 56-year-old lady with virilisation secondary to bilateral ovarian hyperthecosis.

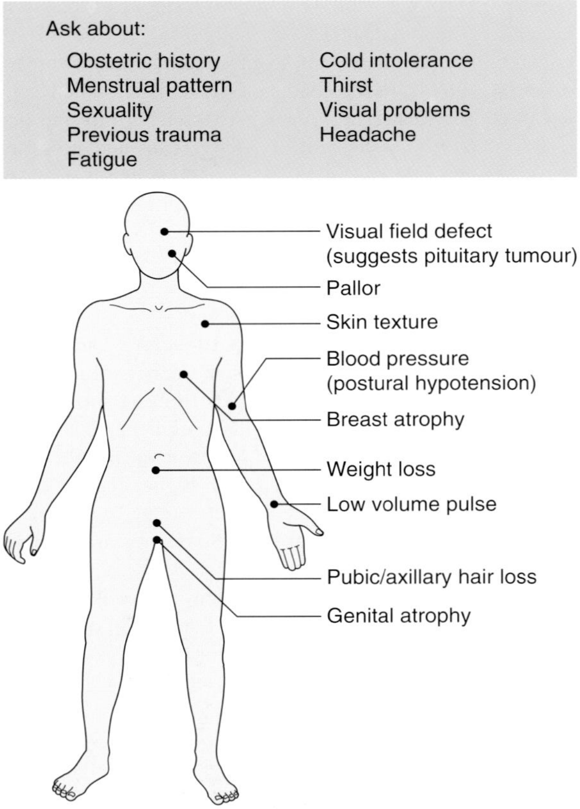

Fig. 2.14 Panhypopituitarism in a woman.

(e.g. minoxidil and cyclosporin), trauma and cutaneous porphyria.

Secondary sexual hair on the face in the male, and in the axillae and on the pubis of both sexes, may fail to develop normally in hypogonadism; it may diminish in quantity in old age or be lost in hypopituitarism or as a result of hepatic cirrhosis. In severe hypopituitarism (Fig. 2.14) the loss is ultimately complete, including the hair follicles, so that the axillae and pubis return to the smooth appearance seen in childhood.

Eyebrows. The amount of hair in the eyebrows varies very widely. Thinning of the outer third of the eyebrows is so common in normal people as to be of little value in the diagnosis of hypothyroidism.

KEY POINTS

- Hirsutism is common, but is rarely associated with underlying disease.
- Thinning of the outer third of the eyebrow is a common feature of normal subjects.

THE SKIN

Anatomy and function of the skin

The skin of an adult weighs an average of 4 kg and covers an area of 2 m^2. It has three layers (Fig. 2.15). The outer avascular epithelium, the epidermis, is firmly attached to, and supported by, a tough fibroelastic dermis. The dermis contains blood vessels, nerves, sweat and sebaceous glands and hair follicles. The third layer, the hypodermis, is of loose connective tissue, often containing abundant fat, which underlies the dermis.

Keratinocytes make up 90% of the epidermal cells. Their primary function is to synthesise insoluble proteins, keratins, which are the main component of the impervious surface of the epidermis, the horny layer. Keratinocytes are generated by division of cells in the basal layers of the epidermis and move outwards, dying in the granular cell layer before being shed at the surface as anucleated horny squames (a significant proportion of common dust). The journey from the basal layer to the surface (epidermal turnover or transit time) takes about 60 days but is greatly accelerated in some skin conditions, for example psoriasis.

Two types of dendritic cell make up most of the remaining epidermal cells. Melanocytes are found mainly in the basal cell layer and are the only epidermal cells to contain tyrosinase, the enzyme essential for the synthesis of melanin from phenylalanine. Melanin is normally formed in the deepest layer of the epidermis and colours the skin brown or black. The amount present is largely determined by hereditary influences. The pigment increases or diminishes in amount with exposure to, or withdrawal from, ultraviolet light. Synthesised melanin is transferred to surrounding keratinocytes in the form of melanosomes. Langerhans cells form a network within the epidermis and are specialised macrophages which circulate between local lymph nodes and the skin. They are capable of presenting antigen to T lymphocytes (e.g. in allergic contact dermatitis), and play a part in immunosurveillance of viral and tumour antigens.

The dermis supports the epidermis both structurally and nutritionally. It is separated from the epidermis by a basement membrane and has three principal components: cells (mainly fibroblasts and a few mononuclear phagocytes, lymphocytes, mast cells and Langerhans cells), fibres (collagen, reticulin and elastin) and an amorphous ground substance (mostly the glycosaminoglycans hyaluronic acid and dermatan sulphate). The functions of the skin are listed in Table 2.7.

Ageing of the skin

Ultraviolet radiation is the main factor speeding the ageing process in skin. This may be very obvious when the wrinkled and inelastic exposed skin of an elderly person

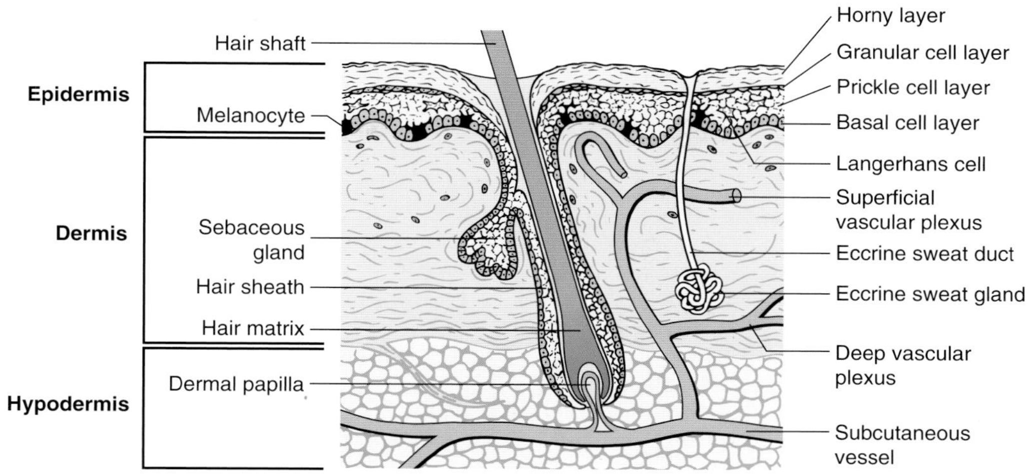

Fig. 2.15 Layers of the skin.

TABLE 2.7 Functions of the skin

Function	Structure/cell involved
Protection against	
Chemicals, particles	Horny layer
Ultraviolet radiation	Melanocytes
Antigens, haptens	Langerhans cells, lymphocytes, mononuclear phagocytes, mast cells
Microbes	Horny layer, Langerhans cells, mononuclear phagocytes, mast cells
Preservation of a balanced internal environment; Prevention of loss of water, electrolytes and macromolecules	Horny layer
Shock absorption; Strong, yet elastic and compliant covering	Dermis and subcutaneous fat
Sensation	Specialist nerve endings
Calorie reserve	Subcutaneous fat
Vitamin D synthesis	Keratinocytes
Temperature regulation	Blood vessels Eccrine sweat glands
Lubrication and waterproofing	Sebaceous glands
Protection and prising	Nails
Body odour	Apocrine sweat glands
Psychosocial display	Skin, lips, hair and nails

who has spent a lot of time out of doors is compared with covered skin (e.g. buttock) of that same person. Ultraviolet rays, especially those of longer wavelength (UVA), damage and destroy the collagen and elastin in the dermis, causing the skin to lose its tensile strength and elasticity. The wrinkled, prune-like faces of elderly Caucasoids living in sunny climates (Fig. 2.16) generate a substantial business in cosmetic surgery; however, prevention of photoageing by reducing excessive exposure to ultraviolet radiation is better than any face-lift.

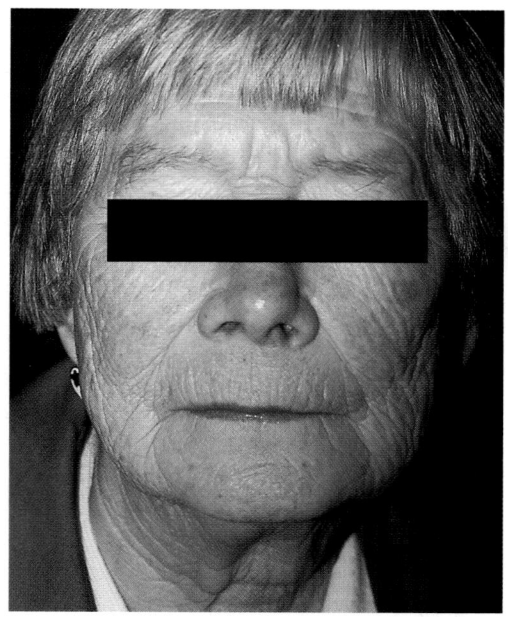

Fig. 2.16 Old face. Note the marked wrinkling and the lentigo on the left cheek.

TABLE 2.8 Some examples of skin lesions and systemic disease

Skin lesions	Associations	Ask about
Erythema nodosum	Sarcoid, tuberculosis, post-streptococcal infection, connective tissue diseases, drugs, etc.	Cough and sputum, breathlessness, sore throat, drugs, etc.
Pyoderma gangrenosum	Ulcerative colitis, rheumatoid arthritis	Rectal bleeding, joint symptoms
Dermatitis herpetiformis	Gluten enteropathy	Family history, change in bowel habit
Generalised purpura	Idiopathic thrombocytopenic purpura and other haematological disorders	Family history, haematuria, fever and weight loss
Dermatitis artefacta	Personality disorders	Stresses or anxieties

THE HISTORY

The ready accessibility of the skin makes it tempting to examine patients with skin disorders without the benefit of a good history. However, the principles of a general medical history should be followed with emphasis on the events surrounding the onset of skin lesions and the progression of the disease. A careful enquiry into drugs (both systemic and topical), a past or family history of skin disease and details of the occupation and any hobbies are especially important.

As in other systems, the more difficult the diagnosis proves to be on examination, the more important the history. Although skin lesions may be caused by an exclusively dermatological problem, sometimes the history, or the lesion itself, may suggest that they are cutaneous

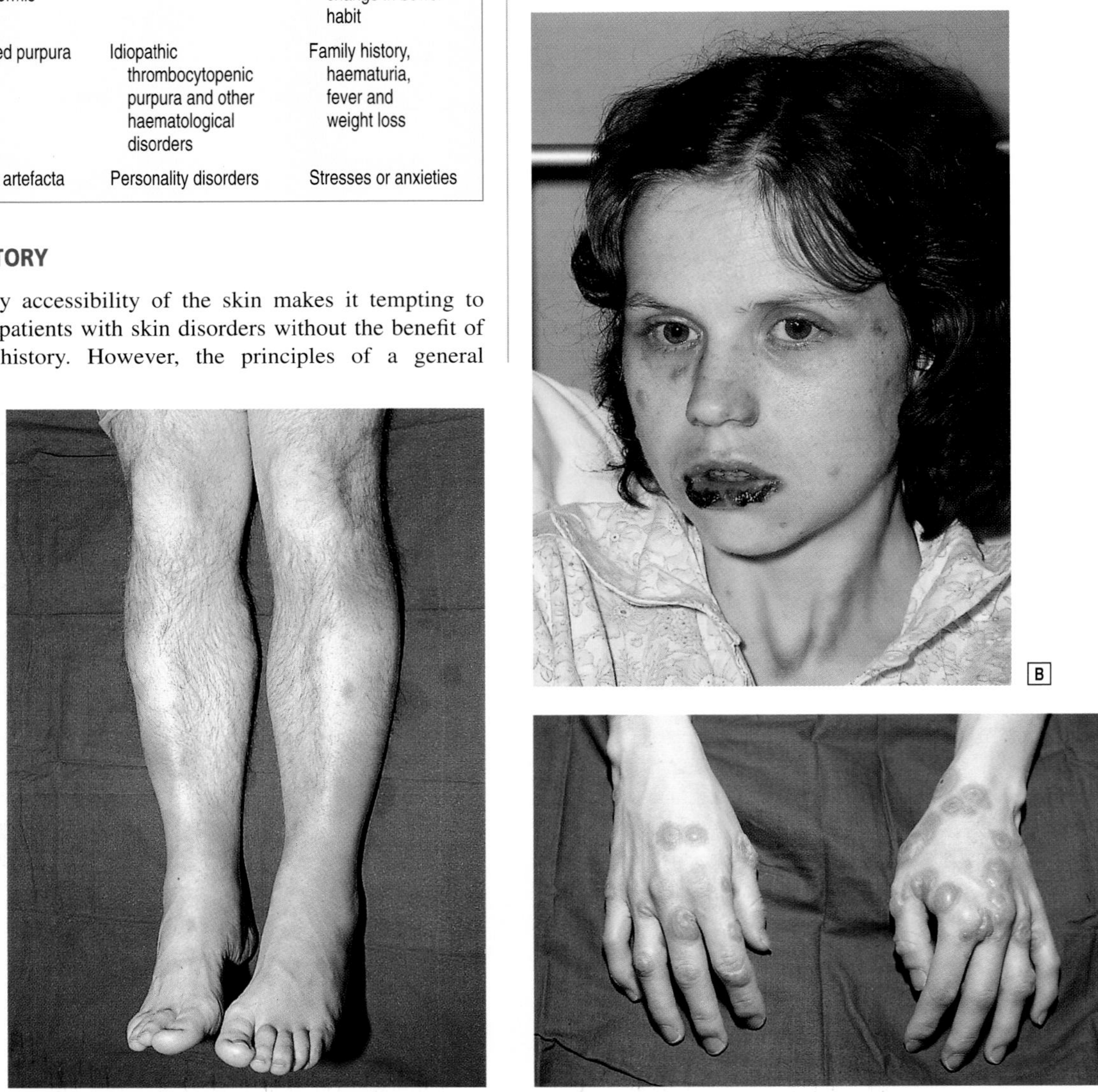

A B C

Fig. 2.17 The skin manifestations of systemic disease. A Erythema nodosum. B Stevens-Johnson syndrome due to mycoplasma pneumonia with C Erythema multiforme ('target lesions') on skin.

manifestations of a more widespread condition (see Table 2.8 and Fig. 2.17).

Examination

Dermatology is primarily a visual speciality, and anything that impairs careful inspection will reduce the chance of making the correct diagnosis. The diagnosis of skin disorders is based on the distribution, morphology and configuration of the skin lesions. Special consideration requires to be shown to the shy or embarrassed patient, but obtaining optimal views is an essential component of the clinical examination. A chaperone is often desirable.

Examination sequence

- ☐ Ask the patient to remove any dressing, wigs and make-up (Fig. 2.18).
- ☐ Examine, using uniform and bright lighting, with the patient undressed if the skin lesions are widespread.
- ☐ First observe the overall distribution of the skin lesions.
- ☐ Then note the morphology of the lesion using a lens if necessary.
- ☐ Note the arrangement and configuration of the lesions.

Common abnormalities

Distribution. The temptation to examine skin lesions closely should be resisted until the distribution of the rash has been noted at arm's length. This may be the most valuable clue to the diagnosis. For example, it is not easy to diagnose herpes zoster by the appearance of the individual lesions, but it becomes simple once the dermatomal distribution is appreciated (Fig. 2.19A). Similarly, a photosensitive basis for a rash becomes obvious when it is noted that only exposed areas are involved and shielded areas spared (Fig. 2.19B). Some skin conditions may affect certain areas (sites of predilection) more than others. Psoriasis preferentially involves the scalp, elbows, knees, natal cleft and nails, atopic dermatitis frequently picks out the antecubital and popliteal fossae in children (Fig. 2.19C) and seborrhoeic dermatitis is seen most often on the scalp, forehead, eyebrows, nasolabial folds and presternal area. The distribution of an eczematous rash may be the main pointer that the problem is due to a reaction from an external contactant (Fig. 2.19D).

Universal and symmetrical eruptions favour systemic or constitutional causes, whereas asymmetrical rashes which spread from a single focus are most often due to fungal, bacterial and some viral infections. Frequently, changes on the soles of the feet may be mirrored by a similar appearance on the palms. Sometimes clues as to the diagnosis may be found at sites distant to the presenting problem, for example a patient may consult the doctor about a solitary perungual fibroma although the diagnosis of tuberous sclerosis becomes evident when ash-leaf depigmented macules on the trunk and adenoma sebaceum on the face

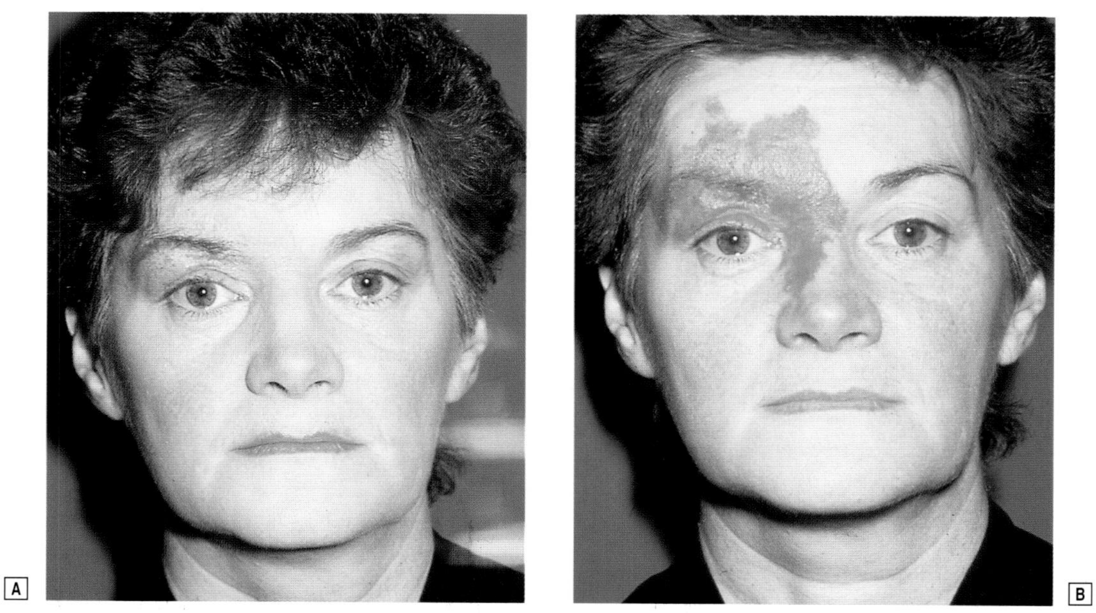

Fig. 2.18 The effect of camouflage make-up in a patient with an extensive port wine stain.

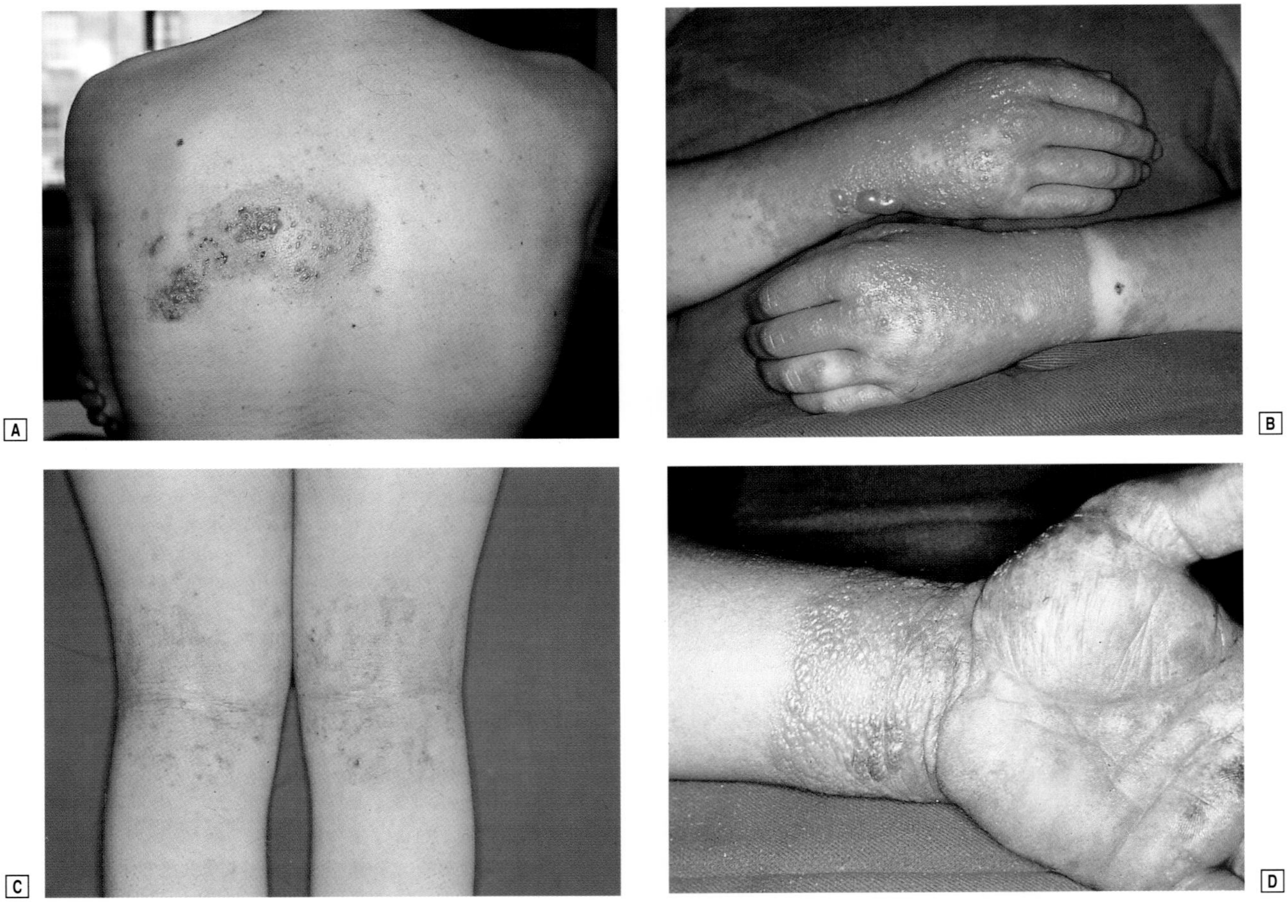

Fig. 2.19 Distribution of rashes as a key to diagnosis. A Herpes zoster. B Griseofulvin photosensitivity eruption. C Atopic dermatitis. D Allergic dermatitis from contact with rubber gloves.

are noted. In summary, before looking at the detail of the individual lesions, stand back from the patient and consider the following questions.

QUESTIONS BOX: DISTRIBUTION OF LESIONS

- Is the rash localised, universal or symmetrical?
- Does the rash follow an anatomical (e.g. dermatomal) pattern?
- Does it affect special sites such as flexures?
- Are areas of predilection for some common disease involved?
- Are certain areas spared?
- Are there other clues to the diagnosis at sites distant to the presenting problem?
- Are there other incidental findings such as skin cancer which the patient has ignored?

Morphology. After the distribution has been noted the morphology of the primary lesions should be defined. Unfortunately, scratch marks, crusting and ulceration may obscure the appearance of early lesions though these should be sought and, when found, inspected closely.

Most types of primary lesions have special names (Table 2.9), and these should be used to describe a skin disease properly. The clinician should not only look at the primary lesions carefully but also record details concisely so that the description can be understood and the rash visualised by others.

With practice, use of the terminology will save much time in describing the rash as well as point to the diagnosis. For example, 'violaceous, shiny, polygonal discrete and flat-topped papules on the fronts of the wrists' are probably due to lichen planus (Fig. 2.20A), but the diagnosis is clinched by recognition of the pathognomonic Wickham's

TABLE 2.9 Terminology of skin lesions

Primary lesions	
Papule	Small solid elevation of skin, less than 0.5 cm in diameter
Plaque	Elevated area of skin greater than 2 cm in diameter but without substantial depth
Macule	Small flat area of altered colour or texture
Vesicle	Circumscribed elevation of skin, less than 0.5 cm in diameter, and containing fluid
Bulla	Circumscribed elevation of skin over 0.5 cm in diameter and containing fluid
Pustule	A visible accumulation of pus in the skin
Abscess	A localised collection of pus in a cavity, more than 1 cm in diameter
Wheal	An elevated white compressible, evanescent area produced by dermal oedema
Angioedema	A diffuse swelling of oedema that extends to the subcutaneous tissue
Nodule	A solid mass in the skin, usually greater than 0.5 cm in diameter
Papilloma	A nipple-like mass projecting from the skin
Petechiae	Pinhead-sized macules of blood in the skin
Purpura	A larger macule or papule of blood in the skin
Ecchymosis	A larger extravasation of blood into the skin
Haematoma	A swelling from gross bleeding
Burrow	A linear or curvilinear papule, caused by a burrowing scabies mite
Comedo	A plug of keratin and sebum wedged in a dilated pilosebaceous orifice
Telangiectasia	The visible dilatation of small cutaneous blood vessels
Secondary lesions (which evolve from primary lesions)	
Scale	A flake arising from the horny layer
Crust	Looks like a scale, but is composed of dried blood or tissue fluid
Ulcer	An area of skin from which the whole of the epidermis and at least the upper part of the dermis has been lost
Excoriation	An ulcer or erosion produced by scratching
Erosion	An area of skin denuded by a complete or partial loss of the epidermis
Fissure	A slit in the skin
Sinus	A cavity or channel that permits the escape of pus or fluid
Scar	The result of healing, in which normal structures are permanently replaced by fibrous tissue
Atrophy	Thinning of skin due to diminution of the epidermis, dermis, subcutaneous fat
Stria	A streak-like linear, atrophic, pink, purple or white lesion of the skin caused by changes in the connective tissue

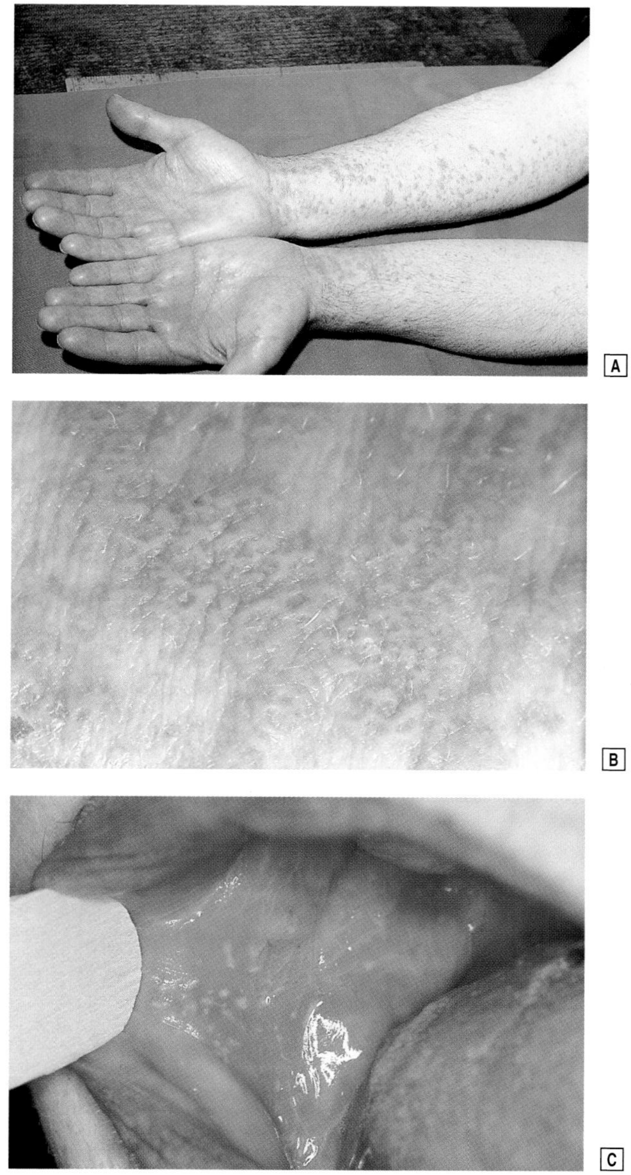

Fig. 2.20 Diagnostic sequence, lichen planus. A Discrete flat-topped papules at the wrist. B Wickham's striae visible on close inspection. C White lacy network of striae on buccal mucosa.

striae on close inspection of the papules (Fig. 2.20B), and made indisputable by the observation of a white lacy network on the buccal mucosa (Fig. 2.20C); a biopsy for diagnostic purposes in this instance would be like checking the engine specification of a car to determine its make rather than looking at the general shape and the name on the body!

Most skin lesions are pink; other colours may help in diagnosis, for example the yellow-orange hue of xanthomata, the violaceous tint of lichen planus, the slate-grey colour of drug-induced pigmentation (Fig. 2.3A). Variation in colour, asymmetry and an irregular outline are key signs in distinguishing some malignant from benign lesions (Fig. 2.21). The surface characteristics of individual lesions may be equally important diagnostic pointers (Fig. 2.22). Finally, a tiny primary lesion, which might only be

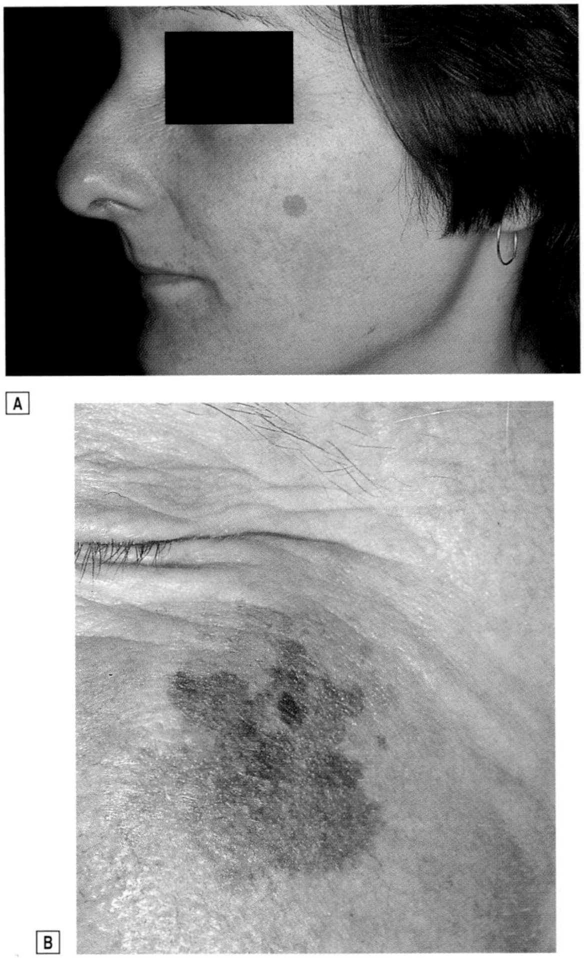

Fig. 2.21 Simple versus malignant lentigo. [A] Simple lesion with well-defined margin. [B] Malignant lesion with irregular margin and pigmentation.

recognised with the help of a lens, may provide the vital clue in diagnosing a widespread and non-specific rash. The best example of this is the burrow caused by the scabies mite (Fig. 2.23).

Close to the patient, perhaps aided by a lens, the clinician should study individual lesions carefully and ask the following questions.

QUESTIONS BOX: SKIN LESION MORPHOLOGY
• What are their shape? • What are their size? • What are their colour? • What are the characteristics of their margin and surfaces?

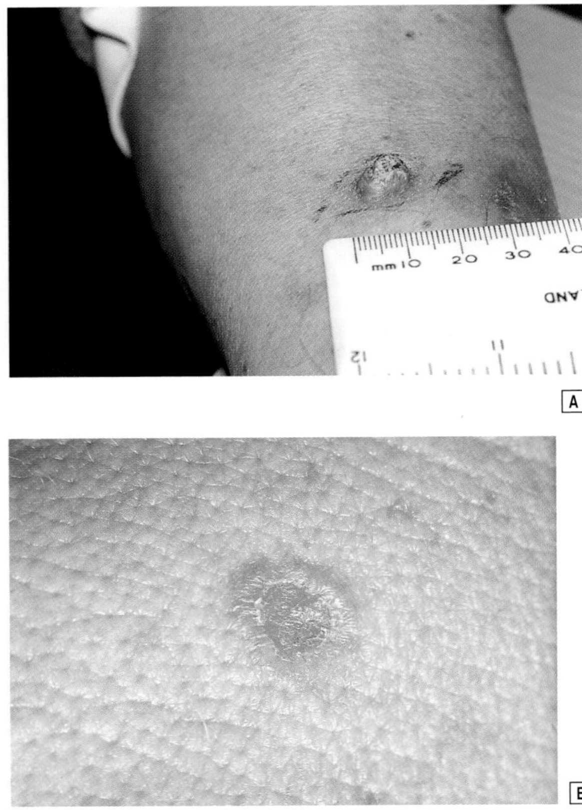

Fig. 2.22 Surface characteristics as a key to diagnosis. [A] Keratoacanthoma. [B] Basal cell carcinoma.

Configuration. Having studied the overall distribution of the rash and the morphology of individual lesions, the clinician should note the arrangement or configuration of the lesion or groups of lesions. Examples in which configuration of lesions aids diagnosis include the Köbner phenomenon in psoriasis and lichen planus, grouping of vesicles in herpes simplex (Fig. 2.24A), the patterning and peripheral spread of urticaria (Fig. 2.24B) and the linear appearance of insect bites (Fig. 2.24C).

KEY POINTS
• Ultraviolet radiation is the main factor speeding the ageing process in skin. • Skin lesions often evolve over a period of time. Several examinations during the period of evolution often facilitate diagnosis. • The overall distribution of a rash may be the most valuable clue to diagnosis. • The morphology of the primary lesion may be obscured by secondary changes but whenever possible should be carefully defined.

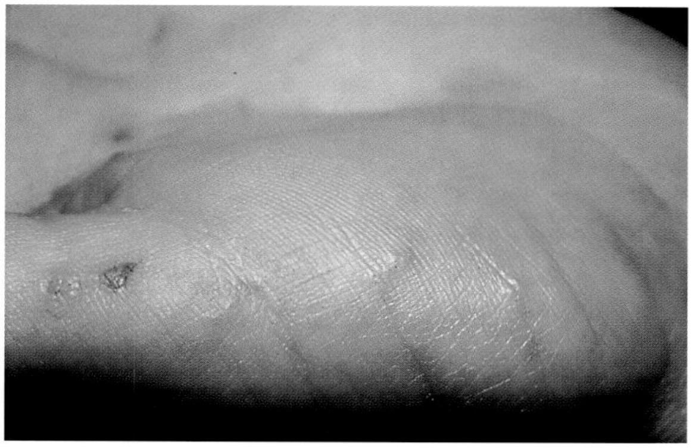

A

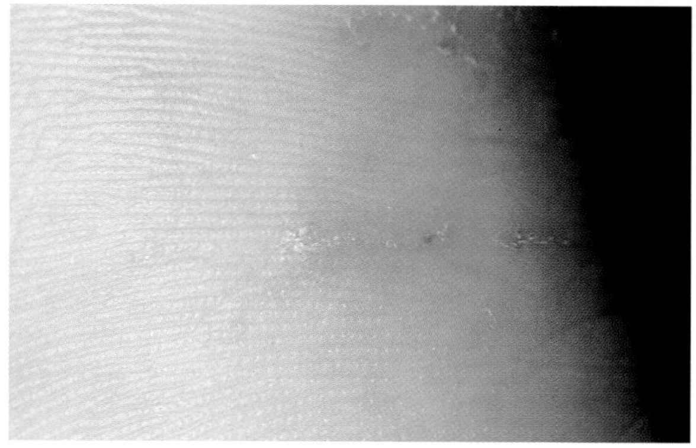

B

Fig. 2.23 Scabies burrow showing lesions on the hand, A and a close-up of a simple lesion, B.

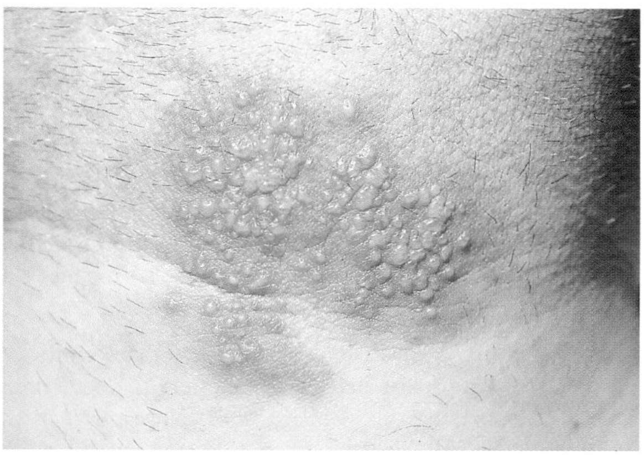

A

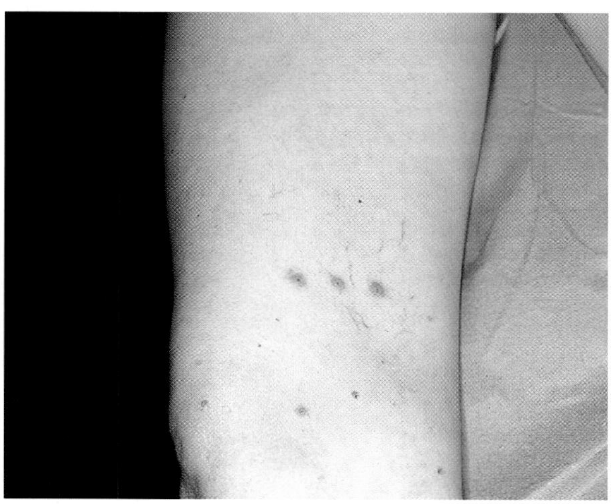

C

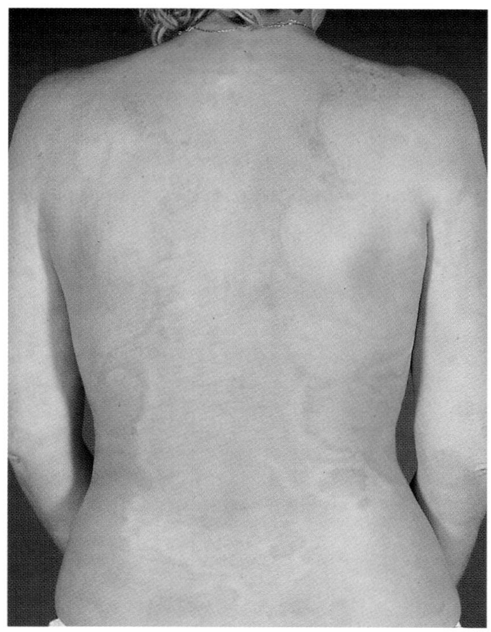

B

Fig. 2.24 Configuration of lesions as a key to diagnosis. A Vesicles of herpes simplex under the chin. B Extensive urticarial reaction. C Insect bites.

THE HANDS

After the initial appraisal of the patient, the formal physical assessment often begins with examination of the hands and pulse.

Anatomy

The hand is a highly developed structure and its area of representation in the cerebral cortex is appropriately extensive. Whilst the palmist may claim to read more from the hand than is justified, critical examination can indeed provide much reliable information. Attention should be paid first to general features and then to detailed consideration of individual structures on an anatomical basis. The examination of the function of the hand is described on page 274, and the significance of right or left handedness on page 231.

The keratinous nail plate is produced mainly in the nail matrix, which lies in an invagination of the epidermis, the nailfold, on the back of the terminal phalanx of each digit. The matrix runs from the end of the floor of the nailfold to the distal margin of the lunula ('half moon'), and from it the nail plate grows forward covering the nail bed (Fig. 2.25). A small part of the nail, the undersurface, is formed from cells in the nail bed. Nails grow throughout life. Fingernails grow more quickly than toenails, the growth in fingernails being approximately 1 cm in 3 months.

Examination sequence

- ☐ Inspect the general features of the dorsal and then the palmar aspects of both hands.
- ☐ Note specific changes in the skin, nails, tendons and joints.
- ☐ Look for evidence of muscle wasting.
- ☐ Assess the temperature and degree of sweating.
- ☐ Test hand function especially power and fine pinch (p. 274) and look for any sensory disturbance (p. 227).
- ☐ Assess the range of joint movements (p. 274).

Common abnormalities

Movements. Some people, including those of Mediterranean origin, 'speak' with their hands. For example, the hand pressed flat on the top of the head accompanying a complaint of headache suggests a psychogenic symptom 'something weighing on the mind'.

Tremors are studied with the hands at rest and then outstretched. Characteristic tremors are described in Table 2.4 (p. 28).

Tetany may be recognised by the presence of carpal spasm, where the hand(s) adopt a characteristic position with flexion of the metacarpophalangeal joints, extension of the interphalangeal joints of the fingers and thumb with opposition of the thumb, so-called *main d'accoucheur*. Latent tetany may be detected by Trousseau's sign (see Fig. 2.26). This is positive where carpal spasm occurs within 4 minutes of inflation of a sphygmomanometer cuff on the upper arm to a level above the systolic blood pressure.

Posture. This may be almost diagnostic. Examples include the flexed hand and arm of hemiplegia, wrist drop or radial nerve palsy and ulnar deviation in long-standing rheumatoid arthritis.

Shape. Trauma is the commonest cause of deformity of the hand. Some diagnostic shapes include the long thin fingers of arachnodactyly, while a short fourth metacarpal, best seen when making a fist, strongly suggests a diagnosis of Turner's syndrome in a girl with primary amenorrhoea. Short metacarpals, especially the fourth and fifth, are found in patients with pseudohypoparathyroidism.

Size. In acromegaly the hands are large and broad. Rings may be difficult to remove or may have been cut off or enlarged. The increase in bulk consists largely of soft tissues.

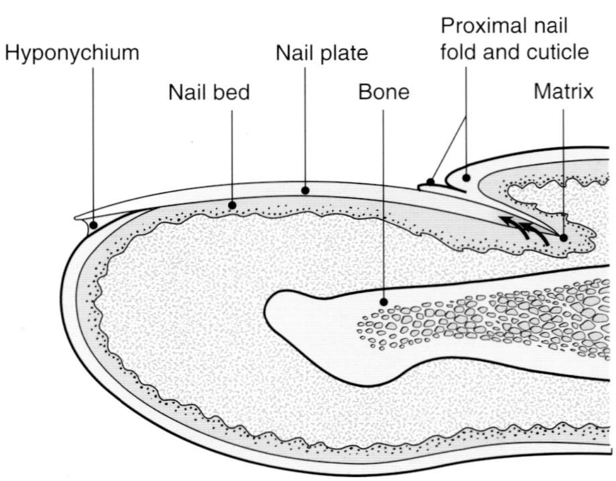

Fig. 2.25 Anatomy of the nail.

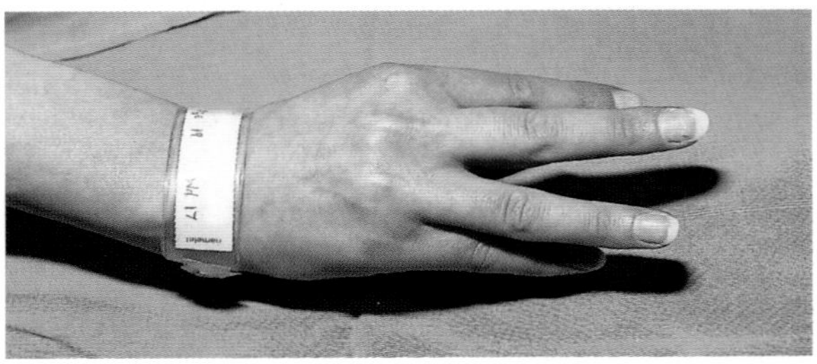

Fig. 2.26 Trousseau's sign.

These are also thickened in myxoedema. Oedema may be part of a generalised process or may arise from local venous or lymphatic obstruction or disuse, as with a hemiplegia.

Colour. By and large changes in the colour of the hands are similar to those of the skin in general (p. 26). The purported cigarette consumption should be reconciled with a degree of nicotine staining of the fingers. Coal miners may have small blue tattoo marks in the skin of their hands and in other sites where particles of coal dust have been embedded in the scars of minor injuries. In miners and in those with professional tattoos, the blue colour in the skin is due to black particles (carbon or Indian ink) changed in appearance by the scatter of light as it passes through and is reflected back from the skin. This explains why veins normally look blue, while in the elderly, with very thin skin, the true red colour of the blood may be seen.

Temperature. In a cold or cool climate the temperature of the patient's hand is a good guide to the blood flow. If the hand is warm and cyanosed, it can be deduced that arterial oxygen saturation is reduced.

The combination of central cyanosis and finger clubbing suggests congenital cyanotic heart disease (Fig. 2.27A). In most patients with heart failure the hands tend to be cold and cyanosed due to vasoconstriction in response to a low cardiac output. If they are warm the cause of the heart failure may be hyperthyroidism or cor pulmonale.

Skin

The smooth, hairless hands of a child become lined and hairy in the adult male unless hypogonadism is present. Manual work may produce specific callosities due to pressure at characteristic sites. In contrast, disuse results in a soft, smooth palmar skin and prolonged recumbency affects the soles likewise.

The skin may feature in a wide variety of specific skin disorders such as contact dermatitis (see Fig. 2.19D, p. 42). Skin changes may also occur as the dermatological manifestation of systemic disease (Fig. 2.27B). Likewise vitiligo may be restricted to the hands or face or widespread (Fig. 2.28). Its presence may indicate underlying autoimmune disease.

Nails

Growth is slowed by acute illness and ischaemia. It is increased in psoriasis. Injury to the nail matrix is by far the most common cause of changes in the nails and may permanently impair their growth. Some important changes in the nails are indicated in Table 2.10.

Longitudinal ridging and beading of the nail plate increases with age and is not abnormal. Similarly, occasional white transverse flecks (striate leuconychia) are seen frequently in normal nails; they are probably caused by minor and repeated trauma to the nail matrix and, contrary to the popular lay belief, are not due to insufficient calcium. Excessively shiny or polished nails are evidence of frequent rubbing of the skin by the nails.

Systemic vasculitis producing splinter haemorrhages (Fig. 2.29A) may also cause haemorrhages in the skin and retina and, occasionally, tender nodules in the fingertips (Osler's nodes). Although one or two are commonly seen under the nails of manual workers, multiple splinter haemorrhages raise the possibility of infective endocarditis.

Onycholysis, separation of the nail plate from the nail bed, may be due to minor trauma (especially if the nails are

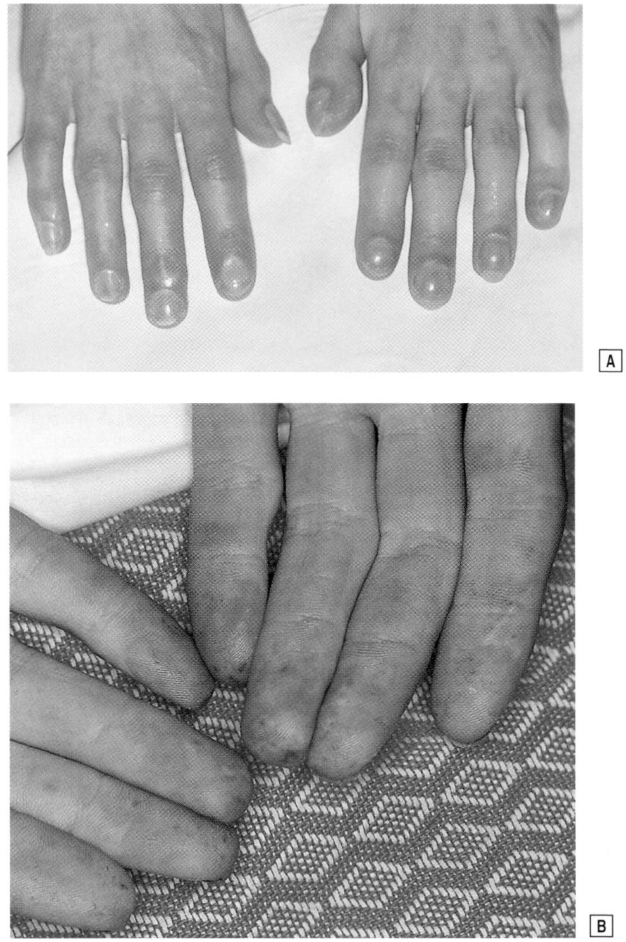

Fig. 2.27 The fingers as a diagnostic aid. A Cyanosis and finger clubbing in a patient with congenital heart disease. B Acute vasculitic lesions in a boy with systemic lupus erythematosus.

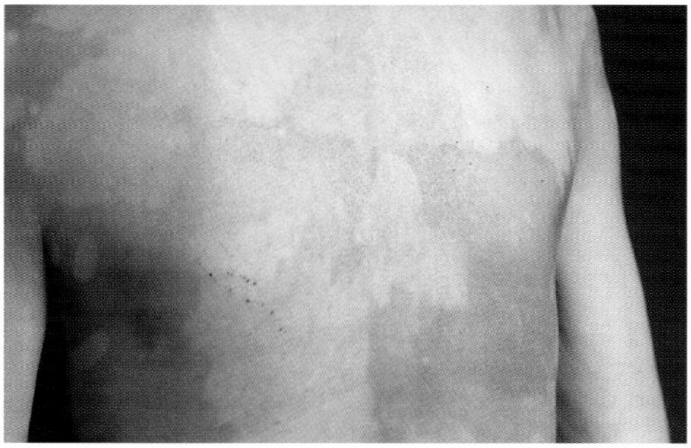

Fig. 2.28 Extensive vitiligo in patient with Addison's disease, primary hypothyroidism, pernicious anaemia and insulin-dependent diabetes mellitus.

TABLE 2.10 Important signs in the nails

Feature	Association
Bitten nails	Anxious personality
Finger clubbing	(See p. 125)
Splinter haemorrhages	Minor trauma, systemic vasculitis
Koilonychia	Chronic iron deficiency anaemia
Pitting	Psoriasis
Onycholysis	Trauma, psoriasis
Striate leuconychia	A 'normal' finding, ? minor trauma
Severe leuconychia (white nails or Terry's nails)	Hypoalbuminaemia, chronic liver disease, other wasting diseases
Transverse ridging (Beau's lines)	Recent acute illness
Fungal infection	Thickening, crumbling and discoloration
Red half-moons	Congestive cardiac failure
Blue half-moons	Hepatolenticular degeneration; Wilson's disease
'Half and half' nails	Chronic renal failure

left long) and psoriasis. It may also occur in thyroid disease. Nail pitting (Fig. 2.29B) is seen commonly in psoriasis though rarely in other conditions, such as alopecia areata and when eczema affects the proximal nailfold. In koilonychia the nails become brittle and flat, and ultimately spoon-shaped. It is a sign of iron deficiency and is seen most often in countries where malnutrition is prevalent. Beau's lines, due to temporary arrest of nail growth (Fig. 2.29C), are transverse grooves which appear at the same time on all nails a few weeks after an acute illness and which move out to the free margins as the nail grows. Colour changes are sometimes seen in nails. Whitening of the nails (leuconychia) is a sign of hypoalbuminaemia, as in cirrhosis of the liver (Fig. 2.29D). Occasionally, 'half and half' nails (white proximally and red-brown distally) are seen in patients with chronic renal failure. Rarely, drugs (e.g. antimalarials and phenothiazines) discolour nails.

The nailfolds

Examination of the nailfolds should accompany examination of the nails. Paronychia is the term used to describe inflamed, bolstered and swollen nailfolds. Chronic paronychia is seen most commonly in those with a poor peripheral circulation, in those involved in wet work, in diabetes and those who are overenthusiastic when manicuring their cuticles. Ragged cuticles and dilated or thrombosed capillaries in the proximal nailfold are an important pointer to connective tissue disease (Fig. 2.29E).

Subcutaneous tissues

In Dupuytren's contracture there is thickening and shortening of the palmar fascia, resulting in flexion deformities, particularly of the fifth and ring fingers. Firm, painless subcutaneous nodules occur in rheumatoid disease; these occur more frequently over the upper end of the ulna than on the hands. Finger clubbing is discussed on page 125.

Joints

Arthritis frequently involves the small joints of the hands. Common conditions include osteoarthrosis, rheumatoid arthritis and psoriatic arthropathy.

Muscles

Wasting is common in rheumatoid arthritis. It also occurs in lesions of the lower motor neurone. Causes include syringomyelia, poliomyelitis, lesions of the first thoracic nerve root, the peripheral neuropathies and motor neurone disease, in which fasciculation is often present. Lesions of the ulnar and median nerves will affect muscle groups, e.g. in leprosy.

In the carpal tunnel syndrome, median nerve compression may result in selective wasting of the thenar muscles. This may occur in rheumatoid arthritis, autoimmune hypothyroidism and acromegaly, or may be associated with premenstrual fluid retention or pregnancy (see Fig 8.14, p. 273).

Tendons

Excessive use of the tendon may result in tenosynovitis. This commonly produces a sensation of local crepitus and swelling over the tendon sheath. A common site is the extensor pollicus tendon at the wrist where it crosses the radial styloid (de Quervain's tenosynovitis). Thickening of a flexor tendon may result in a trigger finger or thumb.

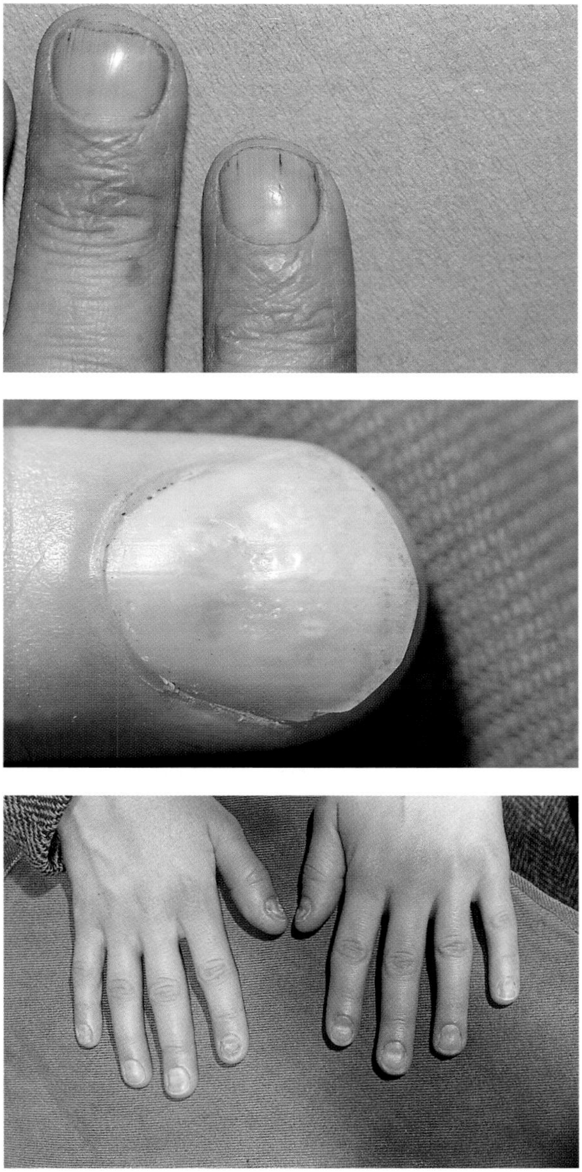

A

B

C

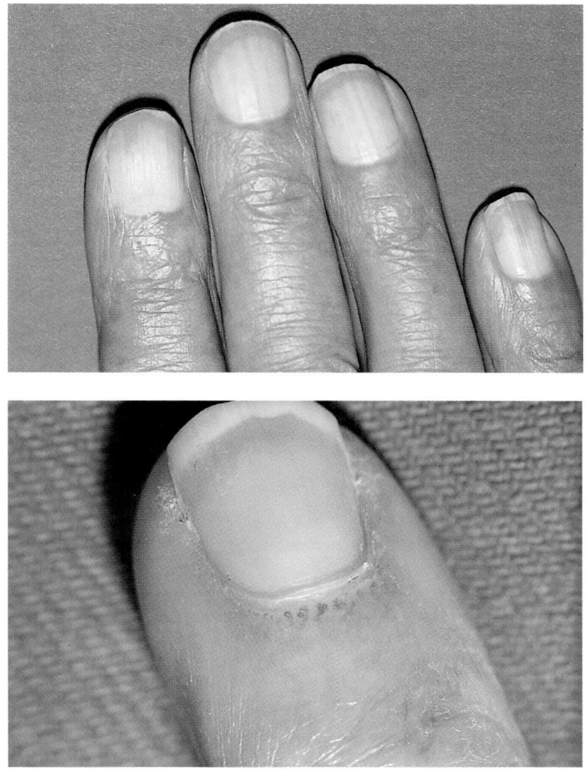

D

E

Fig. 2.29 The nail as a diagnostic aid. A Splinter haemorrhages. B Onycholysis with pitting in psoriasis. C Beau's lines. D Leuconychia. E Dilated capillaries in the proximal nailfold in systemic lupus erythematosus.

Bones

In fractures of the scaphoid the only finding may be tenderness localised in the anatomical snuffbox. Occasionally the bones of the hand, particularly the phalanges, may be involved in granulomatous or other generalised disorders such as sarcoidosis, Paget's disease or hyperparathyroidism. Acute dactylitis is characteristic of sickle cell disease in children. Graves' disease, autoimmune hyperthyroidism, may be associated with finger clubbing and periosteal new bone formation in the phalanges.

Nerves

In sensory polyneuropathy there is a characteristic impairment of a glove distribution affecting both hands; the feet are usually also involved. An example, common in the tropics, is the late result of dimorphous or lepromatous leprosy.

Secondary infection through abrasions leads to deformities from absorption of the phalanges or tissue loss by ulceration. In tuberculoid leprosy the lesions are likely to be asymmetrical or unilateral.

Blood vessels

Palmar erythema is a mottled, bright-red cutaneous vasodilatation seen mainly over the thenar and hypothenar eminences. Though found in normal persons, it is suggestive of liver dysfunction. Arteritis may occur in infective endocarditis and in connective tissue disorders; it may cause small necrotic lesions around the base of the nail and

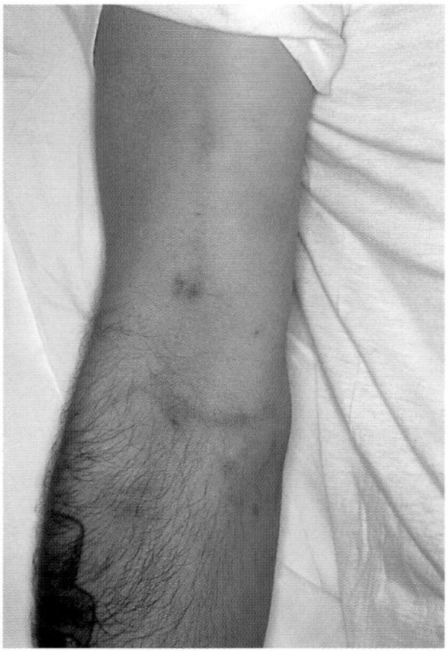

Fig. 2.30 The linear marks of intravenous injection at the right elbow.

on the pulps, most commonly in systemic lupus erythematosus (Fig. 2.27B). Raynaud's phenomenon is described on page 110. Venous abnormalities are seldom seen, but the linear marks caused by the intravenous injection of drugs of addicts ('mainliners') are characteristic (Fig. 2.30).

KEY POINTS

- The importance of the hand is indicated by its area of representation in the cerebral cortex.
- Some people 'speak' with their hands.
- The skin is smooth and soft with disuse, whereas manual work produces distinctive callosities in the hands.
- Trauma is a common cause of changes in the nails.

THE HEAD

The examination of the various components of the head is described in topographical sequence – the hair (p. 36), the cranium, face, eyes, ears, nose and mouth. The examination of the mouth involves the inspection of the lips, teeth, gums, tongue, floor of the mouth, mucosa of the cheeks, palate, tonsils and the oropharynx. In practice, this routine is rarely followed. The examination of the eyes is considered separately in Chapter 7.

Examination sequence

☐ Inspect the general shape of the head. Palpate any abnormalities and auscultate if appropriate (Fig. 2.33).

A

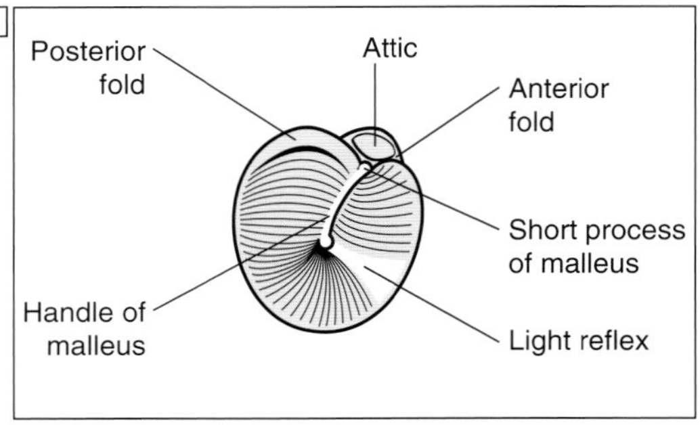

B

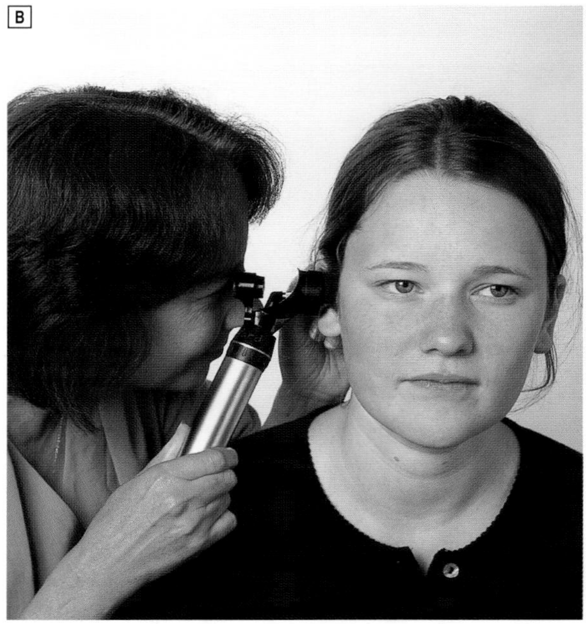

Fig. 2.31 Examining the ear. A The ear drum. B Auroscopic examination.

Ears

☐ Confirm that the light of the auriscope is working.
☐ Select a speculum of appropriate length with the largest diameter that will fit the meatus in comfort.
☐ Gently retract the pinna upwards and backwards to straighten the external meatus (Fig. 2.31B), thereby facilitating insertion of the speculum.
☐ Examine the external meatus, then identify and examine the ear drum (Fig. 2.31A).
☐ If the vision is obscured by wax, remove this using a wax hook or by gentle syringing with warm water.

Nose

☐ Test the patency of the nasal airways by asking the patient to sniff as each nostril is occluded in turn by finger pressure.

- ☐ Using a nasal speculum, examine the state of the mucosa of the nose and identify the anterior ends of the inferior turbinates.
- ☐ If sinusitis is suspected, apply firm finger pressure over the frontal and maxillary areas to identify any localised tenderness.

Mouth
- ☐ Remove any dentures before examining the mouth.
- ☐ Use a pocket torch or other light source with a wooden tongue depressor or similar instrument.
- ☐ Note the symmetry, size and shape of the tongue and look for fasciculation.
- ☐ Carefully inspect the lips, teeth, gums, cheeks, floor of the mouth; use the spatula to separate the cheeks and tongue from the teeth and gums.
- ☐ Inspect the soft palate, tonsils and oropharynx; if a clear view cannot be obtained by asking the patient to say 'Ah', depress the tongue with the spatula.
- ☐ Use a suitable mirror to inspect the nasopharynx.

Common abnormalities

The cranium

The examination of the cranium in infancy and childhood can be very valuable. In the adult, inspection may reveal generalised enlargement in Paget's disease or localised bony bossing overlying a meningioma. The supraorbital ridges often enlarge in acromegaly as a result of increase in the size of the frontal sinuses.

In cranial arteritis the temporal arteries may be visibly or palpably enlarged and tender (Fig. 2.32). On auscultation a bruit may occasionally be detected in the presence of an intracranial arteriovenous malformation (Fig. 2.33).

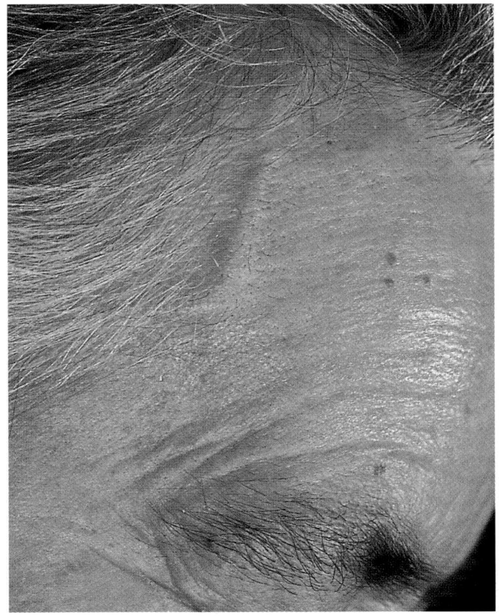

Fig. 2.32 Temporal arteritis showing an enlarged palpable artery.

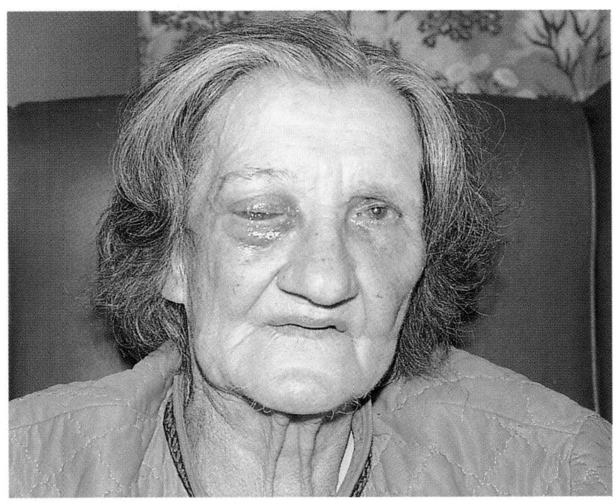

Fig. 2.33 78-year-old lady with 'buzzing noises in head' due to right carotid-cavernous fistula. Periorbital oedema and severe chemosis are present and a bruit was heard over the right forehead and eyelid.

The face and eyes

The face may provide important diagnostic information (Fig. 2.34). Some facial appearances are characteristic of specific diseases (Table 2.11). The eyes are discussed in Chapter 7.

The ears

Normal ears vary widely in size, shape and form. There are some genetic deformities. For example, in Down's syndrome the auricles are usually small and the lobule may be rudimentary or absent. The helix of the ear is a recognised site of gouty tophi – white chalky nodules consisting of sodium biurate crystals deposited in the cartilage (Fig. 2.35). Local trauma to the ear may cause haemorrhage. When frequent, partial organisation can lead to permanent deformity and the features of 'cauliflower ear'.

Acute otitis media usually causes earache, which may be severe, but in infants it may present as an acute febrile illness without local pain and auroscopy is indicated in all such children and any patient with headache or a hearing difficulty.

The normal drum as seen through the auriscope, appears pearly grey, with the handle of the malleus visible and lying almost vertically near the centre of the tympanic membrane.

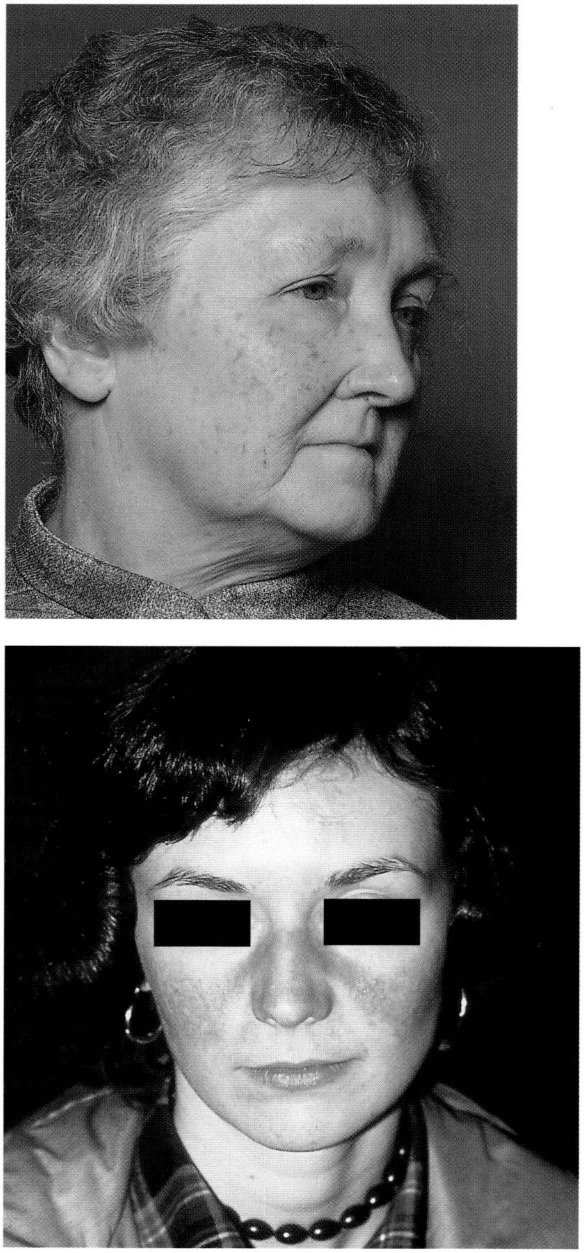

A

B

Fig. 2.34 The face as a diagnostic aid. A Facial telangiectasia in 69-year-old lady with CREST syndrome. B The characteristic rash of systemic lupus erythematosus.

A cone of light is reflected from its lower end downwards and forwards to the periphery of the drum (see Fig. 2.31A).

The common abnormalities on inspection of the drum are acute inflammation and perforation.

TABLE 2.11 Examples of facial appearance characteristic of specific diseases

Endocrine	Hyperthyroidism Hypothyroidism Cushing's syndrome
Genetic	Down's syndrome
Renal	Nephrotic syndrome
Cardiovascular	Superior vena caval obstruction
Infective	Risus sardonicus in tetany
Neuromuscular	Myasthenia gravis VII nerve palsy

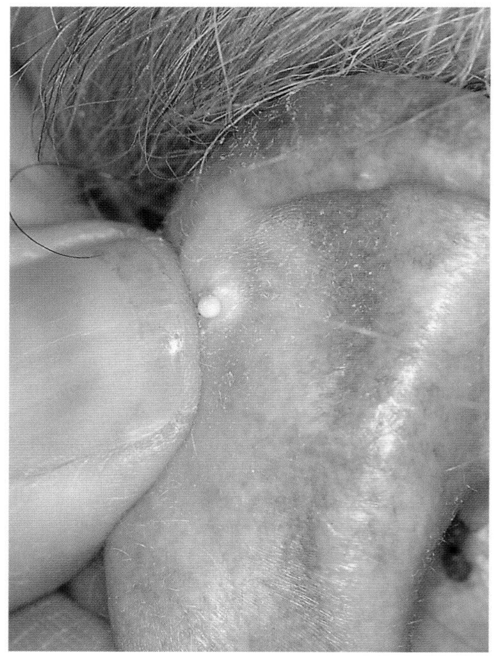

Fig. 2.35 Gouty tophus of the ear (Reproduced by permission of J. Gibson.)

Wax commonly obscures the view and may need to be removed. Hard wax may need to be softened by the application of a few drops of olive oil or an appropriate preparation for 2 or 3 days before removal. Syringing should be undertaken by an expert if there is a history of middle ear disease or in the presence of perforation. Foreign bodies in the external meatus are not uncommon in children.

The nose and sinuses

The nose may be deformed as a result of an old fracture, or enlarged, red and bulbous (rhinophyma) in the late stages of rosacea (Fig. 2.36, p. 53).

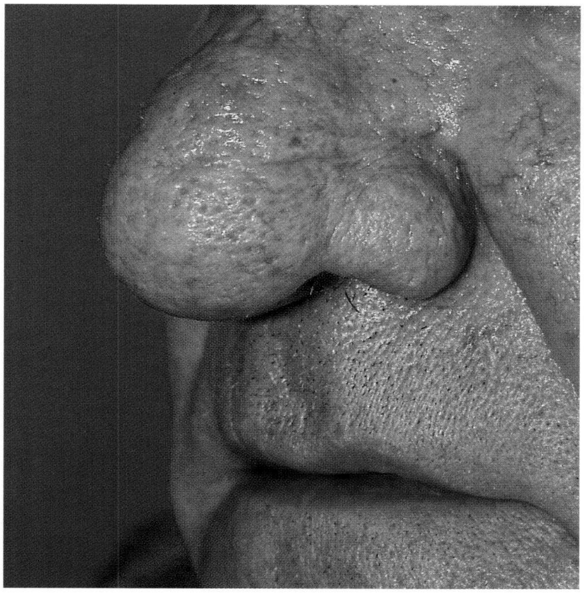

Fig. 2.36 Rhinophyma as a complication of rosacea.

Destruction of the nasal septum may produce flattening of the bridge and a 'saddle-nose' appearance. This is frequently the result of local trauma. Other causes include Wegener's granulomatosis, congenital syphilis or nasal sniffing of cocaine. This may also produce ulceration of the nasal mucosa. Other common mucosal abnormalities include:

- Narrowing of the nose when there is chronic obstruction of the airway in childhood. When associated with mouth breathing this produces the 'adenoidal facies'.
- Widening of the nose, one of the early features of acromegaly.
- Nasal polyps; these are pearly grey in colour and bleeding points can be readily identified on the nasal septum.

Infection of the frontal air sinuses may cause a headache, which characteristically reaches a peak within 2 or 3 hours of rising and then spontaneously subsides as the day proceeds. Involvement of the maxillary sinuses may stimulate toothache. A purulent nasal or postnasal discharge is often present and there may be tenderness on pressure over the affected sinus.

The lips

Exposure to cold commonly causes dryness followed by desquamation and cracking of the lips. Somewhat resembling this is the much rarer cheilosis of riboflavine deficiency causing red, denuded epithelium at the line of closure of the lips, peeling towards the mucocutaneous junction. A similar appearance may result from the use of lipstick to which the patient is hypersensitive.

Angular stomatitis, consisting of painful inflamed cracks at the corners of the mouth, is often caused by ill-fitting dentures allowing saliva to dribble out of the mouth, followed by infection with Candida albicans. Angular stomatitis may also be due to deficiency of iron or riboflavine.

A fissure of the lip in an elderly patient, which fails to heal in spite of treatment, should be regarded as a possible epithelioma and requires biopsy.

The teeth

Inspection of the 32 so-called 'permanent teeth' may reveal important information. There are three common findings:

- *Caries* is related to lack of fluoride and can be kept in check by regular dental care. Extensive caries may be an index of self-neglect.
- *Discoloration* is usually due to staining from tobacco or from poor hygiene, but devitalised teeth also gradually become grey. The teeth may be pitted and mottled yellow in fluorosis.
- *Missing teeth* are most commonly the molars; as these are used for grinding rather than biting, their absence is important in connection with alimentary symptoms.

Notched, separated and peg-shaped upper incisors occur in congenital syphilis (Hutchinson's teeth), and poorly developed teeth are a feature of juvenile hypoparathyroidism. Eruption of the teeth may be retarded as part of any disorder responsible for delayed development, especially rickets.

The gums

Gingivitis is very common. At first bleeding is apt to occur, and a narrow line of inflammation can be seen at the free border of the gum, and the interdental papillae are swollen.

If the condition progresses, food debris, bacteria and pus tend to accumulate between the teeth and the gum margin (pyorrhoea alveolaris). Halitosis may be apparent and the teeth may become loose. Pus or even a tooth may be aspirated into the bronchial tree and initiate pneumonia. Badly affected gums are associated with frequent transient bacteraemia, the usual organism being *Streptococcus viridans*. This may cause infective endocarditis, especially in patients with valvular heart disease. Painful ulceromembranous gingivitis may be due to Vincent's infection (p. 56).

TABLE 2.12 The gums in systemic conditions

Phenytoin treatment	Firm and hypertrophied
Scurvy	Soft, haemorrhagic
Acute leukaemia	Hypertrophied and haemorrhagic
Cyanotic congenital heart disease	Spongy and haemorrhagic
Chronic lead poisoning	Punctate blue line

Changes in the gum may also be a feature of systemic disease (Table 2.12). If phenytoin causes distressing hyperplasia, it is advisable to change to another anticonvulsant.

The tongue

The surface of the tongue normally varies greatly in regard to both colour and appearance. Shades of pink and red or even yellow, brown or almost black may be of no medical significance though they are a potential cause of anxiety to the subject. Variations in colour may be caused by foods, particularly coloured sweets, or they may be due to quantitative or qualitative changes in the haemoglobin. Central cyanosis can best be assessed clinically by inspection of the tongue (p. 81). A clean tongue, often red with prominent papillae, can result from antibiotic treatment. Iron or vitamin B_{12} deficiency causes a smooth clean-looking tongue from diffuse atrophy of the papillae.

The fungiform papillae are small, red, flat elevations on the surface, especially at the tip and edges. The filiform papillae are more numerous at the centre and give rise to the fur. Transient denuded islands (geographical tongue) constitute a symptomless change of no known significance.

Excessive furring occurs in healthy people and in fever or dehydration. Congenital fissuring of the tongue has no pathological significance.

Separating the anterior two-thirds from the posterior third of the tongue are the circumvallate papillae set in a wide V with its apex pointing backwards. Patients who discover these may be alarmed by the thought that they might be cancerous. In contrast, leukoplakia is a precancerous condition. It is characterised by grey opaque areas interspersed with a few red inflamed patches. Ulcers of the tongue may be caused by sharp, damaged teeth, but malignancy should always be considered.

The request 'please put out your tongue' may provide general information. For example, a stuporous patient who responds obviously hears and understands. Neurological disease, a tight frenulum, a painful condition of the mouth or undue modesty may restrict protrusion. Fasciculation (p. 213), within the tongue at rest, is a feature of motor neurone disease. Lesions of the hypoglossal nerve cause wasting of half the tongue (p. 213), which protrudes toward the affected side. The tongue is enlarged in Down's syndrome, acromegaly, myxoedema and in some patients with amyloidosis.

The palate

The hard palate comprises the anterior two-thirds, and the soft palate with the uvula lies posteriorly. Abnormalities include cleft palate and a narrow high arched palate. This is of little importance by itself, but may be associated with other congenital conditions.

The uvula varies greatly in size and shape; it seldom presents clinical problems except to some patients with obsessional anxiety. The examination of movement of the soft palate is described on page 211.

The tonsils

The tonsils are masses of lymphoid tissue that lie beneath the mucous membrane between the pillars of the fauces. In common with lymphoid tissue elsewhere, the tonsils enlarge to reach a maximum between the ages of 8 and 12 years, after which involution takes place. Failure to recognise this normal phase of lymphoid hyperplasia has led to erroneous recommendations for tonsillectomy. In streptococcal tonsillitis the tonsils are swollen and inflamed, often with pus exuding from the tonsillar crypts. Less common causes of sore throat include infectious mononucleosis, Vincent's infection and diphtheria (p. 56).

Tumours of the tonsils may occur either in isolation or as part of lymphatic leukaemia or lymphoma.

The pharynx and buccal mucosa

Small lymphatic nodules can normally be observed on the posterior wall. With infection in the nose or sinuses, mucus or pus may be visible trickling down the back of the throat.

Koplik's spots. In measles small white spots on an erythematous background are distributed over the mucosa of the cheeks opposite the molar teeth and sometimes throughout the mouth. These Koplik's spots are of diagnostic value as they appear before the rash.

Aphthous stomatitis. This is characterised by ulcers on the inner sides of the lips, the edges of the tongue, the insides of the cheek or on the palate. Initially small vesicles form, which quickly burst, leaving shallow ulcers usually surrounded by a red margin. Such ulcers can cause intense discomfort. They may heal quickly in a day or two, or they may progress into deep indurated ulcers which heal slowly (Fig. 2.37) and may leave a small scar. The lesions tend to occur in crops; a patient may be free from ulcers for months only to relapse. The cause is obscure. They are often seen in patients with ulcerative colitis.

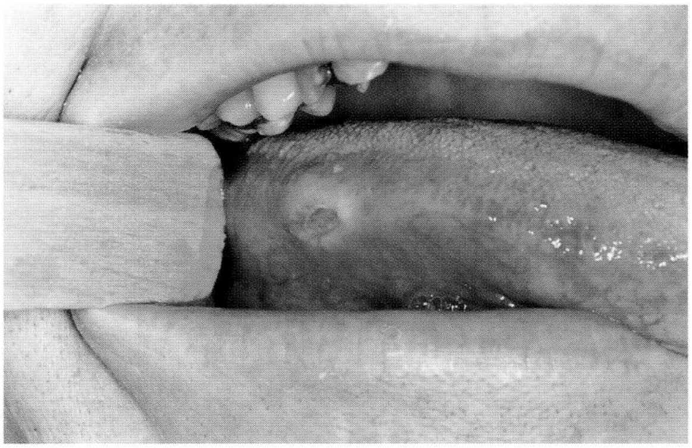

Fig. 2.37 Aphthous stomatitis causing a deep ulcer in a young patient with inflammatory bowel disease.

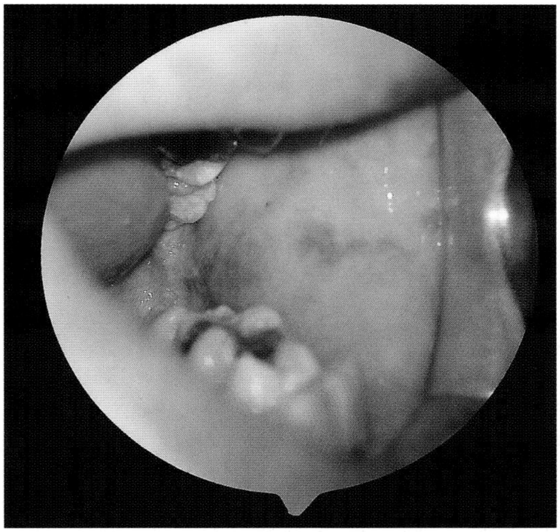

Fig. 2.38 Buccal pigmentation in Addison's disease.

Pigmentation in the mouth. Melanin deposition in the buccal mucosa is normal in black people and is proportionally reduced as the skin becomes lighter. Pathological pigmentation in the mouth occurs in Addison's disease (Fig. 2.38). Other causes are chronic cachexia, the malabsorption syndrome, haemochromatosis or the rare Peutz–Jeghers syndrome. This comprises polyposis of the small intestine with pigmentation around and in the mouth and on the lips and fingers. In patients with black hair and brown eyes buccal pigmentation may be congenital.

The salivary glands

While examining the mouth, the opening of the parotid duct may be seen on the buccal mucosa as a small papilla opposite the second upper molar tooth. The openings of the submandibular salivary gland ducts seldom require identification, but may be found near the midline in the sublingual papilla, adjoining the root of the frenulum of the tongue.

Each of these openings is more readily seen if a free flow of saliva is provoked by something tasty. Purulent infections of the salivary glands may be investigated by culturing pus expressed through these orifices.

Causes of enlargement of the parotid gland include mumps, sarcoidosis, tumour and suppurative parotitis which is often associated with poor oral hygiene. (Fig. 2.39A and B). Obstruction of the duct may produce

A

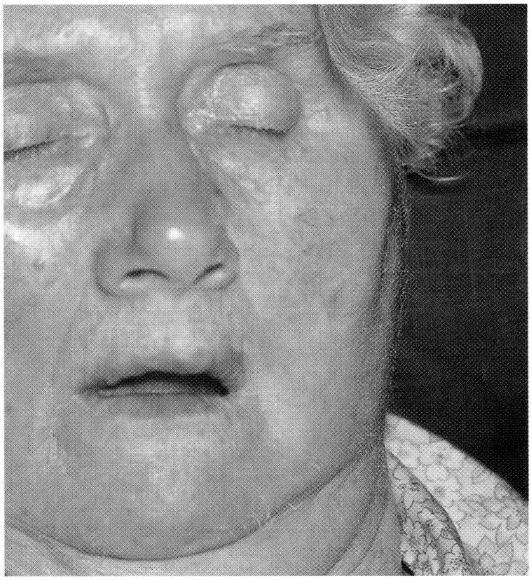

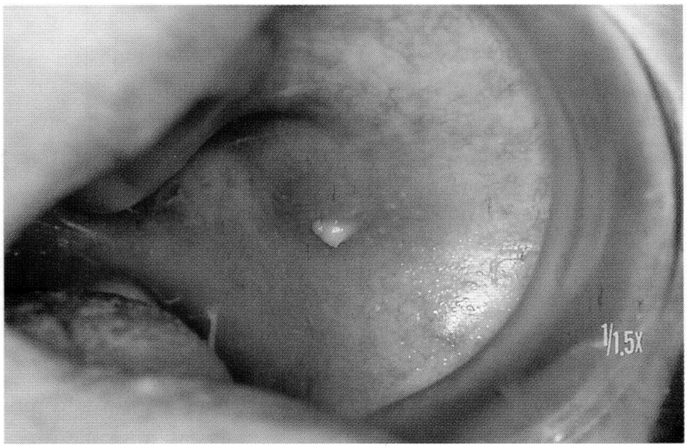

B

Fig. 2.39 A Suppurative parotitis with B pus discharging from parotid duct.

CASE HISTORY

An 80-year-old lady was admitted with a right hemiplegia and difficulty in swallowing. Some 4 days after admission, she had a temperature of 38.5°C and was noted to have a tender enlargement of the left parotid gland (Fig. 2.39A) and a discharge of pus was seen from the left parotid duct inside the mouth (Fig. 2.39B). The clinical picture suggested that relative dehydration and poor oral hygiene had predisposed to the development of acute suppurative parotitis. Staphylococcus aureus was grown and the patient responded to flucloxacillin therapy.

Learning points

- Patients who are compromised for any reason are at increased risk, especially from infection.
- It is important to recognise, and treat, conditions which are treatable.
- The successful management of a 'minor problem' may produce major symptomatic relief.

intermittent swelling with pain while eating. Obstruction due to salivary calculi is very much more frequent in the submandibular ducts. The submandibular glands may sometimes be affected by mumps in the absence of parotid swelling.

Common disorders of the mouth

Ulcerative stomatitis. This is commonly due to the combination of a spirochaete and a fusiform bacillus which can be seen in a smear taken from one of the ulcers (Vincent's infection). The condition is painful and foul smelling.

Ulcerative stomatitis may complicate acute leukaemia or agranulocytosis and immunosuppression. In acute leukaemia the gums often bleed and may be so swollen that the teeth may be largely obscured. Agranulocytosis may present as a sore throat, which may progress to an ulcerative stomatitis.

Thrush. This may occur in the infants of mothers who carry infection with *Candida albicans* in the vagina. It also occurs, particularly in the elderly, in association with febrile or debilitating diseases. It is common in patients being treated with antibiotics, corticosteroids or immunosuppressive drugs (Fig. 2.40). Fungal plaques may be seen as individual or coalescent white deposits adhering to the mucous membrane of any part of the mouth. There is very little evidence of inflammation.

Diphtheria. In this condition an adherent membrane forms on the tonsils or less commonly in the nose or larynx. The affected area bleeds if attempts are made to remove the membrane. The smell is characteristic. The causative organism can be identified on a direct smear and its pathogenicity determined by bacteriological examination. Infectious mononucleosis may also produce a membrane on the tonsils.

Syphilis. In the secondary stages syphilis causes highly

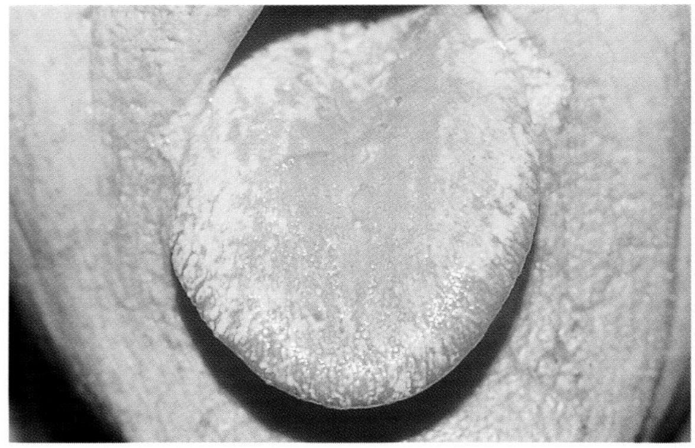

Fig. 2.40 Extensive oral thrush; a feature of previous antibiotic therapy.

infective mucous patches consisting of shallow ulcers with a narrow red margin and a surface covered by a thin white membrane; they resemble snail tracks. The primary ulcer or *chancre* of syphilis may also occur on the lips and sometimes in other parts of the mouth.

Carcinoma. Carcinoma may be found on the lips, the tongue, the fauces, or the floor of the mouth, usually in the form of an ulcer. Any indolent ulcer requires a biopsy. Only in the later stages of disease may other signs of malignant disease appear, such as enlargement of the regional lymph nodes and fixation of the mass.

KEY POINTS

- Auroscopy is indicated in all patients with hearing problems or headache and in children with a febrile illness.
- Removal of wax by syringing should only be performed by an expert if there is disease of the middle ear or perforation of the ear drum.
- Angular stomatitis is often caused by ill-fitting dentures.
- Dental disease may provide an index of self-neglect.
- The colour of the healthy tongue is extremely variable.
- Physiological enlargement of the tonsils occurs during childhood.
- All dentures should be removed before examining the mouth.

SWELLINGS

This section describes the common principles involved in the examination of a swelling.

The 'sudden' finding of a lump by a patient does not necessarily imply that it has only recently developed. It is important to ask if any change in size or other characteristics have been noted since it was first detected and whether there are any associated features such as pain, tenderness or colour changes. The history of preceding events may also be of diagnostic help. Sometimes physical examination will reveal a lump of which the patient is unaware.

Examination sequence

- ☐ Inspect any mass carefully, noting change in the colour or texture of the overlying skin.
- ☐ Gently palpate to elicit any tenderness or change in skin temperature.
- ☐ Without causing undue tenderness (by palpation), define the site and shape of the mass. Measure its size and record the findings diagrammatically.
- ☐ Keep the hand on the mass for a few moments to determine if it is pulsatile.
- ☐ Assess the consistency, surface texture and margins of the mass.
- ☐ Attempt to pick up a fold of skin over the swelling to assess skin fixation and contrast the mobility of the skin with the unaffected side.
- ☐ Determine fixation to deeper structures by attempting to move the swelling in different planes relative to the surrounding tissues.
- ☐ Look for fluctuation by compressing the swelling suddenly with one finger, using another finger to determine if a bulge is created.
- ☐ Confirm the presence of fluctuation in two planes.
- ☐ Auscultate for vascular bruits and other sounds.
- ☐ Elicit transillumination in the dark. Press the lighted end of an electric torch into one side of the swelling. A cystic swelling will light up if the fluid is translucent, provided that the covering tissues are not too thick.

Abnormal features

Position. The site of some swellings such as those in the breast, the thyroid or the parotid glands presents no difficulty. In others, the ease with which the lump can be localised will vary, especially in the abdomen. Features such as shape or mobility may help to identify the anatomical origin and occasionally percussion may also help in defining an abdominal mass.

Size. The size of any swelling requires to be accurately measured and documented. In this way significant changes can be recognised. Vague and misleading statements about size, such as large, medium or small, or comparisons with fruit, eggs or vegetables should be avoided.

Shape. The shape of a mass may be sufficiently characteristic to signify its origin. Examples in the abdomen include an enlarged spleen or liver, a distended bladder or the fundus of the uterus in later pregnancy.

Temperature and colour. The skin over acute inflammatory lesions is usually red and warm. There may also be a rise in skin temperature over a vascular tumour which ranges in colour from red to blue or purple according to the proportions of reduced haemoglobin present and the depth of the layer of skin through which it is seen. In haematomas the pigment from extravasated blood may produce the range of colours so familiar in a bruise. A brown or black colour is common in melanomas (Fig. 2.21, p. 44), though some are not pigmented. A xanthoma is a small skin nodule which may be identified by its yellow colour because of the lipids it contains.

Pain and tenderness. Inflammatory swellings are characterised by tenderness. Some other swellings, such as large lipomas, may be entirely free from pain or tenderness, because they carry no nerve supply and have developed in an area where the mass can be accommodated without subjecting any structure to undue stretching. Tumours eroding bone or growing into nerve roots and plexuses cause severe persistent and intractable pain which is often worse at night.

Movement. A mass may be part of, attached to, or free from adjacent structures, such as skin or bone. Fixation of the skin may be associated with a fine dimpling at the opening of the hair follicles resembling an orange skin when there is lymphatic obstruction ('*peau d'orange*'). Such a change is most commonly due to malignant disease. Fixation to deeper structures may occur. For example, a breast tumour may become fixed to underlying muscle.

The presence or absence of movement on swallowing, respiration and coughing will produce information regarding the nature of the swelling in the neck (p. 62), abdomen (p. 162) and hernial orifices (p. 163) respectively.

Expansile pulsations arise from aneurysmal dilatation of the aorta or other large arteries, or highly vascular tumours. A transmitted pulsation may be detected if a mass is in contact with a major blood vessel. In tricuspid incompetence, the liver is pulsatile.

Consistency. The consistency of a swelling may vary from soft and fluctuant through increasing degrees of firmness until this may merit the term 'stony hard'. Very hard swellings are usually malignant or calcified, or consist of dense fibrous tissue.

Fluctuation indicates a fluid-containing swelling, such as an abscess or a cyst. Soft encapsulated tumours such as lipomas may also show some degree of fluctuation.

Surface texture. The surface of a swelling may vary from the uniformly smooth to the grossly irregular. The texture often provides important evidence of the pathological process. For example, on palpation of the liver the surface is smooth in acute right ventricular failure but is usually grossly nodular in metastatic malignancy.

Margin. The edge or margin may be well delineated or ill defined, regular or irregular, sharp or rounded. The margins

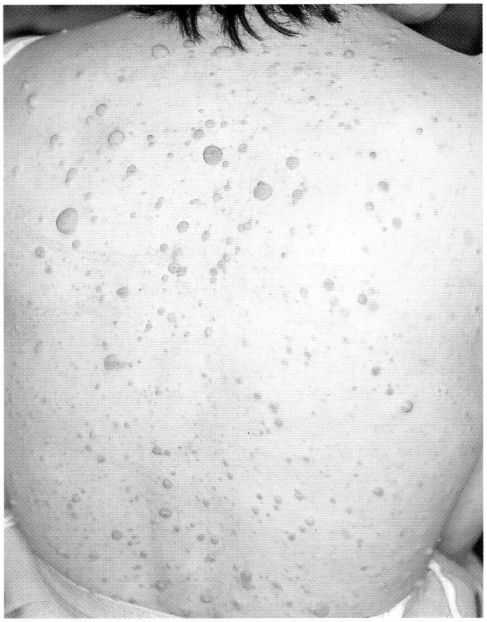

Fig. 2.41 Neurofibromatosis.

of enlarged organs such as the thyroid gland, liver, spleen or kidney can usually be defined more clearly than those of inflammatory or malignant masses. An indefinite margin may suggest an infiltrating malignancy in contrast to the clearly defined edge of a benign tumour.

Associated swellings. Conditions in which multiple swellings occur include neurofibromatosis (Fig. 2.41), lipomatosis, metastases in the skin, lymph nodes in the lymphomas and fibrocystic changes in the breast. If there is suspicion that a tumour is malignant, the lymph nodes draining the area concerned should be thoroughly examined.

Auscultation

Auscultation may be of value. If the blood flow through a tumour is large, a systolic murmur (bruit) may be audible over the swelling and, if it is sufficiently marked, a thrill may be palpable. Systolic murmurs may also be heard over arterial aneurysms, while over the very rare swelling due to an arteriovenous fistula there is a continuous murmur, often accompanied by a thrill, similar to the bruit of a persistent ductus arteriosus (p. 100).

During pregnancy fetal heart sounds may be audible over the uterus after 30 weeks. The noise of blood flowing through extensive vascular formations in the uterus may also be audible (uterine souffle).

Intestine and bowel sounds (p. 170) may be heard over a hernia which contains intestine.

Transillumination

This may be useful in distinguishing between a swelling composed of solid tissue and one consisting of transparent or semitransparent liquid. For example, the sign may help to distinguish a hydrocele from other scrotal swellings (p. 172). It requires to be borne in mind that a testicular tumour may lie within a hydrocele.

KEY POINTS

- A swelling which is suddenly found may not have recently developed.
- The shape and size of any swelling should be defined and measured.

THE LYMPH GLANDS

The lymphoreticular system comprises the spleen, the lymph nodes and lymphatic ducts and lymphoid tissue elsewhere, including the tonsils, adenoids and the Peyer's patches of the ileum. It is important to distinguish between a normal lymph node which may be palpable and a pathological gland. The finding of pathological lymphadenopathy is frequently of considerable diagnostic or prognostic significance, for example in the staging of various lymphoproliferative and other malignancies. Pathological lymphadenopathy may be local or generalised.

History

A patient's attention may be drawn to lymphatic enlargement by the presence of pain. Sometimes pain-free glands are detected on inspection or by palpation, for example when taking a shower or a bath. Their finding may cause understandable but hopefully inappropriate concern.

Frequently the dominant symptoms are those of the underlying pathological process and lymphadenopathy is only discovered during physical examination. Where HIV infection is a possibility, the patient should be asked about possible drug abuse, sexual habits and other risk factors.

Anatomy

The important groups of lymph glands available for clinical examination are shown in Figures 2.42 and 4.1 (p. 125). Other glands can only be assessed by investigation: for example, a chest radiograph may reveal hilar or paratracheal lymphadenopathy and CAT scan the abdominal para-aortic nodes. In healthy subjects palpable glands can usually be detected, especially in the axilla and the groin. They are seldom greater than 0.5 cm in diameter and frequently smaller. They are usually described as soft, rubbery or shotty.

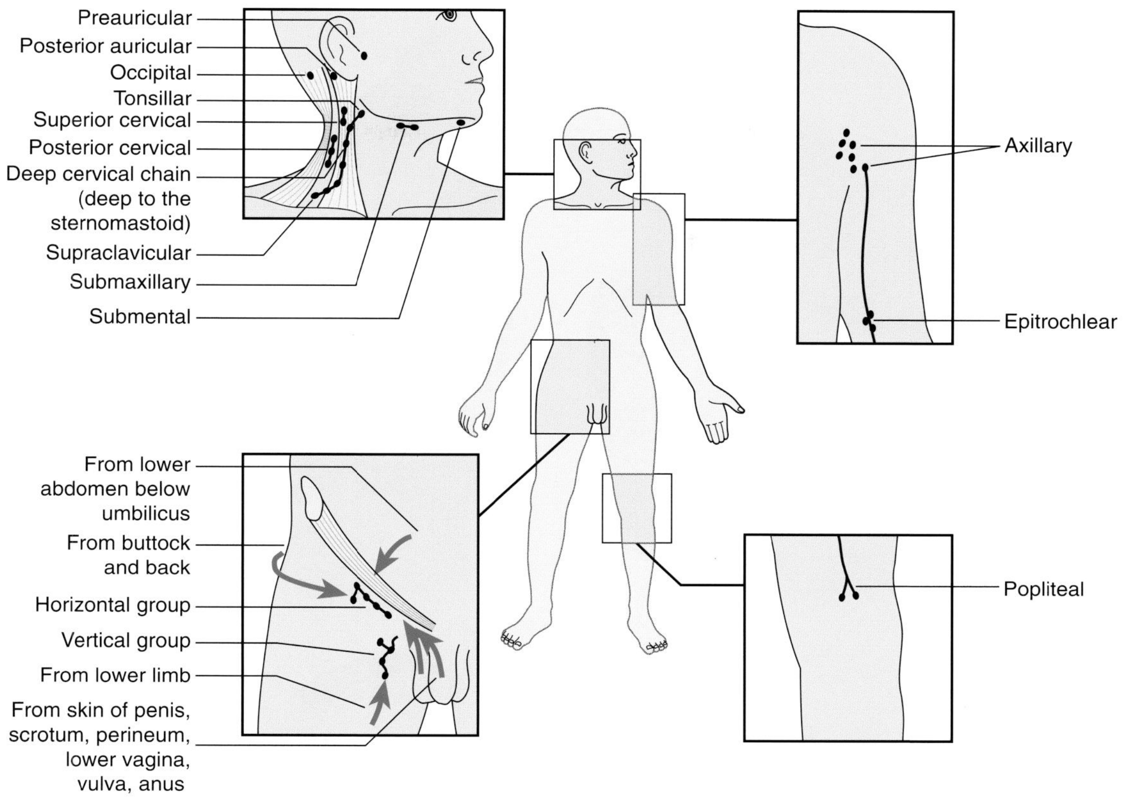

Fig. 2.42 Distribution of palpable lymph glands. The scalene node is not shown in this figure. It is an important gland. Its site is demonstrated in Figure 4.1 (p. 125).

Examination sequence

This involves not only the detection of lymphadenopathy but also an assessment of its significance and the various features as previously described (p. 56). In clinical practice, the lymph nodes are often examined piecemeal and regionally. At this stage, they are considered together.

General principles

- ☐ Inspect for any visible lymphadenopathy.
- ☐ Palpate one side at a time using the fingers of one hand.
- ☐ In turn compare the findings in a group of glands on one side with the contralateral side.
- ☐ Assess the site, size and consistency of any palpable gland. Note tenderness and determine if the gland is fixed to surrounding structures.
- ☐ Examine the cervical and axillary glands with the patient sitting.
- ☐ Lie the patient down to examine for the abdomen, inguinal and popliteal glands.

Cervical glands

- ☐ From behind, examine the submental, submandibular, preauricular, tonsillar, supraclavicular and deep cervical glands in the anterior triangle of the neck (Fig. 2.43A, B and C). Palpate deeply for the scalene nodes (Fig. 4.3, p. 126).
- ☐ From the front of the patient, examine the posterior triangles, up the back of the neck and the posterior auricular and occipital nodes (Fig. 2.43D).

Axillary glands

- ☐ Sit in front of the patient, supporting the arm on the side under examination. Palpate the right axilla with the left hand and vice versa (Fig. 2.44A and B). Insert the fingertips into the vault of the axilla and then draw them downwards while palpating the medial, anterior and posterior axillary wall in turn.

Epitrochlear glands

- ☐ While supporting the patient's right wrist with the left hand, grasp the partially flexed elbow with the right

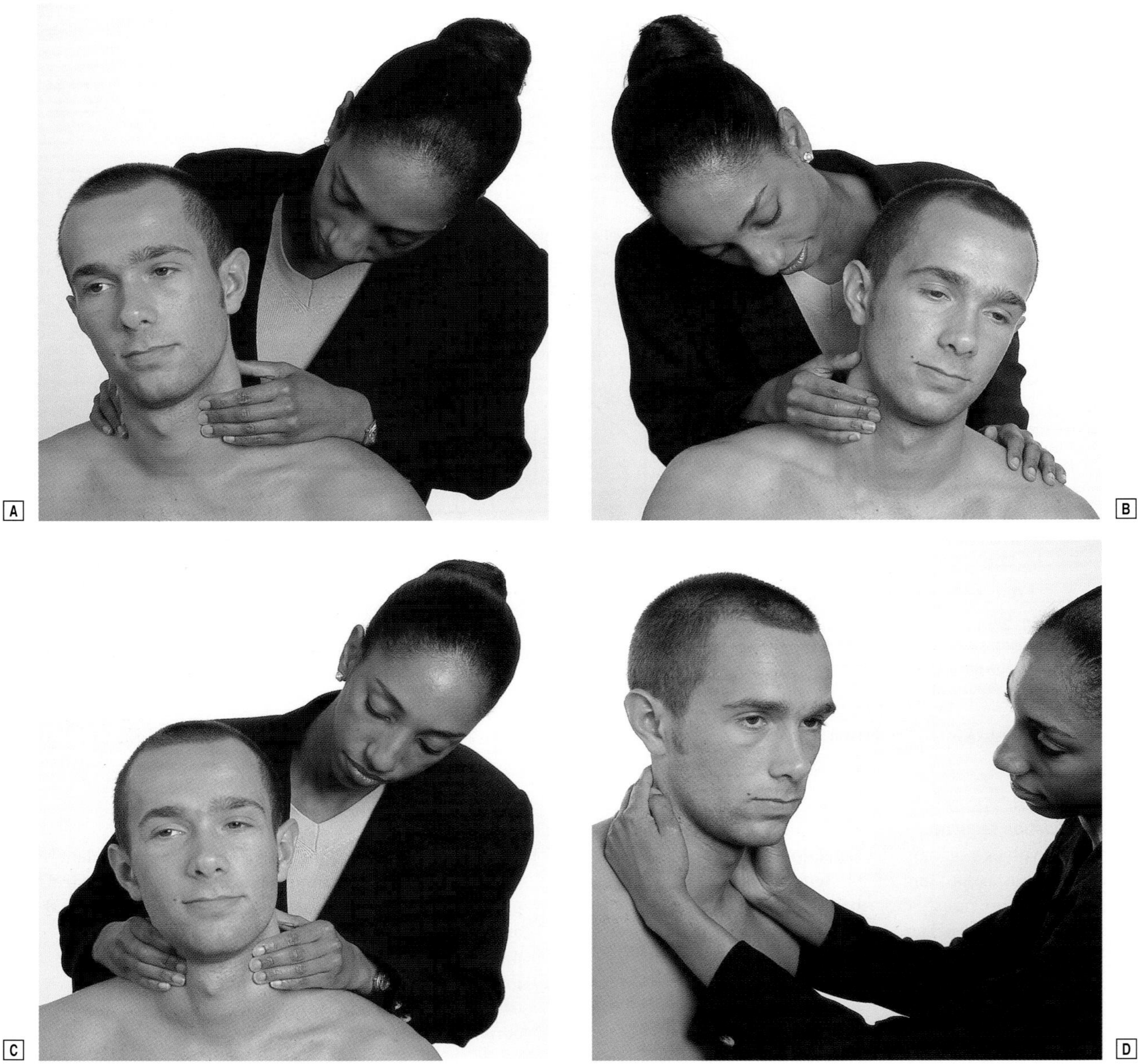

Fig. 2.43 Palpation of the cervical glands. Examine the glands of the anterior triangle from behind (A and B) using one hand at a time or both hands simultaneously (C). Examine the posterior glands from the front (D).

hand and use the thumb to feel for the epitrochlear gland. Examine the left epitrochlear gland with the left thumb (Fig. 2.45, p. 61).

Inguinal glands

☐ Palpate in turn over the horizontal chain, which lies just below the inguinal ligament, and then over the vertical chain along the saphenous veins.

Popliteal glands

☐ Use both hands to examine the popliteal fossa with the knee flexed to less than 45°.

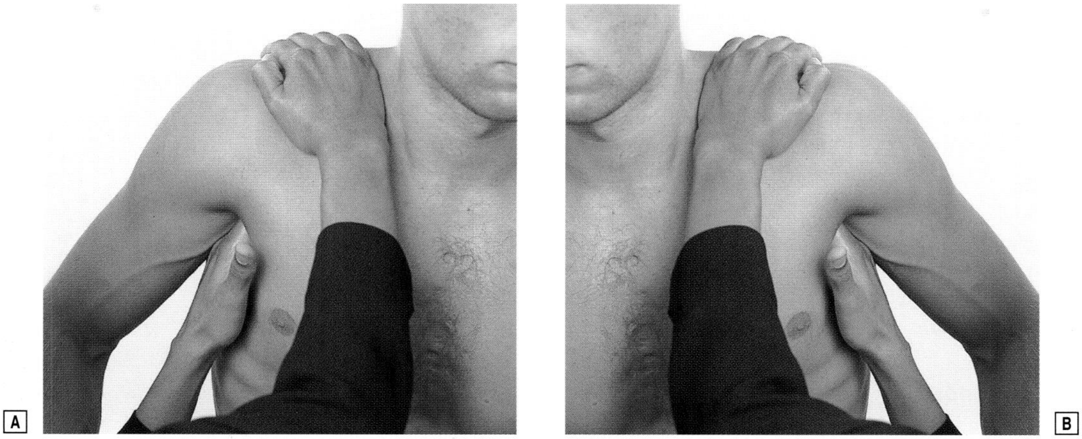

Fig. 2.44 **Palpation of the axillary glands.** [A] Left side. [B] Right side.

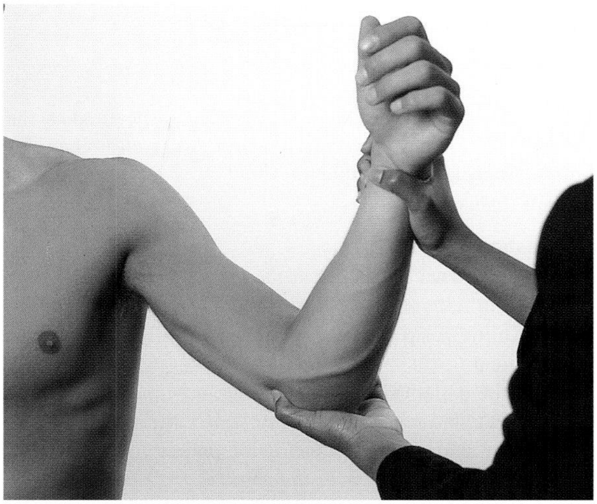

Fig. 2.45 **Palpation of the epitrochlear gland.**

Common abnormalities

Generalised lymphadenopathy can occur in a number of conditions (see Table 2.13). Localised lymphadenopathy is common and usually infective, as in acute tonsillitis. In many instances the precise aetiological factor remains obscure.

In the presence of pathological lymphadenopathy it is important to look for a possible cause, including any possible infection or primary malignancy. Special attention should be paid to the presence or absence of enlargement of the liver and spleen and the haemopoietic system, including features such as bruising, purpura or petechiae.

TABLE 2.13 Some causes of pathological lymphadenopathy

Generalised	
Viral	Epstein–Barr virus, cytomegalovirus and HIV
Bacterial	Brucellosis, syphilis
Protozoal	Toxoplasmosis
Neoplastic	Lymphoma, acute or chronic lymphocytic leukaemia
Others	Rheumatoid arthritis, systemic lupus erythematosus, sarcoidosis
Localised	
Infective	Acute or chronic, including viral, bacterial and other agents
Neoplastic	Secondary metastatic
	Primary haematological, including Hodgkin's and non-Hodgkin's lymphoma

Consistency. The consistency of the glands may provide important information. For example, in Hodgkin's disease the glands are characteristically 'rubbery'. In tuberculosis they may be 'matted' and in metastatic carcinoma they feel 'craggy'. Calcified glands feel stony hard.

Tenderness. Tenderness is usually a feature of acute bacterial infection. With tender cervical lymphadenopathy the possibilities include dental sepsis, tonsillitis and mastoiditis.

Fixation. Glands which are fixed to deep structures or skin are usually malignant.

KEY POINTS

- In healthy subjects small lymph glands can usually be detected in the axilla and groin.
- Localised lymphadenopathy is common and usually infective.
- The lymph glands are best examined one side at a time in turn, comparing the findings with the contralateral side.

THE NECK

Physical abnormalities in the neck are common. In addition to the general inspection of the neck for any skin lesions or visible tumours, various other structures should be examined. These are:

- thyroid gland
- lymph glands (p. 58)
- salivary glands
- neck movements (p. 268)
- carotid and subclavian arteries (p. 83)
- jugular veins (p. 88).

The thyroid gland

History

Disorders of the thyroid gland present in different ways.

Symptoms of thyrotoxicosis. The features include weight loss with increased appetite, heat intolerance, pruritus, emotional lability, excessive sweating and palpitations. There may be a change in the menstrual cycle, either oligomenorrhoea or amenorrhoea, and in bowel habit as a consequence of intestinal hurry. In elderly patients many of these features may be missing and the presenting features may relate to the development of atrial fibrillation (see p. 85).

Symptoms of hypothyroidism. These include weight gain and constipation, apathy and forgetfulness, gruffness of voice and cold intolerance. In the elderly, symptoms tend to develop insidiously and may be unrecognised or wrongly attributed to the ageing process.

Goitre. Significant enlargement of the thyroid gland (goitre) is common. By definition, the lateral lobes of the thyroid have a volume in excess of the terminal phalanges of the thumbs of the subject. Goitre may be noted by the patient or by relatives and friends, but many subjects are unaware of its presence. The vast majority are asymptomatic. Tenderness may be associated with various forms of thyroiditis and acute pain may occur following bleeding into a thyroid cyst. Dysphagia is rare except when there is marked swelling of the gland. Its presence suggests a malignant process.

Anatomy

The thyroid consists of two symmetrical lateral lobes joined together by a central isthmus that normally covers the second and third tracheal rings. Occasionally, the gland may extend into the superior mediastinum, or may be entirely retrosternal. Rarely, the gland may be located along the line occupied by the thyroglossal duct. When situated near the origin on the dorsum of the tongue, it is referred to as a lingual goitre. The gland is normally ensheathed by the pretracheal fascia and moves upwards on swallowing. The normal thyroid is palpable in about 50% of females and 25% of males.

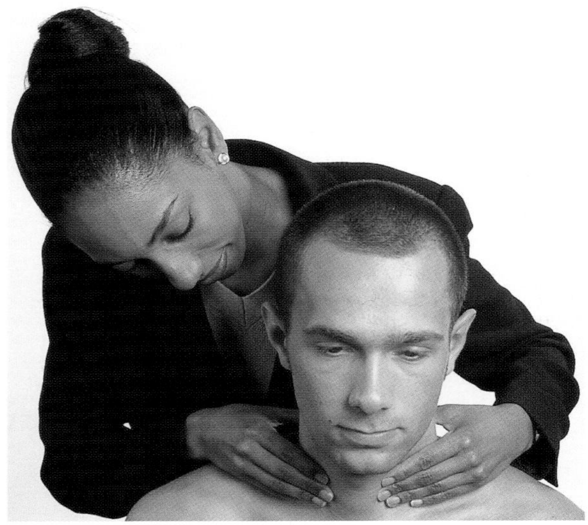

Fig. 2.46 Palpating the thyroid gland from behind.

Examination sequence

- ☐ Inspect the neck from the front.
- ☐ Look for a thyroid swelling while asking the patient to swallow a sip of water with the neck slightly extended.
- ☐ With the patient sitting or standing, now palpate for the thyroid gland from behind (Fig. 2.46). If necessary, confirm its presence by asking the patient to swallow while still palpating over the gland.
- ☐ Note shape, size and other characteristics of any goitre and the presence or absence of a thrill.
- ☐ Auscultate for a thyroid bruit.
- ☐ During the general examination look specifically for systemic features of thyroid disease (see Fig. 2.47).

Abnormal findings

Shape. Simple goitres may be relatively symmetrical in their earlier stages but usually become irregular with time. The gland is usually symmetrical in Graves' disease, whereas it is irregular in multinodular goitre.

Mobility Most goitres move upwards with swallowing; however, an invasive thyroid carcinoma may result in fixation of the gland to other surrounding structures and very large goitres may be immobilised because they expand to occupy all the available space in the root of the neck.

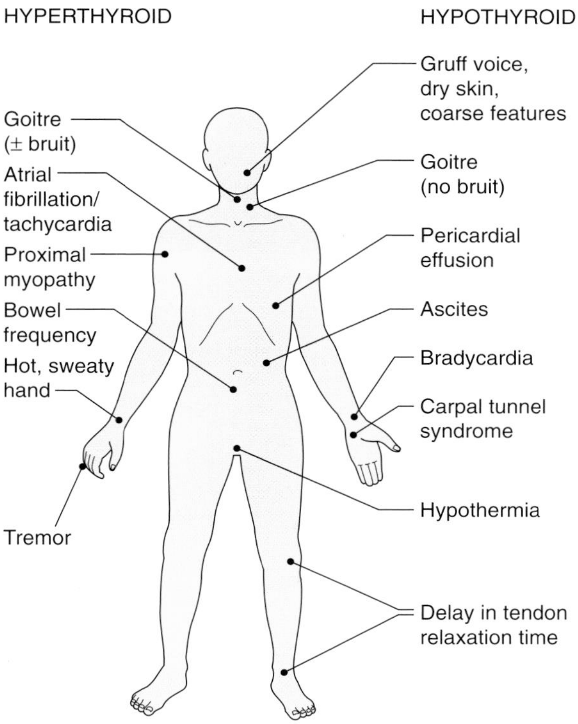

Fig. 2.47 Features of hyper- and hypothyroidism.

Consistency. The consistency, texture and the smoothness of the surface of the gland may vary from one part to another. Nodules in the substance of the gland may be large or small, single or multiple. If the consistency is 'stony hard', carcinomatous change is likely. The presence of large, firm or hard lymph nodes near a goitre also suggests the possibility of a thyroid malignancy.

Tenderness. Diffuse tenderness usually implies thyroiditis; localised tenderness may occur following bleeding into a cyst.

Colour changes. These are most unusual unless the goitre is very big, when distended veins may be responsible for a dusky, blue appearance.

Vascular bruit. This indicates an abnormally large blood flow and is sometimes associated with a palpable thrill. Increased blood flow occurs in hyperthyroidism, but the use of antithyroid drugs may also increase the vascularity of the gland sufficiently to produce a murmur. A thyroid

CASE HISTORY

A 14-year-old schoolboy presented with increasing lethargy over the previous 12 months. Over the past 2–3 years, his performance at school has been noted to deteriorate. On examination he had the characteristic facial features of primary hypothyroidism (Fig. 2.48A). Blood tests confirmed primary hypothyroidism with a normochromic normocytic anaemia (haemoglobin 8 g/dl). The facial change disappeared within 6 months of starting treatment with thyroxine (Fig. 2.48B).

Learning points

- Because the facial and other features of thyroid disease develop over a period of time, they may be overlooked by those in regular contact with the patient.

A

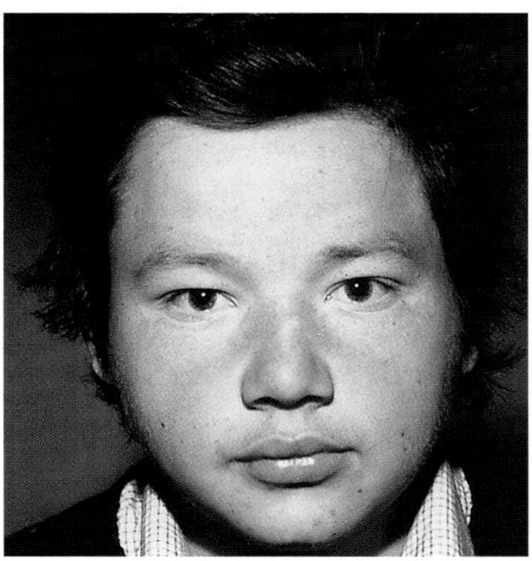

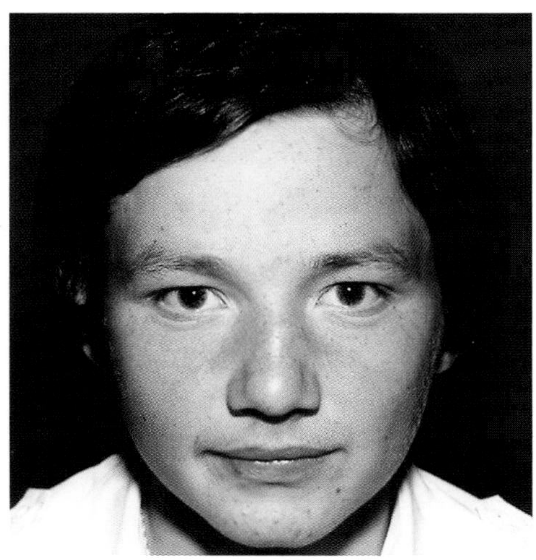

B

Fig. 2.48 Hypothyroid facies A before and B 6-months after thyroxine therapy.

should be distinguished from a murmur arising in the carotid artery or transmitted from the aorta and from a venous hum originating in the internal jugular vein.

Other features. The presence or absence of a goitre is a poor index of thyroid function, but the systemic features and the facial appearance (Fig. 2.48A) may be an excellent guide to the diagnosis. It is necessary, however, not to confuse the signs of thyrotoxicosis with those of autoimmune thyroid disease (Fig. 7.2, p. 245). These may include proptosis, exophthalmos, ophthalmoplegia and pretibial myxoedema. Although these signs are features of Graves' disease, they may be found in subjects who are euthyroid, or even hypothyroid.

Some of the systemic features of thyroid disease are summarised in Figure 2.47.

Thyroid function

Where there is a clinical suspicion of abnormal thyroid function, this should be assessed biochemically. In thyrotoxicosis, the level of thyroid stimulating hormone (TSH) will be suppressed. Total thyroxine and free thyroxine values are usually raised but may be normal in patients with T3 thyrotoxicosis.

Primary failure of the thyroid gland is associated with elevated TSH. Circulating thyroid hormones will be reduced. In secondary hypothyroidism, TSH will be low.

Other investigations of the thyroid gland may be of value in assessing structure:

- *Plain X-ray*. Identifies calcification within the gland and narrowing or displacement of the trachea.
- *Ultrasonography*. To distinguish between cystic and solid 'nodules'.
- *Radionuclide scanning*. Determines the size and site of the gland and whether nodules are 'hot', taking up radioiodine, or 'cold'.
- *Aspiration cytology*. May help in assessing the pathology of cold nodules.

CASE HISTORY

A 69-year-old lady presented with a rapidly enlarging left lobe of the thyroid gland. There was no pain in the neck and she was biochemically euthyroid. The thyroid ultrasound showed a solid nodule within the left lobe (Fig. 2.49) and the radionuclide scan showed that the nodule was non-functioning ('cold'). Fine needle aspiration (FNA) of the nodule showed no malignant cells. A left hemithyroidectomy was performed.

Learning points

- As a general principle, any 'cold nodule' in the thyroid gland should be managed as a potentially malignant lesion.

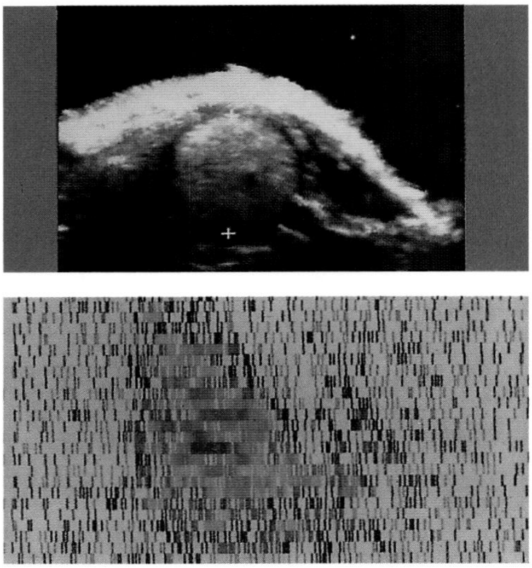

A

B

Fig. 2.49 Thyroid investigations. A Ultrasound scan showing solid nodule within left lobe. B Radionuclide scintogram illustrating a non-functioning left lobe.

KEY POINTS

- The normal thyroid gland is palpable in up to 50% of women, fewer men. The presence or absence of a goitre is a poor guide to thyroid function.
- A thyroid bruit is an indication of increased vascularity of the gland.
- The signs of autoimmune thyroid disease are not features of thyrotoxicosis.

THE BREASTS

The history

The common symptoms of breast disease are lumps, skin changes, nipple inversion, nipple discharge and pain. Breast tumours may present with any of these features and also with symptoms of acute inflammation. The UK Breast Screening Programme invites women between the ages of 50 and 64 to attend for single oblique mammography at 3-year intervals. An increasing number of asymptomatic women present with mammographic abnormalities.

Men may present with gynaecomastia.

Anatomy

The breasts are modified sweat glands. The stages in the development of the female breast are illustrated in Figure 2.50. The commonest site for nipple development is the fourth intercostal space on the midclavicular line, but accessory breast/nipple tissue may develop anywhere down

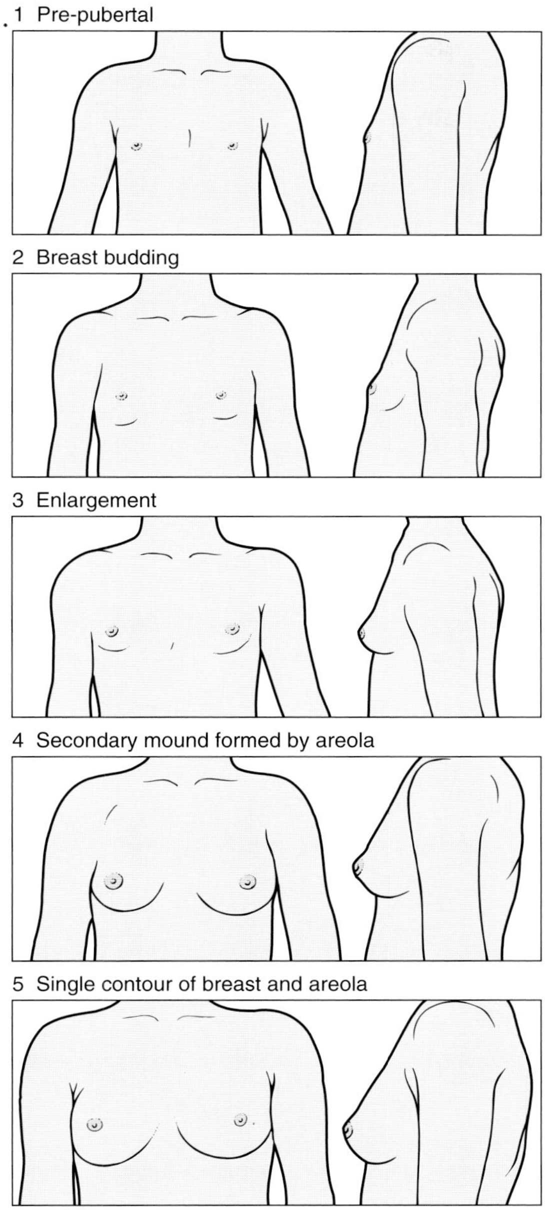

Fig. 2.50 Stages of breast development.

the nipple line (axilla to groin) (Fig. 2.51). The adult breast may be divided into the nipple, the areola and four quadrants, upper and lower, inner and outer, with the axillary tail projecting from the upper and outer quadrant (Fig. 2.52). The nipple consists of erectile tissue covered with pigmented skin, which also covers the areola. The openings of the lactiferous ducts may be seen near the apex

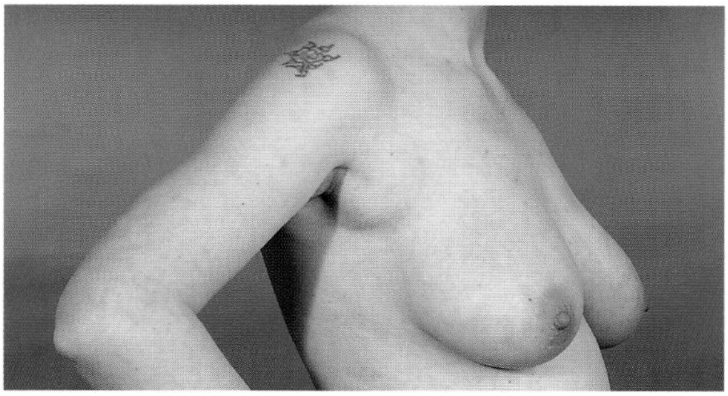

Fig. 2.51 Accessory breast tissue in the axilla.

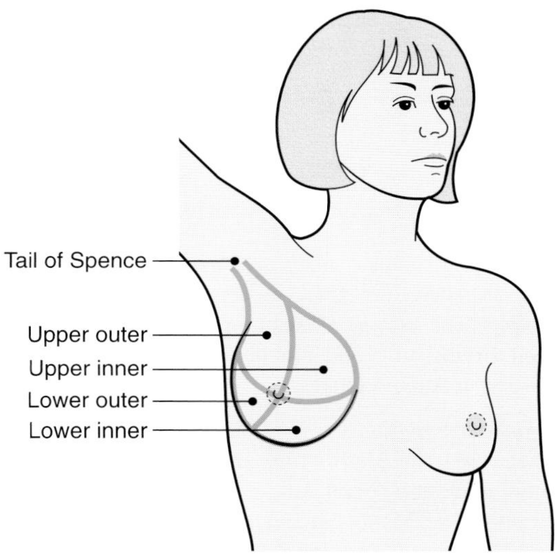

Fig. 2.52 The adult right breast.

of the nipple. The size and shape of the breasts in healthy women vary widely, and are influenced by hereditary factors, sexual maturity, the phase of the menstrual cycle, parity, pregnancy and lactation and the general state of nutrition. The amount of fat and stroma surrounding the glandular tissue largely determines the size of the breast, except during lactation, when the enlargement is almost entirely glandular.

The breast is a hormonally responsive gland, and in premenopausal women its consistency may vary considerably in response to fluctuations in oestrogen and progesterone levels during the menstrual cycle and in pregnancy. Swelling and tenderness due to fluid retention and prominence of the glandular elements of the breast are more common in the premenstrual phase. With age there is a reduction in the amount of glandular tissue with a

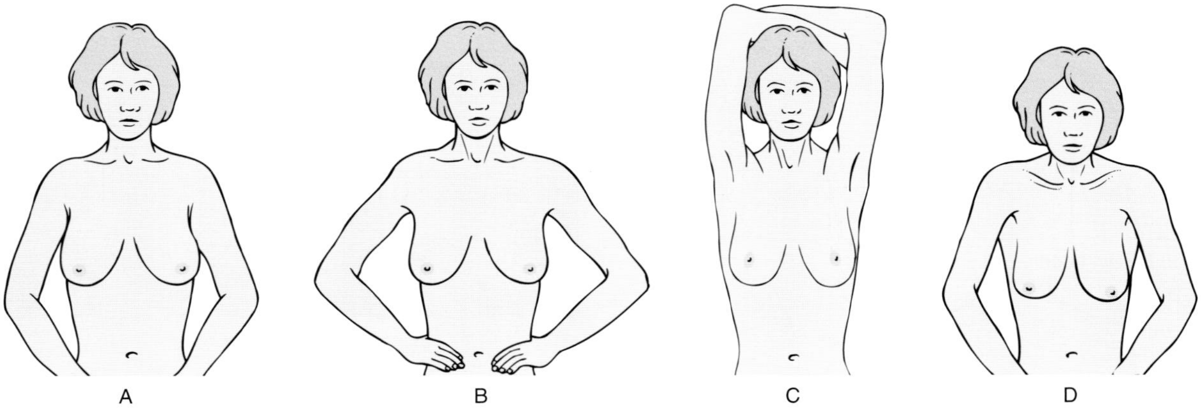

Fig. 2.53 Positions for inspecting the breasts. [A] Hand resting on thighs. [B] Hand pressed onto hips. [C] Arms above head. [D] Leaning forward with breasts pendulous.

corresponding increase in the relative amount of fat. The breasts are therefore softer in consistency and are more pendulous. The breasts of lactating women are swollen and engorged with milk and are best examined after breast-feeding or milk expression.

Examination sequence

☐ Take care to avoid upsetting any patient, particularly the more modest, by explaining the purpose of the examination. Male clinicians should be chaperoned.

☐ Ask the patient to sit upright on a well-illuminated chair, undressed to the waist and with the hands resting on the thighs so that the pectoral muscles are relaxed (Fig. 2.53A).

☐ Sit facing the patient and carefully inspect the breasts for asymmetry, local swelling or changes in the skin or nipples.

☐ Repeat the inspection with the patient's hands pressed firmly on the hips (Fig. 2.53B), thereby contracting the pectoral muscles, then with arms raised above the head (Fig. 2.53C) to stretch the pectoral muscles and the skin over the breasts, and finally leaning forward so that the breasts become pendulous (Fig. 2.53D). Such actions expose the whole breast and exacerbate skin dimpling.

☐ Ask the patient to lie with the head supported on one pillow and with the hand on the side to be examined under the head (Fig. 2.54).

☐ With the hand held flat to the skin, palpate the breast tissue using the palmar surface of the middle three fingers, compressing breast tissue gently against the chest wall.

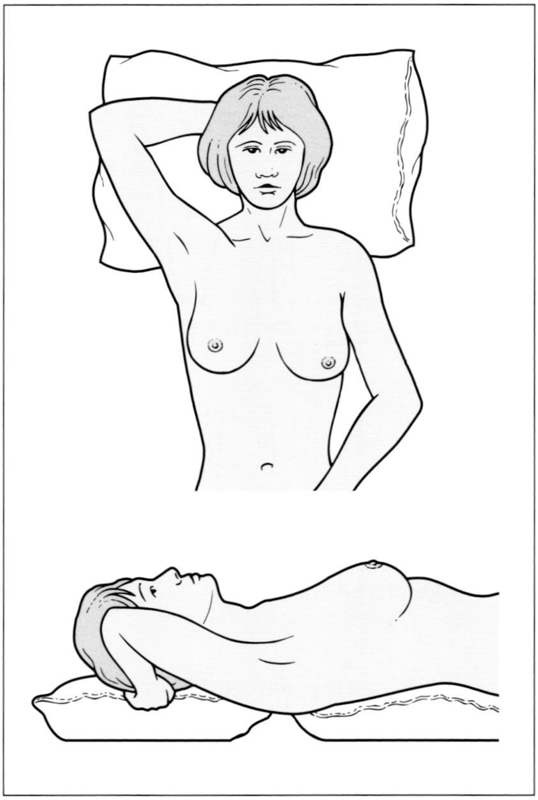

Fig. 2.54 Position for palpating of the right breast.

- ☐ Consider the breast as the face of a clock and carefully examine each hour of the clock from outside towards the nipple, not forgetting the tissue directly under the nipple. Compare the texture of one breast with that of the other.
- ☐ Define the characteristic of any mass, including fixation to underlying tissues or tethering to skin, which may become apparent as a dimpling overlying the tumour when the breast is gently elevated by a hand.
- ☐ To determine if a mass is fixed to underlying tissue, ask the patient to place her hands on her hips. Holding the tumour between thumb and forefinger, then ask the patient to alternately contract and relax the pectoral muscles by pushing into her hips.
- ☐ Examine the axillary tail between finger and thumb as it extends towards the axilla.
- ☐ To palpate the nipple, hold it gently between index finger and thumb and attempt to express any discharge.
- ☐ Complete the examination by palpating the regional lymph nodes, including the supraclavicular group. Examine the axillae with the arms relaxed in order to expose the apex of the axilla and then with the hands on the hips to tense the pectoral fascia and contract the pectoral muscles.

Abnormal findings

Breast lump

The commonest cause of a breast lump varies with age.

Carcinoma of the breast. This is one of the commonest malignancies in women in the UK, affecting 1 in 12 women. Its incidence increases with age, but any mass must be regarded as potentially malignant until proven otherwise. Cancer of the male breast is uncommon and there is a strong genetic factor.

Characteristically carcinomas are solid masses with an irregular outline, often painless but firm or hard, contrasting in consistency with the surrounding breast tissue. The tumour may be confined within the breast tissue or extend into overlying tissues such as skin, pectoral fascia, pectoral muscle or metastasise to intramammary lymphatics, regional lymph nodes or the systemic circulation. When a tumour is fixed to the chest wall, it is fixed when the pectoral muscle is relaxed; when tethered to fascia, but not muscle, it will be mobile when the pectoral muscle is relaxed, and adherent when the muscle is tensed. The current TNM (tumour, nodes, metastases) classification of breast tumours is given in Table 2.14.

TABLE 2.14 TNM malignant classification of breast cancers

Tumour	
Tx	Cannot be assessed
T0	No evidence of primary tumour
Tis	Carcinoma in situ, intraductal carcinoma, lobular carcinoma in situ, Paget's disease of nipple
T_1	Tumour ≤ 2 cm in greatest dimension
	a ≤ 0.5 cm
	b > 0.5 ≤ 1 cm
	c > 1 cm ≤ 2 cm
T_2	Tumour > 2 cm ≤ 5 cm greatest dimension
T_3	Tumour > 5 cm greatest dimension
T_4	Tumour any size with direct extension to chest wall or skin
	a extension to chest wall
	b oedema including peau d'orange or ulceration of skin of breast or satellite skin nodules on same breast
	c 4a + 4b
	d inflammatory carcinoma
Nodes	
Nx	Regional lymph nodes cannot be assessed
N0	No regional lymph node metastasis
N_1	Metastasis with moveable ipsilateral axillary nodes
N_2	Metastases with ipsilateral axillary nodes fixed to one another or to other structures
N_3	Metastases to ipsilateral internal mammary nodes
Metastases	
Mx	Presence of distant metastases cannot be assessed
M0	No distant metastases
M_1	Distant metastases including supraclavicular nodes

This classification with appropriate modification forms the basis for classification of other primary malignancies.

Fibrocystic changes. Fibrocystic change or irregular nodularity of the breast is common, especially in the upper outer quadrant in young women. Usually the tissue is rubbery in texture and varies in size with the hormonal cycle, being at its largest premenstrually. The changes are usually bilateral.

Fibroadenomas. These are abnormalities of normal development and involution due to overgrowth of elements derived from terminal duct lobules. Characteristically they present as smooth mobile discrete rubbery lumps in young women. They are second only to localised benign breast disease as the commonest cause of a breast mass in a woman under the age of 35. The distinction between a juvenile fibroadenoma and phyllodes tumour (giant fibroadenoma) is made on pathological grounds and the two are best regarded as distinct pathological entities.

Breast cysts. The aetiology of breast cysts remains obscure, but they are a feature of the involuting breast which is still subject to hormonal stimulation. They are the commonest cause of a breast lump in women between the ages of 35 and 50. Their clinical picture depends on the intracystic pressure. They present as smooth lumps, which may be soft and fluctuant (or even impalpable) when the intracystic pressure is low, becoming hard and painful when

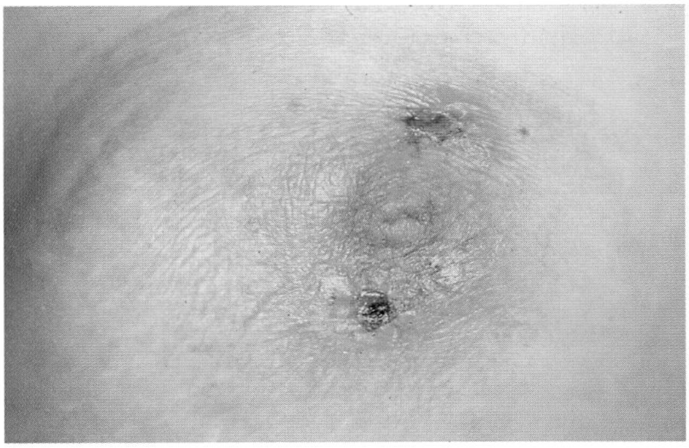

Fig. 2.55 Mammillary fistulae at areolocutaneous border.

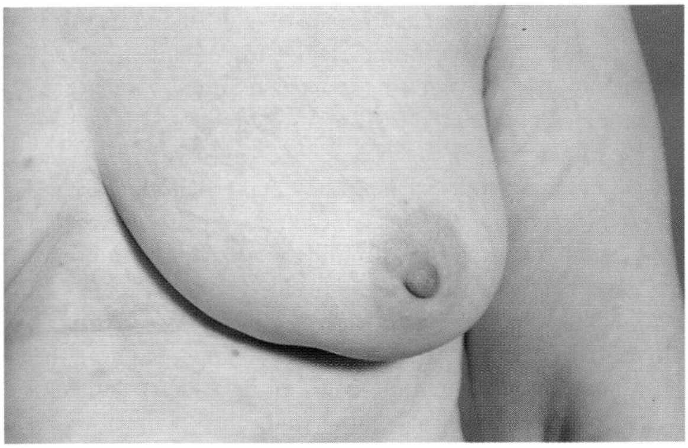

Fig. 2.56 Skin dimpling due to underlying malignancy.

the intracystic pressure is high. Cysts may occur in multiple clusters. Occasionally a cyst may be associated with malignant disease. For this reason any cyst in which the aspirate is blood-stained, in which there is a residual mass following aspiration or which recurs after several aspirations should be excised to exclude malignancy.

Breast abscesses. There are two distinct types of breast abscesses. Lactational abscesses occur in women who are breastfeeding and are usually peripheral in nature. Non-lactational abscesses occur as an extension of periductal mastitis and have a classical distribution at the edge of the nipple, often associated with nipple inversion. They usually occur in young female smokers. Occasionally a non-lactating abscess may discharge spontaneously through an abnormal communication between the inflamed duct and the skin. The classical position of this fistula is at the areolocutaneous border (Fig. 2.55).

Skin changes

It is important to differentiate between simple skin dimpling due to retraction of the skin and indrawing of the skin due to infiltration of the dermis by tumour (Fig. 2.56). In the former the skin remains mobile over the tumour; in the latter the tumour is fixed to the skin. Likewise in tethering to the chest wall the tumour is solid with the chest wall when the pectoral muscle is contracted, but when it is relaxed it is possible to move the lesion separately. Tumours which infiltrate the chest wall are fixed when the pectoral muscle is both relaxed and contracted.

Obstruction of the intramammary lymphatics with tumour results in lymphoedema of the breast. The skin is attached at the hair follicles but swollen in between, giving the appearance of the skin of an orange ('peau d'orange', Fig. 2.57).

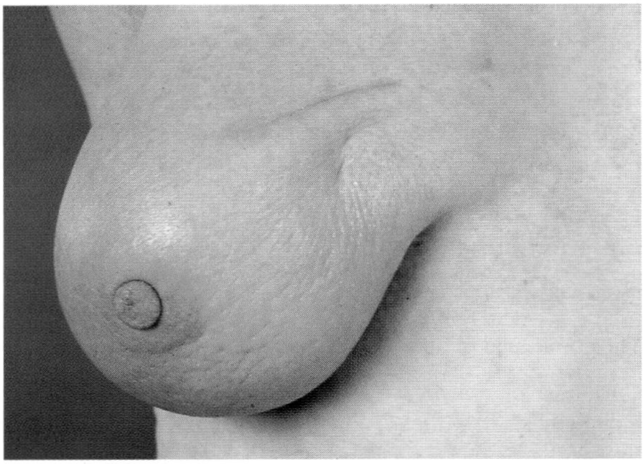

Fig. 2.57 Peau d'orange of the breast.

Eczematous changes of the nipple may be part of a generalised skin disorder; however, when confined to a nipple they should raise the possibility of Paget's disease of the nipple (Fig. 2.58). In this condition there is invasion of the epidermis by cells from an underlying intraductal carcinoma. The diagnosis is established by a skin biopsy.

Nipple inversion

Retraction of the nipple due to shortening of the nipple ducts from periductal inflammation and fibrosis is a common finding. The characteristics of benign nipple inversion are a symmetrical slit-like inversion. Nipple retraction due to malignant disease is asymmetrical and distorting, pulling the nipple away from its central position (Fig. 2.59).

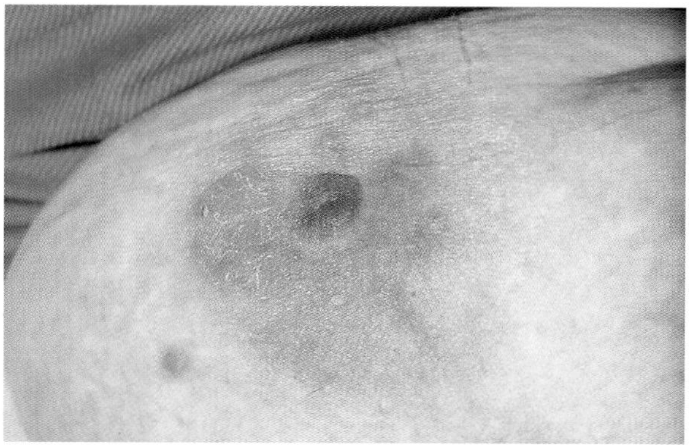

Fig. 2.58 Paget's disease of the nipple.

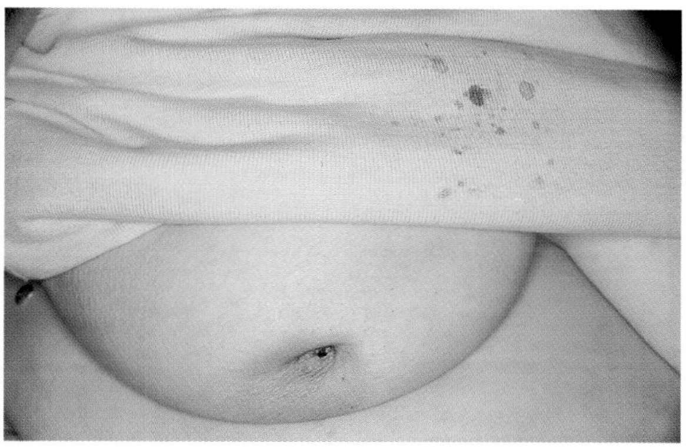

Fig. 2.59 Carcinoma of the breast presenting as indrawing of the nipple. Note the bloody discharge on the underclothing.

Nipple discharge

A small amount of clear fluid expressed from multiple ducts of the breast on massage is normal. Persistent single duct discharge or blood-stained (macroscopic or microscopic) discharge should always be investigated. The differential diagnosis includes duct ectasia, intraduct papilloma or rarely intraduct carcinoma.

Galactorrhoea. Galactorrhoea is characterised by a milky discharge from multiple ducts in both breasts and is a feature of hyperprolactinaemia. There is usually associated Montgomery tubercle hyperplasia. Spontaneous milk production is uncommon and often galactorrhoea is found only by trying to express milk. The causes of hyperprolactinaemia include physiological processes (pregnancy, postpartum), drugs (dopamine antagonists, dopamine-depleting agents), pituitary tumours, hypothalamic and stalk lesions, primary hypothyroidism and renal failure.

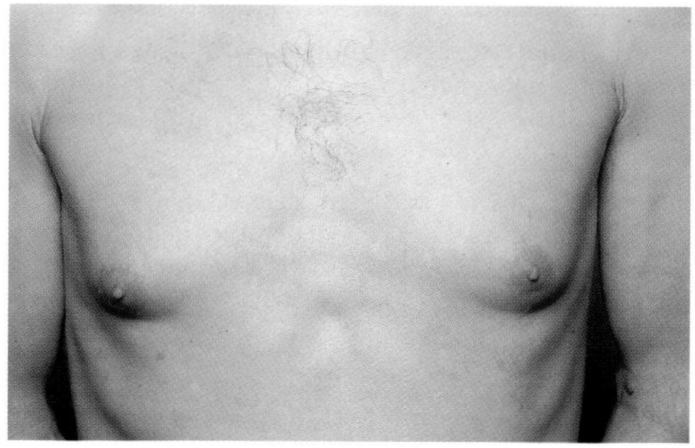

Fig. 2.60 Drug-induced gynaecomastia caused by cimetidine.

Gynaecomastia

Gynaecomastia (enlargement of the male breast) occurs in about 50% of pubertal boys probably because of the relatively high oestradiol levels. Many drugs can cause enlargement (e.g. oestrogens used in the treatment of prostatic cancer, spironolactone and cimetidine) (Fig. 2.60).

Gynaecomastia is also found in cirrhosis of the liver and in conditions associated with increased oestrogen production (interstitial cell tumours of the testis, some adrenal tumours, thyrotoxicosis) or decreased androgen production (hypergonadotrophic hypogonadism, Klinefelter's syndrome, orchitis).

Investigation

Diagnosis of most breast lesions relies on a combination of clinical history and examination, radiological assessment by either mammography and/or breast ultrasound and cytopathological diagnosis, either by fine-needle aspiration cytology or trucut biopsy. In some lesions the ultimate diagnosis requires excision biopsy.

Fine-needle aspiration. This involves the passage of a green needle (21G) on suction through a breast lesion. It allows immediate diagnosis of breast cysts and in experienced hands will yield sufficient cells for the diagnosis of 95% of malignancies and 85% of benign lesions.

Trucut biopsy. Using an automated gun a small match-stick size piece of tissue is taken. Histopathological examination of the tissue will allow differentiation of in-situ from invasive cancer.

Mammography. The classical characteristics of a breast cancer are an irregular opacity with spiculated edges, often in association with irregular microcalcification. Owing to the high fat content mammography is more sensitive in the breasts of older women, in whom it can detect a lesion before it becomes clinically palpable. The mammograms of younger women are more opaque and more difficult to read.

Ultrasound. This is particularly helpful in women under the age of 35. It is possible to differentiate solid from cystic lesions by ultrasound, and also to discriminate between benign and malignant lesions sometimes.

KEY POINTS

- Carcinoma of the breast is one of the commonest malignancies in women. Any breast lump must be regarded as potentially malignant until this possibility has been excluded.
- Examination of the breasts involves careful inspection in various positions as well as a thorough and systematic palpation of the gland and of the regional lymph nodes.

The cardiovascular system

3

J. McMURRAY • D. NORTHRIDGE • A. BRADBURY

THE HISTORY

General considerations

History-taking is at least as important as clinical examination in the evaluation of the patient with cardiac disease. Indeed one of the most common cardiac symptoms, chest pain or discomfort, commonly occurs in the absence of abnormal physical findings.

Presenting complaint

Three general aspects of history-taking are particularly important in assessing the patient with possible heart disease; namely the rate of onset, duration and the severity of the symptoms. Episodes of chest pain or breathlessness of acute onset demand more urgent attention than symptoms that have been present for months. As many cardiac diseases are progressive, it is also important to determine the evolution of symptoms over time. The temporal pattern of symptoms may provide prognostic information and the basis on which to determine the timing of therapeutic intervention (e.g. valve surgery). Likewise, severity provides important prognostic information and helps to determine the urgency of the situation. For example, angina that restricts normal daily activities and persists despite medical treatment is usually an indication for coronary angiography.

Because the principal cardiac symptoms of chest discomfort and breathlessness are effort related, it is important to assess the impact of symptoms on *functional capacity*. The extent of the domestic (e.g. cooking, cleaning, shopping), social (e.g. hobbies, sport) and occupational disability should be established. In particular, occurrence of symptoms while travelling to and from work or the local shops and on the steps or stairs to, or within, the patient's home, should be determined. It is often helpful to determine whether or not patients are able to keep up with their partners or friends of the same age.

Past history

This should include any episode of rheumatic fever and abnormalities found at school or occupational medical examinations, including blood pressure recordings. Specific enquiry about the past history of conditions that may be associated with cardiac disease should be made when appropriate. Examples include the following:

- diabetes and coronary artery disease;
- glomerulonephritis and hypertensive heart disease;
- thyrotoxicosis and atrial fibrillation;
- amyloidosis and cardiomyopathy.

Likewise, because of the association with infective endocarditis, it may be important to specifically enquire about recent dental work and other potential causes of bacteraemia. Other seemingly unrelated problems may also suggest an associated or underlying cardiovascular problem. For example, a patient with Marfan's syndrome may have aortic incompetence.

The knowledge of the obstetric history may be helpful in assessing the significance of a valvular problem or septal defect because these are unlikely to be haemodynamically significant if pregnancy and labour were uncomplicated.

TABLE 3.1 Occupational aspects of cardiovascular disease

Occupational exposure associated with cardiovascular disease	
Organic solvents	Arrhythmias Cardiomyopathy
Vibrating machine tools	Raynaud's phenomenon
Publicans	Alcoholic cardiomyopathy
Occupational exposure exacerbating pre-existing cardiac conditions	
Cold exposure	Angina Raynaud's disease
Deep-sea diving	Embolism through foramen ovale
Occupational requirements for high standards of cardiovascular fitness	
Pilots	
Public transport/heavy goods drivers	
Armed forces	
Police	

Occupational history

A careful occupational history is important. Cardiac disease may impair the patient's physical activity and thus threaten employment. This may be a source of anxiety and an indication for therapeutic intervention. The diagnosis of cardiac disease may also have medicolegal consequences in certain occupations, e.g. commercial drivers, pilots (Table 3.1).

Social history

This is always important. The aetiological role of smoking in coronary and other vascular disease necessitates a detailed smoking history. Consumption of alcohol is also relevant. Although possibly 'cardioprotective' in moderation, excessive alcohol consumption is associated with atrial fibrillation, hypertension and cardiomyopathy (Fig. 1.9, p. 11). Enquiry should also be made into caffeine consumption which, when excessive, can cause palpitation. Some recreational drugs can occasionally be associated with cardiac symptoms (e.g. cocaine and chest pain).

Drug history

The drug history can be very revealing. Medication may be responsible for, or may aggravate, symptoms such as breathlessness, chest pain, oedema, palpitations or syncope (Table 3.2). The introduction of thyroxine may precipitate

TABLE 3.2 Symptoms related to medication

Dyspnoea	Beta-blockers in patients with asthma Exacerbation of heart failure by beta-blockers, some calcium antagonists, non-steroidal anti-inflammatory drugs (NSAIDs)
Dizziness	Vasodilators, e.g. nitrates, alpha-blockers and ACE inhibitors
Angina	Aggravated by thyroxine or drug-induced anaemia, e.g. aspirin or NSAIDs
Oedema	Fluid retention from steroids, NSAIDs Oedema from calcium antagonists (e.g. nifedipine, amlodipine)
Palpitation	Tachycardia and/or arrhythmia from thyroxine, beta-2 stimulants (e.g. salbutamol), digoxin toxicity, hypokalaemia from diuretics, tricyclic antidepressant drugs

TABLE 3.3 Genetically determined cardiovascular disorders

Single-gene defects	Polygenic inheritance
Single-gene defects	Polygenic inheritance
Hypertrophic cardiomyopathy	Ischaemic heart disease
Marfan's syndrome	Hypertension
Familial hypercholesterolaemia	Type 2 diabetes mellitus
Muscular dystrophies	Hyperlipidaemia

or aggravate angina. The drug history should include over-the-counter purchases such as non-steroidal anti-inflammatory drugs (NSAIDs) and alternative medicine and herbal remedies as these may contain ingredients with cardiovascular actions.

The drug history may also reveal the presence of important chronic diseases the patient may have forgotten to mention, e.g. antihypertensive medication and oral hypoglycaemic drugs.

Family history

The family history may be relevant because many cardiac disorders have a genetic component (Table 3.3). It is important to establish if there is a family history of either premature coronary heart disease in a first degree relative (< 55 years in a non-smoking female or < 50 years in a non-smoking male) or of sudden unexplained death at a young age, raising the possibility of a cardiomyopathy or an inherited tendency to arrhythmia.

Cardinal symptoms

Patients with heart disease may be asymptomatic. Their cardiac pathology may be diagnosed during 'routine' examination or because of the development of a complication (e.g. atrial fibrillation in mitral stenosis). However, the cardinal symptoms of heart disease are *chest discomfort, breathlessness, palpitations, syncope* and *peripheral oedema*. None of these symptoms indicate that heart disease is definitely present because they are not specific (see Table 3.4). The probability that a particular symptom is caused by heart disease depends upon many factors, including age, sex, family history, social history, presence or absence of concomitant disease and the physical findings.

TABLE 3.4 Principal symptoms of heart disease

Symptom	Cardiovascular causes	Other causes
Chest discomfort	Angina Pericarditis Aortic dissection	Oesophageal spasm Pneumothorax Musculoskeletal pain
Breathlessness	Heart failure Angina Pulmonary embolism Pulmonary hypertension	Respiratory disease Anaemia Obesity
Palpitations	Tachyarrhythmias	Anxiety Hyperthyroidism Drugs
Syncope/ dizziness	Bradyarrhythmias Postural hypotension Aortic stenosis Hypertrophic obstructive cardiomyopathy Atrial myxoma	Simple faints Epilepsy
Oedema	Heart failure Constrictive pericarditis Venous stasis	Nephrotic syndrome Liver disease Drugs

TABLE 3.5 Types of cardiac pain

Type	Cause	Characteristics
Angina	Coronary stenosis (rarely aortic stenosis, hypertrophic cardiomyopathy)	Precipitated by exertion, eased by rest Characteristic distribution (Fig. 3.1)
Myocardial infarct	Coronary occlusion	Similar sites to angina, more severe, persists at rest
Pericarditic pain	Pericarditis	Sharp, raw or stabbing Varies with movement or breathing
Aortic pain	Dissection of the aorta	Severe, sudden onset, radiates to the back

CHEST DISCOMFORT

Various types of chest discomfort or pain caused by cardiovascular disorders are listed in Table 3.5.

Angina pectoris

The commonest cardiac cause of chest discomfort is angina which is the symptomatic manifestation of myocardial ischaemia. Atypical angina is not uncommon; however, it often has a typical character, distribution and radiation with well-recognised precipitating, aggravating and relieving factors.

Duration

Angina is usually a short-lived discomfort precipitated by conditions which temporarily increase myocardial work and oxygen demand, i.e. anything that increases the heart rate or force of left ventricular contraction. Angina is usually predictable and provoked by a certain level of activity. Sometimes the symptom may be precipitated by emotional upset. Patients quickly learn what provokes their angina and how to relieve it. Angina usually subsides within a few minutes of rest or after taking glyceryl trinitrate, unlike the prolonged chest pain of acute myocardial infarction.

Character

Many patients describe angina as a tightness or heaviness and it is usually not severe, a 'discomfort' rather than a 'pain'. Sometimes the nearest experience patients can relate to the symptom is to describe it as 'breathlessness' or 'like indigestion'. The possibility that symptoms are gastrointestinal may also arise from patients relating the discomfort to meals, or more commonly to exercising after meals (postprandial angina). The patients' body language may be helpful – anginal discomfort is poorly localised and usually indicated using the open hand or a fist (Fig. 3.1).

Severity of angina relates to the degree of functional limitation *not* the intensity of the pain. Changes in the severity of a patient's angina is the principal means of assessing the response to therapy and will influence management decisions. The Canadian Cardiovascular Classification can be used (Table 3.6). It is necessary to establish:

- the degree of functional limitation
- the pattern of symptoms
- the presence of symptoms at night or at rest
- the stability of symptoms.

TABLE 3.6 Canadian Cardiovascular Society: functional classification of stable angina

Grade 1	Ordinary physical activity, such as walking and climbing stairs, does not cause angina. Angina with strenuous or rapid or prolonged exertion at work or recreation
Grade 2	Slight limitation of ordinary activity. Walking or climbing stairs rapidly or after meals, in cold, in wind, or when under emotional stress, or only during the few hours after awakening.
Grade 3	Marked limitation of ordinary physical activity. Walking one to two blocks on the level and climbing less than one flight in normal conditions.
Grade 4	Inability to carry on any physical activity without discomfort – anginal syndrome may be present at rest.

QUESTIONS – To assess the severity of angina

- How far can you walk on the flat before experiencing discomfort?
- Do you get discomfort climbing stairs or hills?
- Do you experience discomfort gardening, making the bed or during other household chores?
- Does sexual intercourse produce discomfort?
- Is the discomfort influenced by meals?
- Is it influenced by cold weather?

The extent of effort limitation is best assessed by identifying those activities that precipitate symptoms. This involves asking specific questions (see Question box).

A patient's activities may appear to be unrestricted because activities that provoke symptoms have been progressively curtailed. It is therefore important to identify activities that have been abandoned, e.g. dancing or playing golf.

Site and radiation

Angina pain is characteristically central and retrosternal. The pain may radiate to either arm, hand or wrist, to the throat or jaw (in which case it may be described as toothache) to the back or the epigastrium. Occasionally pain is experienced in these sites and not in the chest.

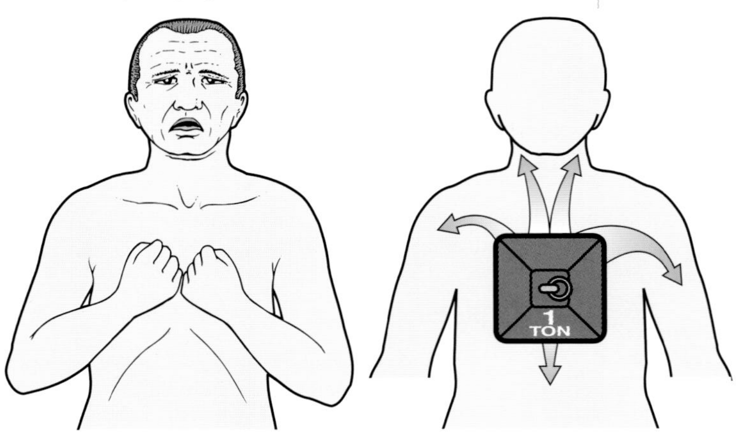

Fig. 3.1 Symptoms of angina.

TABLE 3.7 Factors worsening or relieving angina

Aggravating	Relieving
Exertion	Rest
Emotional excitement	Glyceryl trinitrate
Cold weather	Warm up before exercise
Exercise after meal	

Aggravating and relieving factors

The single most characteristic feature of angina is that it is brought on by exertion and relieved by rest. Other factors which may exacerbate or relieve angina are listed in Table 3.7.

Special types of angina

Unstable or crescendo angina is the term used to describe angina of increasing severity, duration or frequency. The pain may occur on minimal exertion or at rest and glyceryl trinitrate may be less effective than usual. Unstable angina may culminate in myocardial infarction.

Second wind angina occurs on initial exertion but then subsides without the patient resting, only to sometimes recur with continuing exertion. It is not uncommon and may cause diagnostic confusion.

*Nocturnal or decubitus angin*a may occur because of increasing venous return during the night or when short-acting anti-anginal preparations lose their efficacy. It usually indicates severe coronary disease.

Differential diagnosis

Sometimes it is difficult to distinguish between angina and other cardiac or non-cardiac causes of chest pain, including oesophageal pain (Table 3.8). The distinction involves an overall assessment of the clinical situation. Atypical symptoms occurring on exertion and relieved by rest in a 60-year-old man with a strong family history of coronary heart disease and a history of diabetes are probably angina. Conversely, even a characteristic history is unlikely to represent angina if the patient is a non-smoking, young adult female with no relevant family history or past medical history.

Precordial catch is the term that has been used to describe a stabbing pain usually at the cardiac apex. It is a common sensation experienced by many normal subjects which may cause undue anxiety. It is not a feature of organic heart disease.

TABLE 3.8 Differential diagnosis: angina vs oesophageal pain

Angina	Oesophageal pain
Usually precipitated by exertion	Can be worsened by exertion, but often present at other times
Rapidly relieved by rest	Not rapidly relieved by rest
Retrosternal and radiates to arm and jaw	Retrosternal or epigastric, sometimes radiates to arm or back
Seldom wakes patient from sleep	Often wakes patient from sleep
No relation to heartburn (but patients often have 'wind')	Sometimes related to heartburn
Rapidly relieved by nitrates	Often relieved by nitrates
Typical duration 2–10 minutes	Variable duration

Myocardial infarction

Myocardial infarction causes pain which is similar to angina in site, radiation and character but differs in that it is not necessarily precipitated by exertion, persists at rest and is usually much more severe (Table 3.9). Autonomic symptoms such as sweating, nausea and vomiting may be associated with myocardial infarction. Patients may also be breathless, restless and distressed and may experience a sensation of impending death, *angor amini*. Conversely, painless myocardial infarction is not uncommon particularly in elderly patients and those with diabetes. Such patients may present with complications such as cardiac failure or an arrhythmia.

Pericardial pain

Pericarditis causes pain which is retrosternal and may radiate to the shoulders or upper arm. It is accentuated by, or may only be present during, inspiration and varies with posture (Table 3.10). It may be worse on exertion but it is not reliably relieved by rest. It is often described as a stabbing pain or soreness. Rapid and complete resolution with a non-steroidal anti-inflammatory drug (NSAID) is almost diagnostic.

Aortic dissection

Dissection of the aorta causes pain that is usually of sudden onset. It is very severe, often described as tearing in nature and is frequently initially felt in the back between the shoulder blades (Table 3.11).

TABLE 3.9 Differential diagnosis: angina vs myocardial infarction

Angina	Myocardial infarction
Site: retrosternal, radiates to arm, epigastrium, neck	As for angina
Precipitated by exercise or emotion	Often no obvious precipitant
Relieved by rest, nitrates	Not relieved by rest, nitrates
Mild/moderate severity	Usually severe (may be 'silent')
Anxiety absent or mild	Variable anxiety or *angor amini*
No increased sympathetic activation	Increased sympathetic activity
No nausea or vomiting	Nausea and vomiting are common

TABLE 3.10 Characteristics of pericarditic pain

Site	Retrosternal, may radiate to left shoulder or back
Prodrome	May be preceded by a viral illness
Onset	No obvious initial precipitating factor; tends to fluctuate in intensity
Nature	May be stabbing or 'raw' – 'like sandpaper'. Often described as sharp, rarely as tight or heavy
Made worse by	Changes in posture, respiration
Helped by	Analgesics, especially NSAIDs
Accompanied by	Pericardial rub

TABLE 3.11 Characteristics of pain caused by dissection of aortic aneurysm

Site	Often first felt between shoulder blades, and/or retrosternally
Onset	Usually sudden
Nature	Very severe pain, often described as 'tearing' in nature
Relieved by	Tends to persist. Patients often restless with pain
Accompanied by	Hypertension, asymmetric pulses, unexpected bradycardia, early diastolic murmur, syncope, focal neurological symptoms and signs

BREATHLESSNESS

Respiratory causes of breathlessness (dyspnoea) are described in Chapter 4 (p. 120). This chapter deals specifically with dyspnoea of cardiac origin, though respiratory disease may coexist if only because of the common aetiological factor of smoking.

Dyspnoea on effort

Breathlessness on effort is physiological. It becomes a symptom of disease if it occurs at exercise levels below those expected for the patient's age and degree of previous fitness. Dyspnoea on exertion may be the only symptom of heart failure caused by left ventricular systolic dysfunction. Such patients frequently give a history consistent with previous myocardial infarction. Other common cardiac causes of exertional breathlessness include hypertension, valvular heart disease, cardiomyopathies and arrhythmias such as atrial fibrillation.

As with chest pain, it is important to assess the degree of symptomatic limitation caused by exertional breathlessness. This can be graded using the New York Heart Association (NYHA) classification (Table 3.12).

TABLE 3.12 New York Heart Association classification of heart failure symptom severity

Class I	No limitations. Ordinary physical activity does not cause undue fatigue, dyspnoea or palpitation (asymptomatic left ventricular dysfunction)
Class II	Slight limitation of physical activity. Such patients are comfortable at rest. Ordinary physical activity results in fatigue, palpitation, dyspnoea or angina pectoris (symptomatically 'mild' heart failure)
Class III	Marked limitation of physical activity. Less than ordinary physical activity will lead to symptoms (symptomatically 'moderate' heart failure)
Class IV	Symptoms of congestive cardiac failure are present even at rest. With any physical activity increased discomfort is experienced (symptomatically 'severe' heart failure)

Orthopnoea

This is dyspnoea on lying flat. To avoid this unpleasant symptom, the patient will typically try to lie propped up, e.g. using extra pillows. The symptoms may be so distressing that the patient will sleep upright in a chair. Orthopnoea is usually found when cardiac disease is more advanced and rarely occurs in the absence of effort dyspnoea unless it has been precipitated by an acute event such as the onset of a cardiac dysrhythmia. The orthopnoeic patient often experiences paroxysmal nocturnal dyspnoea (PND).

Paroxysmal nocturnal dyspnoea

PND is acute, severe, breathlessness that wakes the patient from sleep. The patient has to sit upright gasping in bed or sitting on the edge of the bed. The patient may even get out of bed, occasionally throwing open the windows in an attempt to relieve the distress. The intensity of the symptom is often described as akin to suffocation. Characteristically, the patient has a cough producing frothy sputum which may be streaked with blood. The mechanism is explained in Figure 3.2, which also lists the causes. Paroxysmal nocturnal dyspnoea has to be distinguished from nocturnal asthma (Ch. 4, p. 139).

Dyspnoea at rest

This represents the most advanced form of cardiac dyspnoea and indicates the presence of severe heart failure. When it occurs in patients with known cardiac disease and is preceded by a history of worsening effort dyspnoea, orthopnoea and PND and perhaps ankle swelling, a cardiac cause is self-evident. However, patients presenting de novo with acute dyspnoea at rest or who have both lung and heart disease may be more difficult to assess. Other causes include pneumothorax and pulmonary embolism. Unlike patients with acute pulmonary oedema, those with pulmonary embolism are often more comfortable lying flat and may even become unconscious if made to sit upright.

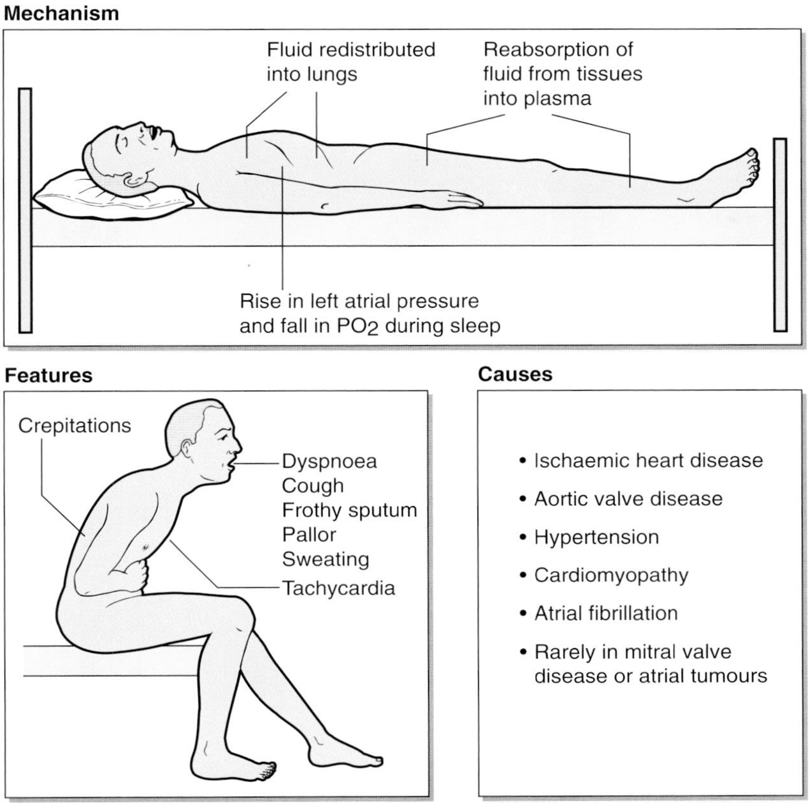

Fig. 3.2 Paroxysmal nocturnal dyspnoea.

CASE HISTORY

A 65-year-old man gave a 6-month history of progressive breathlessness on exertion to such an extent that he had difficulty climbing the stairs to his bedroom. For 2 weeks, he had felt more breathless in bed and had begun to sleep with two extra pillows. On the night of admission, he had woken gasping for breath.

On examination, he was dyspnoeic with a regular tachycardia and a weak thready pulse. There was pitting oedema over the ankles and sacrum. The liver was palpably enlarged and the jugular venous pressure was elevated to 8 cm with a normal waveform. There were fine expiratory crackles at the lung bases. The ECG showed a sinus tachycardia of 120 per minute with evidence of a previous anterior myocardial infarction (Fig. 3.3). The chest X-ray (Fig. 3.4) showed cardiac enlargement with pulmonary oedema. The urea and electrolytes, the haemoglobin and the cardiac enzymes were normal.

He was treated with diuretics and an angiotensin-converting enzyme inhibitor. An echocardiogram subsequently showed significant impairment of left ventricular function with an extensive scar over the anterior wall of the ventricle (Fig. 3.5).

Learning points

- The first priority was to establish that the breathlessness was caused by cardiac failure.
- The second was to exclude any acute precipitating factor, such as a recent myocardial infarct, the development of an arrhythmia or anaemia.

PALPITATIONS

Palpitations are the sensation of the heart beating in the chest. Terms such as thumping, pounding, fluttering, jumping, racing and bumping are often used by the patient. Palpitations may be due to a heightened awareness of the heart beating in sinus rhythm, awareness of occasional irregularities of the heart beat (e.g. ventricular extrasystoles) or awareness of the heart beating in an abnormal rhythm. Most patients complaining of palpitations do not have an arrhythmia and not all patients with arrhythmia have palpitations, e.g. atrial fibrillation is commonly asymptomatic. Although investigation is commonly required to confirm the diagnosis, the history can frequently distinguish between the different types of palpitations (Table 3.13). Important aspects of the history include:

- the mode of onset
- the frequency
- the duration of attacks
- the awareness of the heart beat and its regularity.

The rate and rhythm may be clarified by asking the patient to tap out the sensation experienced during an attack. Additional specific questions may be required to obtain further information

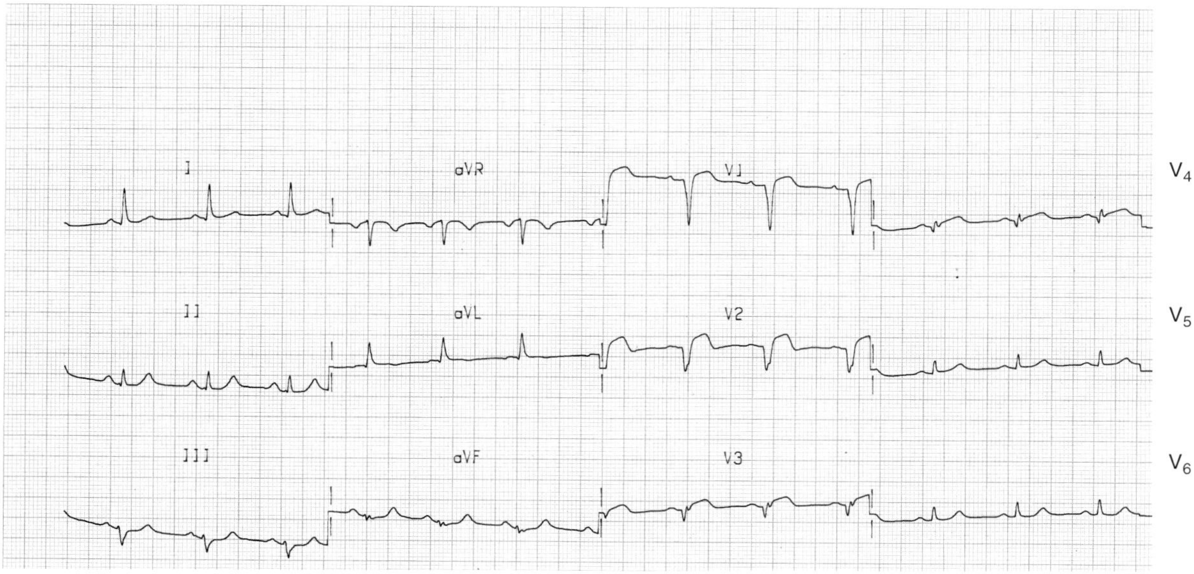

Fig. 3.3 12-lead ECG showing Q waves in leads V1–V4 indicative of established anterior myocardial infarction.

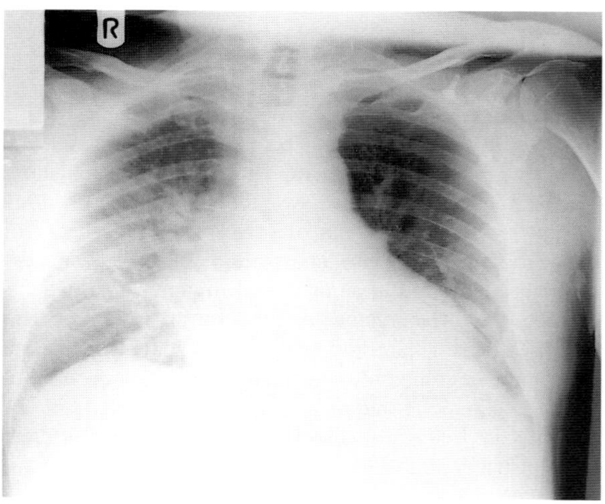

Fig. 3.4 Chest x-ray showing cardiomegaly with left ventricular predominence and fluffy opacification in both lung fields, particularly on the right side, indicative of pulmonary oedema. The veins to both upper lobes are distended.

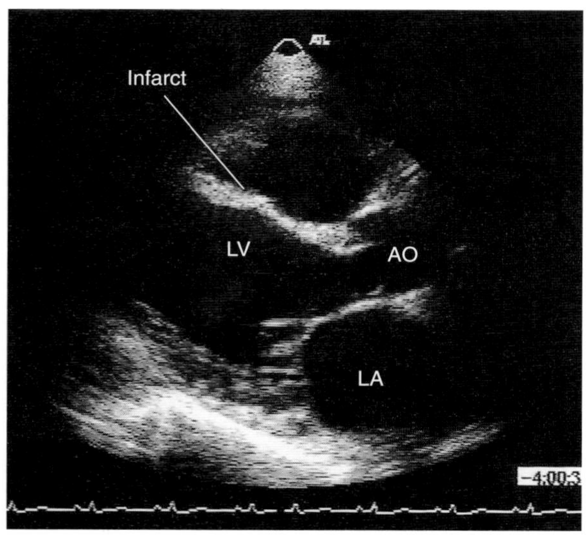

Fig. 3.5 Still frame from the echocardiogram in a parasternal long axis view. This shows thinning of the interventricular septum which has an irregular shape and bright echoes indicating fibrous scarring. This is the site of an old infarct. LA = left atrium, LV = left ventricle, Ao = aortic root.

TABLE 3.13 Descriptions of arrhythmias

Arrhythmia	Patient's description
Ventricular or atrial extrasystoles	'Heart misses a beat' Heart 'jumps' or 'flutters'
Atrial fibrillation	Heart 'jumping about' or 'racing' Associated breathlessness May be unnoticed
Supraventricular tachycardia	Heart racing or fluttering Associated polyuria
Ventricular tachycardia	Heart racing or fluttering. Associated breathlessness
Ventricular tachycardia may present as syncope rather than as palpitation	

QUESTIONS – To ask patients with arrhythmias

- Is there a family history of premature heart disease or sudden death?
- Is there a past history of rheumatic fever, previous heart attacks or other heart disease?
- What is the daily caffeine and weekly alcohol consumption (see p. 12)?
- Are any drugs being taken, whether prescribed, over the counter or recreational?
- Are there any non-specific symptoms of recent ill health (to consider unusual causes such as infective endocarditis or Lyme disease etc.)
- If the attacks are paroxysmal:
  - are there any precipitating factors (e.g. exercise, anxiety or stress)?
  - what is the nature of the onset of the attacks and are there associated symptoms (such as presyncope or chest discomfort)?
  - are there any relieving factors (e.g. breath-holding, exercise).

regarding the nature of the palpitations and also possible underlying pathology.

Awareness of heart beating in sinus rhythm

This is experienced by most healthy subjects at some time. It usually occurs in relation to sympathetic nervous system overactivity, e.g. after strenuous exercise, when given a fright or waiting for an interview or examination. It may be most noticeable in bed at night when external visual and auditory inputs are minimal and visceral sensations more prominent. Similar palpitations occur with excessive caffeine intake in coffee, tea or other drinks. Caffeine (found in tea, coffee, cola, etc.) enhances the action of the sympathetic nervous system by augmenting the concentration of relevant secondary messengers in the myocardium.

Awareness of normal irregularities of the heart beat

Another benign cause of palpitations is ventricular ectopic beats. Very often patients with ectopic beats will have taken their own pulse. As a consequence, they will describe 'missed beats', often followed by a particularly strong heart beat. This is because the premature (ectopic) depolarisation resulted in a low stroke volume producing an impalpable impulse following incomplete left ventricular filling. The subsequent compensatory pause leads to overfilling of the ventricle and a more forceful contraction and greater stroke volume with the next beat. Palpitations of this type occur more often at rest and often subside if the patient gets up and undertakes physical activity.

Palpitations due to arrhythmias

Such palpitations are likely to be of sudden onset, to last for minutes or longer and to be unrelated to anxiety or stress. Specific triggers may be identified such as exercise, and manoeuvres may be found which terminate the arrhythmia, e.g. forced expiration while breath-holding (the Valsalva manoeuvre). It is necessary not only to identify the nature of the arrhythmia but also to determine whether or not it is occurring in the context of structural heart disease. In patients with arrhythmias it is necessary to also establish the nature of the underlying pathology. The questions to ask will depend upon the specific arrhythmia. Examples of useful topics are given in the Question box.

In particular, patients with coronary heart disease or heart failure are at risk of ventricular arrhythmias. Such patients who complain of palpitations or syncope should be considered to have a potentially life-threatening ventricular arrhythmia until proven otherwise.

SYNCOPE AND DIZZINESS

It is uncommon for dizziness to be caused by cardiac disease. However, loss of consciousness (syncope) or the feeling of impending loss of consciousness (presyncope) may be cardiac in origin. The causes can be broadly classified into three groups:

- drug related
- arrhythmias
- left ventricular outflow obstruction.

Drug related

Some of the drugs which may cause palpitations may also produce syncope or presyncope (Table 3.2). Vasodilator drugs (e.g. alpha-blockers) can cause symptomatic postural hypotension. Beta-blockers, verapamil, diltiazem and digoxin can aggravate or cause sinoatrial disease or atrioventricular block. Other cardiac and non-cardiac medications can directly (e.g. tricyclic antidepressants) or indirectly (e.g. diuretics causing hypokalaemia) provoke ventricular arrhythmias in vulnerable patients.

Arrhythmias

Syncope is rarely associated with atrial fibrillation and other supraventricular tachyarrhythmias. However bradycardia related to sick sinus syndrome or atrioventricular block (i.e. Stokes–Adams attacks) and ventricular tachyarrhythmias may cause syncope or presyncope.

Left ventricular outflow obstruction

Severe aortic stenosis and hypertrophic cardiomyopathy associated with muscular obstruction of the left ventricular outflow tract may cause syncope or presyncope, especially on exertion. Clinical examination often reveals a systolic murmur.

Other cardiac causes

Patients may develop recurrent syncope due to an enhanced vagal response (malignant vasovagal syncope). In these patients fainting results from sudden bradycardia in association with vasodilatation. Other rare causes include left atrial myxoma obstructing the mitral valve and carotid sinus hypersensitivity. In the latter, gentle pressure on the carotid sinus may produce the patient's symptoms by causing a profound bradycardia.

OTHER SYMPTOMS OF CARDIAC DISEASE

Symptoms which involve other systems may be the presenting features in patients with cardiac disease. Some of these are listed on Table 3.14. Undue tiredness may be a feature of ischaemic heart disease and the symptoms of infective endocarditis are often non-specific. They include weight loss and tiredness with night sweats.

TABLE 3.14 Cardiovascular disease presenting with 'non-cardiac' symptoms

System	Symptom	Cause
Central nervous system	Stroke	Cerebral embolism Endocarditis Hypertension
Gastrointestinal	Abdominal pain Jaundice	Liver congestion secondary to heart failure Mesenteric embolism
Renal	Oliguria	Heart failure

CASE HISTORY

An 85-year-old man was referred to an outpatient clinic having experienced six syncopal episodes over a 2-year period. On a number of additional occasions he had felt lightheaded without fainting. The attacks had occurred at any time, both standing and sitting, and there were no obvious precipitants. He recovered quickly with no after-effects. Several attacks had been witnessed by his wife. She said that he went pale and showed no features to suggest epilepsy. He had a past history of gout and hypertension treated with a beta-blocker (atenolol).

Examination revealed a bradycardia, 60 per minute, and a blood pressure of 160/80 mmHg. The resting ECG confirmed sinus bradycardia with evidence of left ventricular hypertrophy. Ambulatory ECG monitoring over 24 hours was normal on three occasions while he had no symptoms. During a fourth period of monitoring he felt lightheaded and the ECG showed transient complete heart block (Fig. 3.6). His symptoms resolved when the atenolol was stopped.

Learning points

- An eyewitness account is valuable in assessing the cause of any 'blackout'.
- A negative 24-hour ambulatory ECG does not exclude a dysrhythmia, especially when obtained in the absence of symptoms.
- Many drugs used for cardiac conditions, including beta blockade, may cause cardiac dysrhythmias in susceptible subjects.

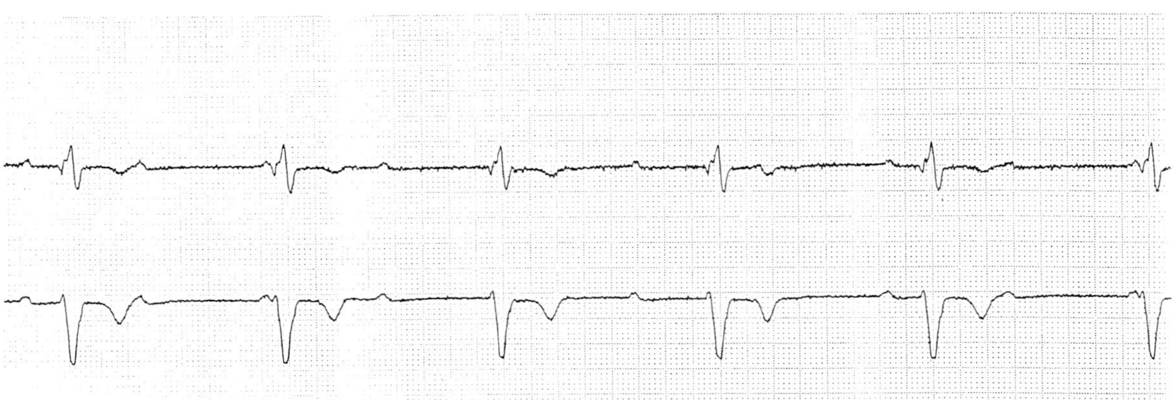

Fig. 3.6 Printout from 24-hour ambulatory ECG recording, showing complete heart block.

PERIPHERAL OEDEMA

Oedema can be both a symptom (ankle swelling) or a sign. Although oedema may occur in heart failure it is also seen in a number of other diseases (p. 33). Even the combination of exertional dyspnoea and oedema is not sufficiently specific to conclude that heart failure is present. A common cause of oedema that is a potential source of confusion is the use of dihydropyridine calcium channel blockers such as nifedipine or amlodipine.

KEY POINTS

- Patients with significant cardiac disease may be asymptomatic.
- The diagnosis of angina is made from the history.
- The characteristic feature of angina is that it is brought on by exertion and relieved by rest.
- Crescendo or unstable angina is a medical emergency.
- The severity of cardiac symptoms often depends upon normal levels of activity; hence the occupational history may exert a major influence on management.
- Paroxysmal nocturnal dyspnoea is commonly due to acute pulmonary oedema.
- Chronic heart failure presents with exertional breathlessness and/or fatigue in association with fluid retention, e.g. peripheral oedema.
- It is important to ask patients to explain what they mean by palpitations; it is often helpful for the patient to 'tap out' the sensation on the table.

THE PHYSICAL EXAMINATION

The approach to physical examination will depend upon the condition of the patient.

Cardiovascular triage divides patients into three categories:

- those with cardiac or respiratory arrest requiring resuscitation
- those who are severely ill and require immediate treatment
- those who are haemodynamically stable.

The management of cardiac arrest is outwith the remit of this book. Examination of severely ill patients requires to be adapted to suit the clinical situation.

In the haemodynamically stable it is valuable to have a scheme or routine of physical examination – an example is shown in Table 3.15.

TABLE 3.15 Scheme of cardiovascular examination

1. Get a general impression of the patient: look for signs of anxiety, breathlessness or pain
2. Shake hands: assess peripheral circulation (warmth), sweating, look for clubbing, splinter haemorrhages
3. Palpate radial pulses: measure rate, assess rhythm
4. Palpate brachial pulses: measure blood pressure
5. Palpate carotid pulses: assess quality and listen for bruits
6. Examine jugular venous pulse
7. Examine face: look for features of hypercholesterolaemia or anaemia, examine tongue for cyanosis
8. Examine chest: assess cardiac impulse, locate apex beat
9. Auscultate the heart
10. Examine back of chest: listen for crepitations. Look for sacral oedema
11. Examine the abdomen especially for hepatomegaly and ascites.
12. Assess femoral pulses: look for radiofemoral delay
13. Examine legs: palpate pulses, assess oedema
14. Examine the optic fundi

THE GENERAL EXAMINATION

The general inspection of patients has been discussed in Chapter 2. In particular, the hands (p. 46), the optic fundi (Ch. 7) and the face (Fig. 3.7) may provide important signs of cardiac disease. Features which are relevant to a cardiac diagnosis include whether or not the patient appears breathless, distressed or anxious or if there is evidence of alcohol abuse (Fig. 1.9) or tobacco consumption (Fig. 1.8), or evidence of anaemia or cyanosis (p. 126). Cyanosis of cardiac origin is usually caused by pulmonary oedema, although cyanosis may be absent even in severe pulmonary oedema. When associated with congenital heart disease, the presence of cyanosis implies the development of a right-to-left shunt. The resultant cyanosis is not corrected when breathing 100% oxygen and is usually associated with finger clubbing.

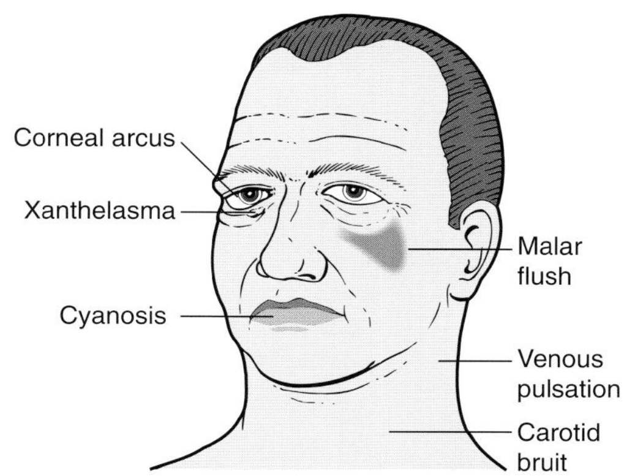

Fig. 3.7 Facial clues to heart disease.

Sometimes signs may be present in the absence of symptoms. For example, hyperlipidaemia is an important risk factor in vascular disease. Evidence to suggest its presence include:

- Palmar or tendon xanthomata (Fig. 3.8).
- Corneal arcus, due to precipitation of cholesterol crystals at the periphery of the cornea. In young people it is associated with hypercholesterolaemia but the association gets weaker with increasing age.

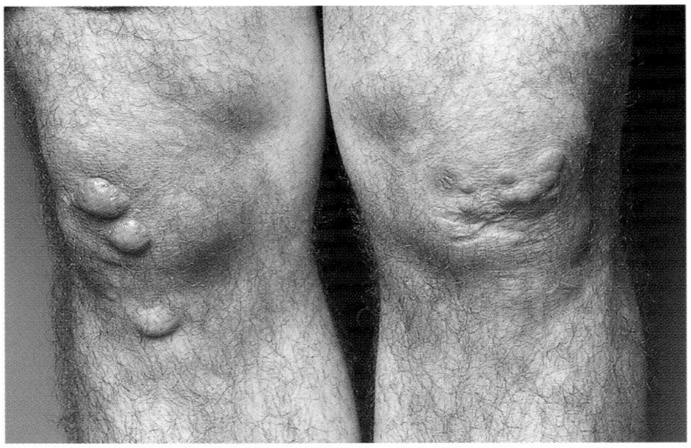

Fig. 3.8 Eruptive xanthomata.

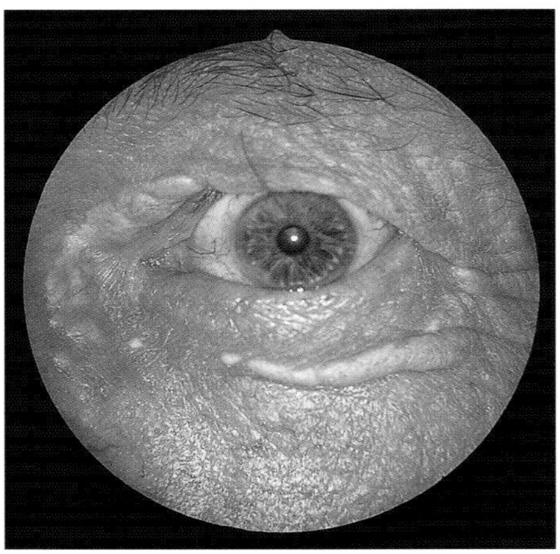

Fig. 3.9 Xanthelasma.

- Xanthelasma, a yellowish eruption at the inner side of the eyelids and periorbital skin, associated with hypercholesterolaemia in people under the age of 50 (Fig. 3.9).

Additional detailed examination to elicit specific signs will be influenced by the history and the presenting features. Examples include the examination of a patient with hypertension (see Fig. 3.18). Less commonly, in patients in whom infective endocarditis is a possibility, various signs may acquire diagnostic significance. These are shown in Figure 3.10. In the hands, possible changes include Janeway lesions, which are non-tender nodules and Osler's nodes on the palms or finger pads (Fig. 3.11). Splinter haemorrhages (Fig. 2.29A) and haematuria both suggest the development of immune complex disease, and finger clubbing only occurs in chronic infection.

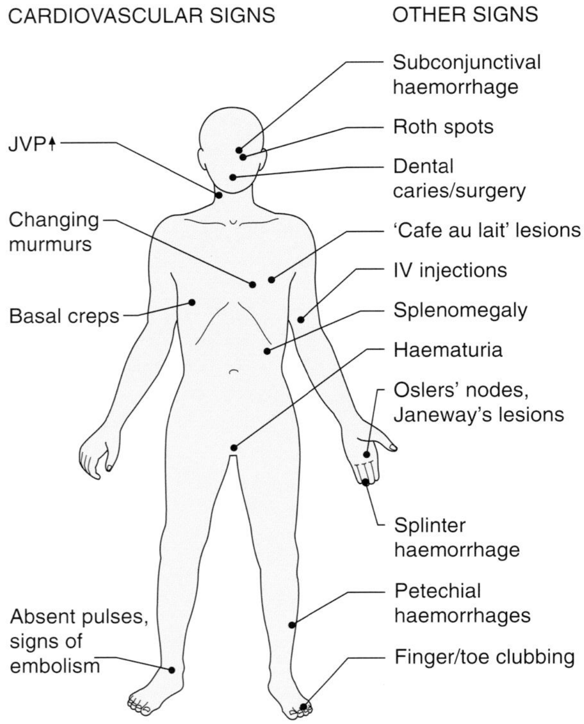

Fig. 3.10 Signs in infective endocarditis.

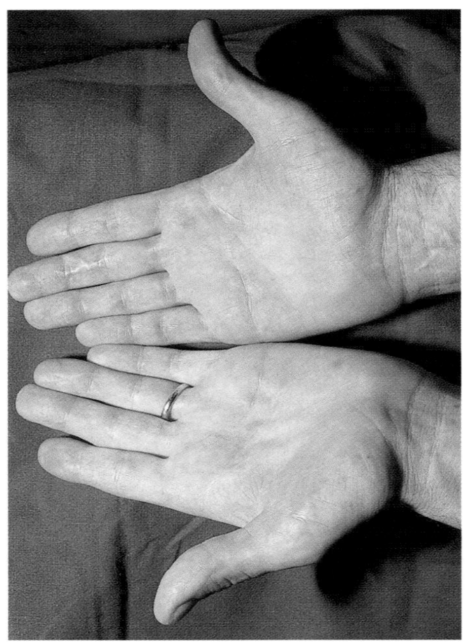

Fig. 3.11 Osler's nodes.

THE PULSES

The pulses are examined for rate, rhythm, volume and character.

Anatomy

The *radial pulse* is readily felt just lateral to the tendon of the flexor carpi radialis muscle (Fig. 3.12). It is particularly useful for assessing the rate and rhythm of the pulse. The *brachial artery* can be felt in the brachial fossa immediately medial to the biceps tendon. The *carotid pulse* is palpable in the neck and provides a better indicator of volume and character than is obtained from the radial pulse.

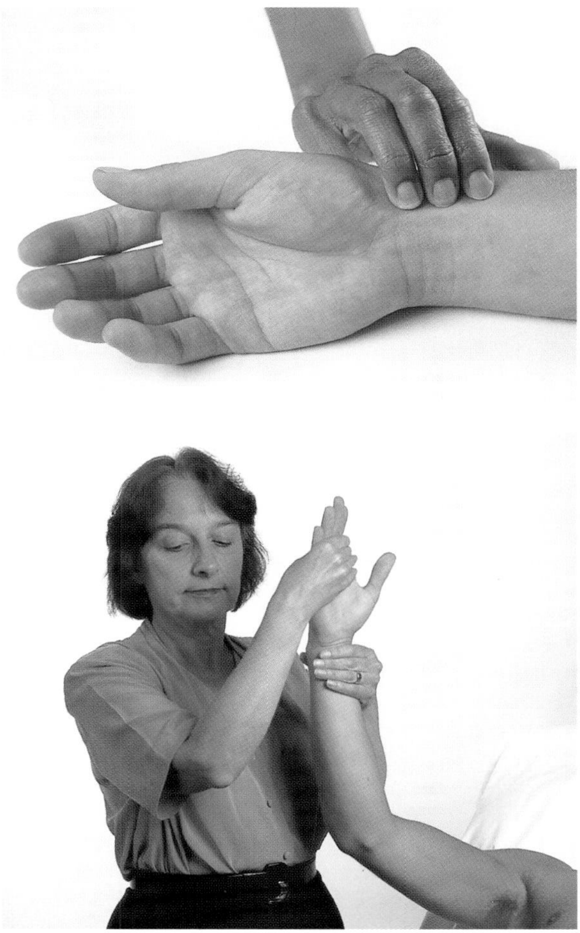
A

B

Fig. 3.12 The radial pulse. [A] Locating and palpating the radial pulse. [B] Feeling for a collapsing radial pulse.

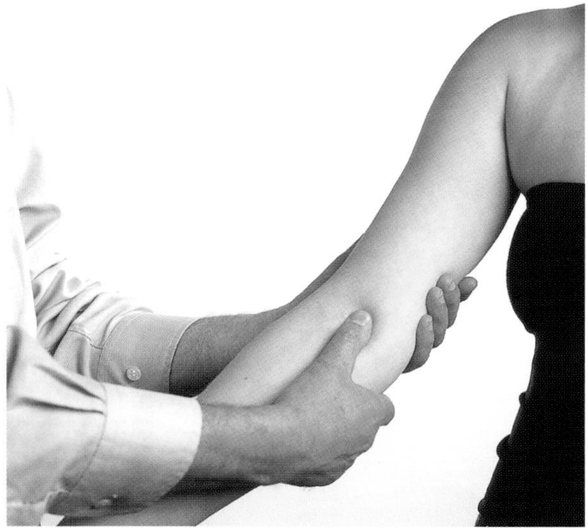

Fig. 3.13 Assessing the brachial pulse with a thumb.

Examination sequence

Radial pulses

- ☐ Apply three fingers over the radial pulse at the right wrist (Fig. 3.12A).
- ☐ Use the pulp of the fingers to assess the rate and rhythm.
- ☐ Count the pulse for 15 seconds and multiply by four to obtain pulse rate in beats per minute (b.p.m).
- ☐ To feel for a collapsing pulse, raise the arm while feeling across the pulse with the fingers of the other hand (Fig. 3.12B).
- ☐ Palpate the left radial pulse. If either pulse feels diminished in volume, confirm any difference by simultaneous palpation.

Brachial pulses

- ☐ Use the thumb (right thumb for right arm and vice versa) with the fingers cupped round the back of the elbow (Fig. 3.13).
- ☐ Feel just medial to the tendon of the biceps muscle to detect the pulse and assess its character.

Carotid pulses

- ☐ Palpate the carotid pulse with the patient lying on a bed or couch.
- ☐ Never compress both carotids simultaneously.
- ☐ Use the left thumb for the right carotid and vice versa.
- ☐ Place the tip of the thumb between the larynx and the anterior border of the sternocleidomastoid muscle.
- ☐ Press the thumb gently backwards to feel the pulse (Fig. 3.14).
- ☐ Auscultate for bruits by 'walking' the stethoscope up the carotid artery using the diaphragm.

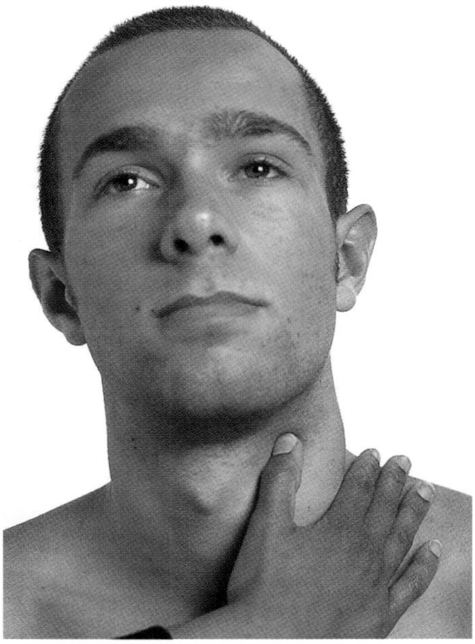

Fig. 3.14 Locating the carotid pulse.

Normal findings

A normal resting pulse rate is between 60–100 b.p.m. in an adult (and 80–200 b.p.m. in a child). Bradycardia is defined as a pulse rate of < 60 b.p.m. and tachycardia as a rate in excess of 100 b.p.m.

The normal rhythm of the heart is called sinus rhythm because it originates from the sinoatrial node. Sinus rhythm is seldom completely regular, because the heart speeds up during inspiration and slows at the beginning of expiration. This sinus arrhythmia is most obvious in children, young people and athletes.

Volume and character. Volume is the term used to indicate the movement imparted to the finger applied gently to the pulse. Character describes the impression of the pulse waveform gained by palpation. Pulse volume and character are best appreciated in a large artery, such as the carotid. Considerable experience is required before characteristic waveforms can be recognised with confidence. Their presence may alert the clinician to a particular valvular or other lesion and also help in determining the severity of such lesions.

Common abnormalities

Rate. The causes of tachycardia and bradycardia are shown in Table 3.16. An important cause of bradycardia is complete heart block (3rd degree atrioventricular block) when the heart rhythm is regular and the rate is often < 40 b.p.m. This may be intermittent and cause the patient to lose consciousness (Stokes–Adams attacks). The commonest cause of tachycardia is sinus tachycardia due to exercise, pain, anxiety or fever.

TABLE 3.16 Causes of a fast or slow pulse

Fast heart rate (tachycardia, > 100/min)	
Sinus tachycardia	Arrhythmia

Exercise
Pain
Excitement/anxiety
Fever
Hyperthyroidism
Medication
  Sympathomimetics
  Vasodilators
	Atrial fibrillation
	Atrial flutter
	Supraventricular tachycardia
	Ventricular tachycardia

Slow heart rate (bradycardia, < 60/min)	
Sinus bradycardia	Arrhythmia

Sleep
Athletic training
Hypothyroidism
Medication
  Beta-blockers
  Digoxin
  Verapamil diltiazem
	Carotid sinus hypersensitivity
	Sick sinus syndrome
	Second degree heart block
	Complete heart block

TABLE 3.17 Causes of an irregular pulse

- Sinus arrhythmia
- Atrial extrasystoles
- Ventricular extrasystoles
- Atrial fibrillation
- Atrial flutter with variable response
- Second degree heart block with variable response

The pulse rhythm. When the pulse is irregular, it is important to identify the nature of the irregularity and to determine whether it is present all the time or only intermittently. Some common causes of an irregular pulse are listed in Table 3.17. An occasional irregularity is commonly caused by ectopic beats or extrasystoles which can be atrial or ventricular in origin (Fig. 3.15A). Frequently the pulse wave produced by the ectopic beat is too weak to be felt at the wrist. The resultant difference between the actual heart rate and the rate palpable at the radial pulse is called the 'pulse deficit'. Ventricular ectopic beats do not 'reset' the sinus node, so there is a delay, or compensatory pause, until the next sinus beat occurs. The prolongation in ventricular filling time leads to an enhanced stroke volume which can be appreciated as an increase in pulse volume. Sometimes ectopic beats occur regularly, e.g. after every normal beat. This is called *pulsus bigemini* and may give the false impression of a very slow pulse (Fig. 3.15B).

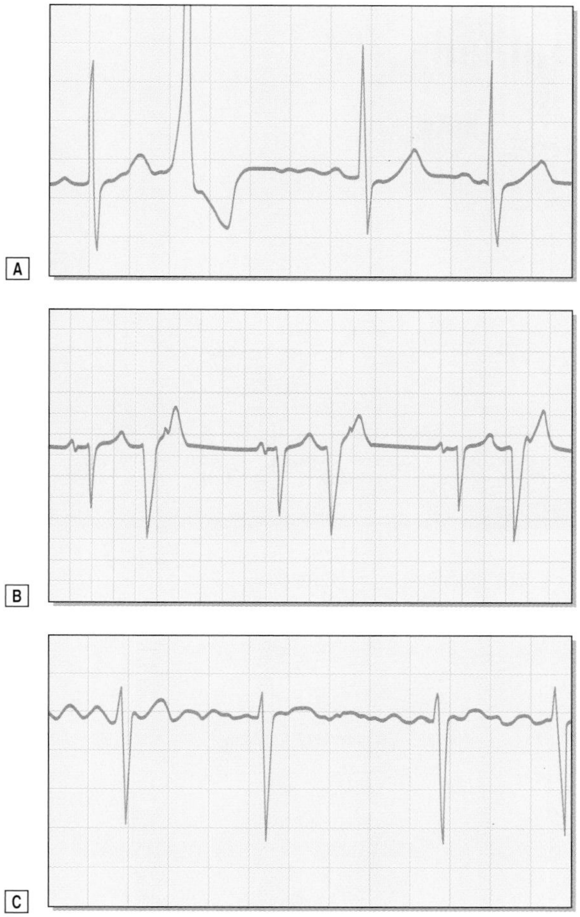

Fig. 3.15 Electrocardiogram showing [A] ventricular ectopic beat, [B] bigeminy, [C] atrial fibrillation with a 'controlled' ventricular response.

Atrial fibrillation causes a totally random heart rhythm leading to a pulse which is irregular in both timing and volume (Fig. 3.15C). This is often described as an 'irregularly irregular' rhythm. Untreated atrial fibrillation usually causes a tachycardia, and the delay between some ventricular contractions may be too short to allow proper filling, leading to a reduced stroke volume and an impalpable pulse. This may produce a considerable pulse deficit. Therefore when the ventricular response to atrial fibrillation is rapid, the heart rate should be measured by listening at the apex and preferably confirmed by counting the rate from an ECG. Common causes of atrial fibrillation are given in Table 3.18. Lone, or idiopathic, atrial fibrillation is unusual; if there is no obvious explanation it is important to positively exclude thyrotoxicosis and alcohol-related disease.

TABLE 3.18 Common causes of atrial fibrillation

- Hypertension
- Cardiac failure
- Myocardial infarct
- Thyrotoxicosis
- Alcohol-related heart disease
- Mitral valve disease
- Acute chest infection
- Following surgery, especially cardiothoracic surgery

Pulse volume. A large volume pulse may be due to aortic regurgitation or vasodilatation. Exercise, emotion, heat and pregnancy are physiological factors causing vasodilatation which also occurs with fever, thyrotoxicosis, anaemia, peripheral AV shunts, Paget's disease of bone, and drug therapy.

A low volume pulse is found in patients with reduced stroke volume due to heart failure, or peripheral vascular disease. The pulse may be thin and thready in the shocked patient.

Coarctation is a congenital narrowing of the aorta usually situated just *after* the left subclavian artery. In children with this condition the upper limb pulses are normal, while all lower limb pulses are reduced or impalpable. In adults, coarctation usually presents with hypertension, and although the femoral pulses are usually palpable owing to the development of collaterals they are diminished in volume and delayed with respect to the radial pulse (see Fig. 3.16).

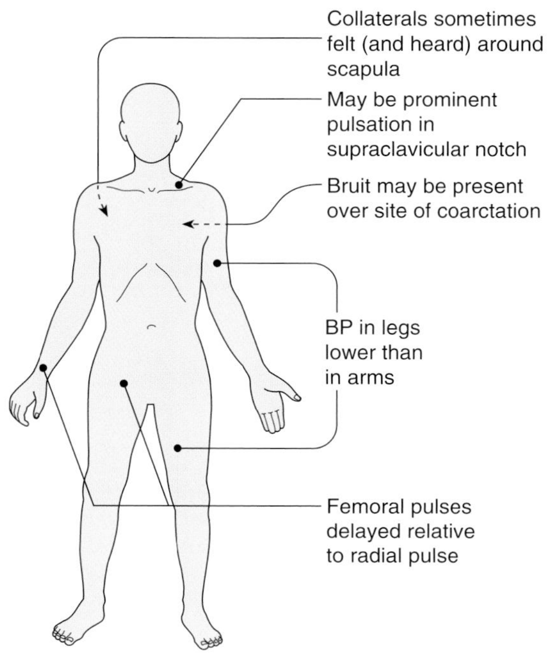

Fig. 3.16 Coarctation of the aorta.

Pulsus alternans is rare and describes alternate variations in the size of the pulse wave. The pulse rhythm is regular. It is a sign of severe myocardial disease and heart failure. It may be first detected when measuring the blood pressure.

Pulsus paradoxus describes a pulse that increases in volume on expiration and decreases in volume in inspiration. Technically the term is a misnomer because this variation is physiological, though not detectable in a normal individual. When respiratory variation is exaggerated to the extent that it is clinically detectable it is an abnormal finding which occurs with severe airways obstruction (e.g. asthma) and pericardial tamponade, due to a tense pericardial effusion. Pulsus paradoxus is most accurately assessed using a blood pressure cuff to measure the difference in systolic pressure between inspiration and expiration. A difference > 15 mmHg is pathological.

The character. A slow-rising pulse characterised by a reduced peak occurring late in systole, sometimes associated with a carotid thrill, is a feature of aortic stenosis. A *bisferiens* pulse, characteristic of combined aortic stenosis and regurgitation, has two systolic peaks separated by a distinct midsystolic dip.

The collapsing pulse. The peak of the pulse wave occurs early and is of brief duration followed by an equally rapid descent. This rapid fall in pulse pressure imparts the 'collapsing' sensation. It is best felt when the patient's arm is raised (see Fig. 3.12B). This pulse is most characteristic of aortic regurgitation.

BLOOD PRESSURE

Blood pressure is usually measured using a sphygmomanometer cuff wrapped round the upper arm. This is shown in Figure 3.17. Attention to detail is needed for accurate blood pressure measurement. A checklist is given in Table 3.19. It is important to use the correct size of cuff. A bladder length of 30–35 cm and width of 12 cm is suitable for most adults.

Examination sequence

- ☐ Support the arm comfortably at about heart level.
- ☐ Apply the cuff to the arm.
- ☐ Identify the brachial pulse.
- ☐ Inflate the cuff until the pulse is impalpable. Note the pressure on the manometer which is a rough estimate of systolic pressure.
- ☐ Now inflate the cuff another 10 mmHg and listen through the stethoscope over the brachial artery.
- ☐ Deflate the cuff slowly until regular heart sounds (called Korotkoff sounds) can be just heard. This is the systolic pressure which should be measured to the nearest 2 mmHg.
- ☐ Continue to deflate the cuff slowly until the sounds disappear.
- ☐ Record the point at which the sounds just disappear as diastolic pressure.

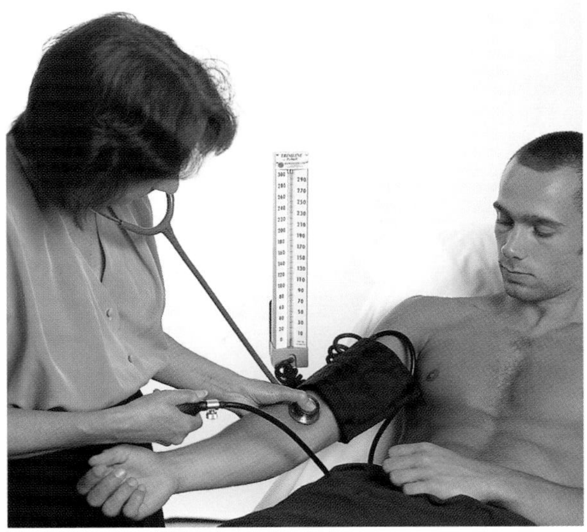

Fig. 3.17 Measuring the blood pressure.

TABLE 3.19 Checklist for blood pressure measurement

Patient	Relaxed Arm supported at heart level Clothing removed from arm
Cuff	Neatly applied Correct size for arm No leaks
Manometer	Well supported Upright If aneroid manometer, regularly calibrated
Operator	Check systolic pressure by palpation Release pressure slowly Avoid parallax error (eye same level as manometer) Avoid end-digit preference: record to nearest 2 mmHg

Normal findings

Usually as the sphygmomanometer cuff is deflated the Korotkoff sounds get gradually louder, then suddenly become muffled just before they disappear. Occasionally the muffled sounds persist, in which case the point at which they first become muffled is the best guide to the diastolic pressure.

Blood pressure is usually recorded as systolic pressure/diastolic pressure, thus 145/92 means that the systolic pressure was 145 and the diastolic 92 mmHg.

Blood pressure varies with excitement, stress and environment. Repeated measurements are required before a patient should be identified as hypertensive. In some patients the very measurement of blood pressure can cause it to rise – so-called 'white coat' hypertension. Ambulatory blood pressure monitoring helps to distinguish these patients from those with true sustained hypertension.

Common abnormalities

Hypertension. Systemic hypertension is common, particularly in the elderly, has no specific symptoms but, if untreated, can lead to death or morbidity from heart disease, cerebrovascular accident or renal failure. Clinical assessment of the hypertensive patient has three aims:

- to seek a specific cause
- to assess the severity of the problem
- to evaluate the extent of damage already done and the overall risk of cardiovascular disease (Fig. 3.18).

The secondary causes of hypertension are all relatively rare but are more likely in younger subjects. Many patients with essential, or primary, hypertension give a family history of the condition. However, the diagnosis is one of exclusion. Other specific questions to ask include a detailed renal history because renal disease is the commonest secondary cause of hypertension. A history of paroxysmal headaches, vomiting, sweating, pallor and weight loss, may suggest phaeochromocytoma. Enquiry should also be made concerning alcohol intake; some secondary causes, e.g. Conn's syndrome, have no specific symptoms.

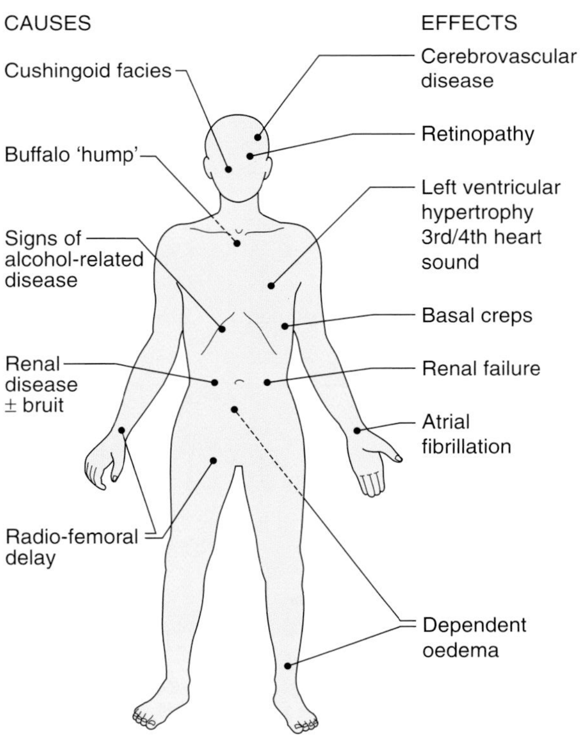

Fig. 3.18 Signs of hypertension.

The severity of the hypertension will influence the need for treatment. This will involve asking questions about cardiac symptoms, particularly dyspnoea and angina, and making an overall assessment of the cardiovascular risk taking into account the patient's age, sex, smoking habit, and family history.

The choice of treatment will also be influenced by the presence or absence of complications. For example beta-blocking agents and calcium channel antagonists may be particularly useful in treating hypertensives with angina but an ACE inhibitor with a diuretic may be preferred if there is significant left ventricular dysfunction.

Examination sequence

- ☐ Make serial recordings of the blood pressure.
- ☐ Check the pulse for atrial fibrillation.
- ☐ Look for radiofemoral delay in patients < 40 years old.
- ☐ Examine the optic fundi for hypertensive retinopathy (p. 256–257).
- ☐ Look for features of Cushing's syndrome (Fig. 2.8A and p. 32) or virilisation.
- ☐ Palpate the abdomen for adrenal masses and for enlarged kidneys (p. 165).
- ☐ Auscultate for bruits over the renal arteries.
- ☐ Examine the heart for features of left ventricular hypertrophy (p. 91).
- ☐ Look for evidence of cardiac failure (p. 101).
- ☐ Perform microscopic examination of the urine (p. 180–181) looking particularly for red cell casts (Fig. 5.27).

JUGULAR VENOUS PRESSURE AND WAVEFORM

Examination of the internal jugular vein provides valuable information regarding the right atrial pressure and the character of the venous waveform.

Anatomy

There are no valves between the right atrium and the internal jugular vein. It follows that the degree of distension in the vein equates to the pressure in the right atrium and the venous waveform provides information about cardiac function.

The internal jugular vein enters the neck behind the mastoid process. It runs deep to the sternomastoid muscle before entering the thorax between its sternal and clavicular heads. Because of its deep position the internal jugular vein can only be examined when the neck muscles are relaxed. Only a diffuse pulsation can be seen and the vein is not visible. The external jugular vein is visible but it is not routinely examined because it is prone to kinking and partial obstruction as it traverses the deep fascia of the neck.

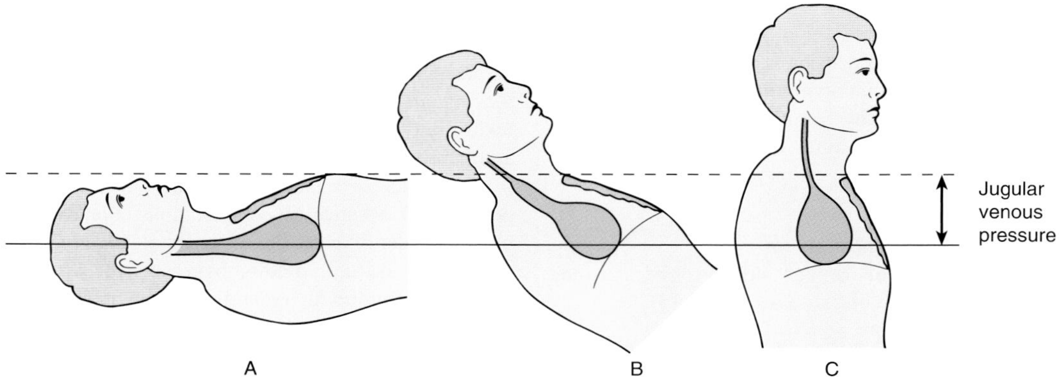

Fig. 3.19 Jugular venous pressure in a normal subject. A Supine: jugular vein distended, pulsation not visible. B Reclining at 45 degrees: point of transition between distended and collapsed vein can usually be seen to pulsate just above the clavicle. C Upright: upper part of vein collapsed and transition points obscured by sternum.

Normal findings

Jugular venous pressure. The normal mean right atrial pressure is < 9 cmH_2O (7 mmHg). Since the sternal angle is approximately 5 cm above the right atrium, the normal jugular venous pulse should extend no more than 4 cm above the sternal angle (Fig. 3.19). When a normal subject sits upright the pulse is hidden behind the clavicle and sternum. When reclining at 45 degrees the top of the pulsation is normally just at the level of the clavicle. If it can not be seen, then a normal right atrial pressure can be confirmed by applying firm pressure over the centre of the abdomen for 5–10 seconds (abdominojugular reflux). This increases the venous return and normally leads to a transient increase in right atrial pressure of 1–3 cm which is reflected in the height of the jugular venous pulse.

Waveform. Identification of the jugular venous pulse waveform requires experience. The normal waveform comprises two peaks, which helps to distinguish the vein from the carotid artery (Table 3.20). The first, or 'a' wave coincides with right atrial contraction and occurs just before the first heart sound. The second is the 'v' wave which is caused by atrial filling during ventricular systole when the tricuspid valve is closed (Fig. 3.20). A third positive wave, the 'c' wave, comprises a transmitted pulsation from the carotid artery and is not normally visible.

Normally the jugular venous pressure falls on inspiration because the fall in intrathoracic pressure is transmitted to the right atrium.

Examination sequence

☐ Position the patient reclining supine at 45 degrees in good light.

TABLE 3.20 Differences between carotid and jugular pulsation

Carotid	Jugular
Rapid outward movement	Rapid inward movement
One peak per heartbeat	Two peaks per heartbeat (in sinus rhythm)
Palpable	Impalpable
Pulsation unaffected by pressure at the root of the neck	Pulsation diminished by pressure at the root of the neck
Independent of respiration	Height of pulsation varies with respiration
Independent of position	Varies with position of patient
Independent of abdominal pressure	Rises with abdominal pressure

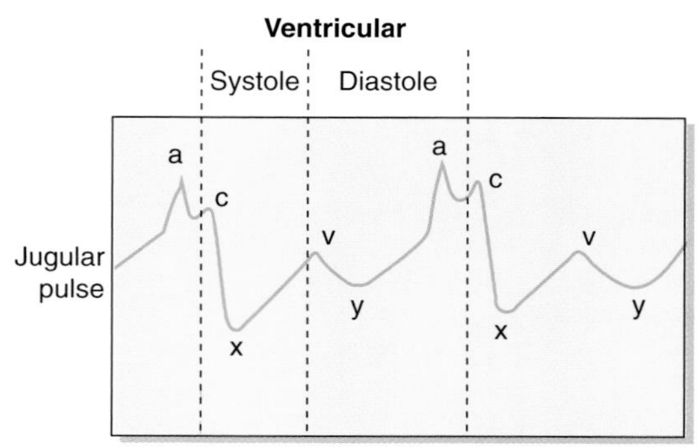

Fig. 3.20 Form of the venous pulse wave tracing from internal jugular vein. a = atrial systole; c = transmitted pulsation of carotid artery at onset of ventricular systole; v = peak pressure in right atrium immediately prior to opening of tricuspid valve; a – x = descent, due to atrial relaxation; v – y = descent at commencement of ventricular filling.

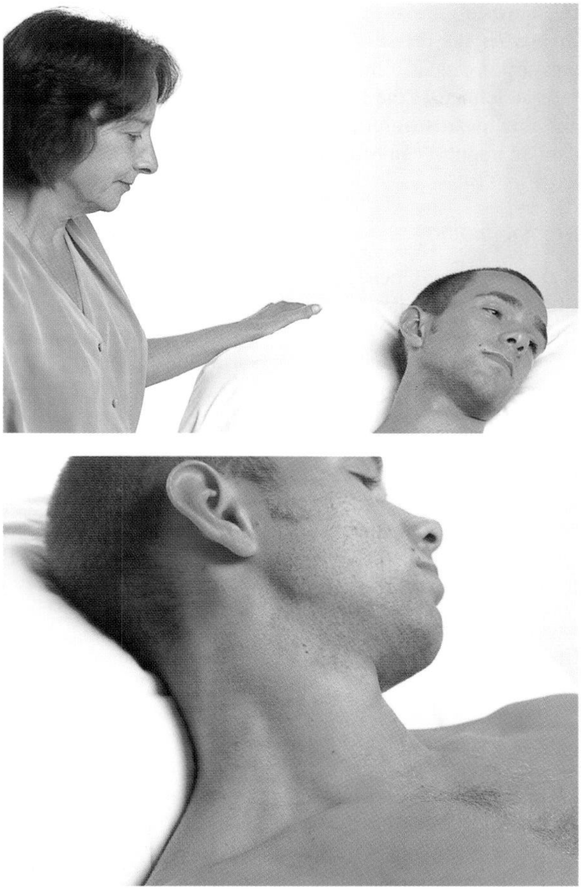

Fig. 3.21 **Inspecting the jugular venous pressure from the side.** (The internal jugular vein lies deep to the sternomastoid muscle.)

- ☐ Ensure that the neck muscles are relaxed by resting the back of the head on a pillow.
- ☐ Inspect by looking across the neck from the side of the patient (Fig. 3.21).
- ☐ Identify the internal jugular pulsation, if necessary, by means of abdominojugular reflux.
- ☐ Measure the vertical height in centimetres between the top of the venous pulsation and the sternal angle to give the venous pressure (Fig. 3.22).
- ☐ If necessary, readjust the position of the patient until the waveform is clearly visible.
- ☐ Now identify the pattern of the pulsation and note any abnormality.

Common abnormalities

Raised jugular venous pressure. Heart failure is the commonest cause of a raised jugular venous pressure (see Table 3.21). In milder degrees of heart failure abdominojugular reflux results in a rise in pressure which is sustained while abdominal pressure is applied. In major pulmonary embolism the JVP may be so elevated that it is missed in a semi-recumbent position. Marked elevation also occurs in SVC obstruction when the vessel is non-pulsatile. In pericardial constriction the JVP is elevated and there is a characteristic paradoxical rise on inspiration (Kussmaul's sign).

Serial estimations of the jugular venous pressure give valuable information regarding response to treatment; e.g. a reduction in the pressure as a result of effective diuretic therapy in the patient with heart failure.

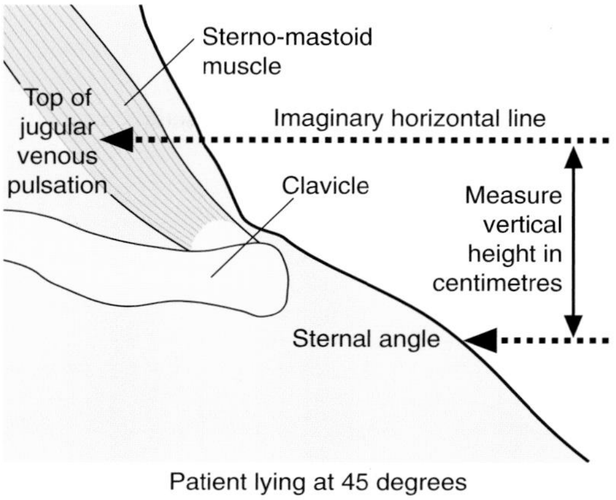

Fig. 3.22 **Measuring the height of the JVP.**

TABLE 3.21 Abnormalities of the jugular venous pulse

Condition	Abnormalities
Heart failure	Elevation, sustained abdominojugular reflux
Pulmonary embolism	Elevation
Pericardial effusion	Elevation, prominent 'y' descent
Pericardial constriction	Elevation, Kussmaul's sign
Superior vena caval obstruction	Elevation, loss of pulsation
Atrial fibrillation	Absent 'a' waves
Tricuspid stenosis	Giant 'a' waves
Tricuspid regurgitation	Giant 'v' waves
Complete heart block	'Cannon' waves

Waveform. Abnormalities of jugular venous pulsation are also given in Table 3.21. In atrial fibrillation there is no atrial systole. This results in the loss of the 'a' wave and the characteristic double impulse.

Prominent 'a' waves are seen in any condition that restricts blood flow from the right atrium to the right ventricle, e.g. pulmonary hypertension and, rarely, tricuspid stenosis.

Cannon waves are giant 'a' waves occurring when the right atrium contracts against a closed tricuspid valve. They are seen as impulses shooting up the neck. Cannon waves occur with complete heart block and in both ventricular and supraventricular tachycardias.

A prominent 'v' wave is characteristic of tricuspid regurgitation. When severe this may be associated with pulsation of the liver.

KEY POINTS

- General examination may reveal features of disorders which can cause, or aggravate, cardiac symptoms, e.g. anaemia, hyperthyroidism.
- Atrial fibrillation produces a pulse which is irregular in both time and volume.
- Pulse character should be assessed from a large artery, e.g. the carotid.
- Use the thumb to palpate brachial and carotid pulses; never palpate both carotids simultaneously.
- Accurate measurement of arterial blood pressure requires care and attention to detail.
- Pulsatile elevation of the JVP is a valuable sign of elevated right atrial pressure.
- A transient rise in the jugular venous pressure during abdominal compression is normal.

THE PRECORDIUM

Examination of the precordium is the central component of clinical cardiology.

Anatomy and function

A knowledge of the surface anatomy of the heart is important (Fig. 3.23). The auscultatory areas do not correspond with the surface markings of the heart valves. The cardiac impulse is the result of the heart rotating, moving forward and striking against the chest wall during systole. The apex beat is defined as the furthermost point outwards (laterally) and downwards (inferiorly) from the sternum at which the cardiac impulse can be palpated.

Normal findings

The normal apex beat lies in the 5th left intercostal space (the space below the 5th rib) within the midclavicular line which, in the male, is the intercostal space immediately below and approximately in line with the left nipple. The intercostal space can be located by counting down from the second rib which is at the level of the sternal angle. The normal apical impulse gently and briefly lifts the palpating fingers and is quite localised. However, in some normal subjects, particularly if overweight or muscular, the apex beat may be impalpable. The apex beat may also be impalpable in patients with asthma or emphysema because the chest is hyperinflated.

Examination sequence

- ☐ Inspect the precordium with the patient sitting at 45° to the upright with the shoulders horizontal, looking for any surgical scars, pulsations or other abnormalities.
- ☐ Lay the whole hand flat on the chest to get a general impression of cardiac activity (Fig. 3.24A).
- ☐ Localise the apex beat (Fig. 3.24B); if necessary ask the patient to roll on to the left side (Fig. 3.24C).
- ☐ Assess the character of the apex beat.
- ☐ Count the rib spaces from the sternal angle.
- ☐ Palpate for the right ventricle using the heel of the hand

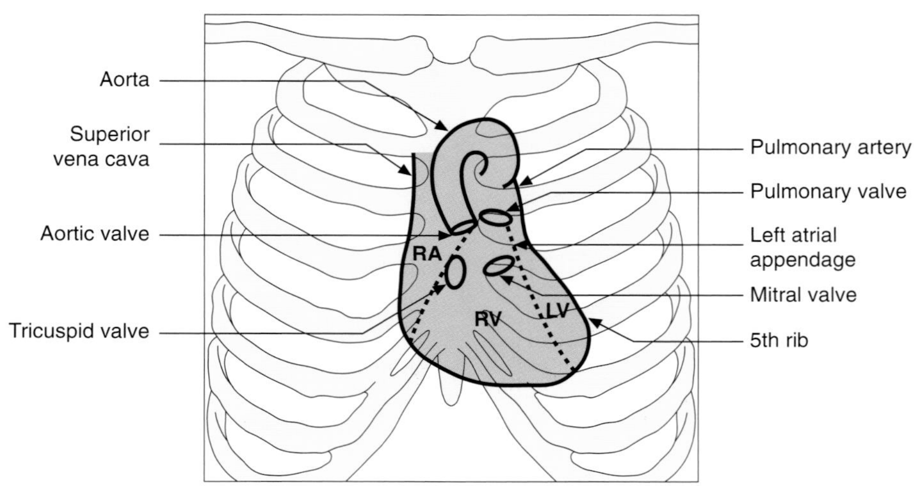

Fig. 3.23 Surface markings of the valves in relationship to the radiological outline of the heart. The directions in which murmurs are preferentially conducted from the valves depend upon the direction of the blood flow producing the murmur.

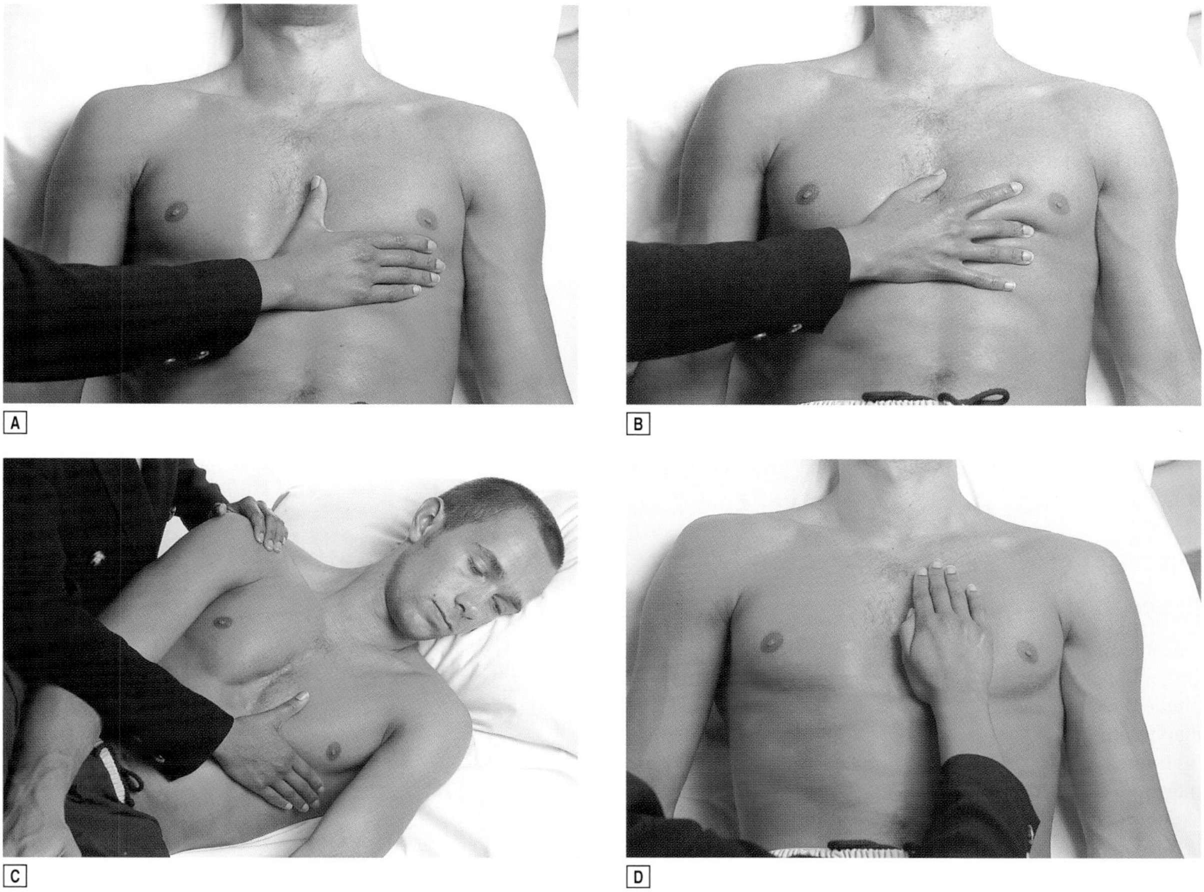

Fig. 3.24 Palpating the heart. [A] Use the hand to palpate the cardiac impulse. [B] Localise the apex beat with a finger. [C] If necessary, roll the patient into the left lateral position. [D] Palpate from apex to sternum for parasternal pulsations.

firmly applied to the left parasternal position while the breath is held in expiration (Fig. 3.24D).

- ☐ Palpate for thrills at the apex and to both sides of the sternum.
- ☐ Where a murmur is audible, palpate again for a thrill using the flat of the fingers while the patient is in the optimum position (see below).

Common abnormalities

Inspection. Much can be learned by inspecting the precordium. Chest deformities including pectus excavatum (posterior displacement of the lower sternum) can affect the rest of the examination. A midline sternotomy scar usually indicates previous coronary bypass surgery, or valve replacement. A left submammary scar is usually the result of a mitral valvotomy.

Pulsations are most readily identified by a combination of inspection (best for inward movements) and palpation (best for outward movements).

Displacement of the apex beat. The apex may be displaced laterally in subjects with chest deformity such as pectus excavatum (p. 131). It may also be displaced because of mediastinal shift secondary to a large pleural effusion, tension pneumothorax or pneumonectomy. In these situations the trachea may also be deviated.

In cardiac disease causing left ventricular dilatation, the apex beat is displaced inferiorly and laterally and it is diffuse, felt over a wide area.

Character of the apical impulse. The character of the cardiac impulse is often more important than its precise position. The so-called 'tapping apex' which is found in mitral stenosis is actually a palpable first heart sound. In pure mitral stenosis the apex is not displaced. Conditions which cause left ventricular pressure overload and consequent hypertrophy, such as hypertension and aortic stenosis, lead to a forceful and sustained apex beat which is usually not displaced. This apical 'heave' or 'lift' is distinguishable from the diffuse impulse of left ventricular dilatation.

A double apical impulse is characteristic of hypertrophic cardiomyopathy.

Heaves are palpable impulses from either the right or left ventricle which feel as though they are 'lifting' the examiner's hand from the chest. A pulsation over the left parasternal area (right ventricular heave) is usually abnormal in adults and indicative of right ventricular hypertrophy, e.g. pulmonary hypertension.

Thrills are palpable murmurs. They feel rather like placing one's hand on a purring cat. The most commonly detected systolic thrill is that of aortic stenosis which may be palpable at the apex, the left or right sternal edge or over the carotid arteries in the neck. The thrill arising from a ventricular septal defect is usually best felt at the left sternal edge. Diastolic thrills are rare; the thrill of mitral stenosis is best felt at the apex with the patient rolled on to the left side; thrills arising from the base of the heart are best felt with the patient leaning forward.

AUSCULTATION OF THE HEART

General considerations

Auscultation of the heart requires a stethoscope with a bell and a diaphragm. The bell is best for listening to low-pitched sounds such as the murmur of mitral stenosis. The diaphragm filters out such sounds and helps to identify high-pitched sounds such as normal heart sounds and the murmur of aortic regurgitation. The earpieces of the stethoscope should fit comfortably and the tubing should be about 25 cm in length and thick enough to reduce external sound.

Knowledge of the surface anatomy of the heart is helpful in understanding the sites which various murmurs radiate to (Fig. 3.23). A basic knowledge of cardiac physiology is also important (Fig. 3.25). This is further discussed on page 104. Normal heart valves make a sound when they close but not when they open. These sounds are readily heard with a stethoscope.

It is advisable to have a fixed routine for auscultation, especially for the inexperienced. Most clinicians first auscultate at the apex. However, it is easier to start at the base, where the heart sounds are more distinct from each other (the second heart sound is louder and higher pitched). Simultaneous palpation of the carotid pulse may also be helpful; the first heart sound precedes the pulse, the second sound follows it.

Auscultation involves identifying and describing the following:

- the first and second heart sound
- extra heart sounds (third and fourth)
- additional sounds, e.g. clicks and snaps
- pericardial rubs
- murmurs.

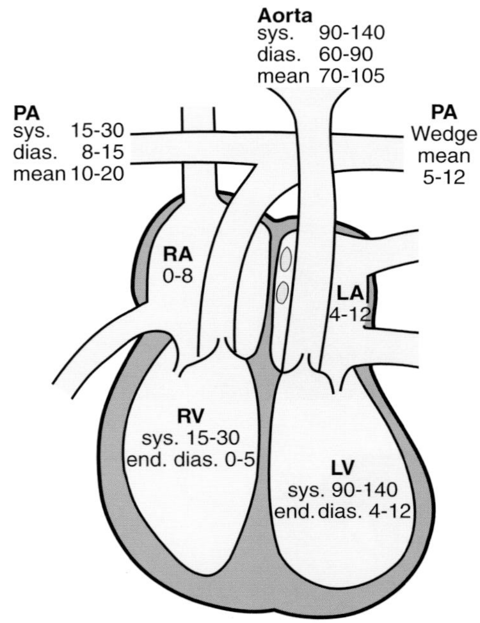

Fig. 3.25 Normal resting pressures in mm mercury in the chambers of the heart.

Heart sounds and added sounds

Normal findings

The first heart sound. The first heart sound is caused by the closure of the mitral and tricuspid valves at the beginning of ventricular systole. It is best heard at the apex.

The second heart sound. This is caused by the closure of the pulmonary and aortic valves at the end of ventricular systole and is best heard at the left sternal edge. It is louder and higher pitched than the first sound and normally the aortic component is louder than the pulmonary one. *Physiological splitting* of the second heart sound occurs because left ventricular contraction slightly precedes right ventricular systole. As a consequence, the pulmonary valve shuts after the aortic valve. This increases at the end of a quiet inspiration because the increased venous filling of the right ventricle further delays pulmonary valve closure. Conversely, the separation disappears on expiration (Fig. 3.26). The resultant splitting of the second sound is best heard at the left sternal edge using the diaphragm of the stethoscope. On auscultation, the clinician hears 'lub d/dub' (inspiration) 'lub-dub' (expiration).

Third heart sound. The third heart sound is a low-pitched sound best heard with the bell of the stethoscope at the apex. It coincides with the phase of rapid ventricular filling

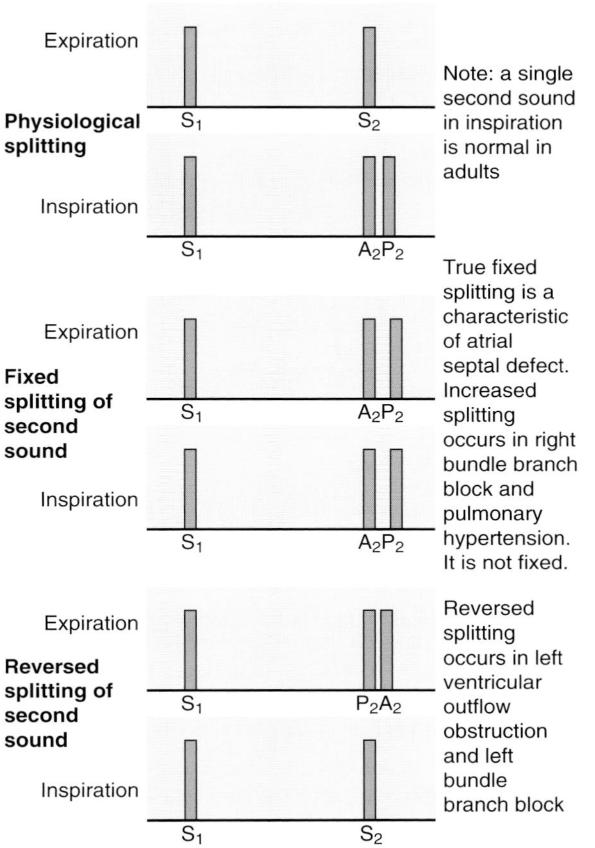

Fig. 3.26 Normal and pathological splitting of the second heart sound.

immediately after opening of the AV valves and therefore occurs at the beginning of mid-diastole. A third heart sound is therefore heard after the second as 'lub-dub-dum'. A third heart sound is a normal finding in children, young adults and during pregnancy.

Examination sequence

- ☐ With the patient sitting semirecumbent auscultate all over the precordium, listening in turn at the base of the heart, apex, right and upper left sternal edges with both bell and diaphragm. Also auscultate over the carotids and, where appropriate, into the axilla.
- ☐ At each site identify the first and second heart sounds and assess the character with regard to intensity and splitting.
- ☐ Then listen specifically during systole and diastole, first for added sounds and then for murmurs.
- ☐ Roll the patient on to the left side and listen at the apex using the bell pressed lightly on to the skin to detect the murmur of mitral stenosis (Fig. 3.27A).
- ☐ Sit the patient up, leaning forward, and listen over the right second interspace and then down at the left sternal edge with the diaphragm for the murmur of aortic incompetence (Fig. 3.27B).
- ☐ Note the features of any murmur heard.

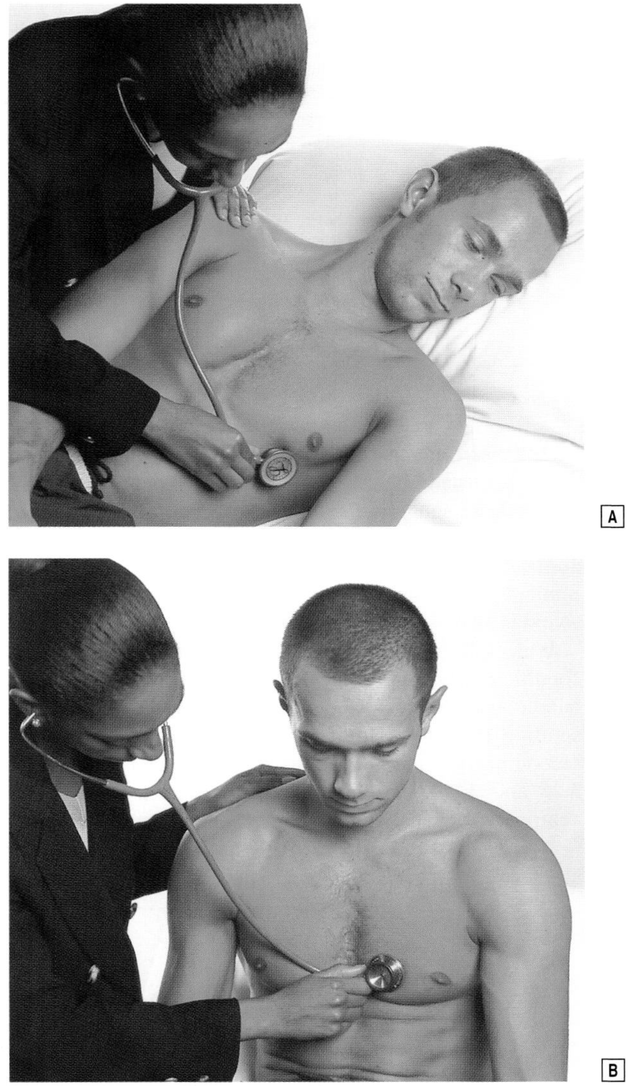

Fig. 3.27 Auscultating the heart. A Listen with the lightly applied bell with the patient in the left lateral position for the murmur of mitral stenosis. B Listen with the diaphragm with the patient leaning forward for the murmur of aortic incompetence.

Common abnormalities

First heart sound. Abnormalities of the intensity of the first heart sound are listed in Table 3.22. In mitral stenosis the intensity of the first heart sound is often increased.

TABLE 3.22 Abnormalities of intensity of the first heart sound

Quiet	Low cardiac output Poor left ventricular function Long P–R interval (first degree heart block) Rheumatic mitral regurgitation
Loud	Increased cardiac output Large stroke volume Mitral stenosis Short P–R interval Atrial myxoma (rare)
Variable	Atrial fibrillation Extrasystoles Complete heart block

TABLE 3.23 Abnormalities of the second heart sound

Quiet	Low cardiac output Calcific aortic stenosis Aortic incompetence
Loud	Systemic hypertension (aortic component) Pulmonary hypertension (pulmonary component)
Split	Widens in inspiration (enhanced physiological splitting) Right bundle branch block Pulmonary stenosis Pulmonary hypertension Ventricular septal defects Fixed splitting (unaffected by respiration) Atrial septal defect Widens in expiration (reverse splitting) Aortic stenosis Hypertrophic cardiomyopathy Left bundle branch block Ventricular pacemaker

Second heart sound. Abnormalities of the second heart sound are listed in Table 3.23. The aortic component of the second heart sound is sometimes reduced in intensity, even absent, in calcific aortic stenosis. It may also be reduced in aortic incompetence. It is loud in systemic hypertension. Similarly the pulmonary component of the second heart sound is increased in pulmonary hypertension.

Wide splitting of the second heart sound occurs in any condition delaying right ventricular emptying, e.g. right bundle branch block and pulmonary hypertension. Such splitting gets wider in inspiration. Fixed splitting of the second heart sound is a feature of atrial septal defect (Figs 3.26 and 3.28). The splitting is wide because the right ventricle is dealing with a larger blood volume than the left and it is fixed because the defect equalises pressure between the atria throughout the respiratory cycle.

Reversed splitting occurs when left ventricle emptying is so delayed that the aortic valve closes after the pulmonary valve. Examples are left bundle branch block and right ventricular pacing. In reverse splitting the two components of the second heart sound come together on inspiration and separate on expiration (Fig. 3.26).

Third heart sound. A third heart sound is usually pathological after the age of 40 (Table 3.24). The commonest causes are a large, poorly contracting ventricle and mitral regurgitation.

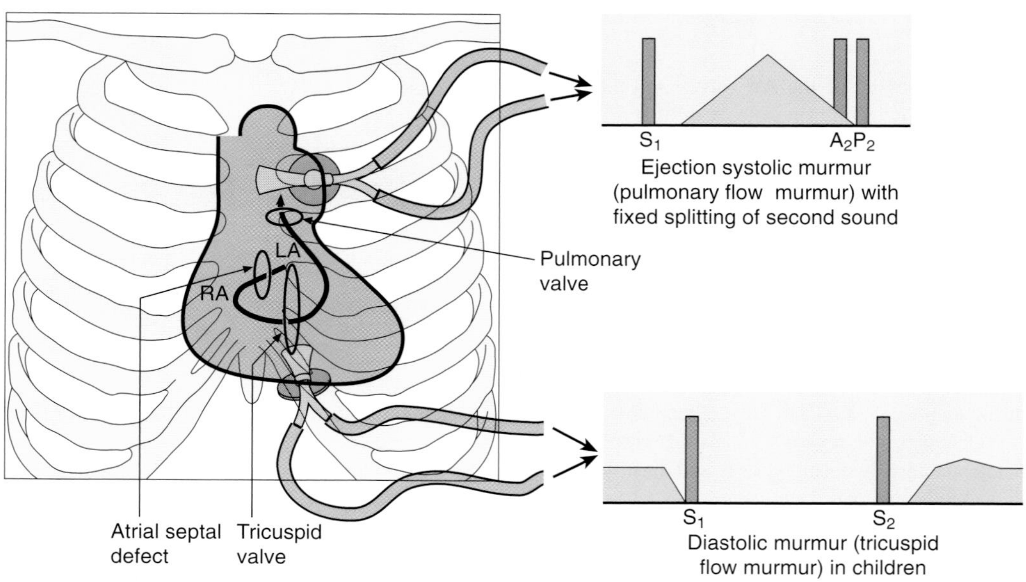

Fig. 3.28 Auscultatory features of atrial septal defect.

TABLE 3.24 Causes of a third heart sound

Physiological	Healthy young adults Athletes Pregnancy Fever
Pathological	Large, poorly contracting left ventricle Mitral reflux

It is often associated with heart failure, when the third heart sound is usually accompanied by a tachycardia and a quiet first and second sound. The resulting 'triple rhythm' is sometimes called a gallop rhythm because it is said to resemble the sound of a galloping horse.

Fourth heart sound. The fourth heart sound is soft and low pitched, best heard with the bell of the stethoscope at the apex. It occurs just before the first sound (da-lub-dub). It is pathological and caused by forceful atrial contraction and therefore occurs during presystole and cannot occur if there is atrial fibrillation. A fourth heart sound may be heard in conditions associated with left ventricular hypertrophy such as hypertension and aortic stenosis.

Added sounds. Added sounds need to be distinguished from other heart sounds described above.

An *opening snap* is commonly heard in mitral (rarely tricuspid) valve stenosis. It results from the restricted opening of a stenosed valve. It is only audible when the valve is mobile. Opening snaps occur in early diastole, just after the second heart sound (Fig. 3.29A). The opening snap of mitral stenosis is best heard at the apex.

Ejection clicks may be heard in early systole just after the first heart sound, in patients with congenital pulmonary or aortic stenosis (Fig. 3.29B). The mechanism is similar to an opening snap. Ejection clicks are not associated with calcific aortic stenosis because the cusps are rigid.

Midsystolic clicks occur in mitral valve prolapse (Fig. 3.29C) and may be associated with a late systolic murmur (Fig. 3.30). They are high pitched and usually best heard at the apex. Their timing is determined by the cessation of posterior motion of the prolapsing leaflet.

Mechanical heart valves make a sound both when they close and on opening, the latter normally being the quieter sound. The sounds are high pitched and 'metallic', loud, commonly palpable and often audible without a stethoscope. A mechanical mitral valve replacement makes a metallic first heart sound and a sound like a loud opening snap (Fig. 3.29D). Mechanical aortic valves have loud, metallic second heart sounds, and an opening sound like an ejection click (Fig. 3.29E). They are associated with a flow murmur.

Pericardial rubs. A pericardial rub is the characteristic physical sign of acute pericarditis (Table 3.25). It is generally best heard at the left of the lower sternum with the patient breathing out, using the diaphragm of the stethoscope. It is a superficial scratching sound which often has systolic and

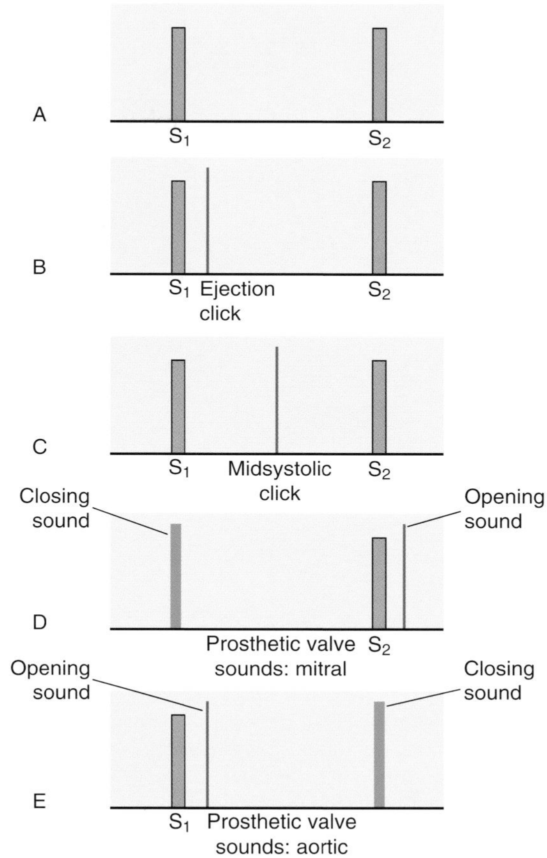

Fig. 3.29 'Added sounds' on auscultation.

TABLE 3.25 Features of pericardial disease

Acute pericarditis	Pericardial pain Pericardial friction rub
Pericardial effusion	Retrosternal 'oppressive' feeling Raised JVP Rub variable or absent
Pericardial tamponade (pericardial effusion under pressure)	Raised JVP Hypotension Paradoxical pulse (pulse volume smaller on inspiration) Postural hypotension Oliguria
Chronic constrictive pericarditis	Exertional dyspnoea Peripheral oedema Raised JVP with exaggerated x descent JVP rises on inspiration (Kussmaul's sign)

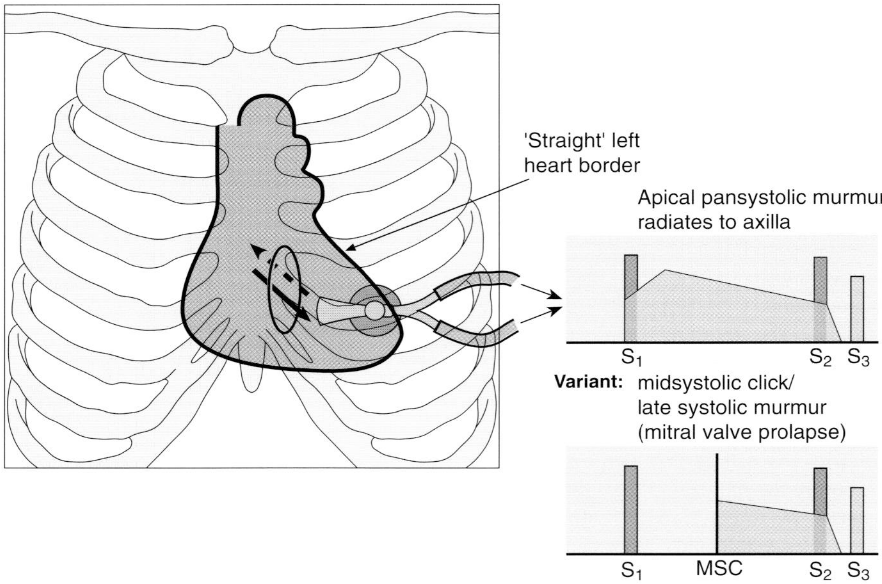

Fig. 3.30 Features of mitral regurgitation.

diastolic components. Like the pain of pericarditis, it may vary from hour to hour in intensity and its intensity may alter with the position of the patient.

A pericardial rub requires to be distinguished from a pleuropericardial rub. In both, the sounds coincide with the cardiac cycle but the pleuropericardial rub is also influenced by respiration and is pleural in origin.

Murmurs

General considerations

Heart murmurs are produced by turbulent blood flow in the heart. They are either caused by abnormal valve function or arise from an increased volume, or velocity, of blood flowing through a normal valve. This may occur in a healthy heart. Such innocent murmurs are more likely to occur when the stroke volume is increased, e.g. during pregnancy and in athletes.

The following characteristics of heart murmurs need to be considered

Timing

Most heart murmurs are either systolic or diastolic. Systolic and diastolic murmurs can, of course, coexist and need to be differentiated from the much less common continuous murmurs.

Systole starts with the first heart sound which is the closure of the mitral and tricuspid valves. This occurs as soon as the initiation of ventricular contraction raises the ventricular pressure above the corresponding atrial pressure. Ventricular pressures continue to rise until they exceed the pressure in the aorta and main pulmonary artery. This results in the aortic and pulmonary valves opening. Systole ends with the closure of these valves producing the second heart sound. At this time there is still a pressure gradient between the ventricle and the atrium. It follows that a mitral or tricuspid valve regurgitant murmur may start with the first heart sound and, being independent of the second heart sound, may continue up to or even beyond this sound. With an ejection systolic murmur, however, there is a short time interval between the first heart sound and the onset of the murmur which invariably stops before the second heart sound.

Diastole is the interval between the second and the first heart sound. Physiologically it can be divided into three phases:

- *Early diastole (isovolumic relaxation)* – the time from the closure of the aortic and pulmonary valves until the opening of the mitral and tricuspid valves
- *Mid-diastole* – the period of passive ventricular filling
- *Presystole* which coincides with atrial systole.

It follows that murmurs of aortic (and pulmonary) incompetence start in early diastole often extending well into mid-diastole. In contrast the murmurs of mitral or tricuspid stenosis cannot start before mid-diastole. Likewise third

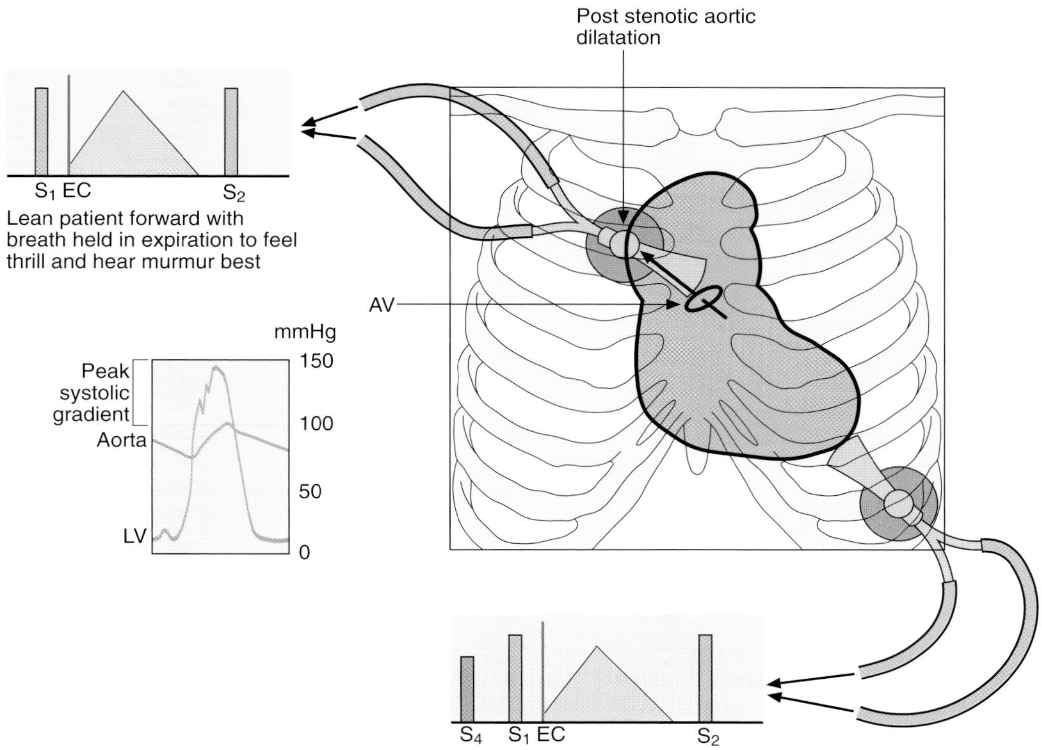

Fig. 3.31 Aortic stenosis. There is a systolic pressure gradient across the stenotic aortic valve (AV). The resultant high-velocity jet (arrow) impinges on the wall of the aorta, and the diaphragm placed near to this on the chest detects the murmur best. Alternatively the bell may be placed in the suprasternal notch. The diagrammatic representation of the phonocardiogram shows the ejection systolic murmur preceded by an ejection sound (EC). A fourth heart sound may be heard at the apex.

heart sounds occur in mid-diastole; fourth heart sounds occur in presystole.

The timing of murmurs is determined with reference to the heart sounds or the carotid pulse. Systolic murmurs coincide with the pulse; diastolic murmurs do not.

Duration

Regurgitant systolic murmurs have the potential to be pansystolic but some may become inaudible in mid- or late systole. Moreover, if the murmur is produced by mitral valve prolapse it will not commence until the valve prolapses during systole (Fig. 3.30). Ejection systolic murmurs begin *after* the first heart sound, reach maximal intensity in mid-systole, then fade, stopping before the second heart sound (Fig. 3.31).

Character and pitch

Quality of murmurs is hard to define. They are often described as harsh, blowing, musical, rumbling, high or low pitched. As a principle, the higher the pitch, the greater the pressure gradient. Thus the murmur of aortic incompetence is high pitched and best heard with the diaphragm, whereas that of mitral stenosis is low pitched and best identified using the bell.

Intensity

There are six grades of intensity (Table 3.26) used to describe murmurs. Diastolic murmurs are rarely louder than grade 4. The severity of valve dysfunction cannot be determined from the intensity of the resultant murmur. However, changes in intensity are often of prognostic significance. For example an increase in the intensity of an aortic early diastolic murmur implies increasing valvular incompetence. A reduction in intensity may also indicate deterioration, the fall in intensity being associated with reversal of flow in a right-to-left shunt or a fall in cardiac output, as in critical aortic stenosis which may be associated with a very quiet murmur.

TABLE 3.26 Grades of intensity of murmur

1. Heard by an expert in optimum conditions
2. Heard by a non-expert in optimum conditions
3. Easily heard; no thrill
4. A loud murmur, with a thrill
5. Very loud, often heard over wide area, with thrill
6. Extremely loud, heard without stethoscope

Optimum conditions require the room to be quiet, the patient to be properly positioned and the clinician to listen with the correct piece of the stethoscope over the correct site

Location

The site on the precordium where a murmur is last heard should be determined. This is most useful in differentiating diastolic murmurs (mitral stenosis at the apex, aortic regurgitation at the left sternal edge). Site can be misleading with systolic murmurs since the murmur of aortic stenosis is often readily heard at the apex.

Radiation

This should not be confused with location. Murmurs radiate in the direction of blood flow responsible for the murmur, to specific sites outwith the precordium, including the upper right sternal edge, the axilla, the back of the chest and over the carotids in the neck. Radiation is useful in differentiating systolic murmurs.

Common abnormalities

Systolic murmurs. The causes of systolic murmurs are listed in Table 3.27.

Ejection systolic murmurs can be caused by an increased stroke volume (flow murmur), or a stenosed aortic or pulmonary valve. Causes of flow murmurs include pregnancy, fever, bradycardia and atrial septal defect.

The murmur of aortic stenosis is usually audible all over the precordium, including the apex (Fig. 3.31). It may be harsh, or high pitched and musical, and radiates to the upper right sternal edge and carotids. The murmur is often loud and may be associated with a thrill. However, in critical aortic stenosis the degree of obstruction and the resultant deterioration in left ventricular function may reduce the cardiac output to such an extent that the intensity of the murmur is diminished.

Pansystolic murmurs are most frequently caused by mitral or tricuspid regurgitation. The murmur of mitral regurgitation radiates to the axilla. It is often loud and blowing in character, best heard at the apex (Fig. 3.30). In some patients the mitral valve prolapses during ventricular systole producing a mid- or late systolic murmur (Fig. 3.30).

Tricuspid incompetence is heard at the left sternal edge and associated with confirmatory signs including a large 'v' wave in the jugular venous pulse and a pulsatile liver.

TABLE 3.27 Causes of systolic murmurs

Ejection systolic murmur

Increased flow through normal valves:
- 'Innocent systolic murmur'
  - Fever
  - Athletes (bradycardia → large stroke volume)
  - Pregnancy (cardiac output maximum at 15 weeks)
- Atrial septal defect (pulmonary flow murmur)

Normal or reduced flow through stenotic valve
- Aortic stenosis
- Pulmonary stenosis

Other causes of flow murmurs
- Hypertrophic obstructive cardiomyopathy (obstruction at subvalvular level)
- Acute regurgitation (aortic flow murmur)

Pansystolic murmurs

All caused by a systolic leak from a high to a lower pressure chamber
- Mitral regurgitation
- Tricuspid regurgitation
- Ventricular septal defect
- Leaking mitral or tricuspid prosthesis
- Mitral valve prolapse

Another cause of a pansystolic murmur is a ventricular septal defect. Even small congenital defects can cause a loud murmur at the left sternal edge, often associated with a thrill. A pansystolic murmur developing in a patient recovering from acute myocardial infarction is most commonly caused by rupture of the ventricular septum. Other possibilities include mitral incompetence caused by rupture of the chordae tendineae, or functional incompetence produced by acute left ventricular dilatation.

Diastolic murmurs. *Early diastolic murmurs* are typified by aortic regurgitation (Fig. 3.32). They are usually best heard at the left sternal edge, but are occasionally louder at the lower right sternal edge. Quiet early diastolic murmurs may be audible only in expiration with the patient leaning forward. Since the regurgitant blood volume must be ejected during the subsequent systole, aortic regurgitation leads to an increased stroke volume and may be associated with an ejection systolic flow murmur.

Pulmonary regurgitation is uncommon. It may be secondary to pulmonary artery dilatation in pulmonary hypertension (Graham Steell murmur).

The *mid-diastolic murmur* of mitral stenosis is a low-pitched rumbling sound which begins after the opening snap, if this is present (Fig. 3.33). It is best heard with the bell of the stethoscope at the apex. The whole cadence sounds like 'lup-ta-ta-roo' where lup is the loud first heart sound, ta-ta the second sound and opening snap and roo the mid-diastolic murmur. If the patient is in sinus rhythm, atrial contraction increases the blood flow across the stenosed valve leading to presystolic accentuation of the murmur.

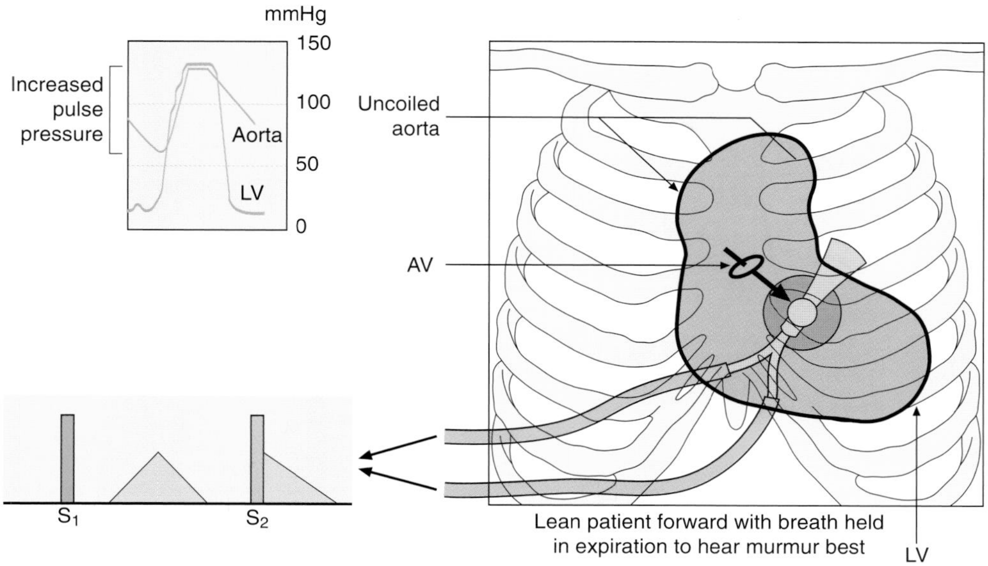

Fig. 3.32 Features of aortic regurgitation. The pulse pressure is usually increased; the jet from the aortic valve (AV) impinges on the interventricular septum (arrow) during diastole, producing a high-pitched murmur which is best heard with the diaphragm. The diagrammatic representation of the phonocardiogram also shows the systolic murmur which is common because of the increased flow through the aortic valve in systole.

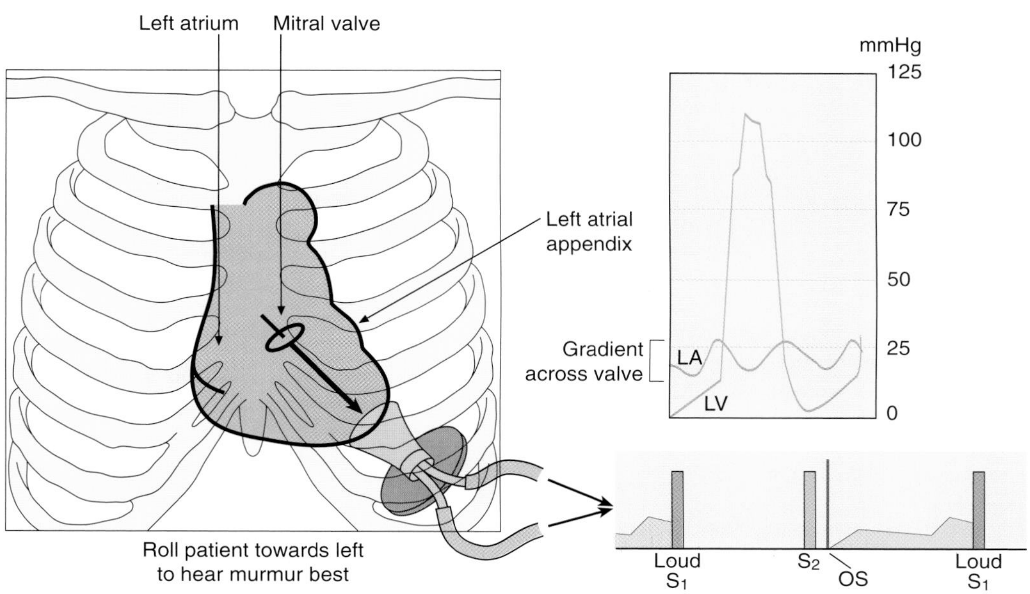

Fig. 3.33 Features of mitral stenosis. There is a pressure gradient across the mitral valve; in this example it continues throughout diastole. This causes a sharp movement of the tethered anterior cusp of the mitral valve at the time when the flow commences, and the opening snap (OS) results. The jet through the stenotic valve (arrow) strikes the endocardium at the cardiac apex. The murmur which results is best heard with the bell lightly applied over the apex.

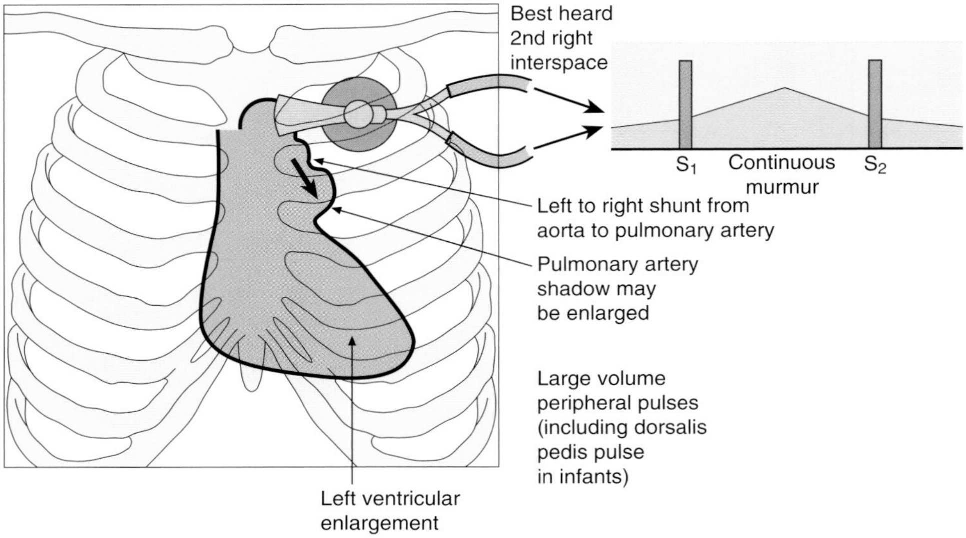

Fig. 3.34 Features of a persistent patent arterial duct.

The murmur of tricuspid stenosis is similar to mitral stenosis, but it is rare. An *Austin Flint* murmur is a mid-diastolic murmur caused by a jet of blood in aortic regurgitation impinging directly on the anterior leaflet of the mitral valve thereby causing it to close and restricting the inflow to the left ventricle.

Continuous murmurs are rare in adults. The commonest cause is a patent arterial duct which connects the upper descending aorta and pulmonary artery, and normally closes just after birth. The murmur is best heard at the upper left sternal edge, radiating to the left scapula. Its continuous character has been described as machinery-like (Fig. 3.34).

Interpretation of findings

In many situations abnormal findings detected on auscultation will be subsequently confirmed by investigations, often echocardiography. However, auscultation is an important clinical skill. The correct interpretation of the signs involves applying as much significance to changes in heart sounds and added sounds as to the murmurs. This is illustrated in Figures 3.30–3.34.

However, these figures indicate the features that may be present in a single valve lesion. Clinically many patients, especially those with rheumatic heart disease, have multiple heart lesions. Here the interpretation is more critical. For example, a patient with mixed mitral stenosis and incompetence will probably have dominant stenosis if the first heart sound is loud; dominant incompetence if there is a third heart sound. This illustrates the need to consider all the auscultatory findings.

KEY POINTS

- Displacement of the apex beat can be due either to cardiac enlargement or mediastinal shift.
- The bell of the stethoscope is used to detect low-pitched sounds, e.g. mitral stenosis. The diaphragm is preferred for high-pitched sounds, e.g. normal heart sounds and the murmur of aortic incompetence.
- A third heart sound may be physiological; a fourth heart sound is always pathological.
- The intensity of the heart murmur is *not* a reliable guide to the severity of the problem. However, changes in intensity may be of considerable prognostic significance.
- Aortic diastolic murmurs are best heard with the patient holding the breath in expiration and leaning forward; mitral diastolic murmurs are best heard with the patient lying on the left side.

ASSESSMENT OF CHRONIC HEART FAILURE

The clinical assessment of a patient with chronic heart failure can be considered to comprise five stages:

1. *The severity of the disability.* Chronic heart failure can cover a wide range of disability, from virtually no limitation to severe symptoms, even at rest. There is a poor correlation between a patient's symptoms and the severity

of the underlying cardiac abnormality. Enquiry is made into the effect of the condition on the patient's employment, activities of daily living, pastimes, sexual function and sleep pattern. Signs of decompensation are sought, especially fluid retention (pulmonary congestion, peripheral or sacral oedema).

2. *The underlying cause*. Heart failure may be the result of any condition which impairs the normal function of the heart, including:
   - myocardial disease secondary to ischaemic heart disease, hypertension or a primary cardiomyopathy
   - heart valve disease, particularly mitral valve disease and aortic stenosis
   - arrhythmias
   - pericardial constriction.

   Features to look for include a history of myocardial infarction, angina or excess alcohol intake, which are associated with myocardial disease, and heart murmurs, which may indicate a valve abnormality. Both tachycardias (especially atrial fibrillation) and bradycardias (e.g. complete heart block) may present with symptoms of chronic heart failure. Certain diseases share some of the clinical features of chronic heart failure, and can lead to confusion. These include anaemia, fluid retention secondary to renal or hepatic failure, and cor pulmonale (pulmonary hypertension secondary to lung disease with secondary dilatation and failure of the right ventricle).

   Initial investigations include a chest X-ray to determine the heart size and look for pulmonary congestion, and an ECG to confirm the cardiac rhythm and look for evidence of previous myocardial infarction. The definitive investigation is often an echocardiogram but will depend upon the nature of the problem (see Table 3.29).
3. *Any aggravating factors*. In addition to the primary cause, other factors may be aggravating the patient's symptoms. Enquiry should be made into:
   - drug therapy (e.g. non-steroidal anti-inflammatory drugs)
   - alcohol consumption
   - symptoms of hypo- or hyperthyroidism
   - dark stools suggesting gastrointestinal blood loss.

   Routine blood tests should include a full blood count to exclude anaemia, urea and electrolytes to check renal function, liver and thyroid function tests.
4. *Changes in lifestyle*. Patients with heart failure may become deconditioned through lack of exercise. This can be reversed, at least partially, by regular exercise. Excess liquid intake should be avoided, and salt intake restricted. Alcohol should be taken only in moderation or avoided completely if the patient has an alcoholic cardiomyopathy.
5. *Drug therapy*. Treatment requires to be tailored to the particular patient, depending on the severity of symptoms, the underlying cause, and the presence of any treatable aggravating factors.

ASSESSMENT OF THE ACUTELY ILL PATIENT

Patients with heart disease may present acutely and need urgent treatment. They may be too unwell to give a coherent history in which case any observations from a friend or relative may be valuable. It is important to make an expeditious assessment. The aim is to treat the acute problem and to prevent, life-threatening events such as cardiogenic shock or ventricular fibrillation. The usual sequence of history, physical examination, investigation and then management will require to be adapted to accommodate the urgency of the problem. The priority given to the examination sequence will depend upon the clinical situation. One sequence is as follows.

Examination sequence

- ☐ Ask about pain. When pain is severe relieve it with an opiate drug given intravenously with an antiemetic.
- ☐ Feel the pulse rate, rhythm and character.
- ☐ When the pulse is irregular, or inappropriately fast or slow, or if the clinical picture raises the possibility of a myocardial infarct, obtain an immediate ECG to determine the cardiac rhythm and thereafter monitor the patient.
- ☐ Take the arterial blood pressure and look for other evidence of shock (Table 3.28). Where there is circulatory failure, assess the severity and initiate treatment.
- ☐ Examine the JVP and waveform.
- ☐ Ask about breathlessness; assess the degree of dyspnoea, look for central cyanosis and where indicated give oxygen therapy.
- ☐ Determine the duration of any chest pain. If relatively short (less than 6 hours) and consistent with acute myocardial infarction, obtain a full ECG and without delay administer a thrombolytic drug if appropriate.
- ☐ Consider other causes of acute chest pain including pneumothorax, pulmonary embolism and dissection of the aorta. If dissection is suspected, compare the peripheral pulses and take the blood pressure in both arms.
- ☐ Listen for heart murmurs.
- ☐ Examine the lungs for signs of pulmonary oedema.
- ☐ Obtain a chest X-ray and look for evidence of pulmonary oedema, widening of the mediastinum, etc.

TABLE 3.28 Characteristics of patients with severe circulatory failure (shock)

Hypotension	Systolic blood pressure < 100 mmHg
Tachycardia	Pulse usually > 100/min
Peripheral vasoconstriction	Cold, pale or cyanosed peripheries
Reduced urine output	< 30 ml/h

CASE HISTORY

A 25-year-old man was brought unaccompanied to casualty by emergency ambulance. He was too ill to give a history. On examination he was pale, malnourished and dirty. He was tachypnoeic (36/min) with a tachycardia (160/min) and hypotensive (84/62 mmHg). The JVP was elevated at 10 cm, with a very prominent 'v' wave. The liver was enlarged, tender and pulsatile. He had a left parasternal heave and a loud pansystolic murmur at the lower left sternal edge, increased during respiration and radiating into the epigastrium. There were multiple injection sites in the arms, particularly in the anterior cubital fossae. Some of the sites were infected.

Swabs were obtained from the injection sites and six sets of blood cultures were taken. Further blood was obtained to assess his haematological status and renal and liver function, including coagulation studies. Blood for hepatitis B virus and HIV serological testing was obtained.

Immediately after taking the blood cultures, treatment was commenced with high-dose antistaphylococcal intravenous antibiotics. He was also given high-flow oxygen, intravenous fluid replacement, paracetamol for his pyrexia and a urinary catheter was inserted to monitor urine output.

A subsequently performed echocardiogram (Fig. 3.35) showed multiple vegetations on the tricuspid valve confirming the clinical diagnosis of tricuspid incompetence secondary to infective endocarditis. Four of the blood cultures were positive to *Staphylococcus aureus*.

Learning points

- The clinical suspicion of septicaemia in a patient with a heart murmur should suggest infective endocarditis.
- In the acutely ill it is necessary to institute urgent treatment before performing a full clinical examination and pending the results of bacteriological investigations.
- The presence of overwhelming infection should suggest the possibility that the patient is immunocompromised.
- Staphylococcal endocarditis is a fulminating condition; many of the physical signs associated with other forms of infective endocarditis take time to develop (see Fig. 3.10).

KEY POINTS

- The condition of the patient determines the approach to the clinical examination.
- Pain relief and monitoring cardiac rhythm are priorities in managing acutely ill patients.
- The assessment of patients in cardiac failure includes determining the underlying cause and the aggravating factors.

COMMON CARDIAC INVESTIGATIONS

The indications for common cardiac investigations are shown in Table 3.29 along with possible findings and their diagnostic interpretation. The investigations most commonly requested are electrocardiography, echocardiography, radionuclide studies and cardiac catheterisation.

Electrocardiography (ECG)

This is a routine investigation. It is inexpensive and non-invasive. The standard 12-lead ECG (Fig. 3.36) comprises

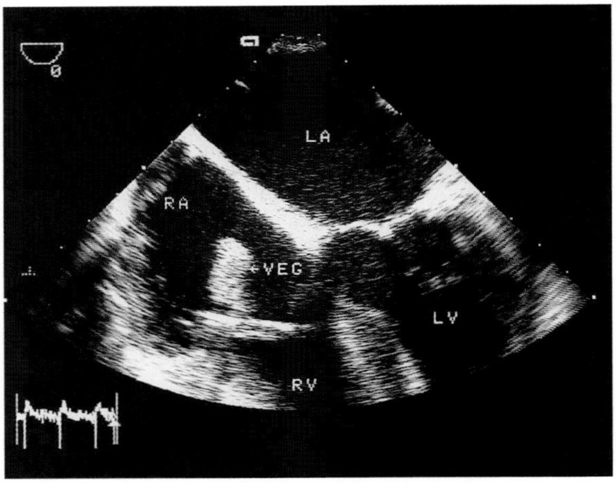

Fig. 3.35 Transoesophageal echocardiography in a 4 chamber view. There is a large vegetation attached to the atrial aspect of the tricuspid valve. LA = left atrium, RA = right atrium, LV = left ventricle, RV = right ventricle, VEG = vegetation.

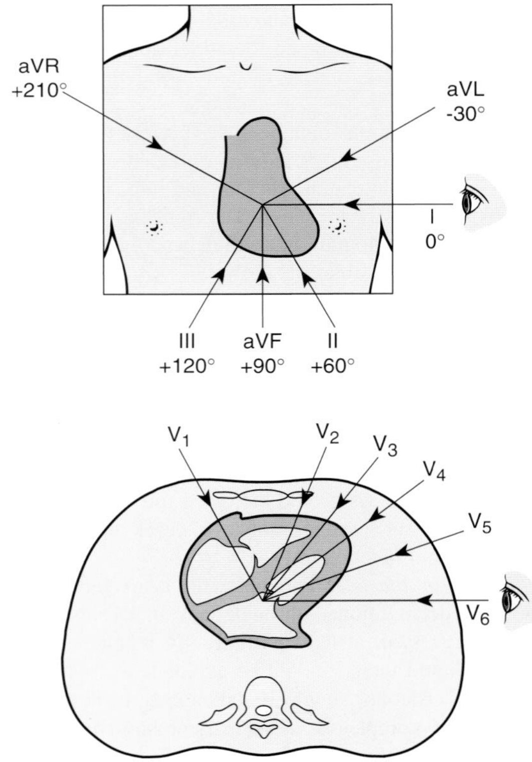

Fig. 3.36 Electrocardiography. Diagram to show the directions from which the 12 standard leads 'look at' the heart. The transverse section is viewed from below like a CT scan.

TABLE 3.29 Common cardiac investigations

Investigation	Indications	Implications
ECG	Numerous (medical and medico-legal)	Confirms the cardiac rhythm and reveals abnormalities in conditions such as LBBB and W.P.W. syndrome Diagnosis of myocardial infarction Assessing abnormalities in left ventricular hypertrophy. May reveal ischaemia; however usually normal in patients with angina
Exercise ECG	Chest pain	Ischaemic changes during exercise, especially when associated with symptoms, support a diagnosis of angina. However, exercise test can be normal in angina patients (false negative) and abnormal in healthy individuals (false positive)
	Post-myocardial infarction	Provides prognostic information
Ambulatory ECG monitoring	Palpitations	Confirms whether patients' symptoms are coincident with cardiac arrhythmia, e.g. ventricular ectopic beats or atrial fibrillation
	Syncope or presyncope	May show intermittent bradycardia or tachyarrhythmia if symptoms occur during monitoring
Chest X-ray	Numerous	Cardiothoracic ratio: maximum width of the cardiac silhouette/widest part of lung fields, usually the base. Increased in heart failure and valve disease Pulmonary oedema in heart failure
Echocardiography	Cardiac murmur	Stenotic valve lesion readily diagnosed and accurately quantified Regurgitation readily detected with semi-quantitative assessment
	Breathlessness	Left ventricular function can be assessed. Impaired in heart failure
	Infective endocarditis	Valve vegetations confirm the diagnosis. Transoesophageal echo is more sensitive
Radionuclide studies	Breathlessness	Blood pool scanning provides an accurate assessment of left ventricular function, usually expressed as ejection fraction (end diastolic volume – end systolic volume/end diastolic volume)
	Chest pain	Myocardial perfusion scan reveals ischaemic deficits in ischaemic heart disease
	Pulmonary embolism	Lung scan shows a perfusion deficit. Usually compared with simultaneous ventilation scan
Cardiac catheterisation	Angina	Coronary angiography reveals the extent and severity of coronary stenoses. This determines the therapeutic approach
	Valve disease	Better evaluated non-invasively by echocardiography. Cardiac catheterisation is only indicated to assess the coronary anatomy in patients who require heart valve surgery
	Heart failure	Right heart catheterisation in patients with severe heart failure helps determine suitability for cardiac transplantation

recordings made from six pericardial electrodes (V1–V6) together with six different pairings from three limb electrodes (left arm, right arm and left leg). The right leg electrode is used as a reference.

Ambulatory ECG monitoring

The most frequently used mobile ECG monitor resembles a small tape recorder with input from three chest electrodes which is normally worn on a belt for periods of 24 or 48 hours. Other monitors are available which are not worn continuously but can be activated by applying them to the precordium while the patient experiences symptoms.

Exercise ECG

Patients with angina usually have a normal resting ECG unless it is recorded during an attack. Patients are therefore exercised on a treadmill or a stationary bicycle and if the symptoms induced are due to angina changes are usually visible on the ECG. The severity of the changes induced, and the degree of exercise required to produce them, may be of prognostic significance.

Echocardiography

Cardiac ultrasound scanners have improved to the point that diagnostic images can be obtained in nearly every patient. The commonest indication is the assessment of left ventricular function. In addition to imaging cardiac structure, blood flow can be displayed (Doppler echocardiography) and quantified. Most scans are performed through the anterior wall of the chest but when high-resolution images of posterior structures (e.g. left atrium or descending aorta) are required transoesophageal imaging is employed. This can be carried out safely in outpatients using topical anaesthesia and intravenous sedation.

Radionuclide studies

Radionuclides can be injected intravenously and then detected using a gamma camera. Technetium-99 is used to label the circulating blood and image the right and left ventricles. Conversely, thallium and sesta-MIBI are taken up by myocardial cells and provide an indication of myocardial perfusion, both at rest and during exercise.

Cardiac catheterisation

This invasive procedure involves introducing fine catheters, approximately 2 mm in diameter into the femoral (or brachial) artery and/or vein, and advancing them to the left or right side of the heart respectively. Originally these techniques were developed to measure pressures in the different cardiac chambers in patients with valve disease. However these patients are now investigated by echocardiography. Cardiac catheterisation is now predominantly used to undertake coronary angiography. Coronary angiography is frequently combined with balloon angioplasty in patients with stenotic lesions suitable for dilatation (Fig. 3.37).

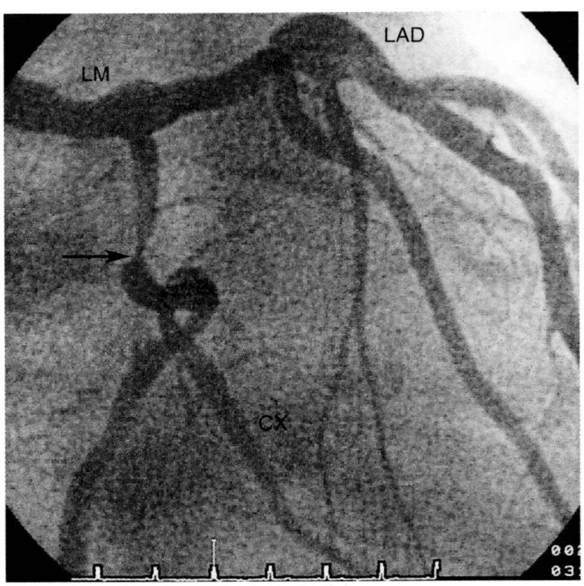

Fig. 3.37 Coronary angiography in an RAO projection. The arrow indicates a severe discreet stenosis in the circumflex coronary artery. LM = left main, LAD = left anterior descending, Cx = circumflex.

PERIPHERAL ARTERIAL DISEASE (PAD)

THE HISTORY

General considerations

In 'developed' countries clinical examination often reveals evidence of peripheral artery disease (PAD) in patients over the age of 60. In the great majority of cases the underlying pathology is atherosclerosis affecting large and medium-sized vessels. The general history should accordingly focus on the family history of premature arterial disease and on the risk factors associated with atheroma. Diabetes is particularly important because it is associated with atheroma that develops early, progresses rapidly, and is widespread in distribution. Furthermore, the clinical manifestations of diabetic arterial disease are frequently exacerbated by coexisting peripheral neuropathy and microangiography.

Although approximately two-thirds of patients with clinically detectable PAD will be asymptomatic, their identification is important:

- The first manifestation of PAD may be with a life-threatening complication.
- Evidence of PAD is a marker for premature cardiovascular and cerebrovascular death and its recognition should provide the stimulus to identify and attempt to modify risk factors.
- The presence of PAD may affect the outcome of medical and surgical treatment for a range of other conditions. For example the prescription of a beta-blocker may precipitate the onset of claudication. Likewise, cardiac surgery performed on bypass in the presence of severe but asymptomatic carotid artery stenosis may lead to stroke.

Presenting complaints

There are four major ways in which patients may present:

1. limb symptoms
2. neurological symptoms
3. abdominal symptoms
4. vasospastic symptoms.

Lower limb symptoms

There are four well defined stages of lower limb ischaemia (Table 3.30).

TABLE 3.30 Classification of lower limb ischaemia

I	Asymptomatic
II	Intermittent claudication
III	Rest pain
IV	Tissue loss (ulceration/gangrene)

Asymptomatic ischaemia. Lower limb ischaemia as defined by a reduced ankle : brachial pressure index (ABPI) is very common in the middle-aged and elderly. They may be asymptomatic either because they choose not to walk very far, or because their exercise tolerance is limited by other pathology. Such patients are at as high a risk from 'vascular' complications as those with symptoms and should be managed as if they have claudication.

Intermittent claudication (IC). This term refers to pain on walking due to arterial insufficiency. It is the commonest symptom of PAD. The pain typically occurs in the calf but may be felt in the thigh and/or buttock if the obstruction to flow is sufficiently proximal. It is often described as a tightness or 'cramp-like'. Characteristically, the pain develops after a relatively constant distance, which will be shorter if walking uphill. On resting, the pain disappears completely within a few minutes but recurs on walking. The claudication distance described by the patient is often misleading with many patients underestimating their walking abilities. Rather than focusing upon absolute distances, it may be more useful to ask patients specific questions. Can they walk to the clinic from the bus stop or car park without stopping? Can they do their own shopping? The impact that claudication has on patients is clearly related to their age and lifestyle. The inability to walk 400 m would be a serious problem for a postman but perhaps not for an elderly man who simply wants to get across the road to the shops and the pub! It is also important to assess claudication in the context of the patient's other medical conditions. There is little point in subjecting patients with intermittent claudication to the risk of vascular surgery, only to find that they are now limited by osteoarthritis of the hip, angina or severe breathlessness.

Male patients with gluteal claudication, due to internal iliac disease, are almost invariably impotent. Enquiry into sexual activity (p. 11) should be made if not volunteered by such patients.

The term claudication is also used to denote pain in the leg on walking due to neurological and musculoskeletal disorders of the lumbar spine (neurogenic claudication) and due to venous outflow obstruction from the leg (venous claudication). However, these are much less common than arterial claudication and can usually be distinguished on history and examination (see Table 3.32, p. 108).

Night/rest pain. Typically this first manifests itself as night pain. The patient goes to bed and falls asleep only to be woken 1–2 hours later by pain in the foot, usually in the instep. This is due to the loss on recumbency of the beneficial effects of gravity on lower limb perfusion. Sleep is also associated with a reduction in heart rate, blood pressure and cardiac output. Patients usually find that they only obtain relief by hanging their leg out of bed or by getting up and walking around. When the patient returns to bed, symptoms recur. The pain and sleep disturbance may be so debilitating that the patient takes to sleeping in a chair. This leads to dependent oedema and the increased interstitial tissue pressure causes further reduction in tissue perfusion, and more pain. Rest pain usually indicates the presence of multi-level disease.

Tissue loss (ulceration and/or gangrene). Patients with rest pain caused by arterial insufficiency are frequently termed as having critical limb ischaemia. In such patients trivial injuries will fail to heal and provide a portal of entry for bacteria leading to gangrene and/or ulceration. Without revascularisation the ischaemia will rapidly progress.

THE PHYSICAL EXAMINATION

General considerations

Much of the general assessment follows the pattern described for the heart and includes looking for evidence of anaemia or cyanosis, for signs of cardiac failure and for direct or indirect evidence of vascular disease (see Table 3.31). A thorough search for these signs should complement the detailed examination of the arterial pulses.

Abnormally prominent pulsation in the neck of the elderly is usually of little clinical significance being caused by arterial tortuosity rather than by a carotid aneurysm or carotid body tumour.

TABLE 3.31 Signs suggesting vascular disease

Sign	Implication
Hands and arms	
Nicotine stains	Smoking
Purple discoloration of the fingertips	Atheroembolism from a proximal subclavian aneurysm
Pits and healed scars in the finger pulps	Secondary Raynaud's syndrome
Calcinosis and visible nailfold capillary loops	Scleroderma and the CREST syndrome
Wasting of the small muscles of the hand	Thoracic outlet syndrome
Face and neck	
Corneal arcus and xanthelasma	Hypercholesterolaemia
Horner's syndrome	Carotid artery dissection or aneurysm
Hoarseness of the voice and 'bovine cough'	Recurrent laryngeal nerve palsy from a thoracic aortic aneurysm
Prominent veins in the neck and over shoulder and anterior chest	Axillary/subclavian vein occlusion
Abdomen	
Epigastric/umbilical pulsation	Aortoiliac aneurysm
Mottling of the abdomen	Ruptured abdominal aortic aneurysm or saddle embolism occluding aortic bifurcation
Evidence of weight loss	Visceral ischaemia

Anatomy

The anatomy of the radial, brachial and carotid pulses have been described (p. 83).

Femoral artery. The femoral artery is situated just below the inguinal ligament, midway between the anterior superior iliac spine and the pubic symphysis (mid-inguinal point). It is immediately lateral to the femoral vein and medial to the femoral nerve. In the obese it can be difficult to feel.

Popliteal artery. At the level of the knee crease, the artery lies deep in the popliteal fossa and the pulse is sometimes difficult to feel, even by the experienced clinician.

Posterior tibial artery. This is located 2 cm below and posterior to the medial malleolus where it passes beneath the flexor retinaculum between flexor digitorum longus and flexor hallucis longus.

Dorsalis pedis artery. This is the continuation of the anterior tibial artery on the dorsum of the foot. It passes lateral the tendon of the extensor hallucis longus and is best felt at the proximal extent of the groove between the first and second metatarsals. It may be absent or abnormally sited in 10% of normal subjects, sometimes being 'replaced' by a palpable perforating peroneal artery.

Individual pulses should be recorded as follows:

normal	+
reduced	±
absent	–
aneurysmal	++

Examination of pulses

If the examiner is in any doubt about which pulse is being felt, it is useful for the clinician to palpate his or her own pulse at the same time. Lack of synchronisation implies that it is the patient's pulse.

Examination sequence

General

- ☐ Examine the radial, brachial and carotid pulses (p. 83). Measure the blood pressure in both arms.
- ☐ Palpate and auscultate over the abdominal aorta in any patient with suspected vascular disease.
- ☐ Inspect the legs and feet for changes of ischaemia including changes in temperature and colour.
- ☐ Note any scars from previous vascular or non-vascular surgery and the position, margin, depth and colour of any ulceration.
- ☐ Specifically look between the toes and at the heels for ischaemic changes.

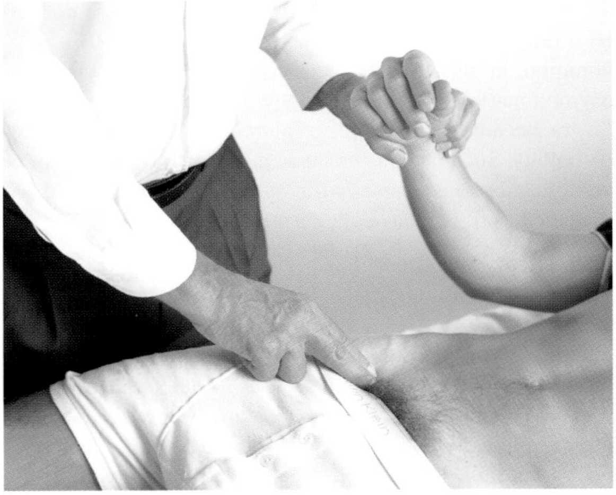

Fig. 3.38 Examine the femoral artery, stimultaneously while checking for radiofemoral delay.

Femoral

- ☐ With the patient supine, firmly press down and cephalad in the groin crease (Fig. 3.38) using two or three extended fingers.
- ☐ Auscultate for a bruit.
- ☐ Check for radiofemoral delay.

Popliteal

- ☐ Flex the knee to 30 degrees and make sure the patient is relaxed.

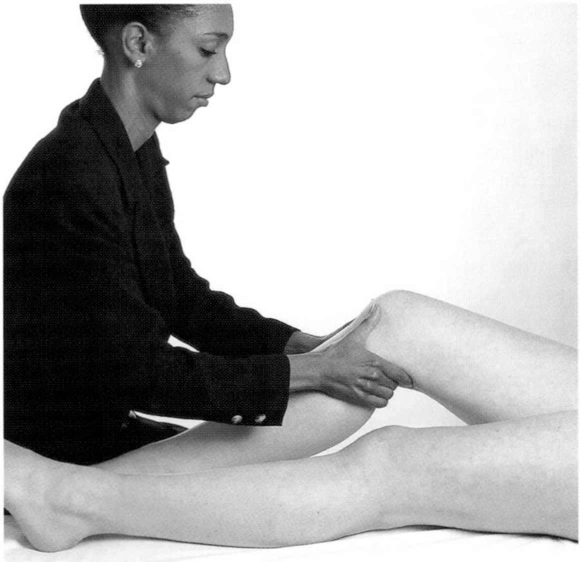

Fig. 3.39 Examination of the popliteal artery. Feel the popliteal artery with the fingertips, having curled both hands into the popliteal fossa.

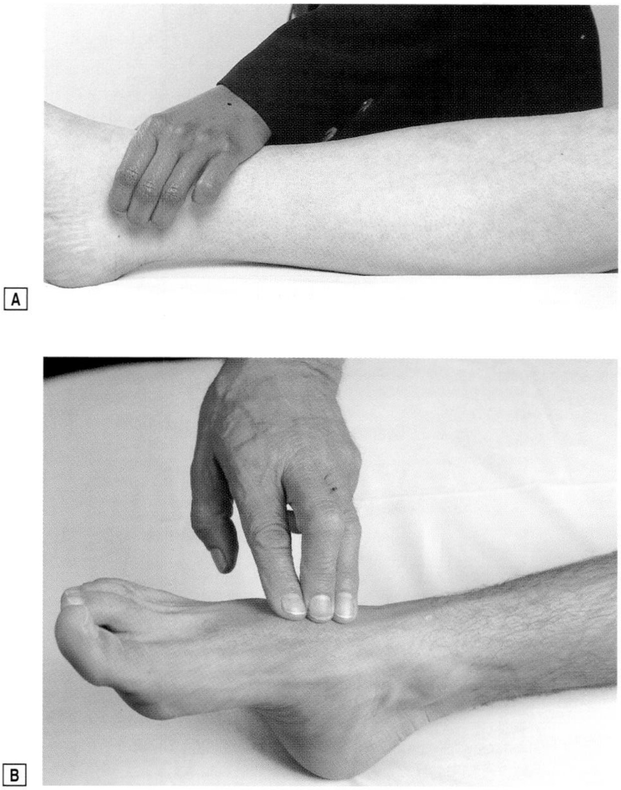

Fig. 3.40 Examination of A the posterior tibial artery and B the dorsalis pedis artery.

- ☐ With the thumbs in front and the fingers behind, press firmly over the popliteal artery.
- ☐ Feel for the pulse in the midline 3–4 cm below the knee crease where the artery can be compressed against the posterior aspect of the tibia as it passes under the soleal arch (Fig. 3.39).

Posterior tibial

- ☐ Feel 2 cm below and 2 cm behind the medial malleolus (Fig 3.40A).

Dorsalis pedis

- ☐ Feel in the middle of the dorsum of the foot just lateral to the tendon of extensor hallucis longus (Fig. 3.40B).

Buerger's test

- ☐ With the patient lying supine, stand at the foot of the bed. Raise the feet and support the legs at 45 degrees to the horizontal.
- ☐ Then ask the patient to sit up and swing the legs over the edge of the bed.

Common abnormalities

Chronic lower limb ischaemia

The leg is affected eight times more commonly than the arm because:

- the arterial supply to the leg is less well developed
- the lower limb is more frequently affected by atherosclerosis.

In many patients the pedal pulses may be absent or diminished. However, the presence of pedal pulses at rest does not exclude a significant lower limb PAD. If the history is convincing ask the patient to walk until the onset of pain. If the symptoms are vascular in origin the pulses will disappear. Additional ischaemic changes may be present; for example, there may be absence of body hair on toes and dorsum of the feet. Other clinical features of arterial claudication are illustrated in Table 3.32.

Changes are more severe once there is critical limb ischaemia. Such patients will have an ankle blood pressure of < 50mmHg and a positive Buerger's test. This is indicated by the presence of rubor of the forefoot (sunset foot) due to reactive hyperaemia within 2–3 minutes of the legs becoming dependent. Severe chronic ischaemia of the limb is associated with the onset of extreme pallor of the sole of the foot and emptying, so-called 'guttering', of the dorsal foot veins with the leg elevated.

Acute limb ischaemia

The features of the acutely ischaemic limb are conveniently known as the 6 Ps (Table 3.33). Of these, loss of motor (ability to wiggle the toes/fingers) and/or sensory function (light touch over the forefoot/dorsum of the hand) are the most important and indicate nerve ischaemia. Once these features are present the limb will become irreversibly damaged unless the circulation is restored within a few hours. Calf muscle tenderness is another grave sign indicating impending muscle infarction.

The common causes of acute limb ischaemia are embolus (usually cardiac in origin) or thrombotic occlusion of a narrowed atherosclerotic arterial segment (Table 3.34).

Acute arterial occlusion is associated with intense spasm in the arterial tree distal to the blockage and the limb will appear 'marble white'. Over the next few hours, the spasm relaxes and the skin fills with deoxygenated blood leading to mottling which is light blue or purple, has a fine reticular pattern and blanches on pressure. As ischaemia progresses, blood coalescing in the skin produces a coarser pattern which is dark purple, almost black, and does not blanch. The final stage is large patches of fixed staining leading on to blistering and liquefaction. Fixed mottling of an anaesthetic, paralysed limb, in association with muscle rigidity and

TABLE 3.32 The clinical features of arterial, neurogenic and venous claudication

	Arterial	Neurogenic	Venous
Pathology	Stenosis or occlusion of major lower limb arteries	Lumbar nerve root or cauda equina compression (spinal stenosis)	Obstruction to the venous outflow of the leg due to iliofemoral venous occlusion
Site of pain	Muscles, usually the calf but may involve thigh and buttock	Ill-defined. Whole leg. May be associated with numbness and tingling	Whole leg. 'Bursting' in nature
Laterality	Unilateral if femoropopliteal, and bilateral if aortoiliac disease	Often bilateral	Nearly always unilateral
Onset	Gradual after walking the 'claudication distance'	Often immediate upon walking or even standing up	Gradual, often from the moment walking commences
Relieving features	On cessation of walking, the pain disappears completely in 1–2 minutes	Eased by bending forwards and stopping walking. May have to sit down to obtain full relief	Usually necessary to elevate leg to relieve discomfort
Colour	Normal or pale	Normal	Cyanosed, Often visible varicose veins
Temperature	Normal or cool	Normal	Normal or increased
Oedema	Absent	Absent	Always present
Pulses	Reduced or absent	Normal	Present but may be difficult to feel owing to oedema
Straight leg raising	Normal	May be limited	Normal

TABLE 3.33 Signs of acute limb ischaemia

Soft signs
Pulseless
Pallor
Perishing cold

Hard signs (indicating a threatened limb)
Paraesthesia
Paralysis
Pain on squeezing muscles

TABLE 3.34 Acute limb ischaemia – embolus vs thrombosis in situ

	Embolus	Thrombosis
Onset and severity	Owing to lack of pre-existing collaterals the onset is acute (seconds or minutes) and the ischaemia profound	Owing to pre-existing collaterals, onset is more insidious (hours or days) and ischaemia less severe
Embolic source	Present (usually AF)	Absent
Previous claudication	Absent	Present
Pulses in contralateral leg	Present	Often absent
Diagnosis	Clinical	Angiography
Treatment	Embolectomy and anticoagulation	Medical, bypass surgery, thrombolysis

CASE HISTORY

This patient was admitted with an acutely painful right hand. On examination, the patient was in atrial fibrillation, the hand was pale and the fingers mottled (Fig. 3.41). Right arm pulses were absent. Arteriography showed occlusion of the right axillary artery consistent with embolus (Fig. 3.42). The patient was heparinised, underwent successful brachial embolectomy under local anaesthetic and was then commenced on warfarin.

Learning points

- Acute embolism is the commonest cause of acute arm ischaemia.
- To avoid amputation, time is critical; all patients with a suspected acutely ischaemic limb should be considered for vascular surgery immediately.

turgor, indicates irreversible ischaemia and amputation is the only option.

Neurological presentation of vascular disease

Vascular disease may present with multi-infarct dementia, strokes or transient ischaemic attacks.

A stroke may be defined as a focal neurological deficit of vascular cause. If symptoms and signs last less than 24 hours then the event is termed a *transient ischaemic attack* (TIA).

Internal carotid artery territory. A significant proportion of strokes and TIAs are due to atheroemboli originating from a tight atherosclerotic stenosis at the origin of the *internal carotid artery*.

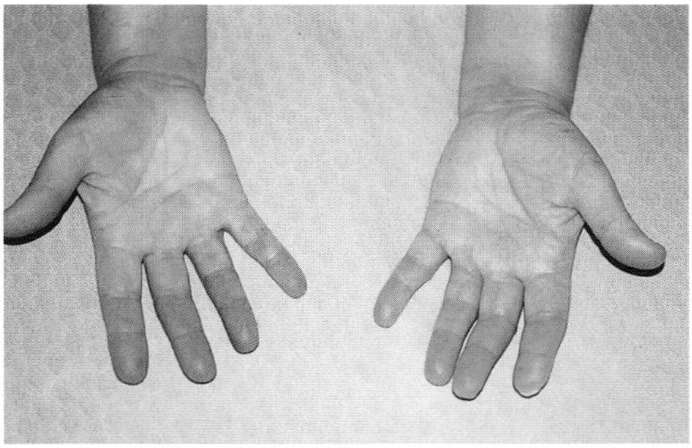

Fig. 3.41 Pallor of the hand with mottling of the fingers following occlusion of the right axillary artery.

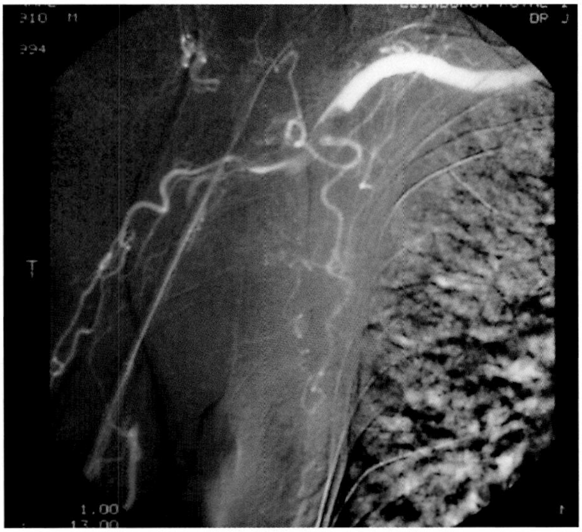

Fig. 3.42 Arteriogram showing axillary embolus.

Arterial insufficiency in the internal carotid territory typically presents with ocular and/or hemispheric features:

- *Ocular*: loss of vision in the ipsilateral eye (amaurosis fugax), often described by the patient as a curtain coming across the field of view, usually lasting a few minutes, due to transient occlusion of the retinal artery or one of its branches. Less commonly, permanent monocular blindness occurs when an embolus causes retinal infarction.
- *Hemispheric*: loss of power and/or sensation in the contralateral arm and/or leg. If the dominant hemisphere is affected there may also be dysphasia.

The presence or absence of a bruit in the neck is an unreliable sign of either the presence or the severity of internal carotid artery stenosis. A bruit may arise from stenosis in other vessels, such as the external carotid artery. Conversely there may be so little blood flowing through a critical internal carotid artery stenosis that no bruit is audible. This consideration is equally applicable over other sites (e.g. the femoral and subclavian arteries).

Vertebrobasilar artery territory. TIAs and strokes arising from vertebrobasilar insufficiency are less common and produce different signs and symptoms. These may comprise giddiness, collapse, with or without loss of consciousness, transient occipital blindness or complete loss of vision in both eyes.

Patients with subclavian artery stenosis or occlusion proximal to the origin of the vertebral artery may experience vertebrobasilar symptoms, as part of the *subclavian steal syndrome*. This happens when the arm is exercised. The increased blood supply to the arm is met by blood travelling up the carotid arteries and then, via the circle of Willis, down the vertebral artery into the arm, so 'stealing' blood from the posterior cerebral circulation. Signs of this include asymmetry of the pulses and blood pressure in the arms and sometimes a bruit over the subclavian artery in the supraclavicular fossa.

Visceral ischaemia

Owing to the rich collateral circulation that exists in the gut usually two of the three major visceral arteries (coeliac axis, superior and inferior mesenteric arteries) are critically stenosed or occluded before a patient begins to experience the symptoms and signs of *chronic mesenteric vascular insufficiency*. Typically, the patient will develop severe central abdominal pain (mesenteric angina) 10–15 minutes after eating. Diarrhoea may also be a feature. This leads to fear of eating and significant weight loss. Visceral ischaemia may mimic a whole range of gastrointestinal pathologies and the patient may have undergone numerous investigations, even laparotomy, before the clinical diagnosis is made, and confirmed by angiography.

Acute mesenteric ischaemia is a surgical emergency. The patient typically presents with severe abdominal pain, shock, bloody diarrhoea and profound acidosis.

Renal angle pain from renal infarction or ischaemia is rare. It is associated with micro- or macroscopic haematuria.

Abdominal aortic aneurysm (AAA)

AAA are present in 5% of men aged over 65 years and are three times commoner in men than women. Patients may present with abdominal and/or back pain or an awareness of pulsation. Many patients are asymptomatic until the aneurysm ruptures. Clinical examination is much less reliable than ultrasonography in detecting AAA, especially if the abdominal girth exceeds 38–40 inches (96–102 cm). As the aortic bifurcation is at the level of the umbilicus, a palpable AAA is felt in the epigastrium. A pulsatile mass below the umbilicus suggests an iliac aneurysm.

The diagnosis of ruptured AAA can be difficult because many patients do not exhibit the classical features of abdominal and/or back pain, pulsatile abdominal mass and hypotension. The commonest misdiagnosis is renal colic. 'Renal colic' presenting for the first time over the age of 60 years is due to a ruptured AAA until proved otherwise.

Atheroembolism may arise from an AAA and cause the 'blue toe syndrome' characterised by purple discoloration of the toes/forefoot usually in association with a full set of pedal pulses.

CASE HISTORY

A 65-year-old male patient presented with a 12-hour history of abdominal pain radiating through to his back. On examination, he was normotensive and there was a pulsatile mass in his epigastrium. Contrast-enhanced computed tomography (CT) of the abdomen confirmed the presence of an 8 cm AAA (Fig. 3.43). The patient subsequently underwent successful emergency AAA repair.

Learning points

- Consider AAA in any patient over the age of 60 years presenting with abdominal pain, especially if the pain radiates to the loins and/or the back.

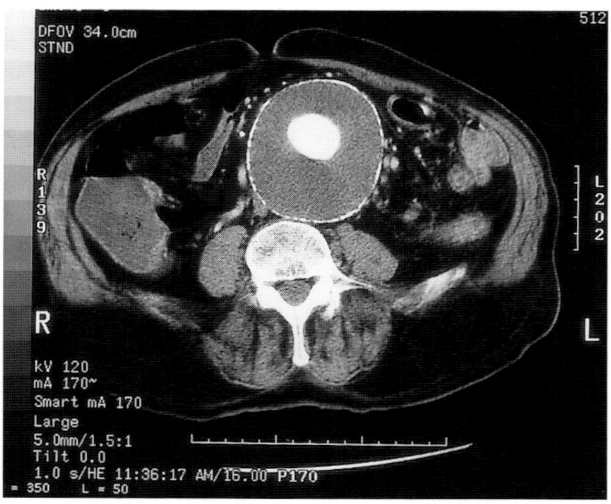

Fig. 3.43 CT scan of the abdomen showing abdominal aortic aneurysm.

Vasospastic conditions

Raynaud's phenomenon (RP) describes digital ischaemia induced by cold and emotion and comprises three phases:

1. pallor due to digital artery spasm and/or obstruction
2. cyanosis due to deoxygenation of static venous blood (this phase may be absent)
3. rubor due to reactive hyperaemia.

RP may be *primary* (Raynaud's disease) owing to idiopathic digital artery vasospasm or *secondary* (Raynaud's syndrome) because of digital artery obstruction caused by:

- connective tissue disease (most commonly systemic sclerosis)
- vibration injury (secondary to the use of power tools)
- atheroembolism from a proximal source such as subclavian artery aneurysm.

Patients presenting with unilateral RP over the age of 40 should be assumed to have underlying PAD unless proved otherwise.

INVESTIGATIONS OF PERIPHERAL ARTERIAL DISEASE

When investigating patients with PAD it is important to choose the test that will provide the most information at the least risk to the patient, and at the least expense. Ultrasound techniques have replaced angiography in many instances (Table 3.35).

Measurement of ankle : brachial pressure index (ABPI)

Measurement of ABPI is performed using a hand-held Doppler (HHD) and a sphygmomanometer. The probe is held over the three pedal arteries (posterior tibial, dorsalis pedis, perforating peroneal) in turn while a blood pressure

TABLE 3.35 Investigation of peripheral arterial disease

Investigation	Common uses
Doppler ultrasound	Ankle pressure; ankle brachial pressure index (ABPI), pulse waveform analysis
B-mode ultrasound	Abdominal aortic aneurysm, popliteal artery aneurysm
Duplex ultrasound	Carotid artery stenosis, vein bypass graft surveillance
Computed tomography	Abdominal aortic aneurysm, detection of cerebral infarct/haemorrhage
Magnetic resonance imaging	Arteriovenous malformations, carotid artery stenosis
Angiography	Acute and chronic limb ischaemia, carotid artery stenosis

cuff wrapped round the ankle is inflated. The pressure at which the Doppler signal disappears denotes the systolic pressure in that artery as it passes under the cuff. The ratio of the highest pedal artery pressure to the highest brachial artery pressure is the ABPI.

In health, the ABPI should be ≥1.0 in the supine position. Typical values in claudication and critical ischaemia are < 0.8 and < 0.4 respectively. Absolute values, however, may be less informative than the trend over a period of time.

Patients with severe lower limb ischaemia, particularly diabetics, may have incompressible, calcified crural arteries. This will falsely elevate the pedal pressures, and thus the ABPI. In such circumstances, an alternative is to 'isonate' the artery while elevating the foot. The height above the bed in centimetres at which the Doppler signal disappears is approximately equal to the perfusion pressure in mmHg.

KEY POINTS

- Widespread PAD may be asymptomatic for many years and then present with life-threatening complications.
- Acute limb ischaemia and chronic arterial insufficiency causing rest pain and/or tissue loss require urgent assessment.
- The ankle : brachial pressure index (ABPI) is useful in assessing the severity of chronic lower limb ischaemia.
- Patients presenting with hemispheric or ocular TIAs should have an urgent carotid ultrasound.
- Visceral ischaemia is frequently overlooked as a cause of 'unexplained' abdominal pain and weight loss.

VENOUS DISORDERS

General considerations

The clinical examination is primarily concerned with:

1. determining the nature and severity of any venous problem
2. identifying any underlying or precipitating factors.

Venous disease is much more common in the legs than in the arms. It usually presents in one of four ways (Table 3.36).

TABLE 3.36 Common venous abnormalities

Deep venous thrombosis (DVT)
Varicose veins
Superficial thrombophlebitis
Chronic venous insufficiency and ulceration

THE HISTORY

Presenting complaints

The severity of the symptoms may bear little relationship to the gravity of the underlying pathology. For example life-threatening, deep venous thrombosis (DVT) may be asymptomatic. There are four cardinal symptoms of lower limb venous disease.

1. *Pain*. Patients with uncomplicated varicose veins may complain of an aching discomfort in the leg, itching and a feeling of swelling. Symptoms are typically aggravated by prolonged standing and are often worse towards the end of the day.

   The pain of deep venous thrombosis is deep-seated and associated with swelling below the level of obstruction. Superficial venous thrombophlebitis produces a red, painful area overlying the vein involved. Varicose ulceration may be painless but if there is pain it may be relieved by elevation of the limb.
2. *Swelling* may be associated with varicose veins, deep venous reflux and deep venous thrombosis.
3. *Discoloration*. Chronic venous insufficiency is associated with deposition of haemosiderin in the skin leading to lipodermatosclerosis (LDS). This may vary from deep blue/black to purple or even bright red. It typically affects the medial aspect of the lower third of the leg but may be laterally placed if superficial reflux predominates in the short saphenous veins.
4. *Ulceration*. Patients with venous ulceration may not seek medical attention for many years. Venous ulceration is always associated with LDS.

Supplementary questions

Relevant further questions will depend upon the nature of the venous problem. They may be particularly important in assessing a patient presenting with a possible pulmonary embolus (p. 122) or suspected of having a deep venous thrombosis (see Question box).

QUESTIONS – Deep venous thrombosis

Ask about:

- recent bed rest or operations (especially to the leg or pelvis)
- recent travel, especially long air flights
- previous trauma to the leg, especially long bone fractures, plaster of Paris splintage and immobilisation
- pregnancy or features to suggest pelvic disease
- previous DVT
- family history of thrombosis
- recent central venous catheterisation injections of drugs etc. (in the upper limb).

In superficial thrombophlebitis, particularly if it is recurrent, questions should be directed to cover the possibility of underlying malignancy.

THE PHYSICAL EXAMINATION

Anatomy

The long saphenous vein passes anterior to the medial malleolus, up the medial aspect of the calf to behind the knee, then up the medial aspect of the thigh to join the common femoral vein in the groin at the saphenofemoral junction. The short saphenous vein passes behind the lateral malleolus and up the posterior aspect of the calf. It commonly joins the popliteal vein at the saphenopopliteal junction which usually lies 2 cm above the posterior knee crease. There are many intercommunications between the long and short saphenous systems and, as with most areas of the body, the venous anatomy of the leg is highly variable.

Examination of venous system

Examination of the venous system largely involves inspection and palpation.

Examination sequence

- ☐ Examine the legs with the patient standing and then lying supine.
- ☐ Expose the patient's limbs and inspect the skin for colour changes, limb swelling and superficial venous dilatation and tortuosity.
- ☐ Palpate for any differences in temperature.
- ☐ Elevate the limb to about 15 degrees above the horizontal and note the rate of venous emptying.
- ☐ If appropriate, perform the Trendelenburg test.

Trendelenburg test for saphenofemoral junction incompetence

- ☐ Ask the patient to sit on the edge of the examination couch.
- ☐ Elevate the limb as far as comfortable for the patient and empty the superficial veins by 'milking' the leg.
- ☐ With the leg still elevated exert digital pressure over the saphenofemoral junction (2–3 cm below and 2–3 cm lateral to the pubic tubercle). If preferred, a high thigh tourniquet can be used instead of finger pressure.
- ☐ Now ask the patient to stand.
- ☐ In the presence of saphenofemoral junction incompetence, the patient's varicose veins will not fill until digital pressure, or the tourniquet, is removed.

Common abnormalities

Deep venous thrombosis

Deep venous thrombosis occurs most often in the leg, but can also affect the arm (axillary vein thrombosis).

TABLE 3.37 Clinical features of deep venous thrombosis of the lower limb

Clinical features	Non-occlusive thrombus	Occlusive thrombus
Pain	Often absent	Usually present
Calf tenderness	Often absent	Usually present
Swelling	Absent	Present
Temperature	Normal or slightly increased	Increased
Superficial veins	Normal	Distended
Risk of pulmonary embolus	High	Low

The leg. The clinical features of leg DVT depend upon its site and extent and whether it is occlusive or not (Table 3.37). The 'classical' features of DVT relate to well-established occlusive thrombus. In contrast, most patients who die from pulmonary embolus have non-occlusive thrombosis and normal legs on clinical examination. Non-occlusive thrombus poses the highest threat of pulmonary embolus as the clot lies within a flowing stream of venous blood, is perhaps more likely to propagate and has not yet induced an inflammatory response in the vein wall which anchors it in place.

The arm. DVT can occur as a *primary* event due to repetitive trauma of the vein, e.g. thoracic outlet syndrome. It is also seen as a secondary thrombotic complication around indwelling catheters in the subclavian vein. Symptoms comprise arm swelling and discomfort which is exacerbated by activity, especially where it involves holding the arm overhead. On examination the arm is swollen and the skin often cyanosed and mottled, especially on dependency. Superficial distended veins acting as collaterals are often seen in the upper arm, over the shoulder region and anterior chest wall.

Superficial venous thrombophlebitis (SVT)

This is a, usually sterile, inflammation of superficial veins associated with intraluminal thrombosis. It affects up to 10% of patients with severe varicose veins and appears to be commoner during pregnancy.

Recurrent superficial thrombophlebitis may be associated with underlying malignancy. SVT at or near the saphenofemoral junction is associated with a high incidence of pulmonary embolism.

Chronic venous insufficiency

Chronic venous insufficiency produces skin changes in the lower leg (varicose eczema, lipodermatosclerosis, ulceration) due to sustained venous hypertension which in turn is due to reflux (90%) and/or obstruction (10%) in the superficial and/or deep veins.

TABLE 3.38 Clinical features of venous and arterial ulceration

Clinical feature	Venous ulceration	Arterial ulceration
Age	Typically first develops at 40–60 years but many do not present to medical attention until many years later; multiple recurrences are the norm	Typically affects patient for the first time > 60 years
Sex	Women predominate, especially in the elderly	Men predominate
Past medical history	Many have a or history of DVT, or give a history suggestive of occult DVT, i.e. leg swelling after childbirth, hip/knee replacement, or long bone fracture	Most have a clear history of previous PAD, cardio- and cerebrovascular disease
Risk factors	Thrombophilia, family history, previous DVT (see above)	Smoking, diabetes, hypercholesterolaemia, and hypertension
Pain	Present in about a third of patients but not usually severe; often improves with elevation	Severe pain is the rule except in diabetics with neuropathy; usually better on dependency
Site	Distal one-third of leg; usually medial in relation to long saphenous veins disease; 20% are lateral related to short saphenous disease	Pressure areas (malleoli, heel, 5th metatarsal base, metatarsal heads) and toes
Margin	Irregular often with neo-epithelium (appears whiter than mature skin)	Regular, indolent, 'punched out'
Base	Often pink and granulating under green slough	Sloughy (green) or necrotic (black) with no granulation
Surrounding skin	Lipodermatosclerosis always present	No venous skin changes
Veins	Full and usually varicose	Empty with 'guttering' on elevation
Swelling (oedema)	Usually present	Absent
Temperature	Warm	Cold
Pulses	Present, but may be difficult to feel	Absent

Chronic leg ulceration

In developed countries, the vast majority of leg ulcers are caused by venous and/or arterial disease. The aetiology of a leg ulcer can usually be ascertained by clinical examination (Table 3.38). However, 1 in 5 patients with a venous ulcer will also have significant arterial disease. Bandaging for a leg ulcer is contraindicated unless there is documented evidence of the adequacy of the arterial circulation, either by feeling the pulses or by measuring the ankle : brachial pressure index.

CASE HISTORY

This patient had suffered recurring episodes of venous ulceration (Fig. 3.44) over many years as a result of a deep venous thrombosis (post-phlebitic syndrome). Venography shows post-phlebitic occlusion of the popliteal vein (Fig. 3.45).

Learning points

- DVT is a common cause of chronic venous insufficiency, which, in turn, is the commonest cause of leg ulceration.

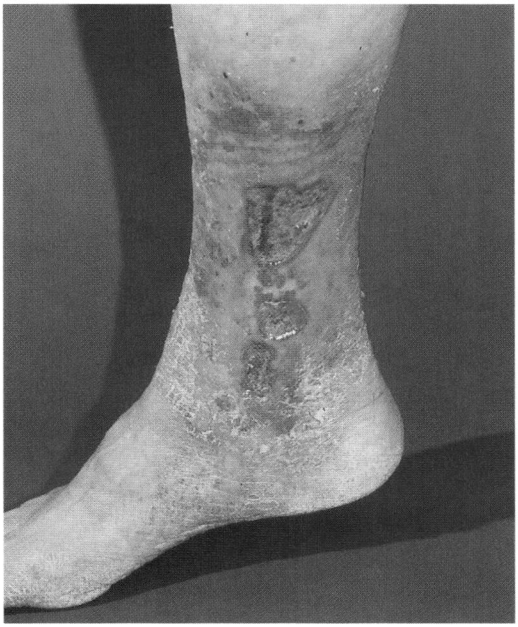

Fig. 3.44 Venous ulceration.

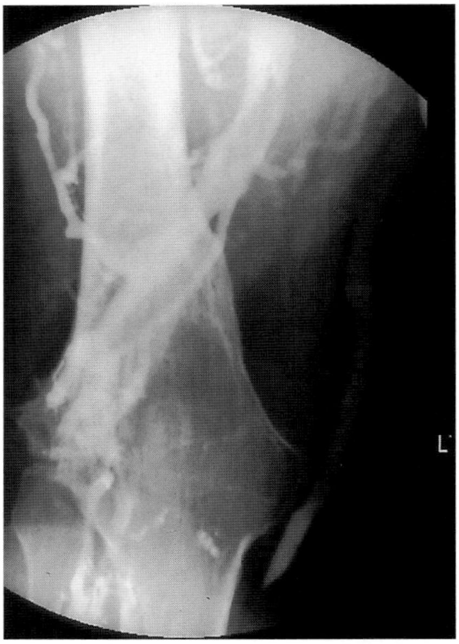

Fig. 3.45 Post-phlebitic popliteal vein stenosis.

KEY POINTS

- The cardinal symptoms of venous disease are pain and discomfort, swelling of the limb and discoloration with ulceration.
- Life-threatening DVT may be asymptomatic.
- Leg ulceration in the elderly is often multifactorial but the commonest single underlying pathology is chronic venous insufficiency.
- Superficial thrombophlebitis, especially in the absence of varicose veins, and where it is migratory in character, often signifies underlying malignancy.

COMMON PITFALLS AND HOW TO AVOID THEM

- It is easy to miss a history of angina if the clinician only asks about chest pain. Most patients do not describe angina as painful. It may be a mild chest discomfort, tightness or heaviness or a sensation of breathlessness. To avoid confusion ask about any discomfort in the chest or other symptoms associated with exertion.
- A typical history of exertional chest tightness may be due to aortic stenosis, not angina. To exclude this possibility, examine the patient specifically for the murmur and the other features of aortic stenosis.
- Peripheral oedema is a non-specific sign. Vasodilating drugs are a common cause. Always obtain a drug history. Only attribute oedema to heart failure if there are confirmatory signs, e.g. elevation of the JVP.
- Acute pulmonary oedema may occur without causing crackles. Moreover, crackles in the lung have causes other than heart failure. Remember, 'all that crackles is not failure' and 'failure does not always crackle'. The chest X-ray is a better indicator of pulmonary oedema.
- The arterial blood pressure rises in response to stress; therefore readings obtained during a first consultation may be unrepresentative of the average. Avoid diagnosing hypertension after only one or two blood pressure measurements, particularly if there is no evidence of end-organ damage, i.e. normal fundi and no left ventricular hypertrophy.
- The heart rate in patients with rapid atrial fibrillation is frequently underestimated, because of the pulse deficit. This mistake is avoided by counting the heart rate while listening at the apex.
- When a systolic murmur is heard at the apex it is often assumed to be mitral regurgitation. However, aortic stenosis is commonly audible at the apex. These two systolic murmurs are best differentiated by their mode of radiation and character. In aortic stenosis there is always a gap after the first heart sound and the murmur ends before the aortic component of the second heart sound. Listen specifically to the relationship between the murmur and the heart sounds.
- Diastolic murmurs may be missed especially when they are accompanied by louder systolic murmurs. Specifically, listen for the murmurs of aortic regurgitation and mitral stenosis, with the patient in the optimum position and using the diaphragm and bell respectively
- Confusion may be caused by the similarity in the timing of a split second heart sound, and either an opening snap or a third heart sound. However, the opening snap is characteristically high pitched and the third heart sound is low pitched. In contrast, the two components may differ in intensity but are of the same pitch. Moreover, a split second heart sound is best heard at the base and splitting is affected by respiration unless caused by an atrial septal defect.
- In a large patient a sizeable AAA may be easily missed. One reason for failing to diagnose an AAA is that it gives rise to a pulsatile mass in the epigastrium, not below the umbilicus. The possibility of a ruptured AAA should be excluded as a cause of abdominal pain, especially in men over the age of 65.
- Raynaud's phenomenon may be associated with vascular disease. Investigate any patient over the age of 40 presenting with unilateral Raynaud's phenomena for PAD.
- Subclavian artery disease may present with apparent vertebrobasilar insufficiency. A difference in systolic pressure > 15 mmHg suggests the diagnosis. Measure the blood pressure in both arms.

- Diabetic patients with rest pain of arterial origin may be misdiagnosed as having the pain of diabetic neuropathy. Both may be worse at night. However, unlike ischaemic pain, the pain of neuropathy is not usually confined to the foot, is often associated with burning and tingling, is not relieved by dependency and is often associated with dysaesthesia (many patients cannot even bear the pressure of bedclothes on their feet).
- Visceral ischaemia is a cause of recurrent and 'obscure' abdominal pain. Consider this diagnosis especially in patients who have already undergone multiple negative investigations of the gastrointestinal tract.
- Disorders of the lumbar spine (neurogenic claudication) and venous outflow obstruction of the leg (venous claudication) may mimic the symptoms of arterial claudication. A careful history and examination should distinguish among these three conditions (Table 3.32).
- 1 in 5 patients with a venous ulcer will have significant arterial disease. Always confirm that the pedal pulses are present and the ABPI normal before prescribing graduated compression bandaging.
- The red discoloration in lipodermatosclerosis may be superficially mistaken for cellulitis, especially if there is venous ulceration. However, these can be readily distinguished because cellulitis, unlike LDS, is associated with the other features of inflammation.
- An aneurysmal popliteal artery may be a sign of widespread vascular disease. If one popliteal artery is unexpectedly easy to palpate, consider abdominal ultrasonography to exclude a co-existent AAA.

The respiratory system

4

G. K. CROMPTON

THE HISTORY

Advances in physiology, pathology, immunology, microbiology, radiology, endoscopy and thoracic surgery have enhanced the precision of diagnosing respiratory disease and resulted in a reappraisal of the value of various clinical investigations. In many instances careful history-taking is more important than the elicitation of physical signs. Indeed, in many disorders the disease process may reach an advanced stage before any abnormal signs can be detected and, unless symptoms are investigated, serious delays in diagnosis and treatment may result.

The approach to history-taking in patients thought to have respiratory disease differs according to the nature of the illness, the main distinction being between an acute or subacute illness and a chronic respiratory disorder. The methods used to obtain a coherent account of the patient's symptoms are, however, the same. Firstly, a narrative history is taken, as outlined in Chapter 1. Specific enquiry is then made about any of the principal respiratory symptoms not mentioned in the narrative history. At this stage the clinician should consider all the conditions that might be responsible for the patient's symptoms. This will seldom be more than three or four options. A series of supplementary questions designed to provide evidence for and against each possible diagnosis should then be asked. This method of integrating and rationalising the history is important because it facilitates the recognition of certain characteristic symptom patterns, such as those presented by chronic bronchitis and bronchial asthma, in which physical signs and specialised investigations may be of limited diagnostic value.

In an *acute respiratory illness* it is important to enquire carefully about the onset of the illness. For example, in pneumococcal pneumonia systemic disturbance (rigor, pyrexia, malaise) seldom precedes the first respiratory symptom (often pleural pain) by more than a few hours, while in viral pneumonia the patient may be generally unwell for several days before there are any symptoms or signs to suggest pulmonary involvement. Pleural pain may be a manifestation of pneumonia, but pulmonary thromboembolic disease should always be considered. Acute breathlessness often demands urgent treatment, and an error in diagnosis, for example between tension pneumothorax, an acute attack of bronchial asthma and left heart failure may have catastrophic consequences. If the patient is too breathless to give a coherent account of the illness, a carefully taken history from a relative may be very important. The nature and effect of any treatment taken before the patient is seen should also be carefully noted.

In *chronic respiratory disorders* history-taking is complex and time-consuming. Care should be taken not only to elicit major incidents in the illness but also to describe and assess the background symptoms. In the case of acute episodes, such as exacerbations of chronic bronchitis, an enquiry should be made into any preceding events and their apparent effects on the course of the disease. Most chronic respiratory disorders pursue a fairly predictable course and, if a patient exhibits symptoms out of line with the established pattern of the illness, the development of another disease should be suspected. The course of disease may also be adversely influenced by the treatment of coexisting disorders, for example a beta-adrenoreceptor blocking drug for hypertension or angina in a patient with chronic asthma. The influence of occupational and environmental factors should be recorded in detail. Such information, in addition to its diagnostic value, may be relevant to prevention and compensation in the case of occupational lung diseases.

SYMPTOMS OF RESPIRATORY DISEASE

The six principal symptoms of respiratory disease are cough, sputum, haemoptysis, chest pain, breathlessness and wheeze. All of these may occur in the absence of primary respiratory disease. In particular, central chest pain may be cardiac, pericardial or oesophageal in origin: breathlessness may be due to pulmonary oedema secondary to left ventricular failure, and haemoptysis may be the presenting symptom in mitral stenosis or disorders of the blood clotting mechanism. Nevertheless, lateral chest pain and the other five principal symptoms are usually indicative of respiratory disease, and will be discussed in that context.

Cough

This is the most frequent symptom of respiratory disease. It may be caused by stimuli arising in the mucosa of the respiratory tract from the pharynx to the smaller bronchi. Stimuli arising in the parietal pleura may, on rare occasions, also produce cough, for example during the aspiration of a pleural effusion. The frequency, severity and character of cough are dependent on several factors including (a) the situation and nature of the lesion responsible, (b) the presence or absence of sputum and (c) coexisting abnormalities such as vocal cord paralysis, impairment of ventilatory function and pleural pain.

Types of cough. Cough can be produced by stimulation of sensory nerves of the mucosa of the pharynx, larynx, trachea and bronchi (see Table 4.1).

In chronic bronchitis cough is accompanied with sputum. In chronic obstructive pulmonary disease (COPD) there is also wheeze, which is predominantly irreversible. In contrast, cough in asthma is associated with reversible wheeze, is usually worse in the early hours, i.e. between 2 and 4 a.m., and causes sleep disturbance in many patients. Prolonged bouts of coughing in chronic bronchitis may give rise to cough syncope (p. 189).

TABLE 4.1 Cough		
Origin	**Common causes**	**Nature/characteristics**
Pharynx	Post-nasal drip	Usually persistent
Larynx	Laryngitis, tumour Whooping cough, croup	Harsh, barking, painful, persistent, associated with stridor
Trachea	Tracheitis	Painful
Bronchi	Bronchitis (acute and chronic, i.e. COPD)	Dry or productive. Worse in mornings
	Asthma	Dry or productive. Worse at night
	Bronchial carcinoma	Persistent (often with haemoptysis)
	Pneumonia	Dry initially, productive later
	Bronchiectasis	Productive. Changes in posture induce sputum production
	Pulmonary oedema	Often at night (may be productive of pink frothy sputum)
	End-stage interstitial fibrosis	Dry, irritant and distressing

The explosive quality of a normal cough is lost in patients with very severe airflow obstruction, respiratory muscle paralysis and vocal cord paralysis. Single vocal cord paralysis, usually the left, gives rise to a prolonged low-pitched inefficient and *bovine cough* – which is accompanied by hoarseness.

Sputum

All patients should be specifically asked about sputum. When present, further information should be obtained as to amount, character, viscosity and taste or odour.

Amount. This can seldom be accurately estimated by the patient, although statements that it is very large (e.g. a teacupful per day) or very small (one or two spits per day) are usually reliable. Most children and some adults swallow their sputum, even large amounts. The sound of the cough, if it is loose or moist, will, however, indicate that sputum is present. Other patients deny cough while admitting to the presence of sputum, saying that they bring it up merely by clearing the throat.

Character. This is seldom described accurately and, wherever possible, a specimen should be inspected. Apart from haemoptysis (coughing up blood), there are four main types of sputum: serous, mucoid, purulent and mucopurulent (Table 4.2). The term 'dirty spit' used by many patients is misleading as it may refer either to purulent sputum or to mucoid sputum containing soot particles. Mucoid sputum may be copious and frothy in COPD and asthma.

Viscosity. Mucoid sputum is often more viscous than purulent sputum and is more difficult to cough up. Sputum is particularly viscous in the early stages of pneumococcal pneumonia and in asthma. Serous sputum is watery with a low viscosity.

TABLE 4.2 Sputum		
Type	**Appearance**	**Cause**
Serous	Clear, watery, frothy, may be pink	Acute pulmonary oedema Bronchioalveolar cell carcinoma (rare)
Mucoid	Clear, grey, white, may be frothy or black (soot)	Chronic bronchitis, COPD Chronic asthma
Mucopurulent or purulent	Yellow, green, brown	All types of bronchopulmonary bacterial infection (eosinophils can cause sputum to appear purulent)
Rusty	Rusty, golden yellow	Pneumococcal pneumonia

Taste or odour. When this is described as 'nasty' the patient may merely be referring to the normal taste of purulent sputum. When sputum is foul tasting/smelling this suggests bronchiectasis, lung abscess or infection with anaerobic organisms. The clinician's own sense of smell should be used to assess odour.

Haemoptysis

Coughing up blood from the lower respiratory tract occurs in many disorders (Table 4.3). Although most patients know whether blood has been coughed up or vomited, haemoptysis is occasionally confused with haematemesis.

Whenever a history of haemoptysis is obtained, questions

TABLE 4.3 Causes of haemoptysis		
Common	**Uncommon**	**Others**
Pulmonary infarction*†	Mitral stenosis	Foreign body inhalation
Bronchial carcinoma*†	Aspergilloma	Chest trauma
Tuberculosis*	Bronchial adenoma	Iatrogenic
Bronchiectasis†	Tracheal tumours	Bronchoscopy
Lung abscess	Metastatic pulmonary malignant disease	Transbronchial biopsy
Acute bronchitis§	Laryngeal tumours	Transthoracic lung biopsy
Chronic bronchitis§		
COPD	Connective tissue diseases	
	Idiopathic pulmonary haemosiderosis	
	Goodpasture's syndrome	
	Blood dyscrasias and anticoagulation	
	Hypertension	

* Most important causes.
† Most common causes of frank/ massive haemoptysis.
§ Diagnosis assumed only after exclusion of other causes.

should be asked about its type, degree, frequency and duration. In some cases the events preceding it may be of importance in diagnosis, e.g. deep venous thrombosis in a lower limb or a respiratory infection.

Unless frank haemoptysis proves fatal, the blood becomes progressively darker for 48 hours or longer after the bleeding ceases. Regular frank haemoptysis or blood streaking of mucoid sputum, sometimes only in the mornings for a week or longer, strongly suggests a diagnosis of bronchial carcinoma. Recurrent episodes of haemoptysis over many years, usually associated with purulent sputum, are a feature of bronchiectasis.

When no cause can be found, the oropharynx should be examined for a source of bleeding. The blood is bright red at first but may later become dark red. It is often frothy and may be mixed with sputum.

Chest pain

Chest pain may be central (retrosternal) or lateral. Retrosternal chest pain is caused by disorders of the mediastinal structures, e.g. trachea, oesophagus, heart and great vessels. The most common medical cause of non-central chest pain is pleural disease. Pleural pain is recognised by its sharp, stabbing character and by its relationship to breathing and coughing. It is always made worse by deep breathing and coughing, in contrast to most causes of central chest pain except tracheitis. Disorders of the chest wall, e.g. fractured rib, often produce pain that is similar to pleural pain, but rib fracture produces localised chest wall tenderness, which is uncommon in pleural disease. Spontaneous pneumothorax can give rise to pleural pain and/or central chest discomfort.

Pleural pain is often excruciating and causes shallow breathing and suppression of coughing.

DISORDERS – Causes of chest pain
Non-central – pleural • Pneumonia • Pulmonary infarction • TB • Malignant disease
Non-central – chest wall • Rib fractures • Direct invasion of chest wall by tumour or rib metastatic lesions • Spinal nerve root involvement by vertebral disease (usually vertebral body collapse) and herpes zoster (p. 41) • Coxsackie B infection (Bornholm disease)
Retrosternal • Tracheitis • Mediastinal tumours • Acute mediastinitis • Mediastinal emphysema • Lesions of heart and great vessels (p. 73) • Oesophageal disorders (p. 151)

Breathlessness (dyspnoea)

Contributory factors

The complaint of shortness of breath (*dyspnoea*) indicates a conscious appreciation of increased work done during breathing and is a natural consequence of strenuous physical exercise. The principal factors contributing to the production of breathlessness are (a) an increase in the work of breathing, (b) increased ventilatory drive and (c) impaired respiratory muscle function. Each has a variety of causes. Several factors may operate in an individual patient to produce breathlessness. The clinical analysis of the breathless patient comprises both an assessment of the severity of breathlessness and identification of its cause.

In general, there is little correlation between the respiratory rate (*tachypnoea* is sometimes used to indicate rapid breathing) and the sensation of breathlessness. While some patients with severely impaired respiratory function may notice only slight breathlessness, others with minor respiratory dysfunction may be distressed by this symptom. Only when hypoxaemia is severe does it contribute to the sensation of breathlessness. Similarly, there is often little correlation between breathlessness and the severity of hypercapnia. Though a rise in arterial $Pa\text{CO}_2$ rapidly induces hyperventilation and breathlessness in healthy subjects, it may fail to do so in patients with chronic type II respiratory failure in whom the brain stem has become less responsive, or unresponsive, to changes of arterial $Pa\text{CO}_2$. Stimulation of pulmonary stretch receptors in the alveolar capillary walls (*J receptors*) may mediate the sensation of breathlessness in diseases such as pulmonary oedema, thromboembolism and pneumonia.

Breathlessness associated with increased work of breathing. The work of breathing is increased by airflow obstruction in either the small or large airways, decreased pulmonary compliance ('stiff lungs') and restricted chest expansion (Table 4.4).

TABLE 4.4 Increased work of breathing
Airflow obstruction Bronchial asthma Chronic bronchitis and emphysema Tracheal obstruction
Decreased pulmonary compliance Pulmonary oedema Pulmonary fibrosis Extrinsic allergic alveolitis
Restricted chest expansion Ankylosing spondylitis Respiratory muscle paralysis Kyphoscoliosis

Breathlessness associated with increased ventilatory drive. An increase in the physiological dead space (ventilation-perfusion mismatch) and increased stimulation of the respiratory centre (hyperventilation) may each contribute to an increase in ventilatory drive either singly or in combination, to produce breathlessness.

Increased physiological dead space occurs when ventilation and perfusion are mismatched. The net result is often an increase in respiratory rate (*tachypnoea*) and in depth of ventilation. Ventilation-perfusion mismatch occurs in a wide variety of disorders such as consolidation, collapse, pulmonary thromboembolism and pulmonary oedema.

Hyperventilation resulting from stimulation of the respiratory centre may occur in response to chemical or neural stimuli (see Table 4.5). Hyperventilation associated with emotional distress may produce respiratory alkalosis with decreased intracellular potassium, magnesium and alkali reserves and decreased ionisation of extracellular calcium. Breathing is often deep, irregular and sighing; patients may describe needing to take an extra breath or to breathe more deeply or an inability to fill the lungs completely. When hyperventilation is acute and sustained, tetany (p. 46) and even epilepsy may occur.

In the chronic hyperventilation syndrome (*effort syndrome*), the metabolic effects on neural and myoneural junctions may explain the spectrum of symptoms that may be observed though usually only a few features are present in any one patient (see Table 4.6).

TABLE 4.5 Chemical and neural stimulation of respiration

Increased arterial hydrogen ion concentration, e.g. metabolic acidosis producing 'air hunger' (*Kussmaul respiration*)

Increased arterial $Paco_2$, e.g. respiratory acidosis

Descreased arterial Pao_2 via aortic, carotid and brain stem chemoreceptors, e.g. pneumonia; impaired oxygen delivery due to anaemia, shock and stroke also stimulates the chemoreceptors

Increased central arousal, e.g. exertion, anxiety, thyrotoxicosis and phaeochromocytoma

Pulmonary J receptor discharge, e.g. pulmonary oedema

TABLE 4.6 Symptoms in chronic hyperventilation syndrome

- Lightheadedness, faintness and dizziness
- Dullness of hearing and tinnitus
- Peripheral and circumoral paraesthesiae
- Cold hands and feet and cold sweats
- Muscle cramps, muscle aches, trembling, shivering
- Constant tiredness and generalised weakness
- Breathlessness at rest with sighing and yawning
- Chest tightness, heaviness and palpitation
- Abdominal 'butterflies', cramps and bloating
- Urgency and frequency of defecation and micturition
- Restlessness, anxiety and panic attacks

TABLE 4.7 Specific factors producing breathlessness

Disorder	Factors
Pneumonia	Pyrexia stimulating respiratory centre Pleuritic pain limiting chest expansion Increased work – 'stiff lungs' Ventilation – perfusion mismatch Stimulation of pulmonary J receptors Hypoxaemia Low $Paco_2$ Septic shock
Pulmonary oedema	Ventilation – perfusion mismatch Increased work – 'stiff lungs' Hypoxaemia Low $Paco_2$ Cardiogenic shock Increased work – bronchiolar obstruction Hyperventilation – fear and anxiety

Breathlessness associated with impaired respiratory muscle function. Neuromuscular disorders may impair the function of the intercostal muscles and diaphragm to produce partial or complete respiratory paralysis. Examples include poliomyelitis, Guillain-Barré polyneuropathy, cervical cord transection, muscular dystrophies and myasthenia gravis.

Breathlessness associated with multiple factors. The pathophysiological mechanisms responsible for the production of dyspnoea in individual disease states are often complex and multifactorial (see Table 4.7).

Although pathophysiological considerations may help to explain the mechanisms of breathlessness, the cause of dyspnoea can often be assessed by obtaining a detailed history (see Table 4.8).

Clinical patterns

The cause of breathlessness is often indicated by the clinical pattern of its onset, duration and progression, variability, aggravating factors, relieving factors and its association with other symptoms.

TABLE 4.8 Checklist for the history of breathlessness

- Mode of onset – acute or gradual
- Exercise tolerance – daily activities
- Associated symptoms
  - Cough, sputum, haemoptysis
  - Wheeze, chest pain
- Past history of allergic, cardiac or respiratory disorder
- Occupation – exposure to dust, pollens, animals, chemicals
- Tobacco consumption – past and present
- Recent travel abroad

DISORDERS – Causes of breathlessness
Physiological ● Exercise ● High altitude
Pathological ● Obesity ● Anaemia ● Respiratory disorders ● Cardiac disorders
Psychological ● Hyperventilation
Pharmacological ● Drug-induced respiratory disorders ● Drug-induced cardiac disorders

TABLE 4.9 Modes of onset, duration and progression

Minutes to hours	Hours to days	Months to years
Pneumothorax	Pneumonia	Pulmonary TB
Acute asthma	Pleural effusion	Chronic bronchitis
Pulmonary oedema	Anaemia	Bronchial carcinoma
Pulmonary embolism	Guillain–Barré syndrome	Fibrosing alveolitis

Mode of onset, duration and progression. The principal patterns of breathlessness comprise rapid onset and progression over minutes, gradual onset and slow progression over days and slow onset and progression over months (see Table 4.9).

Variability, aggravating and relieving factors. Diurnal and day-to-day variability may be characteristic. Breathlessness which improves at the weekend or on holiday suggests occupational asthma or even extrinsic allergic alveolitis. In asthma, symptoms may be particularly striking after coughing or laughing or exertion or following exposure to smoke, dust, animal or plant allergens. Asthmatics usually complain of cough and wheeze as well as breathlessness.

Breathlessness which wakes the patient from sleep is a typical feature of asthma, pulmonary oedema (*paroxysmal nocturnal dyspnoea*) and severe chronic obstructive pulmonary disease (COPD). In cardiac failure and severe COPD, breathlessness is often brought on by lying flat, and many patients have to sleep in the sitting position propped up by pillows.

Associated symptomatology. The common symptoms associated with breathlessness include cough, wheeze, sputum, haemoptysis and chest pain. Their presence or absence associated with the acute onset of breathlessness will help to determine the likely diagnosis (see Table 4.10 and the Case history below).

TABLE 4.10 Acute breathlessness: diagnostic value of associated symptoms

With chest pain If lateralised and pleuritic consider Pneumonia Pulmonary infarction Rib fracture Pneumothorax	*Without chest pain, cough or wheeze* Pulmonary embolism Tension pneumothorax Hypovolaemic shock Metabolic acidosis
If central and non-pleuritic consider Myocardial infarction Massive pulmonary embolism	*Without chest pain but with cough and wheeze* Asthma Pulmonary oedema Pneumothorax

CASE HISTORY

A 55-year-old woman with a history of recurrent episodes of bronchitis as a child until the age of 16 was found on routine clinical examination to have significant hypertension. She had a family history of high blood pressure, hay fever and eczema. Her GP prescribed tablets for the treatment of her hypertension and within hours of taking the first tablet she became breathless, wheezy and developed chest tightness. She contacted her GP who visited her at home. On examination, the patient was sitting upright, obviously distressed and frightened and had a respiratory rate of 30 per minute. She was pale and sweaty, but not cyanosed, and numerous mainly high-pitched rhonchi (wheezes) were heard over all areas of her chest. She was told not to take any more of the tablets prescribed for hypertension, and her breathlessness and wheeze were treated with nebulised salbutamol and intravenous hydrocortisone.

The repeated episodes of 'bronchitis' as a child were likely to be asthma rather than bronchitis, and her history of hay fever, together with the family history of atopic disorders, was ignored when the GP prescribed treatment with beta-blockers for hypertension. Diagnosis: asthma precipitated by beta-blocker therapy.

Learning points

- Recurrent episodes of bronchitis in childhood disappearing during mid-teens are almost certainly asthma and not bronchitis.
- Never treat a patient with asthma or a history of having asthma with beta-blockers. Even the 'selective' beta-blockers can cause death if given to an asthmatic.

Severity

It is important to assess the severity of breathlessness in terms of daily activities. If these are impaired, the precise limiting factor should be identified. For example, the exercise tolerance of an elderly patient may be more limited by intermittent claudication, angina pectoris or osteoarthritic hips than by breathlessness attributable to chronic bronchitis. Though grading systems exist to assess cardiac and respiratory disabilities (see Table 4.11), simple questions about daily activity provide an effective functional assessment of the severity of dyspnoea (see Table 4.12).

TABLE 4.11 New York Heart Association classification: severity of heart failure

Grade I	No dyspnoea at rest or on moderate exertion
Grade II	Dyspnoea on moderate exertion No symptoms at rest or on mild exertion
Grade III	Dyspnoea on mild exertion but minimal at rest
Grade IV	Significant dyspnoea at rest and often bed bound Severe dyspnoea on minimal exertion

Note: Patients with major heart disease may have no, or only minor, symptoms, while patients with only minor heart disease may have major symptoms especially if they are anaemic, pregnant or anxious.

TABLE 4.12 Functional assessment of breathlessness

- Is sleep disturbed by breathlessness?
- Does breathlessness occur at rest?
- Does breathlessness interfere with normal conversation?
- Does dressing or washing produce breathlessness?
- How far can the patient walk on the flat without stopping?
- How many stairs can the patient climb without stopping?
- What activities are avoided because of breathlessness?

Apnoea

Apnoea or cessation of breathing can occur during life in a number of circumstances:

- Breath may be voluntarily held for short periods.
- Periods of apnoea alternate with overventilation in Cheyne-Stokes breathing (p. 132).
- Apnoea during sleep is of two main types:
  1. *Obstructive sleep apnoea* occurs when the upper airway is intermittently obstructed during sleep and is more often seen in obese short-necked adults who snore loudly.
  2. *Central sleep apnoea.* Breathing may occasionally cease for up to 10 seconds in healthy people. Pathological central sleep apnoea is rare but causes prolonged and frequent periods during which there is no activity of the respiratory muscles.

Wheeze

When a patient complains of wheeze it is important to discover what this implies. Some patients use the term merely to describe noisy and laboured breathing, while others apply it to the rattling of secretions in the upper air passages. Wheeze should, however, only be used to describe the musical sounds produced by the passage of air through narrowed bronchi. It is invariably louder during expiration and is often confined to that phase of the respiratory cycle. It is more conspicuous, and sometimes audible only, during deep breathing. Many patients become so accustomed to wheeze that they cease to be aware of its presence. Patients with stridor (see below) may describe it as wheeze. Care must be taken to distinguish between these two sounds because stridor is caused by partial obstruction of a major airway (e.g. laryngeal oedema, tumour or an inhaled foreign body), and requires urgent investigation and treatment.

Upper respiratory tract symptoms

Nose and nasopharynx. The most frequent symptoms of disease in the nose and nasopharynx are obstruction of the nasal airway, and nasal discharge often described by patients as 'catarrh'. These two symptoms often coexist.

Intermittent *nasal obstruction* is frequently caused by mucosal oedema and excessive secretions. Persistent obstruction is usually due to adenoidal enlargement, a deflected septum or to polypi. Bilateral nasal obstruction may lead to chronic mouth breathing, which, in children particularly, is often the reason for seeking medical advice.

Factors which precipitate recurrent nasal obstruction and discharge, e.g. the inhalation of dust or grass pollens, should be identified whenever possible. Enquiry should also be made about excessive *sneezing*, a common feature of allergic rhinitis, and *headache*, which may accompany acute infection of the nasal sinuses.

Epistaxis may give rise to apparent haemoptysis if blood in the posterior nares is inhaled and then coughed up.

Larynx. The two chief symptoms of laryngeal disease are hoarseness and stridor, but lesions of the larynx may also produce cough and pain. Stridor, and hoarseness which persist for more than a few days, should be fully investigated.

Hoarseness (*dysphonia*) may vary in degree from a slight harshness of the voice to complete loss (*aphonia*). The voice may have a croaking quality in hypothyroidism (p. 62). Enquiries should be made about the duration of hoarseness and about events which may have preceded its onset, such as a head cold, abuse of the voice, chronic cough or an operation on the neck or throat. It should be noted whether it is improving, worsening or remaining static.

Cough of a short, dry barking character almost invariably accompanies hoarseness caused by an organic lesion within the larynx. The bovine cough of laryngeal paralysis is described on page 211.

Laryngeal stridor is a high-pitched crowing sound occurring during inspiration. It may be produced by a foreign body lodged between the cords or by laryngeal spasm, exudate or oedema related to acute viral or bacterial infection. The sound is aggravated by coughing.

Laryngeal pain of mild degree occurs transiently in acute laryngitis; constant severe pain is a feature of advanced tuberculous laryngitis and laryngeal carcinoma.

Trachea. Diseases of the trachea may produce pain, cough, stridor and dyspnoea.

Tracheal pain is referred behind the sternal manubrium. In the early stages of acute tracheitis it may be severe and become momentarily intense on coughing but subsides soon after the cough becomes productive.

Tracheal stridor is usually due to obstruction by a malignant tumour and is always accompanied by breathlessness. It is lower in pitch than laryngeal stridor, is heard best during inspiration and is accentuated by coughing. Stridor may also be present when a tumour partially obstructs one or both main bronchi. If stridor is suspected the patient should be asked to cough and then breathe deeply in and out with the mouth wide open. Listening carefully, close to the patient's mouth during the first few breaths after coughing, can often confirm the presence of stridor at an early stage.

HISTORY OF PREVIOUS ILLNESS

Information of considerable value in diagnosis, prognosis and treatment of respiratory illness may be obtained from the past medical history. Important consequences of some previous medical events are shown in Table 4.13.

Previous radiological examination

If an abnormality is present on the chest radiograph, details of previous X-rays should be obtained since comparison with the earlier films, or at least the reports, is often of diagnostic value.

FAMILY, OCCUPATIONAL AND SOCIAL HISTORY

Family history

The family history of patients with respiratory disease may be significant in three ways:

- Certain *infections*, notably tuberculosis, may be transmitted from one person to another. Any history of contact with an infected person is, of course, more important than the family relationship.
- In *allergic disorders*, such as bronchial asthma, there is often an inherited predisposition, and a family history of eczema, hay fever and asthma is not uncommon.
- In *chronic bronchitis*, although an inherited predisposition cannot be excluded, the liability of several members of one family to develop the disease is more likely to be related to their living conditions and smoking habits.

Occupational history

A detailed history of all occupations and hobbies is essential. Numerous chemicals, moulds, organic dusts and animal proteins can cause asthma and allergic alveolitis. Non-organic particles such as silica, coal dust and asbestos are important causes of pneumoconiosis and malignant diseases.

TABLE 4.13 Previous history

History	Consequences and Comments
Tuberculosis	May have relapsed, caused bronchiectasis or a fungus ball (aspergilloma) may have formed in an old TB lung cavity
Pneumonia and pleurisy	May have caused bronchiectasis. Recurrent pneumonia and pleurisy may be caused by bronchiectasis, bronchial tumour, aspiration of oesophageal contents (achalasia of the cardia) or of pharyngeal secretions or vomit (bulbar palsy) and alcoholism. Immunological disorders such as hypogammaglobulinaemia and multiple myeloma should also be considered in patients with recurrent pneumonias
Measles and whooping cough	Can be complicated by pneumonia, particularly in early childhood, and cause 'wheezy bronchitis' or bronchiectasis
Wheezy bronchitis or recurrent bronchitis in childhood	In the past asthma in childhood was often diagnosed as bronchitis. Recurrence of asthma in adults who have a history of childhood asthma or wheezy bronchitis is common
Chest injuries	Traumatic haemothorax can give rise to gross pleural thickening which splints the lung ('frozen chest')
Recent general anaesthetic or loss of consciousness	Inhalation (aspiration) of oropharyngeal secretions or foreign body (e.g. tooth) can give rise to aspiration pneumonia or lung abscess
Pregnancy, recent travel, illness or surgery	Pulmonary embolism
Chest radiograph	Comparison of a recent chest radiograph with one taken in the past may be of great diagnostic value

Social history

A full social history should be taken as described on page 11 including enquiry about pets (mammals and birds) which may be the cause of rhinitis, asthma, allergic alveolitis and pneumonia (psittacosis). Information which should be obtained from all patients with chronic breathlessness includes the physical effort involved in any employment. With the more severely disabled it is vital to know about hills and steps leading to the home and stairs within it.

Cigarette smoking is the most important cause of bronchial carcinoma and COPD. Indeed both are rare in non-smokers though even 'passive smoking' may increase the liability. A smoking history should include the age when regular smoking started, the age when smoking was given up (where applicable) and the average consumption of tobacco (number of cigarettes or cigars per day, amount of tobacco per week). Patients often underestimate the amount;

the number of cigarettes bought each day or week is a useful guide to the number smoked!

KEY POINTS

- Cough causing sleep disturbance is common in asthma, rare in COPD unless it is severe.
- Small but frequent amounts of frank haemoptysis or blood-stained sputum suggest a diagnosis of bronchial carcinoma.
- Pleuritic pain is stabbing in nature and is aggravated by deep inspiration and coughing.
- Listening carefully close to the patient breathing deeply through an open mouth during the first few breaths after coughing can often confirm the presence of stridor at an early stage.
- The past history often provides valuable information regarding current respiratory symptoms.
- A smoking history should be obtained from all patients.
- A full history of present and previous occupations should be obtained from all patients.

THE PHYSICAL EXAMINATION

EXTERNAL FEATURES OF RESPIRATORY DISEASE

On first meeting the patient and during the history-taking process, a number of features may be evident which indicate or suggest the presence of respiratory disease. These include the features of hypoxia, evidence of dyspnoea or abnormalities in the state of hydration and nutrition. Examination of the skin may also yield information of considerable value in the diagnosis and assessment of respiratory problems. The cervical glands in general, and the scalene lymph nodes in particular, require careful examination. The latter group of nodes is within a pad of fat on the surface of the scalene anterior muscle, just in front of its insertion into the scalene tubercle of the first rib (Fig. 4.1). Other external features of respiratory disease may be found by examining the eyes and the hands in particular.

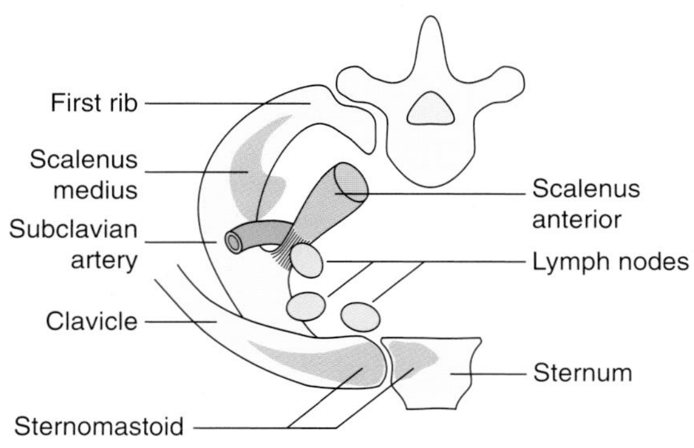

Fig. 4.1 Relation of lymph nodes to scalenus anterior.

Examination sequence

General

- ☐ Note the patient's general appearance, observe the rate and nature of breathing.
- ☐ Note any cough, wheeze or stridor and abnormality of the voice.
- ☐ Look for cyanosis, anaemia or polycythaemia and also for evidence of hypoxia and/or carbon dioxide retention.
- ☐ Look for other systemic features of respiratory disease including peripheral oedema and signs of right heart failure.

Finger clubbing

- ☐ Inspect the fingers laterally for loss of nail bed angle.
- ☐ To elicit fluctuation, place the finger on the pulp of the examiner's two thumbs and hold in this position by gentle pressure with the tips of the middle fingers over the proximal phalyngeal joint.
- ☐ Then palpate the finger over the base of the nail with the tips of the examiner's two index fingers (Fig. 4.2).

Cervical lymphadenopathy

- ☐ Examine for cervical lymphadenopathy as previously described (p. 59).
- ☐ Warn the patient of possible discomfort before examining for the scalene node. Then, with the patient's neck slightly flexed towards the side under examination, examine for the scalene node by dipping the palpating finger behind the clavicle, through the clavicular insertion of sternomastoid (Fig. 4.3).

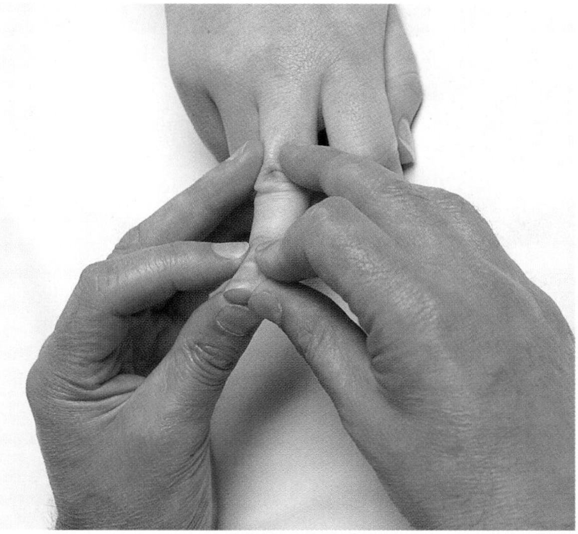

Fig. 4.2 Testing for fluctuation of the nail bed.

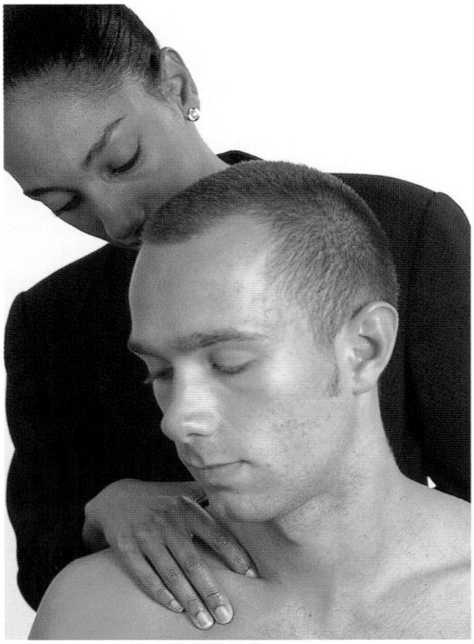

Fig. 4.3 Palpation of the right scalene lymph node. The patient should tilt the head forwards and to the right to relax the sternomastoid during the examination.

Abnormal findings. The speed with which a patient can dress or undress is often a useful index of respiratory disability. Evidence of recent weight loss may suggest malignancy or a chronic infective condition such as tuberculosis. Abnormality of the voice will occur in patients with a laryngeal nerve palsy (p. 211) and where there is chronic lung sepsis, e.g. bronchiectasis, there may be fetor of the breath.

Cyanosis. Central cyanosis of respiratory origin is most frequently seen in chronic obstructive pulmonary disease. In such cases peripheral vasodilatation due to carbon dioxide retention (type II respiratory failure) leads to warm blue hands, but the colour of the tongue is a more reliable indicator of central cyanosis. Central cyanosis may occur in many other diseases, including pneumonia, bronchial asthma, pulmonary infarction, allergic alveolitis and any disease causing pulmonary fibrosis but only when these conditions are severe or extensive. Peripheral cyanosis affecting the face and neck, and sometimes the upper limbs, is one of the features of superior venal caval obstruction (see below). Severe chronic hypoxia of either pulmonary or cardiac origin is often associated with polycythaemia and extreme degrees of cyanosis, partly central and partly peripheral.

The cardiac causes of cyanosis are described on page 81.

Oedema. The presence of peripheral oedema in patients with chronic obstructive airways disease suggests right ventricular failure as a consequence of pulmonary hypertension. Oedema of a different distribution is seen in *superior vena caval obstruction*. This is most commonly a complication of bronchial carcinoma. When the superior vena cava is obstructed, the jugular veins become grossly distended but no venous pulsation is visible in the neck. After a few days, dilated superficial veins and venules appear on the anterior and lateral aspects of the chest wall from the clavicles to below the costal margins (Fig. 4.4). These veins convey blood from the territories of the subclavian and axillary veins to the drainage area of the inferior vena cava. The face and neck become swollen and puffy – although the tissues seldom pit on pressure – and conjunctival oedema (chemosis) is often present. There may be pitting oedema of the hands and forearms. The dilated veins on the dorsum of the hand remain full when lifted well above the level of the suprasternal notch.

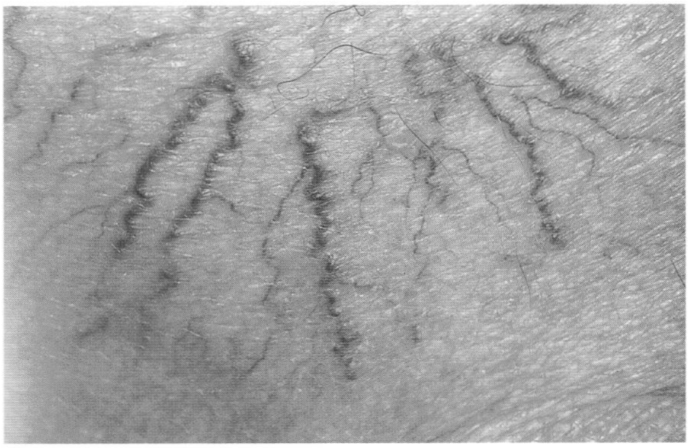

Fig. 4.4 Dilated superficial veins and venules in superior venal caval obstruction.

The hands. Clubbing of the fingers occurs in a variety of respiratory, cardiovascular and alimentary diseases (see Disorders box, p. 127). The swelling of the terminal phalanges in clubbing, which usually, but less obviously, affects the toes also, is due to interstitial oedema and dilatation of the arterioles and capillaries. The early features of clubbing comprise loss of the normal angle between the nail and nail bed and fluctuation of the nail bed.

The test is positive when the sensation of movement of the nail is greater than the very slight degree of fluctuation which can be detected in normal fingers. When fluctuation is marked, palpation of the nail itself may give the impression that it is floating free on its bed.

With more advanced degrees of clubbing, various visible changes develop progressively (Fig. 2.27A):

1. Swelling of the subcutaneous tissues over the base of the nail causes the overlying skin to become tense, shiny and red, with obliteration of the skin creases.

DISORDERS – Some causes of finger clubbing
Respiratory • Bronchial carcinoma • Intrathoracic suppuration – Bronchiectasis – Empyema – Lung abscess • Fibrosing alveolitis
Cardiovascular • Cyanotic congenital heart disease • Bacterial endocarditis
Alimentary • Hepatic cirrhosis • Ulcerative colitis • Crohn's disease • Coeliac disease
Congenital • Familial clubbing

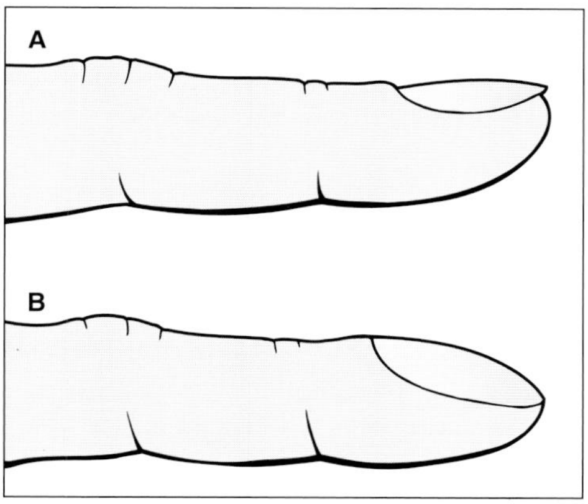

Fig. 4.5 Inspecting the nail bed angle. Note the difference between [A] normal and [B] clubbing, with loss of nail bed angle and increased curvature of the nail.

2. Later, as the swelling involves the nail bed, the curvature of the nail, especially in its long axis, increases (Fig. 4.5).
3. Finally, swelling of the pulp of the finger in all its dimensions occurs in fully developed clubbing. In a few cases there may also be *hypertrophic pulmonary osteoarthropathy* causing pain and swelling of the hands, wrists, knees, feet and ankles, with radiographic evidence of subperiosteal new bone formation.

Increased curvature of the fingernails may occur in normal subjects and, as an isolated phenomenon without other evidence of clubbing, is of no significance.

The neck. When a node is found it should be assessed as indicated on page 58. Nodes which are > 0.5 cm in diameter, firm in consistency and round in shape are usually pathological, a common cause being metastases from a bronchial carcinoma. Large, fixed masses are present in some cases. Hard, craggy nodes may, however, be caused by healed and calcified tuberculosis; in such cases calcification is visible on radiographic examination. Other pathological processes include lymphoma or sarcoidosis.

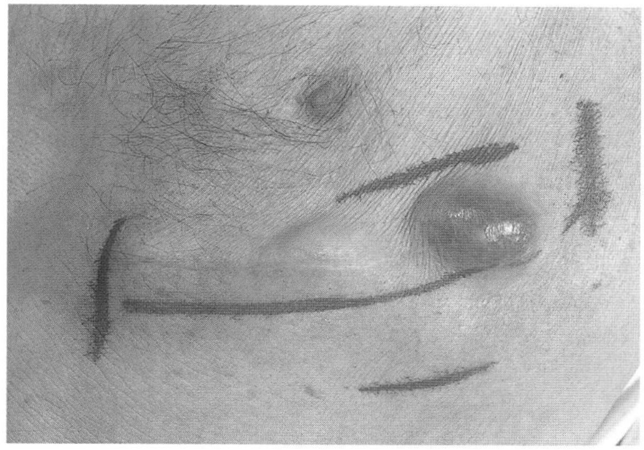

Fig. 4.6 Metastatic nodes of bronchial carcinoma over the left chest. (The red linear marks have been applied as radiotherapy markers.)

Other features. Some of the cutaneous and subcutaneous lesions associated with respiratory disease are listed in Table 4.14. Metastatic subcutaneous tumour nodules from bronchial carcinoma are shown in Figure 4.6. Examination of the eyes may reveal conditions implicating respiratory disease (see Table 4.15) such as Horner's syndrome (Fig. 6.9, p. 198). Where there is CO_2 retention, ophthalmoscopy may show either venous dilatation or, in extreme cases, papilloedema (see p. 255). In patients with severe type II respiratory failure, a flapping tremor of the hand is often present. When the arm is held outstretched with the wrists cocked upwards, a downward intermittent flap of the hands is noted.

TABLE 4.14 Skin lesions which may yield information of diagnostic importance

Erythema nodosum (Fig. 2.17A)	May be the initial clinical manifestation of tuberculosis and sarcoidosis
Metastatic tumour nodules (Fig. 4.6)	May be derived from a primary bronchial carcinoma
Cutaneous sarcoids and lupus pernio (Fig. 4.7)	May occur in association with intrathoracic sarcoidosis
Lupus erythematosus (Fig. 4.8)	May be associated with pulmonary or pleural manifestations
Herpetic vesicles (Fig. 2.19A)	May identify the cause of unilateral chest pain

TABLE 4.15 Examples of eye conditions in respiratory disorders

Condition	Disease
Horner's syndrome	Carcinoma of the bronchus
Phlyctenular keratoconjunctivitis	Primary tuberculosis
Iridocyclitis	Tuberculosis Sarcoidosis
Choroidal tubercles	Miliary tuberculosis
Chemosis, conjunctival and retinal vein dilatation (may develop papilloedema)	Hypercapnia Superior vena caval obstruction

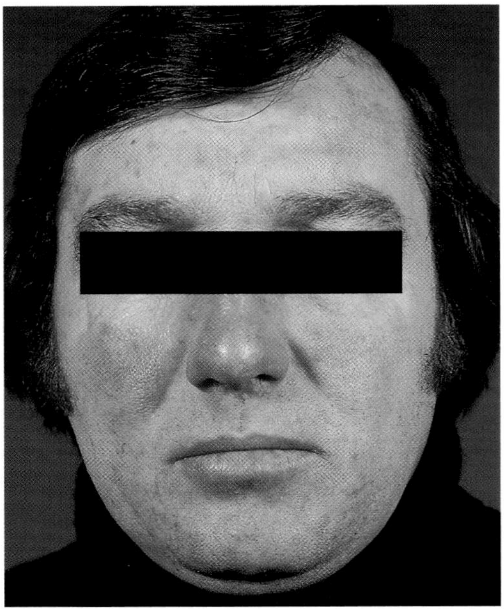

Fig. 4.7 Sarcoidosis associated with bilateral parotid swelling. The skin of the nose and right cheek is also involved ('lupus pernio').

THE UPPER RESPIRATORY TRACT

Anatomy

The upper respiratory tract extends from the external nares to the junction of the larynx with the trachea. It includes the nasal cavity, the nasopharynx, the nasal sinuses, the oropharynx and the larynx. Clinical examination of the nose, throat and mouth is an essential part of the assessment of patients with respiratory disease.

In normal subjects, the upper 4–5 cm of the trachea can be felt in the neck between the cricoid cartilage and the suprasternal notch, but in thick-set or obese subjects it may be so deeply placed that it is difficult or even impossible to feel.

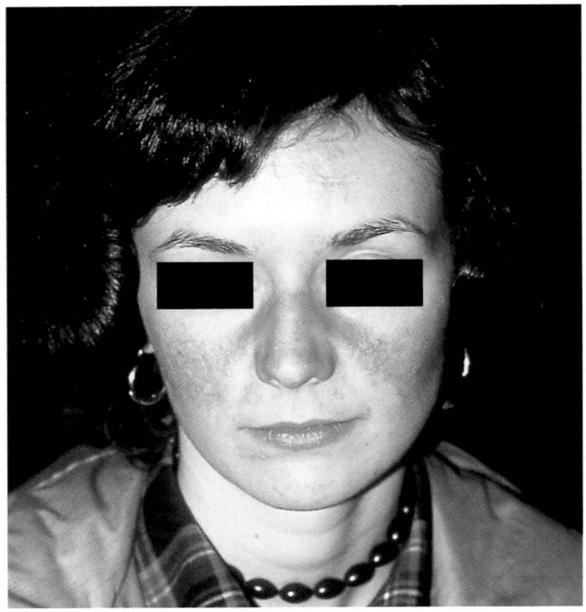

Fig. 4.8 The characteristic rash of systemic lupus erythematosus.

Examination sequence

- ☐ Examine the nose, throat and mouth as previously described (pp. 51 and 53).
- ☐ To examine for sinusitis, press over the frontal and maxillary sinuses in turn, asking the patient to report any tenderness.

The trachea

- ☐ Examine the thyroid gland before localising the trachea.
- ☐ To identify the position of the trachea, gently introduce the tip of the index finger into the suprasternal notch exactly in the midline and press gently against the trachea (Fig. 4.9). If the trachea is deviated the finger will slip partially or completely past it on the side opposite to the displacement.
- ☐ To measure the cricosternal space/distance, insert one or two fingers between the cricoid cartilage and the suprasternal notch.

Abnormal findings

Infective and allergic disorders of the upper respiratory tract are very common and infection may produce or aggravate disease of the bronchi and lungs. Oral sepsis, particularly suppurative gingivitis, may cause pulmonary disease, such as lung abscess. Tenderness over the nasal sinuses often indicates infective sinusitis.

A

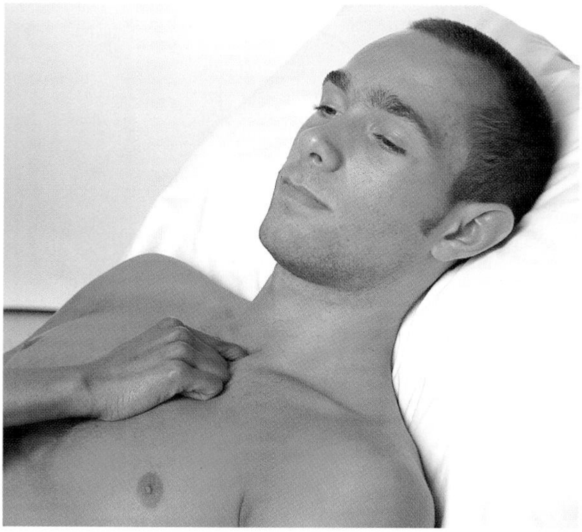

B

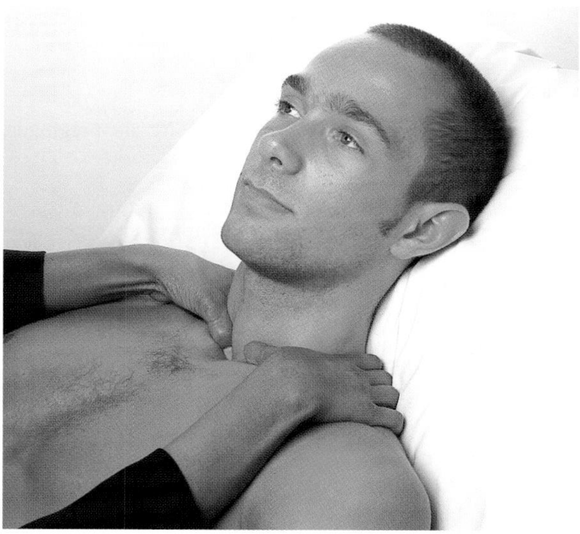

Fig. 4.9 Examining the trachea. [A] Using one finger. [B] Using both thumbs, a technique which is **not** recommended by the chapter author.

The larynx

External examination of the larynx seldom yields useful information, but swelling of the lips, the tongue, around the eyes and in the front of the neck caused by a hypersensitivity reaction (angioneurotic oedema) may be associated with oedema involving the larynx (see Fig. 2.11A). This may give rise to breathlessness and stridor which may proceed to complete respiratory obstruction. Examination of the larynx is best undertaken by fibreoptic laryngoscopy. It is an essential step in the investigation of hoarseness. Lesions that can be detected include laryngeal tumours, laryngeal

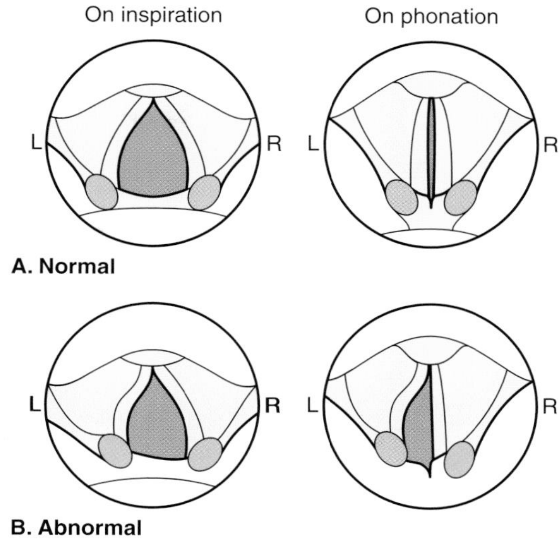

Fig. 4.10 The vocal cords. Diagrammatic representation of the laryngoscopic views of vocal cord movements showing: [A] normal movements; [B] movements in the presence of recurrent laryngeal nerve paralysis most commonly caused by bronchogenic carcinoma. Note that the paralysed left cord is in the cadaveric position (between inspiration and expiration).

tuberculosis and vocal cord paralysis. Paralysed cord adopts a position midway between abduction and adduction and fails to adduct on phonation (Fig. 4.10). Paralysis of abduction may precede complete cord paralysis. Unilateral vocal cord paralysis causes hoarseness and bovine cough. Bilateral cord paralysis causes stridor.

The trachea

Tracheal displacement by an enlarged thyroid gland should be excluded before attributing any tracheal deviation to intrathoracic disease. Sometimes the trachea is displaced by a superior mediastinal mass including lymphoma and carcinoma, or by a massive effusion. More frequently, tracheal deviation is caused by collapse of the lung or upper lobe, or fibrosis pulling the trachea towards the pathological side. Apical fibrosis is most commonly caused by tuberculosis. In patients with chronic airflow obstruction there is a downward movement of the trachea during inspiration. This may greatly reduce the distance between the cricoid cartilage and the suprasternal notch (the cricosternal space).

KEY POINTS

- Loss of the nail bed angle and increased fluctuation are early signs of finger clubbing.
- In patients with possible respiratory disease, the neck should be examined from the back, one side at a time, for lymphadenopathy with special attention to the scalene regions.

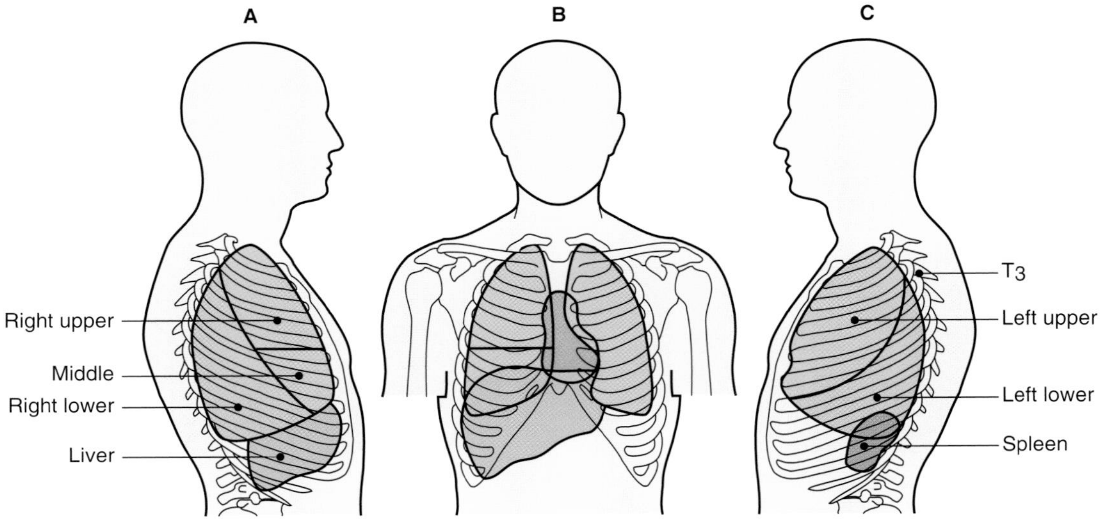

Fig. 4.11 Surface markings of the lungs and underlying viscera: A right lateral; B anteroposterior; C left lateral.

THE CHEST

Physical examination of the chest makes use of the techniques of inspection, palpation, percussion and auscultation.

Surface anatomy

In health, the trachea is central and the apex beat is in the normal place (see p. 90).

The surface markings of the lungs are shown in Figure 4.11. The upper lobes are primarily in the front of the chest and the lower lobes are predominantly posterior, with the apex of the lower lobes at the level of the 4th thoracic vertebra, 3rd spinous process.

Respiratory movements

In normal subjects the two sides of the chest move to an equal extent with respiration.

Respiratory frequency at rest in a healthy adult is about 14 respirations per minute. The depth of respiration is difficult to assess clinically because movements of the chest and diaphragm, on which it is dependent, cannot be accurately measured. Indeed, chest expansion does not correlate well with vital capacity, probably because some subjects' breathing is predominantly diaphragmatic. A difference of more than 5 cm between full expiration and full inspiration can, however, be regarded as normal.

Most women make more use of the intercostal muscles than of the diaphragm and, therefore, respiratory movements are predominantly thoracic. Men rely more on the diaphragm and their respiratory movements at rest are mainly abdominal. Babies of both sexes are also predominantly diaphragmatic breathers.

Examination sequence

- ☐ Examine the patient with chest and upper abdomen fully exposed and evenly illuminated.
- ☐ Surreptitiously count the number of breaths in a full minute by observing the chest movements with the fingers held on the pulse.
- ☐ Examine the front and sides of the chest with the patient lying in a semirecumbent position on a bed or couch and with the arms sufficiently abducted to allow access to the axillary regions.
- ☐ Note the mode of breathing and the presence of any abnormal inspiratory or expiratory movements.
- ☐ Compare the range of respiratory movements on the two sides during normal and deep breathing.
- ☐ To compare the range of movement in the infraclavicular regions, position the patient supine, shoulders relaxed and symmetrical with the head resting on a pillow and the head and trunk in a straight line. Then ask the patient to take deep steady breaths while viewing the infraclavicular regions tangentially.
- ☐ Examine breathless patients semirecumbent or sitting if they are made more dyspnoeic when lying flat.
- ☐ Assess lower anterior movements by inspecting the patient semirecumbent and breathing deeply.
- ☐ Examine the posterior aspect of the chest with the patient sitting upright with arms folded across the chest and remove any pillows to allow unimpeded access to the whole of the back.

- ☐ Allow patients too weak to maintain this position to lean forward with arms resting on pillows or hold them forward for assistance.
- ☐ Assess chest movements posteriorly with the patient sitting erect. Careful inspection gives at least as much information as trying to assess chest expansion by palpation.
- ☐ Palpate the chest wall for localised skin and bony lesions and to determine the cardiac apex and the position of the trachea.
- ☐ Record with a tape measure the maximum inspiratory/expiratory difference in the lower chest.

Common abnormalities

Abnormalities in the shape of the chest

Those of clinical importance are as follows.

Increase in anteroposterior diameter. In some patients with emphysema, the posterior AP diameter is increased and the two measurements may approximate (barrel chest). The degree of chest deformity in emphysema is not a reliable guide to the severity of the functional defect. An increase in anteroposterior diameter may also be due to thoracic kyphosis unrelated to respiratory disease (Fig. 4.12).

Thoracic kyphoscoliosis. This ranges in degree from the minor changes in spinal curvature seen in many otherwise healthy subjects to grossly disfiguring and disabling deformities (Fig. 4.12). Thoracic scoliosis may alter the position of the mediastinum in relation to the anterior chest wall, with the result that abnormalities in the position of the trachea and the apex beat may be mistakenly attributed to heart or pulmonary disease. Severe kyphoscoliosis may have profound effects on pulmonary function, as the chest deformity reduces the ventilatory capacity of the lungs and increases the work of breathing (p. 120). Such patients may develop hypoxaemia, hypercapnia and heart failure at an early age.

Pectus carinatum (pigeon chest). This is a common sequel of chronic respiratory disease, usually asthma, in childhood (Fig. 4.13). It consists of a localised prominence of the sternum and adjacent costal cartilages, often accompanied by indrawing of the ribs to form symmetrical horizontal grooves (*Harrison's sulci*) above the costal margins, which are themselves usually everted. These deformities are thought to result from lung hyperinflation with repeated strong contractions of the diaphragm while the bony thorax is still in a pliable state. Pectus carinatum deformity may also be caused by rickets or be present for no obvious reason.

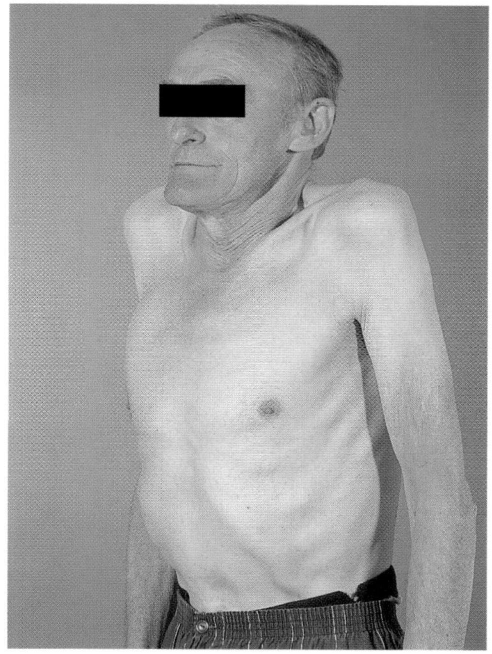

Fig. 4.12 Kyphoscoliosis.

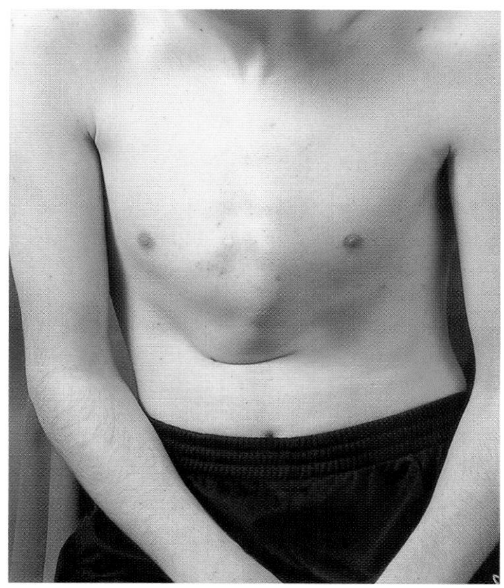

Fig. 4.13 Pigeon chest deformity (pectus carinatum).

Pectus excavatum (funnel chest). In this developmental defect there is either a localised depression of the lower end of the sternum (Fig. 4.14), or, less commonly, depression of the whole length of the body of the sternum and of the costal cartilages attached to it. Pectus excavatum is usually asymptomatic, but, when there is a very marked degree of depression of the sternum, the heart may be displaced to the left, and the ventilatory capacity of the lungs restricted.

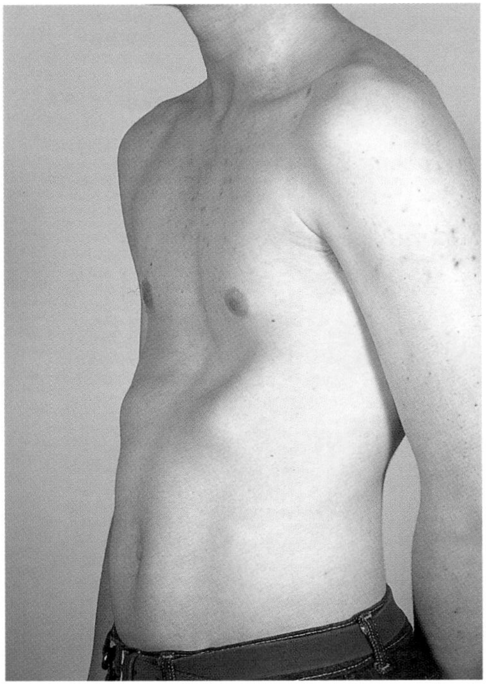

Fig. 4.14 Funnel chest deformity (pectus excavatum).

Thoracic operations. Surgery may result in varying degrees of chest deformity as may severe chest trauma.

Lesions of the chest wall

Abnormalities which may be detected by combined inspection and palpation of the chest wall are listed in Table 4.16. The nature of skin and subcutaneous nodules may have to be determined by aspiration or biopsy.

Subcutaneous emphysema (air in subcutaneous tissues) is recognised by the characteristic crackling sensation elicited by palpation of the air-containing tissues. It may cause diffuse swelling of the chest wall, neck and face. Subcutaneous emphysema is a common complication of intercostal tube drainage of a pneumothorax. In severe asthma, air may track into the mediastinum (mediastinal emphysema) via ruptured alveoli or bronchioli. The air usually escapes innocuously into the neck, and even when there is marked mediastinal and subcutaneous emphysema it is not in itself dangerous. When air is present in the mediastinum, the heart sounds may be obscured by a churning noise accentuated during cardiac systole.

Abnormalities of respiratory movements

Respiratory frequency. Respiratory rate is increased in a variety of pathological states, including pyrexia, acute pulmonary infections, chest wall and pleural pain, and conditions in which there is an increase in the work of breathing, e.g. bronchial asthma and acute pulmonary oedema.

TABLE 4.16 Lesions of the chest wall

Cutaneous lesions	Skin eruptions, sarcoid nodules, purpuric spots (Fig. 2.1D), bruises, scars, discharging sinuses
Subcutaneous lesions	Inflammatory swellings, metastatic tumour nodules, sebaceous cysts, sarcoid nodules, neurofibromas (Fig. 2.41), lipomas
Subcutaneous emphysema	Pneumothorax, severe asthma
Vascular anomalies	Spider naevi, enlarged vascular channels (arterial in coarctation of the aorta; venous in superior vena caval obstruction)
Localised prominences and deformities	Clavicles, scapulae, sternum, ribs, costochondral junctions, spinous processes
Localised tenderness	Fractured rib, tumour involving chest wall, spinal nerve root disorders
Lesions of breast (p. 67)	
Enlargement of axillary lymph nodes (p. 59)	

Respiratory depth. Although difficult to assess accurately, it is usually possible to recognise marked degrees of overventilation and underventilation. The latter may be of considerable importance in the recognition of type II respiratory failure.

In massive pulmonary embolism and in metabolic acidosis, usually due to diabetic ketoacidosis or uraemia, pulmonary ventilation at rest may be considerably raised. This can be recognised by an increase in the depth of respiration (*air hunger*) which may give rise to the subjective sensation of breathlessness. In *periodic* or *Cheyne-Stokes breathing* there is a cyclical variation in the depth of respiration, with overventilation alternating with periods during which breathing ceases (apnoea). This occurs in certain neurological conditions, particularly those involving the medulla, and in some patients with cardiac failure.

Chest expansion. A measured maximum chest expansion of 2 cm or less is definitely abnormal. Chest expansion is diminished in almost every type of diffuse bronchopulmonary disease, e.g. bronchial asthma, emphysema and pulmonary fibrosis, and in conditions which restrict movement of the ribs, such as ankylosing spondylitis.

Mode of breathing. If respiratory movements are exclusively thoracic, this may be because diaphragmatic movement is inhibited by abdominal pain or restricted by increased intra-abdominal pressure caused by ascites, gaseous distension of the bowel, a large ovarian cyst or pregnancy. If respiratory movements are exclusively abdominal, ankylosing spondylitis, intercostal paralysis or pleural pain may be responsible for the lack of chest expansion.

Reduced expansion. Unilateral reduction of chest wall expansion occurs in many types of respiratory disease. In pleural effusion (see Fig. 4.20) and empyema, expansion may be absent. If the condition is chronic and has resulted in pleural thickening and fibrosis, retraction of the ribs and intercostal spaces may produce flattening of the affected side of the chest. This is sometimes described as a 'frozen chest'. Less marked reduction of expansion occurs in pulmonary consolidation and collapse. In pneumothorax (see Fig. 4.22D) the limitation of expansion is related to the amount of air in the pleural space; in tension pneumothorax, the affected side of the chest may be immobilised in a position of almost full inspiration. In pulmonary tuberculosis, even extensive lesions may have little effect on chest wall expansion during the early stages of the disease, but when fibrosis develops there may be severe restriction of expansion, with flattening of the affected side of the chest.

In bronchial asthma, emphysema and diffuse pulmonary fibrosis, expansion of the chest wall is symmetrically reduced. In the first two conditions this results from overinflation of the lungs. In diffuse pulmonary fibrosis, on the other hand, inspiratory movement is restricted by the reduced distensibility of the lungs. In severe cases, this may bring each inspiration to an abrupt halt and produce the phenomenon of 'doorstep' breathing.

Increased movements. Although breathlessness is a subjective sensation, it is usually accompanied by objective evidence of respiratory difficulty or distress. There is often an increase in respiratory frequency, which may be accompanied by dilatation of the alae nasi during inspiration. This may be observed in the absence of breathlessness and is not reliable evidence of respiratory distress. A much more useful clinical guide is the presence of abnormal increase of respiratory movements of the following types:

- *Abnormal inspiratory movements* produced by contraction of the cervical muscles (principally the sternomastoids, scaleni and trapezii), by which the whole thoracic cage is, in effect, lifted off the diaphragm with every inspiration. Patients breathe in this way if adequate pulmonary ventilation cannot be achieved by normal inspiratory efforts, for example when there is gross overdistension of the lungs in advanced emphysema and severe bronchial asthma. More violent inspiratory movements of a similar character are observed in patients with obstruction of the larynx or trachea. Indrawing of the suprasternal and supraclavicular fossae, the intercostal spaces and the epigastrium with each inspiration invariably accompanies airways obstruction of this type, which is also seen, although usually less conspicuously, in COPD and severe asthma.

  A much more striking degree of localised indrawing of the chest wall is seen in patients who have sustained double fractures of a series of ribs or of the sternum. The portion of the thoracic cage between the fractures become mobile and is sucked in with every inspiration. Paradoxical movement of this type interferes seriously with pulmonary ventilation and may cause grave respiratory distress and hypoxaemia.
- *Abnormal expiratory movements* are produced by powerful contractions of the abdominal muscles and latissimus dorsi. These are observed if the elastic recoil of the lungs is insufficient to complete the expulsion of air from the alveoli, as in emphysema, or when severe expiratory airflow obstruction is present as in bronchial asthma and some cases of COPD. Patients with a severe degree of expiratory obstruction prefer to be upright, grasping a bed table or the back of a chair. This enables them to fix the shoulder girdle so that the latissimus dorsi can be used to augment the expiratory efforts. Many patients, especially those with emphysema and with acute

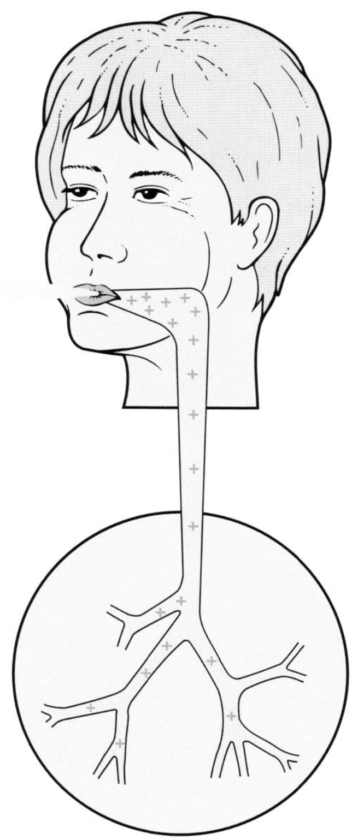

Fig. 4.15 Purse-lip breathing.

exacerbations of COPD, exhale through their mouths with pursed lips (Fig. 4.15). This manoeuvre helps to keep the intrabronchial pressure above that within the surrounding alveoli and reduces or prevents collapse of the bronchial wall which would otherwise result from the unopposed pressure of air trapped in the alveoli.

KEY POINTS

- Chest deformity in emphysema is not a reliable guide to the severity of the functional disability.
- Severe kyphoscoliosis may have a profound effect on pulmonary function.
- Much more reliance should be given to inspection than palpation in detecting differences in the range of expansion on the two sides of the chest.
- Localised impairment of respiratory expansion is usually caused by underlying lung or pleural disease.
- Chest expansion is often much diminished in patients with increased vertical chest movements, e.g. exacerbation of severe COPD.

Percussion

The object of percussion is to compare the degree of resonance over equivalent areas on the two sides of the chest, and to map out any area of abnormality to the percussion note (Table 4.17).

Anatomical considerations

The regions of the thorax over which a resonant percussion note is normally found correspond approximately to the surface marking of the lungs (Fig. 4.11). Percussion over the heart or the liver will elicit a dull note, but the area of dullness is less extensive than would be expected from anatomical surface markings, since aerated lung is interposed between part of the viscus and the chest wall.

TABLE 4.17 Percussion note

Type	Detected over
Tympanitic	Hollow viscus
Hyperresonant	Pneumothorax
Resonant	Normal lung
Impaired	Pulmonary consolidation Pulmonary collapse Pulmonary fibrosis
Dull	Pulmonary consolidation Pulmonary collapse Pulmonary fibrosis
Stony dull	Pleural effusion

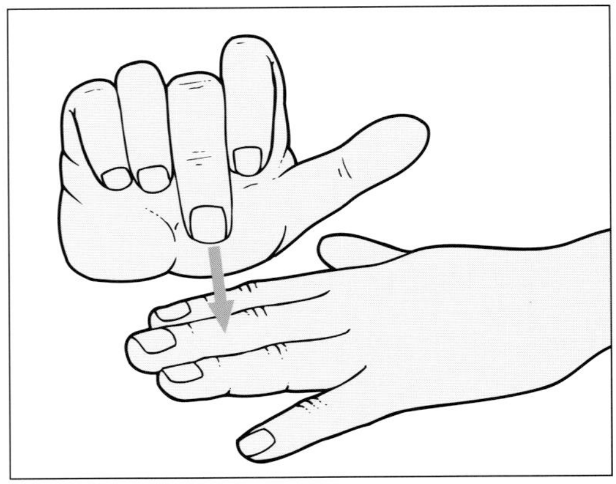

Fig. 4.16 Technique of percussion.

Examination sequence

The basic technique of percussion for a right-handed clinician is as follows:

- ☐ Place the left hand on the chest wall, palm downwards, fingers slightly separated with the second phalanx of the middle finger over the area to be percussed, usually an intercostal space.
- ☐ Firmly press the left middle finger against the chest wall.
- ☐ Strike the centre of the second phalanx with the tip of the right middle finger held at a right angle (to produce a 'hammer' effect) and with the entire movement coming from the wrist joint (Fig. 4.16).
- ☐ Compare the note obtained from identical sites on the two sides.
- ☐ Map out any area of impaired resonance (including cardiac and hepatic dullness, p. 167) by percussing from a resonant to a dull area.

Practical considerations

The positions in which the percussion note on the two sides should be compared are as follows:

- Anterior chest wall (Fig. 4.17): (a) clavicle; (b) infra-clavicular region; (c) second to sixth intercostal spaces.
- Lateral chest wall (Fig. 4.17): fourth to seventh intercostal spaces.
- Posterior chest wall (Fig. 4.18): (a) trapezius, percussing downwards over the lung apex; (b) above the level of spine of scapula; (c) at intervals of 4–5 cm from below the level of spine of scapula down to the eleventh rib.

The lung apices are percussed by placing the left middle finger across the anterior border of the trapezius muscle, overlapping the supraclavicular fossa, and directing the percussion downwards (Fig. 4.19). Percussion over the

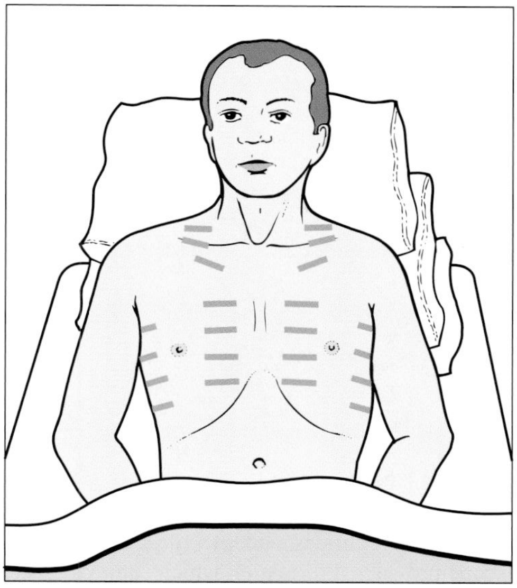

Fig. 4.17 Sites for percussion – anterior and lateral chest wall.

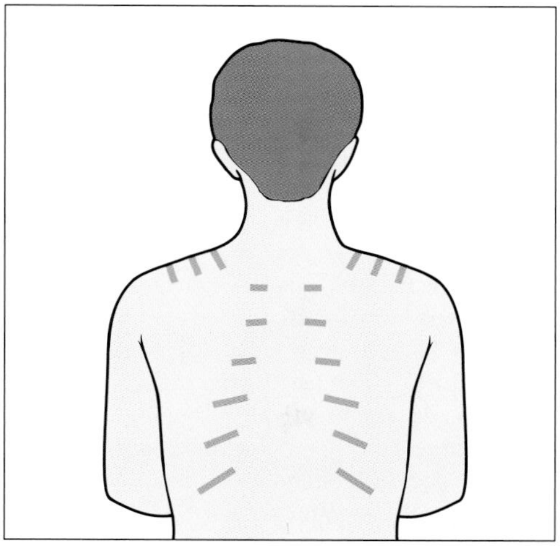

Fig. 4.18 Sites for percussion – posterior chest wall.

clavicle may be of value in detecting lesions of the upper lobe using the same technique of percussion of the chest wall because direct percussion of the clavicle may cause pain. The correct situation for percussion is within the medial third of the clavicle just lateral to its expanded medial end. Percussion more laterally will merely elicit the dullness produced by the muscle masses of the shoulder.

Tidal percussion. A crude impression of the range of diaphragmatic movement can be obtained by measuring the distance between the lower border of pulmonary resonance at the back of the chest in full inspiration and forced expiration, but this procedure is of little practical value.

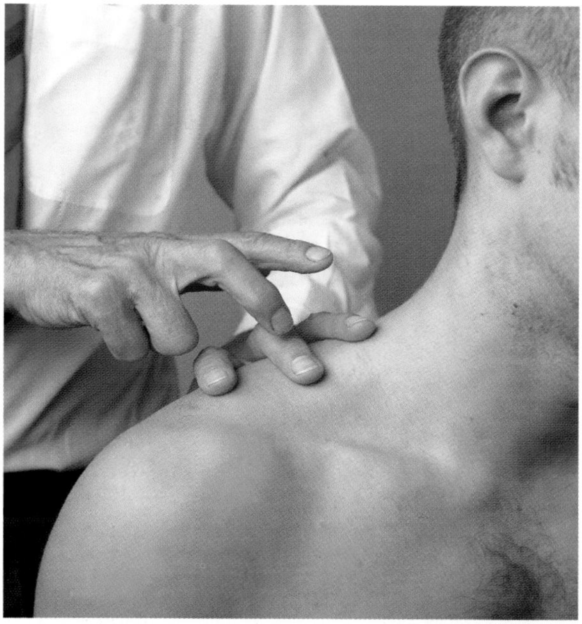

Fig. 4.19 Percussing the right apex from behind.

Common abnormalities

The terms used to describe different types of percussion notes are shown in Table 4.17.

Hyperresonance. Hyperresonance may be found over the lung which is markedly emphysematous, over a large thin-walled pulmonary cavity and also over a pneumothorax, particularly if the pleural pressure is above atmospheric level. An apparent finding of generalised hyperresonance should be accepted only with reservation, since a change in the absolute pitch of a percussion note is difficult to recognise and may depend mainly upon the thickness of the chest wall. It is not usually advisable to attempt to distinguish between normal resonance and hyperresonance when the percussion note is equally resonant on the two sides.

Dullness. The percussion note loses its normal resonance whenever aerated lung tissue is separated from the chest wall by pleural fluid or thickening, or when lung tissue is rendered airless by consolidation, collapse or fibrosis. Over such lesions the percussion note is impaired or dull. The most marked degree of dullness on percussion is associated with a large pleural effusion.

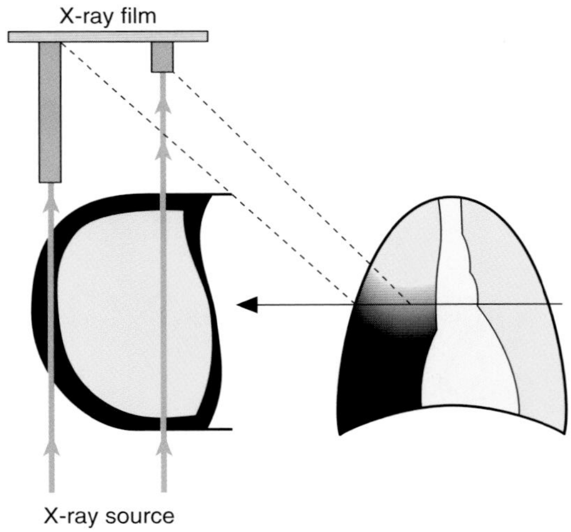

Fig. 4.20 Radiographic appearances of a right pleural effusion. A horizontal section of hemithorax close to the upper margin of the effusion (represented by the horizontal arrow) shows that there is at this site a similar amount of liquid anteriorly, posteriorly and laterally. However, because of the shape of the hemithorax, the X-ray beams traverse more fluid laterally than they do centrally. This produces the characteristic radiographic shape of a pleural effusion shadow with a curved upper margin ascending towards the axilla.

When an abnormality of the percussion note is due to pulmonary consolidation or collapse it is usually possible to identify the lobe or lobes involved by reference to the surface marking of the fissures but, unless a lobe is totally consolidated, the area over which the percussion note is impaired is often much smaller than would be expected from its surface marking. This is even more striking when a lobe is collapsed. With a pleural effusion the area of dullness on percussion is unrelated to the surface anatomy of the lobes. Except with loculated effusions, it is situated over the lower part of the hemithorax with the patient in the upright position. Pleural effusions of considerable size may not be detected during examination of the anterior chest when the patient is in a semirecumbent position because gravity causes the pleural liquid to accumulate posteriorly. When there are no pleural adhesions the radiograph shows an effusion to have a curved upper border, which misleadingly suggests more fluid being present laterally (Fig. 4.20).

In localising the position of a pulmonary or pleural lesion, use should be made of the breath sounds and voice sounds in addition to the percussion note. However, small lesions, such as areas of segmental consolidation or collapse, may not produce any abnormal physical signs. Even with larger lesions the signs may be partly or completely obscured if the lungs are emphysematous.

KEY POINTS

- Always compare identical sites on the two sides.
- The percussion note is impaired or dull whenever aerated lung is separated from chest wall by pleural fluid or thickening, or when lung tissue is rendered airless by consolidation, collapse or fibrosis.
- General hyperresonance on both sides is rarely of diagnostic significance.
- Areas of impaired percussion are often smaller than anticipated from the surface markings.
- Map out areas of impaired resonance by percussing from resonant to dull.

Auscultation

Auscultation of the lungs is important in the diagnosis of certain respiratory diseases, but is of little or no value in others. In the alveolitides and pleurisy, for example, the stethoscope provides information which cannot be obtained in any other way. In contrast, auscultation is unhelpful in the early diagnosis of pulmonary tuberculosis, which may reach an advanced stage before any abnormality can be detected.

The information which should be obtained from auscultation is listed in Table 4.18.

Technique of auscultation

The design of the stethoscope recommended for routine clinical use provides the choice of a bell or diaphragm. As most of the sounds reaching the chest wall from the bronchi and lungs are in the low-frequency range, the bell with a rubber rim cover should normally be used in preference to the diaphragm. Another reason for selecting the bell is that stretching of the skin and hairs under the diaphragm during deep breathing is apt to produce sounds which may be difficult to distinguish from a pleural rub and/or crackles. It is also impossible in some thin patients to achieve full contact between the diaphragm and the skin of the chest wall and where this is the case, nothing may be heard.

Breath sounds and voice sounds

Breath sounds are produced by vibrations of the vocal cords caused by the turbulent flow of air through the larynx

TABLE 4.18 Information obtained from auscultation

- The type and amplitude of breath sounds
- The type and number of any added sounds and their position in the respiratory cycle
- The quality and amplitude of the conducted voice sounds

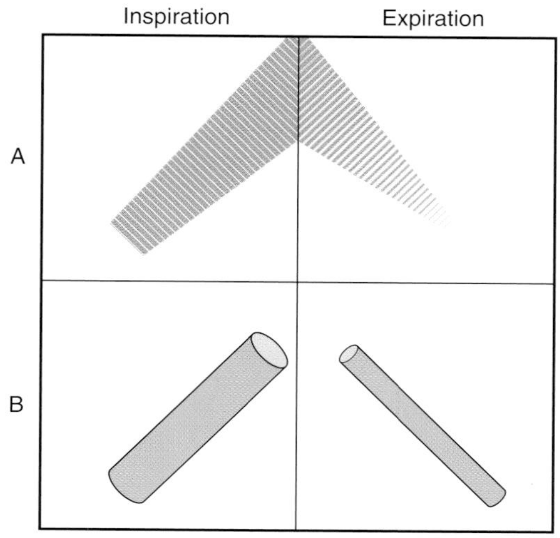

Fig. 4.21 Diagrammatic representation of breath sounds. [A] Vesicular; [B] Bronchial.

during breathing. The sounds so produced are transmitted along the trachea and bronchi and through the lungs to the chest wall. In their passage through normal lungs the intensity and frequency pattern of the sounds are decreased since normal alveoli transmit sounds poorly. When they are heard through a stethoscope on the chest wall they have a characteristic rustling quality to which the term *vesicular* is applied. The intensity of the sounds increases steadily during inspiration and then quickly fades away during the first one-third of expiration (Fig. 4.21).

Speech and other voice sounds are also conducted and are audible through a stethoscope. Auscultation within 2–3 cm of the midline, either anteriorly or posteriorly, may give misleading information in regard to the type of breath sounds and voice sounds, particularly in the upper half of the chest where the stethoscope may pick up sounds transmitted directly from the trachea and main bronchi to the chest wall. It follows that bronchial breath sounds (see below) heard in these situations should be disregarded in the absence of other pathological signs.

Examination sequence

- ☐ Perform auscultation with the patient relaxed and breathing deeply and fairly rapidly through the mouth.
- ☐ Avoid prolonged deep breathing, which may cause giddiness or even tetany.
- ☐ Avoid auscultation within 2–3 cm of the midline.
- ☐ Auscultate the two sides alternately, comparing findings over a large number of equivalent positions to ensure that small localised abnormalities are not missed.
- ☐ Auscultate in two stages; compare first the amplitude of breath sounds and then the vocal resonance.
- ☐ Auscultate anteriorly from above the clavicle down to the sixth rib, laterally from the axilla to the eighth rib and posteriorly down to the level of the eleventh rib.
- ☐ In each area listen in turn to the quality and amplitude of inspiration of the inspiratory phase and then to the expiratory phase. Identify if there is a gap between the two and listen for added sounds.
- ☐ If necessary, repeat after coughing.
- ☐ Assess the quality and amplitude of vocal resonance by asking the patient to say 'one, one, one' and, if resonance is increased, ask the patient to whisper (whispering pectoriloquy, p. 139).

Special situations

- ☐ If there is difficulty in distinguishing between a low-pitched wheeze, coarse crackles and a pleural rub, repeat auscultation after the patient has been asked to cough forcefully.
- ☐ Do not ask a patient with severe pleural pain to take frequent deep breaths or to cough. Test the vocal resonance first. If an area is found in which the voice sounds are increased, ask the patient to take one or two deep breaths and bronchial breath sounds will usually be heard in the same area.
- ☐ When abnormal breath sounds are heard, map out the extent of the lesion by moving the bell of the stethoscope with each breath from the normal towards the abnormal zone and note the level at which the breath sounds changes.

Abnormal findings

Disease of the bronchi, lungs and pleura may alter breath sounds in two main ways: namely diminished vesicular breathing or bronchial breath sounds. There are three types of added sounds which may be heard on auscultation: wheezes (rhonchi), crackles (crepitations) and pleural sounds (Table 4.19).

Diminished vesicular breathing. If the conduction of the breath sounds to the chest wall is attenuated, they remain

TABLE 4.19 Added sounds

• Rhonchi (wheezes)	Musical sounds produced by air passing through narrowed airways, e.g. asthma
• Crackles (crepitations)	Non-musical sounds mainly heard during inspiration caused by: Reopening of occluded small airways (e.g. fibrosing alveolitis, pulmonary oedema). Air bubbling through secretions (e.g. bronchiectasis)
• Pleural friction rub	Leathery or creaking sounds produced by movement of roughened pleural surfaces, e.g. pleurisy caused by pneumonia, pulmonary infarction. Usually associated with pleural pain

vesicular but are diminished in amplitude (see Table 4.20). This change in the breath sounds is invariably accompanied by a reduction in the amplitude of the conducted voice sounds. Asking the patient to cough may help when the breath sounds are diminished or absent over a lobe or segment thought to be involved in pneumonia. If the changes

TABLE 4.20 Causes of diminished vesicular breathing

Reduced airflow	*Reduced conduction*
Generalised (e.g. emphysema)	Thick chest wall
Localised (e.g. bronchial obstruction by tumour)	Pleural effusion/thickening
	Small pneumothorax

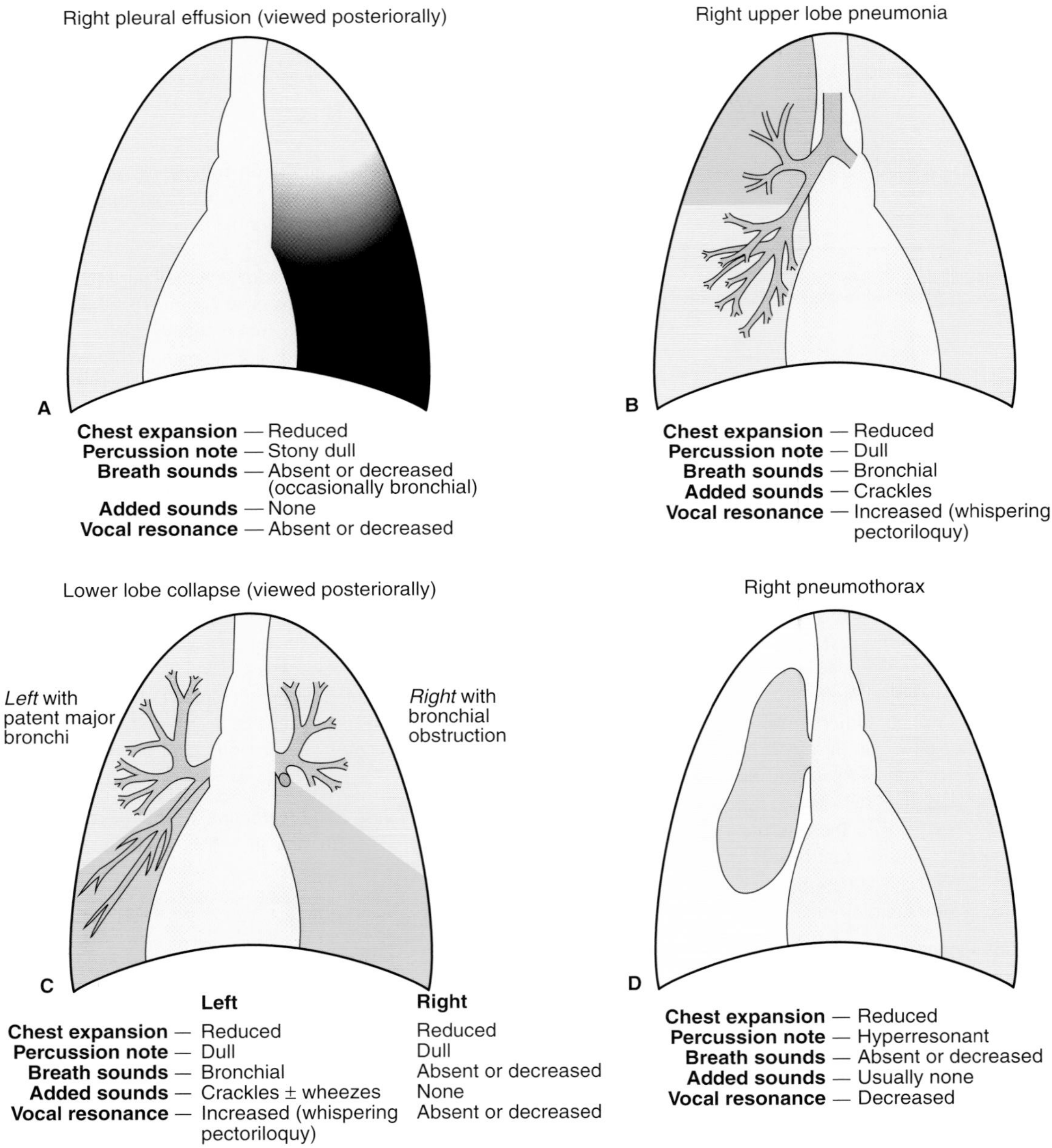

Fig. 4.22 Clinical findings in [A] right-sided effusion, [B] right-sided consolidation, [C] collapse, with bronchial obstruction on the right side and with patent bronchi on the left side, and [D] right pneumothorax.

TABLE 4.21 Bronchial, diminished or absent breath sounds	
Auscultatory findings	**Disease process**
High-pitched bronchial breath sounds	Pneumonic consolidation (Fig. 4.22B) Large superficial pulmonary cavity Collapsed lung or lobe when large bronchi are patent (Fig. 4.22C) Lung compressed by pleural effusion (sometimes) Tension pneumothorax (sometimes)
Low-pitched bronchial breath sounds	Localised areas of pulmonary fibrosis, e.g. chronic pulmonary tuberculosis, chronic suppurative pneumonia
Diminished or absent breath sounds	Pleural effusion (Fig. 4.22A) Marked pleural thickening Collapsed lung or lobe when large bronchi occluded (Fig. 4.22C) Pneumothorax (Fig. 4.22D) Emphysema (symmetrical diminution over both lungs)

are due to bronchial obstruction by secretions, bronchial breath sounds may become audible when these secretions are dislodged by coughing. Breath sounds are characteristically absent over large effusions and may also be inaudible where there is a significant pneumothorax (see Fig. 4.22A and D).

Some clinical causes of diminished or absent vesicular breathing are given in Table 4.21.

Bronchial breathing. If the lung tissue through which the breath sounds are transmitted from the air passages to the chest wall has lost its normal spongy consistence and has become firm or solid, e.g. in consolidation or fibrosis, the sounds are transmitted more readily to the chest wall and when picked up by the stethoscope resemble more closely those produced at the larynx than those heard over normal lung. Such bronchial breath sounds are found whenever (a) normal lung tissue is replaced by a uniform conducting medium, be it consolidation, fibrosis or collapse, and (b) the relevant major bronchus remains patent.

The criteria for the recognition of bronchial breathing are strict and unambiguous. Four conditions require to be satisfied (see Table 4.22).

TABLE 4.22 Bronchial breath sounds

- Both the inspiratory and expiratory sounds are blowing, sometimes called tubular, in character
- The expiratory sound is as long and as loud as the inspiratory sound and usually of high pitch
- There is a pause between the end of inspiration and the beginning of the expiratory sound
- Vocal resonance is increased to allow whispering pectoriloquy to be heard

Some of the pathological processes which produce bronchial breathing are detailed in Table 4.21 (please also see Fig. 4.22).

Bronchial breath sounds (Fig. 4.21) resemble more closely those produced at the larynx than those heard over the normal lung.

The pitch of bronchial breath sounds varies according to the nature of the pulmonary changes. As high-frequency sounds are selectively conducted through consolidated lung tissue, high-pitched bronchial breath sounds are heard in lobar or segmental pneumonia (Fig. 4.22B). Fibrotic lung tissue, on the other hand, transmits sounds of lower frequency and thus produces lower-pitched bronchial breath sounds. With voice sounds, there is a similar selective conduction of certain frequencies. It follows that when bronchial breathing is audible the voice sounds are louder than normal and whispering pectoriloquy is usually present.

When bronchial breath sounds traverse air-containing cavities in their passage to the chest wall, they may occasionally acquire a resonating *amphoric* quality, resembling the sound produced by blowing across the top of a bottle. Breath sounds may be intermediate in type between vesicular and bronchial, for example vesicular with prolonged expiration.

Abnormal vocal resonance. Voice sounds conducted through consolidated lung tissue, extensive fibrosis and pulmonary collapse associated with a patent bronchus resemble more closely those produced at the larynx than those heard over normal lungs in that they are louder and more distinct. In some cases a whispered voice may be transmitted almost without distortion so that individual syllables can be clearly recognised (*whispering pectoriloquy*).

Wheezes (rhonchi). These are musical sounds of high, medium or low pitch produced by the passage of air through narrowed bronchi. Rhonchi caused by mucosal oedema or spasm of the bronchial musculature are usually superimposed upon the expiratory phase of the respiratory noise, which is always prolonged when rhonchi are present. Rhonchi heard during inspiration are more often due to secretions in the large bronchi and may disappear, or at least become less numerous, after coughing.

Wheezes are heard diffusely over both lungs in bronchial asthma and in most cases of COPD. In asthma, wheezes are medium to high pitched and are mainly heard during expiration, which is prolonged. In COPD they are usually low or medium pitched and both inspiratory and expiratory. A localised wheeze may be heard over a partially obstructed large bronchus. If the obstruction is caused by a fixed lesion, such as a tumour or foreign body in a large bronchus, the wheeze is usually louder during inspiration, is not altered by coughing (fixed wheeze or rhonchus) and is often accompanied by stridor. If the obstruction is due to secretions, these are usually removed by coughing, which causes the wheeze to disappear.

Crackles (crepitations). These non-musical sounds are mainly audible during inspiration. When assessing the significance of crackles it is important to note their timing in the respiratory cycle and whether or not they are affected by coughing. Attempting to distinguish between moist and dry, or even between fine, medium and coarse crackles serves no clinically useful purpose.

Crackles may be caused by the bubbling of air through secretions in major bronchi, dilated bronchi (bronchiectasis) and pulmonary cavities. In these circumstances they sound coarse and the presence of secretions is confirmed by the observation that the crackles either decrease in number or disappear temporarily after coughing. Crackles caused by secretions within the large bronchi in acute or chronic bronchitis and COPD, or in resolving bronchopneumonia, are widespread and bilateral, while those audible over resolving lobar or segmental pneumonic consolidation, dilated bronchi (bronchiectasis), lung abscesses or tuberculous cavities are localised to the site of the lesions. In all these conditions they are audible throughout inspiration.

A much more frequent cause of crackles is the explosive reopening, during inspiration, of peripheral small airways which have become occluded during expiration. These are most numerous during the second half of inspiration and in some cases confined to its last part (end-inspiratory crepitations). Crackles of this type are not influenced by coughing, and are more conspicuous over the lower parts of the lungs because in the upright position small airway closure is more liable to occur there than in the upper lobes.

They occur in parenchymal lung conditions, such as interstitial pulmonary oedema, allergic and fibrosing alveolitis, and perhaps early pneumonic consolidation and miliary tuberculosis and are audible mainly during the second half of inspiration.

Pleural sounds. A *pleural* rub is a leathery or creaking sound produced by movement of the visceral pleura over the parietal pleura, when both surfaces are roughened as by fibrinous exudate. It is usually heard at two separate stages in the respiratory cycle, towards the end of inspiration and just after the beginning of expiration. A pleural rub may be inaudible during normal breathing but can be heard when the patient is asked to breathe deeply.

A pleural rub is heard over areas of pleurisy. It disappears as soon as the visceral and parietal pleura are separated by fluid, but often remains audible above an effusion. If pleurisy involves the pleura adjacent to the pericardium, a pleuropericardial rub may also be heard. This is a rather misleading term since the pericardial element in the sound is not due to pericarditis. It is caused merely by roughened pleural surfaces adjacent to the pericardium being moved across one another by cardiac pulsation. A pleuropericardial rub may, in some cases, be impossible to distinguish from a pericardial rub.

A *pneumothorax click* is a rhythmical sound, synchronous with cardiac systole, which may be heard with or sometimes without the aid of a stethoscope. It is produced when there is air between the two layers of pleura overlying the heart.

Examples of common disorders that give rise to abnormal clinical findings which are usually easily detected by inspection, percussion and auscultation are shown diagrammatically in Figure 4.22.

KEY POINTS

- Vesicular breathing is diminished if there is reduced airflow or impairment of conduction from the lung to the chest wall.
- Bronchial breathing occurs when the relevant major bronchus remains patent and normal lung tissue is replaced by a uniform conducting medium.
- A fixed low-pitched wheeze usually indicates partial obstruction of a major bronchus.
- Crackles are usually caused by explosive reopening of peripheral airways during inspiration. These are more conspicuous over the lower lung fields and are not influenced by coughing.
- Crackles caused by bronchial secretions may decrease or even disappear on coughing.
- Patients with pleuritic pain should not be asked to cough or take deep breaths until effective analgesia has been given.
- Auscultate the chest using the bell with a rubber rim cover.
- Avoid auscultating within 2–3 cm of the midline.
- It is often helpful to repeat auscultation after asking the patient to cough.

INTEGRATION OF PHYSICAL SIGNS

Certain groups of physical signs are typically associated with certain pathological changes in the lungs and pleura. Such changes are not necessarily specific for one particular disease. For example, the physical signs of consolidation may occur in pneumonia, pulmonary infarction or tuberculosis, and those of pleural effusion may be present in malignant disease, empyema or cardiac failure. Each group of physical signs therefore gives an indication only of the gross pathology of the lesion, and not of its precise nature, the diagnosis of which depends on an analysis of all the clinical and other evidence. The characteristic physical signs of the more common lesions are shown in Figure 4.22, namely pleural effusion, consolidation, collapse and pneumothorax. All of the signs are not necessarily present in every case. An area of consolidation or collapse may, for example, be too small to give rise to the classical pattern of physical signs. Furthermore, the picture may be confused by the coincidence of two groups of signs, as when consolidation is accompanied by pleural effusion. Difficulties are also apt to arise when the differential diagnosis rests on the observer's estimate of the position of the mediastinum. In patients with pulmonary collapse or pleural effusion mediastinal displacement is an inconstant feature and, even when present, may be difficult to detect especially if the apex is impalpable.

FURTHER INVESTIGATIONS

In many cases it is possible to make a reliable diagnosis from the history and clinical examination. This applies, for example, to conditions such as bronchial asthma, chronic bronchitis and to some cases of pneumonia and pulmonary infarction. At other times clinical examination fails to reveal any abnormality and the diagnosis depends entirely on specialised investigations, particularly radiology.

Pulmonary tuberculosis and bronchial carcinoma are two important diseases which may not give rise to any clinical abnormality in the early stages. It is therefore essential to advise chest radiological examination whenever one of these conditions is suspected from the history. It is not possible to determine accurately the site of most abnormalities visible on posteroanterior or anteroposterior radiographs and a lateral should be used to elucidate any abnormality shown on a PA film (Fig. 4.23). A comparison between current and previous films, if they can be obtained, may provide vital diagnostic information:

- If a pulmonary opacity has not increased in size over a period of a year or longer, a diagnosis of bronchial carcinoma is highly improbable.
- If an opacity has become smaller or less dense in the course of a few days or weeks, pneumonia or pulmonary infarction is its most likely cause.
- If a lesion was not present on an earlier film, or has become larger, it is almost certainly a tumour or an active tuberculous infection.

By means of radiology the precise anatomical position of a lesion can be determined, and from this and other features its pathology may be deduced.

Even when a precise diagnosis has been made, it is usually desirable to measure the effect of the disease on respiratory function. This is useful for the assessment of fitness for work and suitability for certain forms of treatment, such as surgery for bronchial carcinoma.

The important symptom of haemoptysis (Tables 4.24 to 4.26) is used to illustrate how the nature of the presentation influences the likely diagnosis and hence the choice of investigations.

A full account of all the special methods of investigation cannot be given here, nor is it possible to indicate in any detail the information they can be expected to provide. The summary in Table 4.23 is therefore intended to serve only as a guide to the value of each investigation and the indications for its use.

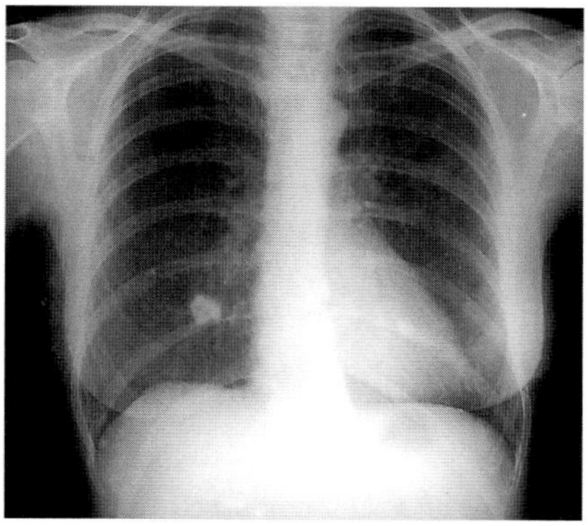

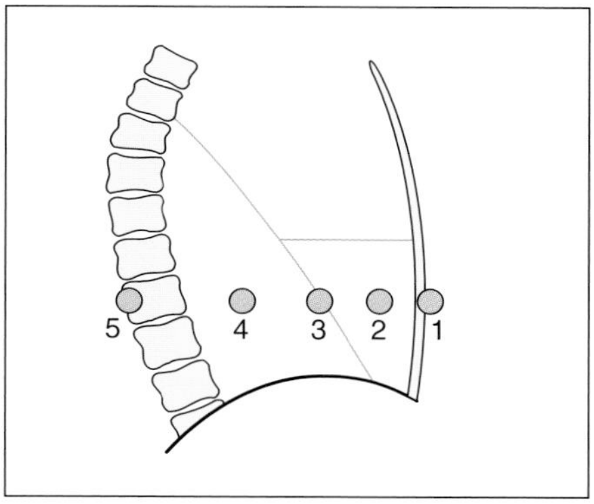

Fig. 4.23 Chest radiographs. For descriptive purposes the straight X-ray is divided into zones – upper, mid and lower – separated by imaginary horizontal lines between the anterior ends of the second and fourth ribs. There is a round shadow in the right lower zone of the straight X-ray. The lateral view shows five possible sites of the abnormality: **1.** anterior chest wall or pleura; **2.** right middle lobe; **3.** fissure between the lobes; **4.** right lower lobe; **5.** posterior chest wall or pleura.

KEY POINTS

- Groups of physical signs are typically associated with certain pathological changes but are not necessarily specific for any particular disease.
- Tuberculosis and bronchial carcinoma are two conditions in which there may be no abnormal physical signs.
- A chest radiograph is an essential investigation in all patients with suspected pulmonary or pleural disease.
- Comparison of the present and a previous chest radiograph may provide vital information.
- Once a diagnosis has been established it is often important to complete the investigations by assessing respiratory function.

TABLE 4.23 Summary of respiratory investigations

Sputum	Should be examined in all cases of suspected pulmonary infection and most patients with bronchial infection. Specific requests for examination of separate specimens for tubercle bacilli and fungi (including *Pneumocystis carinii*) must be made
Induced sputum	In patients who cannot produce sputum the inhalation of nebulised hypertonic saline can induce sputum production
Skin tests	Tuberculin test: chiefly of value in excluding present or past tuberculous infection
	Kveim test: a positive reaction confirms a diagnosis of sarcoidosis
	Skin sensitivity tests (usually common inhaled allergens, e.g. house dust mite, pollens, animal danders) confirm presence or absence of atopy. Not usually used for diagnostic purposes
Blood tests	Total and differential white cell count is helpful in cases of pulmonary bacterial infection and in diseases in which there is pulmonary radiographic shadowing and a high peripheral blood eosinophil count (pulmonary eosinophilia). Blood culture should be a routine investigation in all cases of acute pneumonia
	Examination of serum for viral and other antibodies may be of value in determining the cause of 'atypical' pneumonia
Nasal sinus radiograph	Integral part of the investigation of chronic upper respiratory tract infection and of some pulmonary infections
Chest radiograph	Essential in initial investigation of all patients in whom pulmonary or pleural disease suspected
Lateral chest radiograph	Essential to localise the site of an abnormality visible on the posteroanterior (PA) radiograph (Fig. 4.23)
Previous radiograph	May be invaluable in determining whether a radiographic abnormality is new or old, or increasing or decreasing in size
Tomography	Allows an opacity or part of an opacity to be visualised clearly in different planes or cuts. Can be of help in differentiating between a pulmonary tumour and a tuberculous lesion. Now rarely used if computed tomography is available
Computed tomography	Provides accurate information about single or multiple pulmonary lesions. Allows assessment of structures in the mediastinum including lymph nodes. High-resolution CT is useful in the investigation of diffuse interstitial lung disease. It has replaced bronchography for the diagnosis of bronchiectasis. Spiral CT now used in suspected major pulmonary embolism
Screening	Allows diaphragm movement to be observed. Can detect unilateral diaphragmatic paralysis. Ultrasonography is now used more often for this purpose
Ultrasonography	Used in localisation of loculated pleural effusions. Can be used to aid needle aspiration of lesions invading the chest wall. Also can assess diaphragm movement
Pulmonary angiography	Outlines pulmonary vascular bed. Used in the assessment of pulmonary embolism and in some cases of pulmonary hypertension
Radionuclide scanning	Accurate assessment of lung perfusion (*Q* scan) and ventilation (*V* scan). Its main use is in the diagnosis of pulmonary embolism/infarction. A *Q* scan can be used in patients with previously normal lungs and heart. A *V/Q* scan is necessary in patients with chronic lung disease
Bronchoscopy	Diagnosis and assessment of operability of bronchial carcinoma (biopsy, brushings and bronchial washings)
	Diagnosis of pulmonary infections (diffuse and localised) in patients who cannot produce sputum (bronchial washings/brushings)
	Assessment of diffuse interstitial lung diseases, e.g. fibrosing/allergic alveolitis, sarcoidosis, etc. (transbronchial biopsy and differential cell counts of bronchoalveolar lavage fluid)
Pleural aspiration and biopsy	Aspiration of pleural liquid from pleural effusions and 'blind' biopsy of parietal pleura. Diagnosis of malignant and tuberculous pleural effusion usually established in this way
Thoracoscopy	Allows visualisation of pleural space and biopsy of abnormal tissue. Mainly used in the investigation of pleural effusions when diagnosis has not been made by pleural needle aspiration and biopsy. Also allows video-assisted lung biopsy to be performed
Lymph node aspiration/biopsy	Allows cytological/histological examination of supraclavicular lymph glands (carcinoma, sarcoidosis and tuberculosis)
Mediastinoscopy	Allows visualisation of structures in anterior mediastinum and biopsy of lymph glands. Used in the diagnosis and assessment of operability of bronchial carcinoma
Tests of respiratory function	
Arterial blood gas analysis	Essential investigation in all ill patients with respiratory problems. Partial pressure of oxygen (Pa_{O_2}) low in severe asthma, pneumonia, pulmonary embolism and oedema (type I respiratory failure). Partial pressure of carbon dioxide also elevated in very severe asthma, severe chronic bronchitis and emphysema (type II respiratory failure). Hydrogen ion concentration or pH allows assessment of degree of respiratory acidosis caused by carbon dioxide retention
Pulmonary function tests	Forced expiratory volume in one second (FEV_1) and forced vital capacity (FVC) measured by spirometry provide an accurate assessment of the degree of airflow obstruction in asthma and chronic bronchitis. The FEV_1/FVC ratio is less than 70–75% in all patients with diffuse airflow obstruction. Serial measurements of peak expiratory flow (PEF) are invaluable in the diagnosis and management of asthma
Lung volumes and transfer factor	Used in the assessment of diffuse interstitial lung diseases (e.g. fibrosing alveolitis) in which lung factor volumes are decreased (restrictive defect) and transfer factor is often low. Lung volumes are increased in emphysema and transfer factor is decreased

TABLE 4.24 Causes of haemoptysis

Common causes	Uncommon causes
Pulmonary thromboembolism Bronchial carcinoma Tuberculosis Bronchiectasis Chronic bronchitis Pulmonary oedema Suppurative pneumonia	Bronchial adenoma Aspergilloma Alveolar haemorrhage (Gooodpasture's syndrome, idiopathic pulmonary haemosiderosis) Anticoagulant therapy Blood dyscrasias

With the exception of chronic bronchitis and some cases of bronchiectasis all the common causes usually result in an abnormal chest radiograph at the time of presentation

TABLE 4.25 Relating the presentation of haemoptysis to the common causes

Nature of presentation	Consider
Massive haemoptysis	Tuberculosis Bronchiectasis Pulmonary thromboembolism Bronchial carcinoma Suppurative pneumonia
Scanty haemoptysis	Bronchial carcinoma Pulmonary thromboembolism Chronic bronchitis
Haemoptysis and purulent sputum	Bronchiectasis Chronic bronchitis Suppurative pneumonia
Recurrent haemoptysis	Pulmonary thromboembolism Bronchial carcinoma Bronchiectasis Chronic bronchitis

COMMON PITFALLS AND HOW TO AVOID THEM

- Stridor is caused by partial obstruction of a major airway. In an adult, if the onset is gradual, the cause is usually carcinoma of the larynx, trachea or main bronchus. Early stridor in adults is often missed or thought to be wheeze. Ask the patient to cough and then to breathe in and out deeply with the mouth wide open.
- Pigeon chest deformity becomes irreversible once the bones of the thoracic cage have fused during puberty. In prepubertal asthmatics, its development implies a history of severe disease and indicates the need for maximum therapy since the chest deformity is reversible in some children treated before puberty.

TABLE 4.26 Relating the investigations to the suspected diagnosis

Suspected diagnosis	Possible further investigations
Pulmonary thromboembolism	Ventilation–perfusion lung scan Ascending venography Pulmonary angiography
Bronchial carcinoma	Sputum examination for malignant cells Bronchoscopy Transthoracic needle aspiration
Tuberculosis	Sputum examination for tubercle bacilli. If no sputum, bronchoscopy to obtain bronchial washings Tuberculin test
Bronchiectasis	Sputum examination for bacterial pathogens CT scan if chest radiography not diagnostic Bronchography (rarely necessary if CT available)
Chronic bronchitis	Sputum for malignant cells Bronchoscopy often necessary to exclude bronchial carcinoma
Pulmonary oedema	Electrocardiography Echocardiography
Suppurative pneumonia	Sputum examination for bacterial pathogens, tubercle bacilli and fungi

- Chest movement should not be confused with chest expansion. In exacerbations of COPD or during episodes of severe asthma, chest movement is marked owing to accessory muscles of respiration lifting the hyperinflated chest up and down in an attempt to improve ventilation. This may mislead the unwary. Always specifically check chest expansion which may be negligible.
- Patients with severe emphysema lose weight. Do not investigate such patients unnecessarily for a cause of their weight loss.
- The absence of clinical abnormalities in patients with pulmonary tuberculosis is the rule rather than the exception, even when there are gross radiographic abnormalities. A chest X-ray should be performed in all patients where the history could suggest the diagnosis of tuberculosis.
- Open tuberculosis is an infectious disease. Patients with tuberculosis should be notified immediately in order that contact tracing can be performed. If a patient with sputum smear positive has been in contact with children under the age of 5, these children should be examined without delay.
- Bronchial carcinoma in an adult smoker who has had haemoptysis is not excluded by absence of abnormal clinical findings and a normal chest radiograph. Bronchoscopy may be required to be performed.

- The majority of patients with pulmonary thromboembolic disease do not have clinical evidence of deep venous thrombosis. Indeed, the history, clinical findings and radiographic abnormalities in pulmonary infarction are often similar to those of pneumonia. Many patients with pulmonary thromboembolism are treated, at least initially, with an antibiotic. Where there is doubt, give anticoagulants until the possibility of thromboembolic disease has been excluded.

The alimentary and genitourinary systems

5

M. J. FORD • A. D. CUMMING

THE HISTORY

The diagnosis of intra-abdominal disease is more often dependent upon a careful history than on the presence of physical signs. Pain is prominent among the symptoms encountered in the alimentary system, and may also be present in genitourinary diseases. When pain is present, taking an accurate history usually indicates the probable diagnosis and the best method of investigating the problem. If the history is inadequate, unnecessary tests may result in the discovery of asymptomatic abnormalities such as hiatus hernia or gallstones, leading to inappropriate management and even unnecessary surgery. Conversely, some important conditions, such as chronic renal failure, may only be detected on biochemical screening, in the absence of symptoms or signs.

ALIMENTARY SYMPTOMS

Disorders of the alimentary tract may present with a wide range of symptoms including painful mouth, difficulty in swallowing (dysphagia), nausea and vomiting, abdominal pain, heartburn, indigestion (dyspepsia), loss of appetite (anorexia), weight loss, abdominal distension, altered bowel habit, rectal bleeding and jaundice (Table 5.1). Sometimes, alimentary disease is suggested only by the occurrence of a secondary feature such as anaemia. Occasionally patients may conceal important symptoms such as rectal bleeding because of embarrassment, a belief that the cause is trivial or fear of serious illness. The clinician should not only listen carefully to the patient's presenting complaints but also enquire systematically about the other principal symptoms of abdominal disease. It is important to remember that alimentary symptoms may develop in response to emotional distress.

TABLE 5.1 Gastrointestinal symptoms

Dry mouth (xerostomia)
Excess salivation (waterbrash)
Painful lips, tongue, mouth
Altered taste sensation (dysgeusia)
Foul taste in mouth (cacageusia)
Bad breath (halitosis)
Feeling of a lump in the throat (globus)
Heartburn and acid reflux
Painful swallowing (odynophagia)
Difficulty in swallowing (dysphagia)
Retrosternal chest pain
Indigestion (dyspepsia)
Belching and flatulence
Hiccups
Nausea and vomiting
Anorexia and weight loss
Vomiting blood (haematemesis)
Black tarry stools (melaena)
Rectal bleeding (haematochezia)
Abdominal pain
Abdominal distension
Constipation
Diarrhoea
Jaundice
Itch (pruritus)
Dark-coloured urine (bilirubinuria)

TABLE 5.2 Common causes of a painful mouth

Idiopathic	Recurrent aphthous mouth ulcers
Infections	Candidiasis Dental sepsis Herpes simplex virus (HSV1) Coxsackie A virus, herpangina, hand–foot–mouth disease Vincent's angina (ulcerative gingivitis) Glandular fever
Miscellaneous	Trauma from teeth/dentures Leukoplakia, carcinoma
Associated with systemic disorder	Drug allergies, e.g. sulphonamides, gold, cytotoxics Iron, folate, vitamin B_{12} deficiency Leucopenia, acute leukaemia Reiter's syndrome, Behçet's disease Crohn's disease, ulcerative colitis, coeliac disease
Associated with skin disorder	Lichen planus, erythema multiforme Pemphigoid, pemphigus vulgaris

Painful mouth

Soreness of the lips, tongue or buccal mucosa has a wide variety of causes, including iron, folate or vitamin B_{12} deficiency, dermatological disorders, chemotherapy, aphthous ulceration and infective stomatitis (Table 5.2). Gastrointestinal disorders particularly associated with mouth ulcers include inflammatory bowel disease and gluten enteropathy. A history of recurrent painful tiny mouth ulcers with its onset at the menarche, exacerbations during menstruation and a family history of mouth ulcers suggests idiopathic aphthous ulceration.

Difficulty in swallowing (dysphagia)

The swallowing mechanism involves the brain stem, the glossopharyngeal and vagal nerves and the enteric nervous system of oesophageal smooth muscle. The swallowing reflex begins with an oral phase which drives the food bolus into the pharynx; the pharyngeal phase ensues with closure of the larynx, relaxation of the upper pharyngeal sphincter (cricopharyngeus) and sequential contraction of the pharyngeal constrictors to propel the bolus into the oesophagus. The oesophageal phase comprises oesophageal peristaltic contractions associated with relaxation of the lower oesophageal sphincter.

Retrosternal chest pain experienced during swallowing, *odynophagia*, is characteristic of inflammatory disorders of the oesophagus, e.g. peptic ulceration, candidiasis, herpes simplex oesophagitis. Food sticking during swallowing is an important symptom of oesophageal disease for which an explanation should always be sought. The important features in the history of dysphagia are shown in the symptom checklist (Table 5.3) and some common causes of dysphagia in the box below.

TABLE 5.3 Symptom checklist in dysphagia

Is dysphagia painful or painless? (impact pain)
Is dysphagia intermittent or progressive?
How long is the history of dysphagia?
Is there a previous history of dysphagia or reflux dyspepsia?
Is dysphagia for solids or liquids or both?
At what level does food appear to stick?
Does regurgitation usually occur or does food eventually pass down?

DISORDERS – Common causes of dysphagia

Painful mouth/throat
- Recurrent aphthous mouth ulcers
- Glandular fever, tonsillitis, quinsy

Neurological
- Pseudobulbar palsy, bulbar palsy

Neuromuscular
- Myasthenia gravis, achalasia, systemic sclerosis

Obstruction
- Oesophageal carcinoma, gastric carcinoma, peptic stricture
- Extrinsic obstruction, e.g. bronchial carcinoma

Dysphagia is usually first apparent for solids and progresses to affect the swallowing of fluids. Difficulty in initiating swallowing fluids, rather than solids, accompanied by coughing and spluttering suggests a neurological disorder. Dysphagia localised to the level of the cricoid cartilage may result from tumour, stricture, pharyngeal pouch or from a reflex effect resulting from disease in the lower oesophagus. Dysphagia localised to the level of the lower sternum suggests disease of the lower oesophagus, e.g. tumour, achalasia or peptic oesophagitis. Dysphagia may be slowly progressive or intermittent, occurring only with a large food bolus such as meat. Dysphagia may be painful or painless. Food sticking at the level of narrowing may produce severe *impact pain* and suggests an intact sensory innervation. It is relieved when food is either regurgitated or passes through the stricture into the stomach. Painless dysphagia suggests denervation of the oesophagus and is often due to tumour. In patients with a pharyngeal pouch or long-standing oesophageal obstruction, recognisable food may be regurgitated long after it was eaten. Achalasia of the cardia and chronic oesophageal obstruction may produce bouts of nocturnal cough and dyspnoea as a result of the reflux of oesophageal contents into the trachea and major bronchi, sometimes resulting in an aspiration pneumonia.

Dysphagia should not be confused with *globus*, a symptom in which there is a feeling of a lump in the throat often associated with suppressed emotional distress; it is not associated with eating, does not interfere with swallowing and is rapidly relieved by the release of pent-up emotions, e.g. crying.

Nausea and vomiting

The combination of nausea and vomiting usually suggests an upper gastrointestinal disorder but may also be a prominent feature of non-alimentary disorders (see Disorders box). In most instances, vomiting is preceded by nausea, but in some cases, e.g. intracranial tumour, the vomiting can occur without warning. Vomiting may also result from severe pain, as in renal or biliary colic or myocardial infarction, from systemic disease, metabolic disorders and drug therapy. Vomiting may be self-induced in patients with peptic ulceration (for pain relief) or with bulimia nervosa.

Gastric outlet obstruction is associated with the projectile vomiting of large volumes of gastric content, the vomitus also being noteworthy for the absence of bile-staining. Obstruction distal to the pylorus produces bile-stained vomiting; the lower the level of intestinal obstruction, the more marked are the accompanying symptoms of abdominal distension and intestinal colic. Vomiting also occurs in other gastrointestinal disorders, e.g. acute gastroenteritis, acute cholecystitis, acute pancreatitis and hepatitis.

Enquiry should be made about the frequency of vomiting, the time of day at which it occurs and the taste, colour, quantity and smell of the vomitus (Table 5.4). A yellow colour and bitter taste indicate the presence of bile

DISORDERS – Non-alimentary causes of vomiting

Pharmacological
- Digoxin, opiates, alcohol, theophyllines

Neurological
- Fear, severe pain, shock, vasovagal syncope
- Migraine, acute labyrinthine disorders
- Intracranial hypertension (tumour, haemorrhage, meningitis)

Psychological
- Anorexia nervosa, bulimia

Metabolic
- Pregnancy, hyperparathyroidism, hypoadrenalism
- Diabetic ketoacidosis, renal failure, hepatitis

TABLE 5.4 Symptom checklist in vomiting
What medications has the patient been taking? Is vomiting heralded by nausea or does it occur without warning? Is vomiting associated with dyspepsia or abdominal pain and, if so, does vomiting relieve the symptoms? Is vomiting related to meal-times, early morning or late evening? Is the vomitus bile-stained, blood-stained, faeculent?

TABLE 5.5 Symptom checklist in haematemesis
Is there a previous history of dyspepsia or upper GI bleeding? Is there a history of alcohol abuse? Has the patient recently taken corticosteroid or NSAID therapy? Did the vomitus comprise fresh blood or coffee-ground stained fluid? Was blood-staining of the vomitus apparent in the first vomit? Was the haematemesis preceded by intense retching?

and imply regurgitation of duodenal content into the stomach. If the taste and smell are inconspicuous, this suggests either the presence of achlorhydria or that the vomitus has been regurgitated from the oesophagus. Foul-smelling vomitus suggests pyloric obstruction, carcinoma of the stomach or gastrocolic fistula. Faeculent vomiting may occur in distal small bowel or colonic obstruction and in gastrocolic fistula. Special attention should be paid to the presence of blood in the vomit (*haematemesis*) (Table 5.5). Bright red blood usually arises from pharyngeal or oesophageal lesions. Dark red vomitus, sometimes containing liver-like clots of blood, is due to profuse bleeding as may occur from oesophageal varices or peptic ulcer. In less acute upper gastrointestinal bleeding, the vomitus is often blackish or dark brown and can contain sediment like 'coffee grounds' resulting from the conversion of the haemoglobin to acid haematin by gastric acid. Whenever possible, the patient's description should be supplemented by inspection of the vomitus. Table 5.6 indicates the common causes of upper gastrointestinal bleeding.

Anorexia and weight loss

Loss of body fluid for any reason, e.g. diuretic therapy, can produce rapid and dramatic weight loss (1 litre of water = 1 kilogram). Otherwise, weight loss arises from a reduction in both adipose and fat-free mass. Weight loss is more commonly the result of reduced energy intake than of increased energy expenditure. Reduced energy intake arises from dieting, loss of appetite or malabsorption. Energy loss occurs in marked glycosuria. Increased energy expenditure occurs in hyperthyroidism, fever or a change to a more energetic lifestyle. Since 7000 kcal is the equivalent of 1 kg of human adipose tissue, a net calorie deficit of 1000 kcal per day will produce a weight loss of approximately 1 kg per week. Greater weight losses during the initial stages of energy restriction arise from loss of fat-free mass especially salt and water loss and depletion of hepatic glycogen stores.

Significant weight loss occurring as an isolated symptom is rarely associated with serious organic disease. However, a careful history may elicit other symptoms and alert the clinician to the underlying cause. While some patients can accurately quantify their weight loss, many cannot. The patient may assess the rate and severity of weight loss from ill-fitting clothes. Whenever possible such subjective assessment should be confirmed objectively. Review of previously documented weights from case records may avoid needless investigation in patients who mistakenly believe they are losing weight. The significance of weight loss relates to its duration and extent together with the presence or absence of anorexia (loss of appetite) or deliberate reduction in food intake. Weight loss of less than 3 kg in the previous 6 months is rarely of significance. Weight loss accompanied by severe anorexia or other alimentary symptoms may not necessarily be due to intra-abdominal disease; such features may occur, for example, in depression. Weight loss may result from physical, psychological or social factors. Grief, depression and chronic

TABLE 5.6 Common causes of haematemesis and melaena

Cause	Frequency %
Gastric ulcer	30
Duodenal ulcer	20
Erosive gastritis or duodenitis	30
Oesophagitis or Mallory–Weiss tear	15
Oesophageal/gastric varices	2
Upper GI malignancy	2

CASE HISTORY

A 14-year-old girl presented with a history of weight loss of 6 kg over the previous year. Though menarche had occurred at the age of 12, menstruation had stopped 6 months previously, raising the possibility of anorexia nervosa. On further questioning it emerged that 1 year previously she had developed generalised aches and pains with arthralgia associated with a painful skin rash over the lower limbs. She remembered the date of onset as her grandfather had returned to Jamaica following his visit to the UK. For 3 months she had complained of night sweats and a dry cough. The probability of pulmonary tuberculosis was suggested by a family history of TB, presumed erythema nodosum, persistent febrile symptoms and the absence of BCG inoculation. The diagnosis was rapidly confirmed by chest radiograph and sputum microscopy.

Learning points

- Weight loss >3 kg in 6 months is significant.
- Weight loss from any cause may result in cessation of menstruation.
- Eliciting a history of illness in other family members is important.
- Presenting symptoms may not relate to the organ or system most affected.

alcohol abuse are commonly associated with weight loss. Weight loss with amenorrhoea in an adolescent female suggests the possibility of anorexia nervosa. In addition to a search for serious underlying disease, the physician should enquire of changes in the social well-being and lifestyle of the patient.

Abdominal pain

This is a common symptom. After listening to the patient's history, additional questions may be necessary (see Table 1.6, p. 8). Pain from unpaired intra-abdominal structures is usually in the midline. The patient should be asked to demonstrate the exact site and also any areas to which the pain may radiate. The character of the pain should be noted, e.g. 'stitch-like'. Frequency, duration and timing of attacks may be of diagnostic significance, as may be the associated features. In Table 5.7 the typical features of four common disorders are listed to illustrate the value of an analytical approach to diagnosis. Abdominal pain, sometimes of great intensity, may result from disorders outwith the alimentary system. Associated features such as pain aggravated by movement and coughing usually help to indicate the likely origin of the pain. Table 5.8 illustrates some non-alimentary causes of abdominal pain.

Patterns of presentation:

Site of pain. Visceral abdominal pain results from distension of hollow organs, mesenteric traction or excessive smooth muscle contraction. The sympathetic innervation of the abdominal viscera (spinal cord segments T5–L2) is responsible for the conduction of visceral pain; parasympathetic afferents do not convey pain sensation. Accurate localisation of somatic pain due to irritation of the parietal peritoneum is provided by intercostal (spinal) nerves, which innervate the parietal peritoneum and the overlying abdominal wall.

Some acute disorders are nearly always unilateral, while others are usually bilateral. In young males, when unilateral acute epididymo–orchitis is suspected, torsion of the testis

TABLE 5.7 Analysis of abdominal pain

	Disorder			
	Peptic ulcer	Biliary colic	Acute pancreatitis	Renal colic
Main site	Epigastric	Epigastrium/right hypochondrium	Epigastrium/left hypochondrium	Loin
Radiation	Into the back	Beneath right scapula Right shoulder tip	Into the back May become generalised	Into genitalia/inner thigh
Character	Gnawing	Constant	Constant	Constant with small fluctuations
Severity	Mild to moderate	Severe	Severe	Severe
Duration	$\frac{1}{2}$–2 h	4–24 h	> 24 h	4–24 h
Frequency and periodicity	Remission for weeks/months	Unpredictable – can enumerate attacks	Unpredictable – can enumerate attacks	Usually a discrete episode
Special times of occurrence	Nocturnal Especially when hungry, e.g. between meals		After heavy drinking	Following periods of dehydration
Aggravating factors	Stress, spicy foods, alcohol, smoking, aspirin	Unable to eat during bouts of pain	Alcohol Unable to eat during bouts of pain	
Relieving factors	Food, antacids, vomiting		Eased by sitting upright	
Associated phenomena	Family history, GI bleeding, perforation	Restlessness, vomiting, jaundice	Vomiting, jaundice, paralytic ileus	Restlessness, vomiting, haematuria, dysuria
Causes	Helicobacter pylori associated gastritis	Bile salt disorders, obesity, haemolytic anaemia	Gallstones, drugs, e.g. diuretics, alcohol Hypercalcaemic states	Dehydration, hyperuricaemia, hypercalcaemia

TABLE 5.8 Non-alimentary causes of abdominal pain

Disorder	Clinical features
Myocardial infarction	Cardiac arrhythmia Hypotension, angor animi (feeling of impending doom)
Dissecting aortic aneurysm	Hypotension, hypertension Asymmetry of femoral pulses
Acute vertebral collapse	Lateralised pain restricting movement Marked tenderness overlying the involved vertebra
Cord compression	Pain on percussion of thoracic spine Hyperaesthesia in dermatomal distribution Spinal cord signs
Pleurisy	Lateralised pain on coughing Chest signs, e.g. pleural rub
Herpes zoster	Hyperaesthesia in dermatomal distribution Vesicular eruption
Diabetic ketoacidosis	Cramp-like pain Vomiting, air hunger Tachycardia, ketotic breath
Salpingitis or tubal pregnancy	Suprapubic and iliac fossa pain and tenderness Nausea and vomiting, fever
Torsion of the testis/ovary	Lower abdominal pain Nausea, vomiting Localised tenderness

should always be the first diagnosis to be excluded. In young females, when unilateral salpingitis is suspected, an ectopic pregnancy is often the more likely diagnosis. Similarly, in patients with acute right iliac fossa pain, appendicitis should never be omitted from the differential diagnosis.

Speed of onset. A sudden onset of severe abdominal pain which progresses rapidly, becomes generalised in site and constant in nature, in a previously asymptomatic patient, suggests either perforation of a hollow viscus, a ruptured aortic aneurysm or a mesenteric arterial occlusion. Prior symptoms may help the differential diagnosis; preceding constipation suggests colonic carcinoma or diverticular disease as the cause of the perforation, and preceding dyspepsia suggests a perforated peptic ulcer. Coexisting peripheral vascular disease, hypertension, cardiac failure or atrial fibrillation suggest a vascular disorder, e.g. aortic aneurysm, mesenteric ischaemia. The development of peripheral circulatory failure (shock) following the onset of the pain, strongly suggests intra-abdominal bleeding, e.g. ruptured aortic aneurysm or ectopic pregnancy. The rapid onset of abdominal pain may also occur if an organ twists – known as *torsion* – and occludes its blood supply. Torsion of the testis or ovary produces severe abdominal pain and often nausea. Torsion of the caecum or sigmoid colon (*volvulus*) commonly presents with sudden abdominal pain associated with the development of acute intestinal obstruction.

A slower onset and progression of abdominal pain over hours or days suggests inflammatory disorders such as acute cholecystitis, appendicitis or diverticulitis.

Symptom progression. The development of shoulder tip pain indicates peritoneal inflammation immediately below the diaphragm. In some patients during the first hour or two after a perforation, a 'silent interval' may occur when abdominal pain resolves transiently. There is an initial chemical peritonitis, which then begins to subside, before bacterial contamination and peritonitis ensues.

In appendicitis, pain is initially localised around the umbilicus (visceral pain) and is vague; as the inflammatory response progresses to involve the parietal peritoneum, the main site of pain shifts to the right iliac fossa (parietal or somatic pain). If rupture of the appendix occurs, generalised peritonitis may then develop. If not, the patient may develop a localised abscess, but this in turn may subsequently rupture to produce generalised peritonitis.

A change in the pattern of symptoms should alert the clinician to the possibility that either the initial diagnosis was wrong, or that complications have developed. In a patient with acute small bowel obstruction, a change in the pain from typical intestinal colic to persistent pain with

CASE HISTORY

An 86-year-old man presented with central abdominal pain of 12 hours' duration, associated with vomiting and constipation. The pain occurred every 5–10 minutes, in waves lasting 2–3 minutes suggesting small intestinal obstruction. There was no previous history of abdominal surgery. The patient was pyrexial and the abdomen was distended, tympanitic to percussion and without localising tenderness on palpation.

Treatment with intravenous fluid replacement and nasogastric tube suction was instituted. Plain abdominal radiographs confirmed obstruction of the distal small bowel with gaseous distension and no air visible in the colon. Abdominal examination was repeated and a rectal examination performed. A more careful examination of the hernial orifices revealed a small mass lying below and medial to the mid-inguinal point. The mass was irreducible with no discernible cough impulse. At laparotomy, a strangulated femoral hernia containing ischaemic small bowel was found, necessitating resection of a section of small bowel.

Learning points

- Intestinal obstruction is suggested by the presence of typical central, colicky pain.
- Meticulous clinical examination is essential to avoid missing signs.
- The site of pain may not indicate the site of the problem.

abdominal tenderness suggests intestinal ischaemia, as for example in a strangulated hernia, and is an indication for urgent surgical intervention.

Heartburn

Most healthy individuals have experienced heartburn: the sensation of a hot, burning retrosternal discomfort often accompanied by the reflux of bitter-tasting gastric fluid into the mouth. It commonly occurs after meals or on bending or lying on the left side and is particularly frequent during pregnancy or following recent weight gain. Heartburn is caused by the reflux of acid, pepsin or bile into the oesophagus and is attributable to a combination of relaxation of the lower oesophageal sphincter and increased intra-abdominal pressure. Many patients with heartburn have no evidence of oesophagitis on oesophagoscopy. However, oesophagitis may develop resulting in pain on swallowing (*odynophagia*) or food sticking during swallowing (*dysphagia*). Heartburn is also commonly experienced by patients with duodenal ulceration. When accompanied by reflex salivation, known as *waterbrash*, the mouth fills with tasteless saliva, in contrast to the bitter taste of acid reflux; waterbrash is an uncommon symptom which if present, strongly suggests duodenal ulcer disease.

Dyspepsia (indigestion)

'Indigestion' is a common complaint. It is essential that the patient explains in detail what is meant by this vague term. Indigestion might describe nausea, heartburn, epigastric discomfort, abdominal pain, belching or a feeling of post-prandial bloating. It may even be used to describe angina pectoris. Peptic ulcers usually produce characteristic symptoms, as shown in Table 5.7. Differentiation between oesophageal, gastric or duodenal ulcers on the basis of symptoms alone is often unreliable.

Functional dyspepsia, i.e. persistent dyspepsia for which no structural or biochemical cause can be found, is common; it is commonly classified on the basis of subsets of symptoms though many patients with functional dyspepsia have more than one symptom subset (Table 5.9).

TABLE 5.9 Functional dyspepsia

Type	Symptom subset
Reflux-like	Acid reflux and heartburn relieved by antacids
Ulcer-like	Localised epigastric pain and nocturnal pain Relief with vomiting, food or antacids
Dysmotility-like	Nausea, belching, premature satiety, bloating and abdominal distension

Wind (flatulence)

Repeated belching, excessive or offensive rectal flatus, abdominal distension and even borborygmi (audible bowel sounds) may all be called 'wind', a term which the patient should be asked to clarify. Belching often results from air swallowing (aerophagy) which occurs without the patient's awareness. Belching itself is of no major significance, although it may indicate anxiety, and sometimes occurs in an attempt to relieve abdominal pain or discomfort. The normal volume of flatus per rectum varies greatly from person to person, in the range of 200–2000 ml per day. It consists of a mixture of gases derived principally from swallowed air together with gases derived from colonic bacterial fermentation of poorly absorbed carbohydrates. Excessive flatus is particularly troublesome in lactase deficiency and intestinal malabsorption. Absence of flatus is a feature of intestinal obstruction. Borborygmi result from the movement of fluid and gas along the bowel; though often no more than a source of embarrassment, they may indicate disordered small bowel motility.

Abdominal distension (bloating)

The principal causes of abdominal distension are *fat, flatus, faeces, fluid* and *fetus* (Table 5.10). Increasing abdominal girth is usually due to adiposity and should alert the clinician to the possibility of alcohol abuse. Its development in a patient who is otherwise becoming thinner suggests intra-abdominal disease.

Ascites, the accumulation of fluid in the peritoneal cavity, is usually due to cirrhosis of the liver, malignancy, nephrotic syndrome, tuberculous peritonitis, cardiac or pericardial disease. The acute development of tense ascites suggests intra-abdominal malignancy, infective peritonitis or the onset of hepatic or portal vein obstruction.

Painless abdominal distension in women may be the presenting symptom of an ovarian cyst or of an undisclosed pregnancy. It is also a feature of *pseudo-obstruction*, i.e. non-mechanical obstruction, often seen in neuropathy affecting the gastrointestinal tract, and in elderly patients

TABLE 5.10 Causes of abdominal distension

Factor	Consider
Fat	Excessive alcohol consumption
Flatus	Pseudo-obstruction, obstruction
Faeces	Subacute obstruction, constipation
Fluid	Ovarian or uterine mass Bladder enlargement Ascites
Fetus	Date of the last menstrual period

taking drugs with anticholinergic effects, such as tricyclic antidepressants. Painless abdominal distension and constipation from early childhood in the absence of faecal soiling suggests the possibility of Hirschsprung's disease. Fluctuating abdominal swelling which develops during the day but resolves overnight is particularly common in women and is rarely if ever due to organic disease. It usually occurs with other symptoms of the irritable bowel syndrome, namely abdominal pain relieved by defecation and altered bowel habit. Painful abdominal distension suggests intestinal obstruction associated with intestinal colic. Chronic simple constipation rarely produces painful distension unless associated with the irritable bowel syndrome.

Altered bowel habit

The normal bowel habit varies between several evacuations per day to one every 3 days or so. Changes in bowel habit may be the first symptom of serious underlying disease. Constipation may be used by the patient to describe hard pellety stools, infrequent defecation or excessive straining at stool with difficulty in evacuation (*dyschezia*). Similarly, diarrhoea may be used to describe frequent defecation, loose or fluid stools, urgency of defecation, the persistent desire to defecate or faecal incontinence. *Tenesmus*, the feeling of incomplete rectal evacuation with a persistent desire to defecate, is common in infective colitis, rectal carcinoma, rectal prolapse and the irritable bowel syndrome.

The irritable bowel syndrome is a common cause of altered bowel function in patients under the age of 50 years. The principal symptoms include episodic constipation and diarrhoea associated with abdominal distension, intermittent abdominal pain relieved by defecation and often accompanied by non-specific symptoms including dyspepsia, urinary frequency, backache and tiredness (Table 5.11).

The important questions in the clinical history of patients with diarrhoea and the common causes are shown in Tables 5.12 and 5.13.

TABLE 5.11 Criteria for the diagnosis of irritable bowel syndrome

Continuous or recurrent abdominal pain or discomfort, relieved by defecation or associated with altered stool frequency or consistency, together with either or both of the following features:

Altered pattern of defecation for at least 25% of the time, i.e. **two** or more of the following:
- altered stool frequency (> 3/day or < 3/week)
- altered stool form (lumpy, hard, loose, watery)
- altered stool passage (straining, faecal urgency, feeling of incomplete emptying)
- passage of mucus

Abdominal distension or a feeling of abdominal bloating

TABLE 5.12 Symptom checklist in patients with diarrhoeal disorders

- Is the diarrhoea acute, chronic or intermittent?
- Is there tenesmus, urgency or incontinence?
- Is the stool watery, unformed or semisolid?
- Is the stool of large volume and not excessively frequent suggesting small bowel disease?
- Is the stool of small volume and excessively frequent suggesting large bowel disease?
- Is there blood, mucus or pus associated with the stool?
- Does diarrhoea occur during the night, suggesting organic disease?
- Is there a history of contact with diarrhoea or of travel abroad?
- Does the sexual history provide a clue (gay bowel syndrome, HIV)?
- Is there a history of alcohol abuse or relevant drug therapy?
- Is there a past medical history of GI surgery, GI disease or inflammatory bowel disease?
- Is there a family history of GI disorder, e.g. gluten enteropathy, Crohn's?
- Are there any other GI symptoms, e.g. adominal pain and vomiting?
- Are there symptoms of systemic disease, e.g. rigors or arthralgia?

TABLE 5.13 Important causes of diarrhoea

Acute
- Infective gastroenteritis
- Drug therapy, e.g. antibiotics, mefenamic acid

Chronic
- Irritable bowel syndrome
- Inflammatory bowel disease
- Parasitic gut infections
- Drug therapy, e.g. laxatives
- Malabsorption
- Bowel resection
- Autonomic neuropathy
- Faecal impaction
- Colorectal malignancy
- Metabolic disorders, e.g. thyrotoxicosis

The nature of any medication, prescribed or self-administered, should be established. Patients may be unaware of the laxative effects of some agents, e.g. magnesium-containing antacids, mefenamic acid; or the constipating effects of others, e.g. aluminium-containing antacids, codeine phosphate or tricyclic antidepressants.

Questions to ask patients complaining of constipation, and some of its possible causes, are shown in Tables 5.14 and 5.15. Constipation and faecal incontinence or soiling may coexist, especially with faecal impaction in children or the elderly. It is important to determine the timing and frequency of defecation, any association with abdominal, rectal or anal pain and any difficulty, urgency or tenesmus experienced during evacuation. In addition, the patient should be asked to describe the appearance, colour, consistency and characteristics of the faeces. Sometimes words like 'stools' or 'faeces' are not understood and if there is doubt it is best to use colloquial phrases.

Special enquiry should be made about the presence of blood and pus or mucus, often described by the patient as

TABLE 5.14 Symptom checklist in patients with constipation

Has constipation been lifelong or is it of recent onset?
How often do the bowels empty each week?
How much time is spent straining at stool?
Is there associated abdominal pain, anal pain on defecation or rectal bleeding?
Has the shape of the stool changed, e.g. become pellet-like?
Has there been any change in drug therapy?

TABLE 5.15 Important causes of constipation

Dietary fibre deficiency
Irritable bowel syndrome
Drug therapy, e.g. opiates
Intestinal obstruction
Immobility and lack of exercise
Metabolic disorders, e.g. hypothyroidism, hypercalcaemia

TABLE 5.16 Characteristic abnormalities of stool colour

Tarry black	Upper gastrointestinal haemorrhage (melaena) (proximal to the transverse colon), e.g. peptic ulcers, caecal angiodysplasia Iron or colloidal bismuth therapy
Bloody	Ulcerative colitis Colorectal tumours Colonic diverticulitis
Pale	Fat malabsorption (steatorrhoea) from either small bowel or pancreatic disease
Silvery	Combination of steatorrhoea and gastrointestinal haemorrhage, e.g. pancreatic carcinoma

'slime'. Since many patients do not normally inspect their faeces, only positive observations should be accepted; if necessary, the clinician should confirm the description by inspection of the stools. Abnormalities such as threadworms, roundworms or segments of tapeworms may also be present. Examples of abnormal stool colour are given in Table 5.16.

Rectal bleeding

The cause of this important symptom should always be determined. Though frequently due to haemorrhoids or an anal fissure, these are so commonplace that their presence in a patient with rectal bleeding should not lead to the assumption of cause and effect. The differential diagnosis includes colorectal carcinoma, ulcerative colitis, infective colitis and complicated diverticular disease (Table 5.17). Bleeding from the anal canal is bright red; it is usually clearly separate from the faeces and often seen only on the toilet paper. Haemorrhoidal bleeding may be profuse and splash the toilet bowl and/or continue following defecation. Bleeding from an anal fissure is usually associated with anal pain which occurs during and after defecation. Colitis is commonly associated with the symptoms of urgency of defecation and the passage of unformed stools with blood, mucus and pus. Both colonic adenomas and carcinomas may cause excessive mucus production. Bleeding from any site along the gastrointestinal tract may also present with syncope, peripheral circulatory failure or the symptoms of chronic anaemia.

TABLE 5.17 Causes of bright red rectal bleeding

Haemorrhoids
Anal fissure
Colorectal polyps
Colorectal malignancy
Inflammatory bowel disease
Complicated diverticular disease
Ischaemic colitis

CASE HISTORY

A 45-year-old woman presented with breathlessness on exertion, tiredness and aches and pains in the back and limbs. Systemic enquiry revealed painless abdominal bloating, occasional loose stools, weight loss of 6 kg over 12 months and more recently, intermittent dysphagia. Ever since the menarche, she has had recurrent crops of mouth ulcers occurring especially at menstruation. As a teenager and subsequently during two pregnancies, she had been found to have an iron-deficiency anaemia for which no cause had been found.

Clinical examination findings were unremarkable except for pallor of the mucous membranes and tests for occult blood in the stools were negative. Investigations confirmed recurrence of her iron-deficiency anaemia together with a decrease in the serum concentrations of calcium and phosphate to suggest vitamin D deficiency. Upper GI endoscopy of the oesophagus, stomach and duodenum was unremarkable.

The diagnosis of gluten enteropathy (coeliac disease) was confirmed by the presence of high titres in the serum of endomysial antibodies and total villous atrophy on duodenal biopsy. 3 months after strict adherence to a gluten-free diet, all of her symptoms had resolved completely. Dysphagia was attributed to the mucosal changes associated with severe iron deficiency (sideropenic dysphagia) and the musculoskeletal symptoms attributed to osteomalacia.

Learning points

- GI disorders may present with non-specific and/or non-alimentary symptoms.
- Recurrent mouth ulcers are a typical feature of gluten enteropathy and inflammatory bowel disease.
- The symptom of dysphagia requires direct visualisation of the oesophagus to exclude sinister causes.
- In the absence of GI bleeding, recurrent iron deficiency suggests a malabsorption syndrome.

Jaundice

Jaundice is the result of excess bilirubin circulating in the blood. Most bilirubin originates from the catabolism of

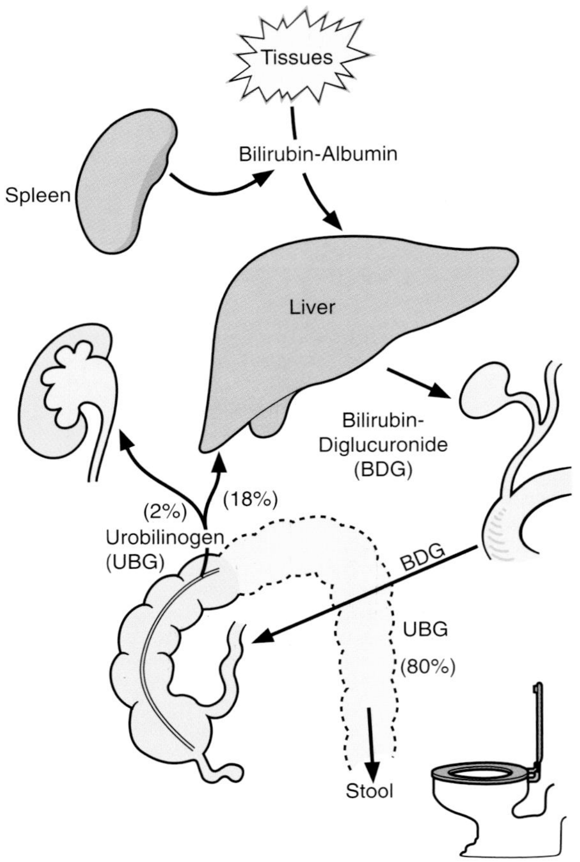

Fig. 5.1 Bilirubin metabolism.

haemoglobin in the reticuloendothelial system. Unconjugated bilirubin bound to albumin cannot be excreted into the urine. Following hepatic glucuronidation, bilirubin diglucuronide enters the gut lumen via the biliary tree and is metabolised by the gut microflora to urobilinogen (Fig. 5.1). Urobilinogen is then reabsorbed and enters the enterohepatic cycle; in health, it is excreted in the urine as a colourless compound in small quantities. In biliary tract obstruction (intrahepatic or extrahepatic in origin), the water-soluble compound bilirubin diglucuronide refluxes into the blood and is excreted in the urine to produce a brownish discoloration (bilirubinuria).

Jaundice may therefore be *haemolytic, hepatocellular* or *obstructive* in origin. A checklist for patients with a history of jaundice is shown in Table 5.18.

Haemolytic jaundice. Unconjugated hyperbilirubinaemia such as in haemolytic anaemia may occur without either symptoms or urine discoloration (hence the term acholuric jaundice).

TABLE 5.18 Checklist for the history of jaundice

Past medical history (pancreatitis, biliary surgery)
Previous jaundice or hepatitis
Blood transfusions (hepatitis B or C)
Family history (congenital spherocytosis)
Sexual and contact history (hepatitis B or C)
Travel history and immunisations (hepatitis A)
Drug and alcohol history
Skin tattooing (hepatitis B or C)
Pruritus, dark urine, rigors
Appetite and weight change
Abdominal pain, altered bowel habit
Gastrointestinal bleeding

Hepatocellular jaundice. Characteristic symptoms include anorexia with impairment of taste, nausea, vomiting and upper abdominal pain (often associated with hepatic tenderness). Common causes include viral hepatitis and chemical hepatitis, e.g. alcohol abuse and drug therapy.

Obstructive jaundice. Typical symptoms include itching (pruritus), dark urine and pale stools. Obstruction of the biliary tract is usually extrahepatic in origin and caused by either gallstones or pancreatic carcinoma. The former is suggested by a history of fever, rigors, biliary colic or previous biliary surgery; in the latter, chronic persistent back pain, aggravated by recumbency, and palpable enlargement of the gall bladder may occur. Intrahepatic obstruction is most often due to alcohol abuse, drug therapy and primary biliary cirrhosis (a disorder of middle-aged women often preceded by marked pruritus).

KEY POINTS

- The first history should be as detailed as possible because acutely ill patients tire easily and accuracy may be lost on repetition.
- Symptom progression and symptom patterns are often of diagnostic value.
- Weight loss as an isolated symptom is rarely the result of serious underlying organic disease.
- Depression may present as weight loss or even weight gain.
- Melaena indicates upper gastrointestinal haemorrhage and is usually associated with significant haemodynamic changes resulting from loss of blood volume.
- Haemorrhoids are so common that their presence in a patient with rectal bleeding should not lead to the assumption of cause and effect.
- Dysphagia is a cardinal symptom which requires prompt investigation even when transient.
- Difficulty in swallowing fluids rather than solids, associated with spluttering and coughing, suggests neurological disorders.
- Vomiting and anorexia are common manifestations of non-alimentary disorders.
- Changes in bowel habit may be the first symptom of serious underlying disease.

GENITOURINARY SYMPTOMS

As part of a general history, all patients should be asked about the cardinal symptoms of genitourinary disorders (Table 5.19) even though this may be embarrassing for some patients to discuss.

Renal disease may present with non-specific symptoms such as tiredness or breathlessness due to renal failure and the associated anaemia, or the observation of oedema due to fluid retention. It may also be detected following the finding of hypertension, microscopic haematuria, or proteinuria on routine assessment, such as insurance medical examinations.

Dysuria, frequency and urgency

These are cardinal symptoms of *urinary tract infection*, the commonest condition to affect the urinary tract. Dysuria is pain experienced prior to, during or following micturition, usually in the urethra or suprapubic region. When due to urinary infection, it is often described as a burning sensation, even akin to passing broken glass. Urinary frequency describes an increased frequency of micturition without implying any increase in the total urine volume. Urgency is a strong desire to pass urine which may be followed by incontinence if the opportunity to urinate is not available.

In general, dysuria, frequency and urgency are associated with disorders of the lower urinary tract – bladder, prostate and urethra. Although commonly due to urinary tract infection, tumours, urinary calculi or urinary tract obstruction should also be considered. Dysuria alone may be due to infection of the urethra, as in gonorrhoea, when there may also be urethral discharge.

TABLE 5.19 List of genitourinary symptoms

General	Pain passing urine (dysuria) Severe suprapubic pain associated with inability to pass urine (strangury) Passing urine more often than usual (frequency) A sudden need to pass urine (urgency) Passing a larger volume of urine than normal (polyuria) Passing a smaller volume of urine than normal (oliguria) Passing urine during the night (nocturia) Total absence of urine output (anuria) Blood in the urine (haematuria) Air bubbles in the urine (pneumaturia)
Females	Stress or urge urinary imcontinence Menstrual irregularities Obstetric difficulties Vaginal bleeding following intrauterine erosions, polyps, malignancy Vaginal discharge (e.g. candidiasis or sexually acquired infection) Altered sexual function, e.g. dyspareunia (painful intercourse)
Males	Delay in initiating urine flow (hesitancy) Impaired urinary flow Post-micturition dribbling Dribbling incontinence Urethral discharge (suggesting sexually acquired infection) Altered sexual function (e.g. impotence)

Frequency alone, particularly in young adults, may be due to anxiety. In the elderly, it is more often the result of abnormally high bladder muscle tone (detrusor instability). Urgency alone may occur in pregnancy, owing to extrinsic pressure on the bladder, or weakness of the pelvic floor muscles or uterine prolapse. It may also be a feature of neurological disease affecting the motor control of the bladder, such as multiple sclerosis. Patients with multiple sclerosis often present with bladder symptoms, including a false sensation of needing to pass urine.

The term strangury is used when the patient experiences suprapubic pain associated with a repeated and urgent desire to urinate every few minutes, often associated with severe dysuria or inability to pass urine. It is usually due to acute bladder neck obstruction by a stone or blood clot.

Haematuria

Haematuria is the presence of blood in the urine attributable to bleeding from the urinary tract. It requires to be distinguished from contamination of the urine by bleeding from the female genital tract. Less commonly, it may also be confused with haemoglobinuria and myoglobinuria. Sometimes urinary discoloration may also be confused with haematuria (Table 5.20). Most often, haematuria is detected on routine chemical testing of the urine and is termed microscopic haematuria (see p. 180). Macroscopic haematuria is visible to the naked eye and is a serious symptom which requires investigation. The various conditions in Table 5.21 and Figure 5.2 can cause either microscopic or macroscopic haematuria, the difference simply reflecting the severity of blood loss.

Painless haematuria in the adult is usually due to a benign bladder papilloma or to renal, bladder or prostatic carcinoma. Haematuria associated with severe loin pain suggests a renal or ureteric origin, commonly due to the presence of a calculus. When haematuria is accompanied by dysuria or frequency, the source is usually in the

TABLE 5.20 Abnormalities of urine colour

Orange-brown	Bilirubin (conjugated) Rhubarb, senna Concentrated, normal urine (e.g. due to very low fluid intake)
Red-brown	Blood, myoglobin, haemoglobin, porphyrins Rifampicin, phenolphthalein Beetroot, blackberries
Brown-black	Bilirubin, melanin, methaemalbumin L-Dopa, homogentisic acid (alkaptonuria)

bladder, possibly bacterial infection of the bladder wall (cystitis). Haematuria which clears rapidly during micturition is usually urethral in origin.

TABLE 5.21 Causes of haematuria

Painless	Urinary tract infection Tuberculosis Schistosomiasis Urogenital tumours Glomerulonephritis Renal cystic disease Hypertension Chronic renal vascular disease
Painful	Renal calculi Urinary tract infection Reflux nephropathy Renal papillary necrosis Acute renal vascular disease, e.g. embolism

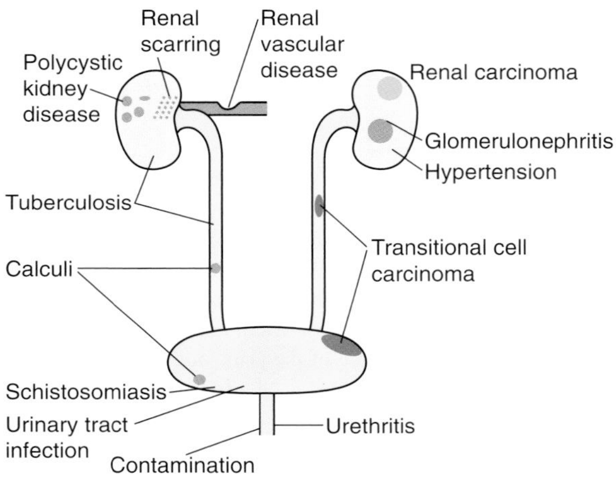

Fig. 5.2 Principal sources of haematuria.

CASE HISTORY

A 65-year-old man presented with an 8-week history of passing blood in the urine without pain. He had noticed slowing of the urinary stream with difficulty initiating micturition though this had changed little over the previous year. He was a lifelong heavy smoker and had worked all his life in the dyeing industry. Clinical examination was normal and rectal examination revealed smooth enlargement of the prostate. Urinalysis confirmed macroscopic haematuria and intravenous urography (IVU) was normal. Cystoscopy showed a large bladder tumour at the trigone.

Learning points

- Many older patients have prostatism; in only a minority is this due to prostate cancer.
- Uroepithelial tumours are associated with cigarette smoking and occupational exposure to dyes.
- Both direct visualisation of the bladder and an IVU are required in the investigation of haematuria.

Polyuria

Polyuria is an increase in urinary volume, regardless of the frequency of micturition. The patient's assessment of urine volume can be misleading and should be confirmed by 24-hour urinary collections. The most common cause of polyuria is an abnormally high fluid intake. In extreme cases, this may be a manifestation of psychiatric disease; it is termed *psychogenic polydipsia* (polydipsia = excessive thirst) and may result in urine flows of up to 12 litres daily. In other cases, polyuria is the primary problem, and thirst is a secondary symptom. Such causes include an increased load of solute, producing an osmotic diuresis, as occurs in untreated diabetes mellitus. Alternatively, there may be impairment of the renal concentrating ability, i.e. the capacity of the kidney tubules to reabsorb water in response to antidiuretic hormone (ADH) is impaired. In its most severe form this is known as nephrogenic diabetes insipidus, and is usually genetic or due to drugs such as lithium. Lesser degrees of ADH resistance can be associated with most types of chronic tubulointerstitial renal damage, including reflux nephropathy and analgesic nephropathy. Polyuria is also seen when ADH is absent or reduced (central diabetes insipidus). In untreated chronic adrenal insufficiency, polyuria is a consequence of renal salt wasting.

Nocturia

The need to rise at night to pass urine may be a lifelong habit. When of recent onset, it may reflect insomnia, polyuria or prostatic obstruction. Nocturia is also a common symptom of cardiac failure, the diuresis resulting from the improvement in renal blood flow which occurs with recumbency.

Oliguria and anuria

Oliguria is a reduction in the urine volume to less than 800 ml/day. A reduction in urine volume may be an appropriate response to a very low fluid intake, or may indicate an acute loss of kidney function. The minimum urine volume needed to excrete the daily solute load varies with the diet, physical activity and the metabolic rate, but in general, normal kidneys do not concentrate the urine to less than 400 ml/day, and values below this usually indicate some degree of renal failure. Acute renal failure is defined as the inability to effectively handle a solute load and maintain a normal blood urea. It is usually associated with oliguria but not invariably; excessive solute loads from hypercatabolic states, e.g. severe burns or infections, may induce renal failure even in the absence of impaired renal function. Non-oliguric acute renal failure accounts for up to 20% of instances and may be overlooked by clinicians unaware of the possibility. Anuria, the total cessation of urine production, is uncommon and should raise the suspicion of urinary tract obstruction. Often, the complaint of being unable to pass urine is due to urinary retention, as a result of bladder neck or urethral obstruction. A mechanical explanation, such as marked prostatic enlargement, or a neurological explanation such as spinal injury, should be sought.

Pneumaturia

This rare symptom consists of passing air bubbles in the urine. It is most often caused by a fistula between the bladder and the colon, usually as a result of a diverticular abscess or a malignant tumour.

Impaired force of micturition and other symptoms of prostatism

Reduced force of the urinary stream in males suggests bladder outlet obstruction due to prostatic hypertrophy or, less commonly, a urethral stricture. Other features of prostatic bladder neck obstruction (often termed *prostatism*) include hesitancy (difficulty in initiating the urine flow), double voiding (the need to pass urine again within a few minutes of micturition), urinary dribbling after micturition, frequency and nocturia due to incomplete bladder emptying or complete urinary retention.

Urinary incontinence

This is categorised as *urge incontinence* when an urgent need to urinate cannot be resisted, and *stress incontinence* when leakage of urine occurs in response to coughing, sneezing or laughing; some patients have both. An information checklist is shown in Table 5.22.

Many parous women experience stress incontinence because of weakness of the anterior wall of the vagina, often accompanied by a degree of uterine prolapse. Incontinence may also arise from neurological disorders of bladder function. In sensory denervation of the bladder, dribbling incontinence results from painless overdistension of the bladder, as in diabetic autonomic neuropathy. Loss of motor control results in urgency. If the desire to urinate is not met promptly, because of immobility or severe urgency, incontinence ensues. Combined motor and sensory damage occurs in spinal cord lesions, e.g. spinal trauma, multiple sclerosis. The bladder fills to a certain pressure and then empties reflexly. The patient may learn to control bladder emptying by raising the intravesical pressure by manual compression of the lower abdomen. Mechanical obstruction may also cause incontinence; in men this is usually due to benign prostatic hypertrophy or prostate carcinoma. Nocturnal bed-wetting (enuresis) is common in childhood and may persist into adult life.

TABLE 5.22 Causes of urinary incontinence

Incoordination of bladder sphincter function in old age
Spinal cord trauma or compression
Multiple sclerosis
Females: Pelvic floor damage during childbirth
Males: Benign prostatic hypertrophy, prostatic carcinoma

Urogenital pain

Renal pain is usually due to stretching of the renal capsule or renal pelvis. A chronic dull aching discomfort in the loin and renal angle may occur in renal scarring or infection and in hydronephrosis. Intermittent pain can occur in polycystic disease from infection or spontaneous bleeding into a cyst. In acute pyelonephritis, renal pain is often accompanied by dysuria, fever and sometimes rigors.

Severe pain, known as *renal colic*, can be caused by acute distension of the renal pelvis and ureter, resulting from obstruction by calculus or blood clot. Renal colic is not a true colic; the pain is severe, sustained and

CASE HISTORY

A 49-year-old woman presented with an 8-hour history of severe left-sided loin pain radiating into the groin and associated with vomiting. The past medical history revealed a previous right nephrectomy for 'chronic pyelonephritis' and long-standing headaches for which she had been taking ibuprofen, a non-steroidal, anti-inflammatory drug (NSAID) on a daily basis for over 20 years. Her last menstrual period had been 2 weeks ago. She had not passed urine for 6 hours.

She was restless and distressed by pain necessitating intravenous opiate therapy before clinical examination could proceed. Tenderness was noted in the left renal angle and left iliac fossa. The bladder was not palpable. Rectal and vaginal examination were normal.

An immediate ultrasound examination of the urinary tract revealed marked dilatation of the left renal pelvicalyceal system. A percutaneous nephrostomy drain was inserted into the left renal pelvis, resulting in rapid restoration of urine flow via the drain. The following day she passed a large fleshy 'stone' per urethra. Pathological examination of the 'stone' revealed a necrotic renal papilla and review of the histopathology of the previous nephrectomy confirmed the diagnosis of NSAID-induced renal papillary necrosis due to analgesic nephropathy.

Learning points

- The pain of ureteric colic is usually sustained and associated with vomiting.
- Anuria strongly suggests complete obstruction of the urinary tract.
- A careful history often elicits key pointers to the underlying diagnosis.
- Look first for a single unifying diagnosis before considering multiple unrelated diagnoses.

unremitting and the patient is restless, nauseated and often vomits. The pain may radiate from the renal angle and loin to the iliac fossa, the groin and into the genitalia. Once the stone reaches the bladder, it is often asymptomatic until it enters the urethra and causes dysuria. In patients with renal colic, specific questions should be asked to try to determine any underlying cause for stone formation (see Fig. 5.3).

Most conditions causing bladder pain also cause frequency and dysuria. In males, perineal and rectal pain with associated dysuria suggest prostatic inflammation or infection (*prostatitis*) and may be associated with symptoms of bladder neck obstruction. Testicular and epididymal pain may be felt in the groin and lower abdomen to such an extent that its testicular origin may be obscured. Its occurrence in pubertal boys and young men is most often the result of torsion of the testis and demands urgent intervention. The onset is frequently at night with pain in the iliac fossa. Tenderness and swelling of the testis may need to be distinguished from a strangulated hernia or acute epididymo-orchitis.

Ovarian pain is also felt in the iliac fossa and may be episodic and cyclical, as in endometriosis, or more constant, as in malignant tumours. Uterine pain is felt centrally in the hypogastrium and may radiate to the lumbosacral area, e.g. labour pains and dysmenorrhoea.

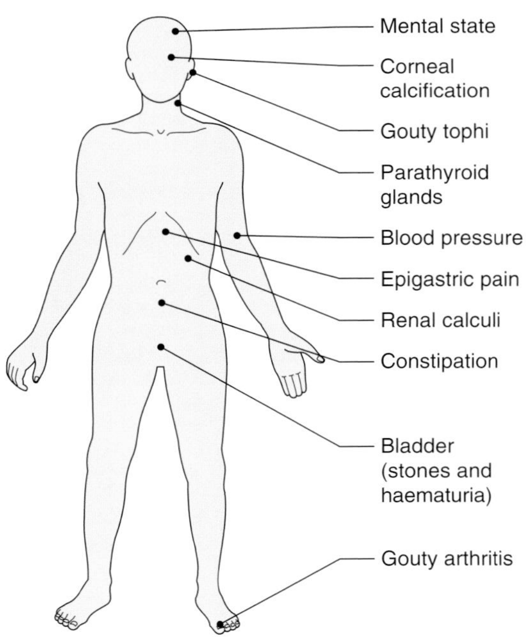

Fig. 5.3 Checklist in patients with renal colic.

Menstrual and obstetric history

The menstrual history should include the age at onset of menstruation (menarche) and of cessation of menstruation (menopause) as appropriate. Details of the menstrual cycle should also include the date of the first day of the last menstrual period and the duration of menses (Table 5.23). The normal age of the menarche varies from the ages 10–15. Thereafter, patients who fail to menstruate at all, primary amenorrhoea, should be investigated for possible gynaecological or endocrinological abnormalities.

The normal age of the menopause varies considerably within the age range 45–55. Secondary amenorrhoea is commonly due to pregnancy. If this is not the case, organic causes such as severe systemic illness, hyperprolactinaemia, androgen excess or hypopituitarism should be excluded before attributing it to a psychological disorder. Useful questions in the menstrual history are shown in Table 5.23.

The obstetric history comprises details of all pregnancies, successful or otherwise, and any problems experienced during pregnancy, such as high blood pressure or urinary infection (Table 5.24). If a woman has never been pregnant, it may be appropriate to enquire whether this was by choice or whether difficulties in conceiving have been experienced.

The presence of a vaginal discharge requires to be assessed and note made of its colour, consistency and smell; for example, particularly strong odour may indicate anaerobic bacterial infection. Vaginal bleeding occurring after intercourse is usually caused by local pathology, e.g. cervical erosions, polyps or carcinoma. The presence of a vaginal discharge or intermenstrual, postcoital or postmenopausal bleeding, is an indication for a gynaecological assessment and examination.

TABLE 5.23 Checklist of the menstrual history
Age at onset of the first period (menarche)
Age at cessation of menstruation (menopause)
Use of contraceptive drugs or hormone replacement therapy
Date of the first day of the last menstrual period
Frequency, regularity and duration of menstruation
Is menstrual blood loss unusually heavy?

TABLE 5.24 Checklist of the obstetric history
Number of pregnancies and live births, miscarriages and terminations
Any health problems during pregnancies or after delivery?*
Were the previous deliveries vaginal or caesarean?
Were forceps or episiotomy used?
*NB: Remember to ask about medical disorders complicating pregnancy, including anaemia, hypertension, diabetes mellitus, thyroid disease or urinary infection.

TABLE 5.25 Checklist for the sexual history

How many sexual partners have you had in the last 12 months?
How many of your partners have been male and how many female?
How many of your partners have been casual relationships?
Do you use a condom most of the time, all of the time or not at all?
Have you ever had a sexually transmitted disease?
Males: Have you had any problems with sexual drive, erections, penetration, ejaculation, or orgasm?
Females: Have you had any problems with sexual drive, pain during intercourse or orgasm?

CASE HISTORY

A 30-year-old female schoolteacher was admitted for investigation of 7 kg weight loss, tiredness and malaise of 3 months' duration. Systemic enquiry was otherwise normal. She had two children by her partner in a stable relationship of 5 years' duration. There was no history of drug use and physical examination was initially normal. The diagnosis was unclear until after complaining of a sore throat, she was found to have oral candidiasis. Suspecting an immunodeficiency disorder, a sexual history was then taken and revealed that 2 years previously, while her partner was abroad, she had unprotected sexual intercourse with a bisexual friend. An HIV test was performed and was positive; her partner and her second child were also later found to be HIV-positive.

Learning points

- An inadequate history may delay both the diagnosis and treatment.
- HIV infection should be considered in patients with unexplained immunodeficiency states even if risk factors are not immediately apparent.

KEY POINTS

- Renal disease may be asymptomatic or present with non-specific symptoms, e.g. tiredness.
- Genitourinary complaints can be embarrassing and need specific enquiry to avoid overlooking important problems.
- Painless visible haematuria in the adult is most often due to a bladder papilloma or carcinoma.
- Symptoms of prostatism are common and develop slowly; in consequence, patients often underestimate their significance.
- Complete anuria is rare; most patients who stop passing urine have bladder neck obstruction.
- Testicular pain may be referred to the groin and lower abdomen.
- The commonest cause of secondary amenorrhoea is pregnancy, but it may indicate severe systemic illness, an endocrinological disorder or a psychological problem.
- Sexual dysfunction and sexually transmitted disease occurs at any age and in any social setting.

The sexual history

Sexual dysfunction and sexually transmitted diseases are common; they are not confined to young adults, or to promiscuous individuals. Although such topics are often avoided by patients because of embarrassment, it is particularly important to ask patients about sexual function and activity and if they have any of the disorders known to predispose to sexual dysfunction. These include diabetes mellitus, alcohol abuse, chronic renal failure, marital difficulty or psychological disorder. Similarly, when sexually transmitted diseases are suspected, e.g. HIV, hepatitis or pelvic inflammatory disease, a careful sexual history should be undertaken. In females, dyspareunia (pain related to sexual intercourse) or failure to achieve an orgasm are common and are frequently caused by, or lead to, psychological difficulties. In males, loss of libido, premature ejaculation and inability to maintain an erection may also be primarily psychological. Questions should be asked objectively with tact and sensitivity in a non-judgemental manner using a non-medical vocabulary to facilitate better communication. One approach would be to start by asking if sexual intercourse is satisfactory and, if it is not, enquire further. Some useful questions to ask are shown in Table 5.25. With practice, the clinician will become more comfortable taking a sexual history and patients should then feel less uncomfortable answering the questions. Even so, a sexual history may prove embarrassing and an alternative method is to ask patients to complete a confidential questionnaire detailing explicitly their sexual history and any problems they may have experienced. This may allow the clinician to identify the main problem earlier and to achieve a better rapport.

THE PHYSICAL EXAMINATION

MOUTH, THROAT AND OESOPHAGUS

The examination of the mouth and throat is described on page 51. It is important to assess whether the teeth provide an adequate chewing surface or, if the patient is edentulous, to know if dentures fit and are used for eating.

When there is a complaint of dysphagia it can be helpful to watch the act of swallowing solids and liquids. This may reveal the organic nature and the site of the lesion. If swallowing is immediately followed by a distressing bout of coughing, either a neuromuscular disturbance such as bulbar or pseudobulbar palsy or more rarely a fistula between the trachea and the oesophagus should be suspected.

ABDOMEN

It is conventional for descriptive purposes to divide the abdomen into nine regions by the intersection of imaginary

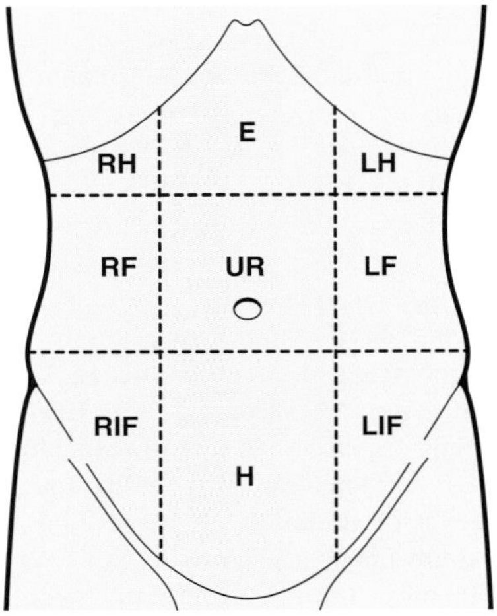

RH	Right hypochondrium	**LH**	Left hypochondrium
RF	Right flank or lumbar region	**LF**	Left flank or lumbar region
RIF	Right iliac fossa	**LIF**	Left iliac fossa

E Epigastrium
UR Umbilical region
H Hypogastrium or supra-pubic region

Fig. 5.4 Regions of the abdomen.

planes, two horizontal and two sagittal. The upper horizontal plane (transpyloric) lies at the level of the first lumbar vertebra, midway between the suprasternal notch and the symphysis pubis. The lower plane passes through the upper borders of the iliac crests. The sagittal planes are indicated on the surface by lines drawn vertically from the mid-inguinal points towards the mid-clavicular points (Fig. 5.4).

The resultant regions are artificial but are helpful in localising most lesions. An alternative description is to refer to the right and left upper and lower quadrants of the abdomen, using vertical and horizontal lines passing through the umbilicus. The contents of the abdomen are illustrated in Figures 5.5 and 5.6.

Anatomy and normal structures

- Quiet respiration is predominantly diaphragmatic, particularly in males, so that the abdominal wall moves out during inspiration.
- In healthy subjects, it may be possible to feel the colon in the left iliac fossa. The caecum and sometimes the transverse colon may also be palpable, especially if the latter contains hard faeces. The aorta, the liver edge and the lower pole of the right kidney are often palpable (Fig. 5.9). Faeces are commonly palpable in the sigmoid colon. The distended bladder and gravid uterus may also be palpable.
- The liver and gall bladder, spleen and kidneys move

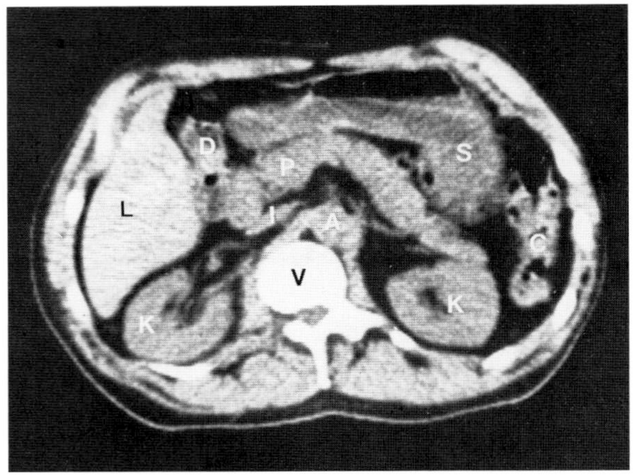

Fig. 5.5 Contents of the abdomen and pelvis shown by CT scan. A, aorta and renal arteries; C, colon and faeces; D, duodenum; I, inferior vena cava; K, kidney; L, liver; P, pancreas; S, stomach; V, vertebra (the apparent deformity of which is due to the scan passing through the pedicle and lamina on the left side and through the foramen on the right. (Courtesy of Dr Andrew R. Wright.)

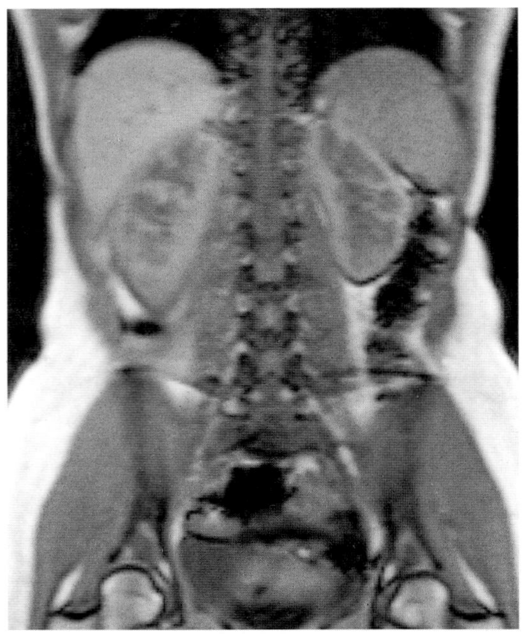

Fig. 5.6 Contents of the abdomen and pelvis demonstrated by magnetic resonance imaging (MRI) scan obtained in an angled coronal-type plane to demonstrate the various structures. (Courtesy of Dr Andrew R. Wright.)

downwards during inspiration, as a result of the downward movement of the diaphragm.

- As the liver descends 1–3 cm on inspiration, it can normally be palpated in adults below the right costal margin during deep inspiration.
- The normal spleen lies against the posterolateral wall of the abdominal cavity, beneath ribs 9–11. The anterior border of the spleen extends to the mid-axillary line. It follows that the healthy spleen is not palpable. As the spleen enlarges, it expands forwards, downwards and medially, the tip emerging beneath the left costal margin.
- A normal kidney has a firm consistency and smooth surface. The lower pole of the normal right kidney is often palpable, especially in thin subjects. The normal left kidney is less often palpable.
- McBurney's point, which is typically the point of maximum tenderness in acute appendicitis, is situated one-third of the distance along a line from the anterior superior iliac spine to the umbilicus.

Inspection

Examination sequence

General principles

- ☐ Whenever possible, examine the patient in good light and in warm surroundings.
- ☐ Position the patient comfortably supine with the head but not the shoulders resting on one or two pillows in order to relax the muscles of the abdominal wall.
- ☐ Use extra pillows to support a patient with severe kyphosis.
- ☐ Do not ask a patient with severe breathlessness to lie flat.
- ☐ Remove the patient's clothes so that there is complete exposure from the xiphisternum to the pubis, leaving the chest and legs suitably covered and respectful of patients' sensitivities.
- ☐ When examining a patient in bed, pull down all bed clothing except for a sheet and then fold back the sheet to the pubis; draw up the night clothes to the chest.

Inspection

- ☐ Observe the shape and symmetry of the abdomen. Identify scars and note any other abnormalities, such as indwelling catheters, e.g. for peritoneal dialysis.
- ☐ Inspect the abdomen tangentially looking for any movements including the slow waves of gastric peristalsis passing from the rib margin on the left, across the midline and subsiding beneath to the right of the midline.
- ☐ Attempt to stimulate peristalsis by giving the patient a fizzy drink or flicking the skin over the area.

Abnormal findings

Skin. In elderly patients seborrhoeic warts, ranging from pink to brown or black, and haemangiomas (*Campbell de Morgan spots*) are so common that they could be considered normal changes. The presence of striae requires explanation. Any abnormality of the skin should be noted, including surgical scars, and the nature of the surgery undertaken should be identified. Laparoscopic incisions are usually immediately below the umbilicus and may be difficult to see. The common sites of surgical incisions are shown in Table 5.26 and illustrated in Figure 5.7. Other transverse incisions are used for access to the aorta, kidneys, adrenals, ureters, sympathetic chain or stoma closures. The common types of stoma are illustrated in Figure 5.8. The effluent from a colostomy is solid with a faecal odour; in an ileostomy there is a fluid, odourless effluent.

TABLE 5.26 Surgical incisions

Non-specific incisions	
Vertical incisions	Midline or paramedian
(used for general access)	Upper, lower or full length
Specific incisions	
Subcostal	Gall bladder
Suprapubic	Bladder, prostate, gynaecology
McBurney's point	Appendix
Inguinal	Hernia

Hair. Secondary sexual hair appears at puberty; its absence after this time suggests the possibility of hypopituitarism or hypogonadism (p. 38). Virilism in the female leads to a male distribution of pubic and body hair, whereas cirrhosis in the male may produce a female distribution of body hair.

Veins. Collateral veins may be visible if the inferior vena cava is obstructed or if there is portal hypertension. These are usually tortuous dilated superficial epigastric veins; in obstruction of the inferior vena cava, the blood flows upwards in the lower abdomen instead of downwards towards the groins. In cirrhosis, dilated collateral veins may also radiate from the umbilicus (*caput Medusa*), blood flowing away from the umbilicus as the portal vein drains through collateral vessels along the falciform ligament.

Shape. A sunken abdomen (*scaphoid abdomen*) may be due to starvation or wasting diseases. Protuberance may be due to obesity, gaseous distension, ascites, pregnancy or other swellings. In obesity the umbilicus is usually sunken, whereas in the other conditions it is flat or even projecting. Visible enlargement of the bladder, uterus or ovary may be evident as a characteristic shape arising from the pelvis, the swelling being predominantly central in contrast to the bulging of the flanks in ascites. Visible bulges may also be due to gross enlargement of the liver, spleen or kidneys or to large tumours. Distension of the stomach due to pyloric obstruction causes bulging of the upper part of the abdomen.

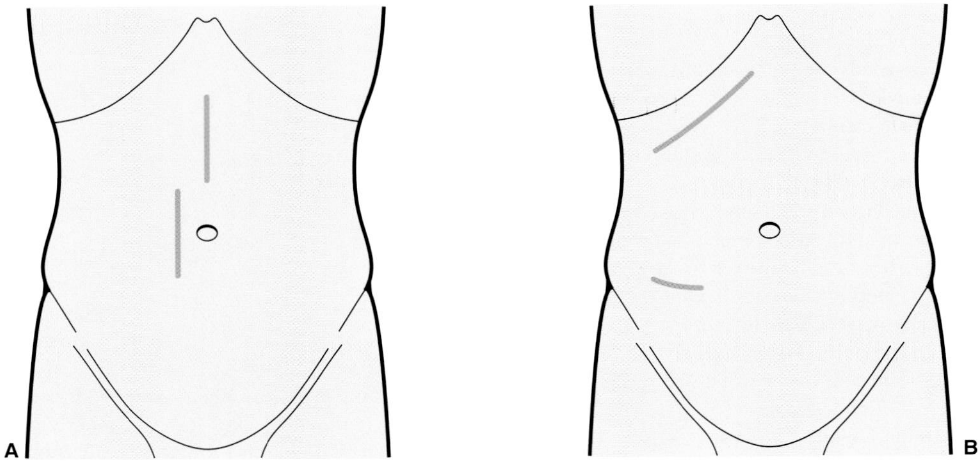

Fig. 5.7 Surgical incision. A Vertical incisions may be midline or paramedian and are used for general access. B Specific incisions may indicate the nature of operation, e.g. biliary or appendix. Note also that McBurney's point is situated one-third of the distance along a line from the anterior superior iliac spine to the umbilicus.

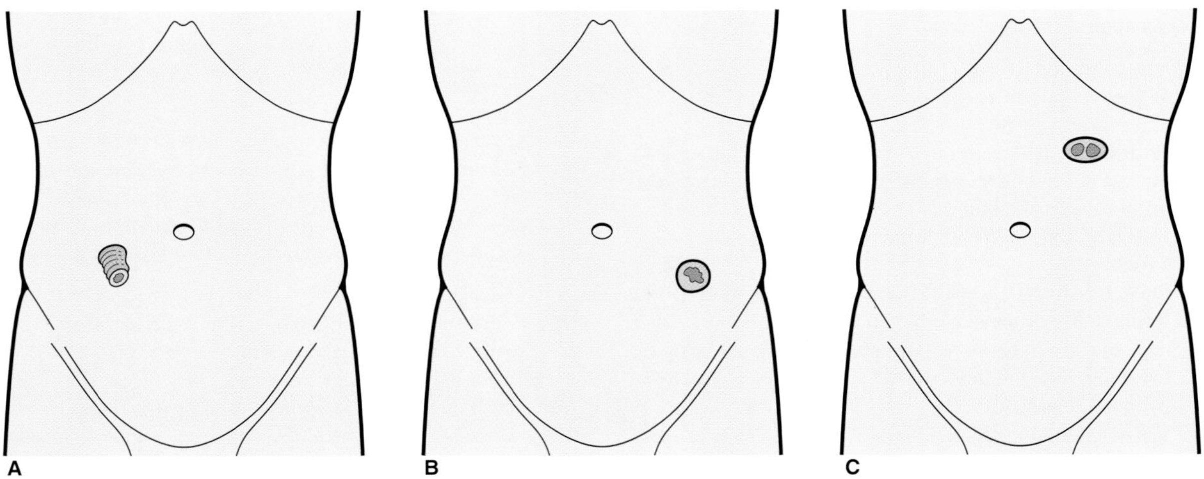

Fig. 5.8 Surgical stomas. A An ileostomy is usually in the right iliac fossa and is formed as a spout. B A colostomy may be terminal, i.e. resected distal bowel. It is usually flush and in the left iliac fossa. C A loop colostomy may be created for temporary defunctioning of the distal bowel. It is usually in the transverse colon and has afferent and efferent limbs.

Movements. Respiratory movements of the abdomen usually cease in the presence of acute peritonitis.

Pulsation in the epigastrium is usually transmitted from the abdominal aorta. Less frequently it is caused by the right ventricle, the liver or an abdominal aneurysm. It may sometimes be difficult to distinguish pulsation of the aorta transmitted through an abdominal mass from pulsation of an aneurysmal aorta. Expansile pulsation favours the latter. The distinction is best confirmed by abdominal ultrasonography.

Small intestinal peristalsis may be seen through a thin abdominal wall, or if there is divarication of the recti abdominis or an incisional hernia. It may become unduly prominent in small intestinal obstruction. It is recognised as writhing movements in the centre of the abdomen.

Hernias. Hernias are common causes of localised swellings and should be distinguished from divarication of the recti abdominis. Divarication of the recti, common in the multiparous, becomes more obvious as the supine patient attempts to sit upright; the intra-abdominal pressure rises and the region of the linea alba bulges between the recti. An *umbilical hernia* bulges through the navel. It is very common in babies and usually disappears spontaneously. An *epigastric hernia* is visible as a small swelling, usually not more than 1 cm in diameter. It is due to herniation of extraperitoneal fat through a defect in the linea alba. By gentle massage with the fingertip it is often possible to reduce such a hernia and then the small defect can be felt. An *incisional hernia* may form at the site of any operation on the abdomen, especially if the wound has been complicated by sepsis. *Femoral* and *inguinal hernias* are considered on page 170.

Palpation

Palpation can be conveniently divided into three phases: light, deep and palpation during respiration. The tendency to contract the abdominal muscles may be minimised by ensuring that the patient is warm and comfortable and by gaining the patient's confidence with a gentle approach. The *dipping technique* may be useful during deep palpation in patients with marked ascites to detect the presence of hepatic or splenic enlargement and map the outlines of enlarged organs or of tumours that might otherwise have been missed because of the ascites. The sudden displacement of liquid gives a tapping sensation over the surface of the liver or spleen similar to a patellar tap (p. 284).

Examination sequence

General principles

- ☐ Ensure that the examining hands are warm.
- ☐ If the patient is in a low bed, sit on, or kneel beside, the bed.
- ☐ Ask the patient to place the arms alongside the body to help relax the abdominal wall.
- ☐ Ask the patient to report any tenderness elicited during the examination.
- ☐ During palpation, observe the patient's face for any grimace indicative of local discomfort.

Light palpation

- ☐ Place the examining hand on the abdomen and thereafter maintain continuous contact with the patient's abdominal wall.
- ☐ Test muscle tone by light dipping movements over symmetrical areas commencing at a point remote from the site of any pain.
- ☐ To elicit rebound tenderness, press the examining hand gently but firmly into the abdomen and then swiftly release the pressure.

Deep palpation

- ☐ Palpate the abdomen more deeply with the flat of the hand.
- ☐ Examine each region in turn, starting remote from any area of tenderness. The predominant use of fingertips should be avoided as it is apt to induce muscular resistance.
- ☐ When indicated, perform the dipping technique by placing the examining hand flat on the abdomen and make quick dipping movements of the fingers.

Abnormal findings

Generalised resistance is commonly due to anxiety in a patient unable to relax. The associated increase in muscle tone can be confirmed by the finding of a reduction in resistance to palpation during the early phase of expiration. Resistance also accompanies intra-abdominal disease, particularly when pain is present. It may be restricted to one site according to the organ affected and the extent of the peritoneal involvement, e.g. McBurney's point in appendicitis. Deep-seated inflammation not causing localised guarding may be revealed by *rebound tenderness*. Although the initial pressure of palpation may fail to elicit a painful response, the abrupt withdrawal may cause the sudden movement of a deeply placed, inflamed organ, resulting in pain. Generalised 'board-like' rigidity implies peritonitis; the abdomen does not move on respiration and bowel sounds are absent. Attempts to elicit other signs such as rebound tenderness are inappropriate. It should, however, be remembered that pelvic peritonitis may be advanced before the signs are apparent abdominally and may only be revealed by rectal examination. The elasticity of the skin provides only a rough index of the degree of hydration and redundant skin folds are evidence of weight loss.

In severe constipation, faeces can be palpable in any part of the colon. Indentation of a lump by finger pressure is evidence that it is faecal. Sometimes, however, a hard, craggy lump of faeces can only be distinguished from malignancy by re-examination following defecation. Enlargement of the bladder, ovary or uterus, suspected from inspection, may be confirmed as a dome-shaped swelling rising from the pubis. An upper abdominal mass which does not move on respiration is either a fixed retroperitoneal structure (e.g. aorta or pancreas) or is attached to the abdominal wall. Masses which are situated within the abdominal wall continue to be palpable when the muscles are contracted, for example by raising the head off the pillow. Tightening the abdominal muscles in this way identifies the intersections of the recti abdominis (Fig. 5.9). An intersection may mislead the beginner into believing that a tumour or the liver edge has been felt. Masses situated more deeply within the abdominal cavity are less easily palpable when the muscles are contracted. The characteristics of any mass found should be assessed systematically with respect to its size, position, attach-

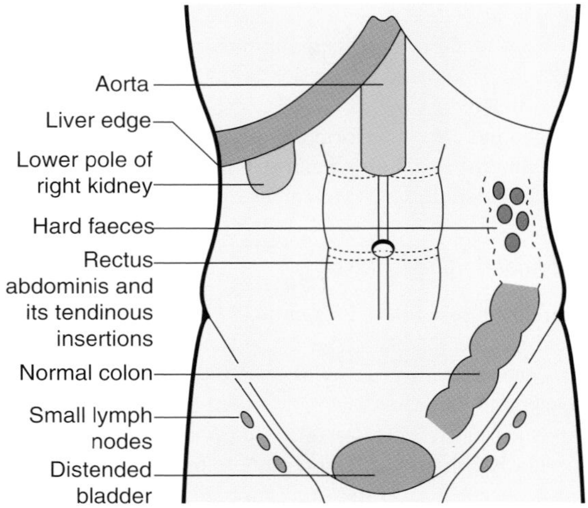

Fig. 5.9 Palpation of the abdomen. Diagrammatic representation of some findings which may be normal and are often misinterpreted.

ments, surface, edge, consistency, thrills, signs of inflammation and transillumination and illustrated diagrammatically, as in Figure 5.10.

Palpation during inspiration

The liver, gallbladder, spleen and kidneys should be examined in turn during deep inspiration. The key to success is to keep the examining hand still and wait for the organ to descend. One common error is to begin palpation of the liver too close to the costal margin, thereby missing the liver edge.

Examination sequence

Liver

- ☐ Place the hand flat on the abdomen with the fingers pointing upwards and position the sensing fingers (index and middle) lateral to the rectus muscle so that the fingertips lie on a line parallel to the expected liver edge (Fig. 5.11). Start palpation from the transumbilical plane.
- ☐ Press the hand firmly inwards and upwards and keep it steady while the patient takes a deep breath through the mouth.
- ☐ At the height of inspiration, release the inward pressure on the hand while maintaining the upward pressure. With this movement, the tips of the fingers should slip over the edge of a palpable liver.
- ☐ Note whether the edge is sharp as is normal, or whether it is rounded, firm, irregular or tender.
- ☐ Trace the surface and edge of a palpable liver across the abdomen and examine it for irregularities using the fingertips, keeping them steady in a new position each time the patient takes a deep breath. Irregularities may be felt as the liver slides under the fingertips with each inspiration.

Gall bladder

- ☐ Place the examining fingers over the gall bladder area and ask the patient to take a deep breath. Inspiration may be sharply arrested with tensing of the abdominal muscles because of a sudden accentuation of pain suggesting acute cholecystitis (Murphy's sign).

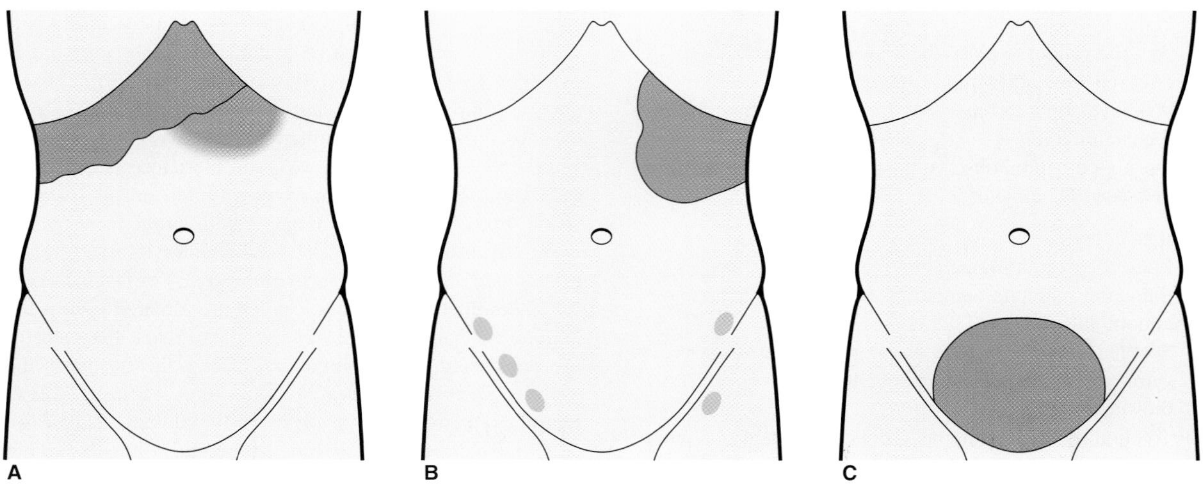

Fig. 5.10 The use of diagrams in case recording. [A] An abdominal mass and enlarged liver in a patient with gastric carcinoma and hepatic metastases. [B] Splenomegaly and lymphadenopathy in a patient with Hodgkin's lymphoma. [C] Tumour arising from the pelvis. This could be a bladder, uterine or ovarian swelling.

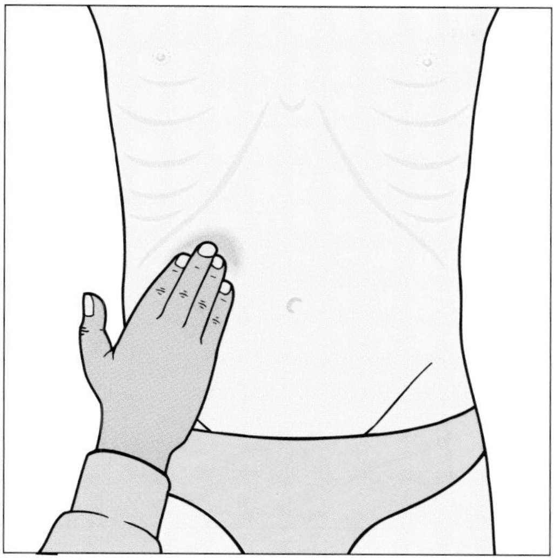

Fig. 5.11 Palpation of the liver.

Spleen

- ☐ Place the examining hand on the anterior abdominal wall with the fingertips well below the left costal margin, pressing inwards and upwards (Fig. 5.12A).
- ☐ Ask the patient to breathe in deeply. If the spleen is significantly enlarged, it will bump against the fingertips.
- ☐ At the height of inspiration, release the pressure on the examining hand so that the fingertips slip over the lower pole of the spleen, confirming its presence and surface characteristics.
- ☐ If the spleen is not palpable, move the examining hand upwards after each inspiration until the fingertips are under the costal margin.
- ☐ Repeat this process along the entire rib margin as the position of the enlarging splenic tip is variable.
- ☐ If still not palpable, position the patient in the right lateral position with the left hip and knee flexed, and repeat the examination.
- ☐ Alternatively, examine the patient from the left side, curling the fingers of the examining hand under the left costal margin as the patient breathes in deeply (Fig. 5.12B).

Kidneys

- ☐ Use a bimanual technique to palpate the kidneys.
- ☐ Place one hand posteriorly below the lower rib cage and the other over the upper quadrant.
- ☐ Push the two hands together firmly but gently as the patient breathes out.
- ☐ Feel for the lower pole moving down between the hands as the patient breathes in deeply.
- ☐ Push the kidney back and forwards between the two hands – this is known as ballotting. It helps to confirm that the structure being palpated is the kidney.
- ☐ Assess the size, surface and consistency of a palpable kidney.
- ☐ Examine the left kidney from either side (Fig. 5.13).

Abnormal findings

Common causes of hepatomegaly in adults in Britain are shown in Table 5.27. Physical signs that may occur in hepatobiliary disorders are illustrated in Figure 5.14.

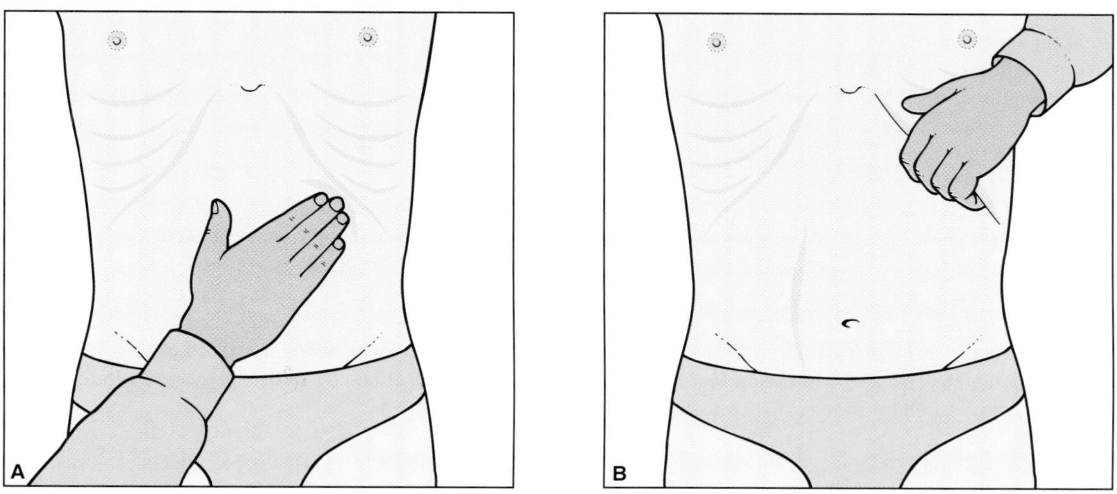

Fig. 5.12 A Palpation of the spleen. B Alternative method for palpation of the spleen.

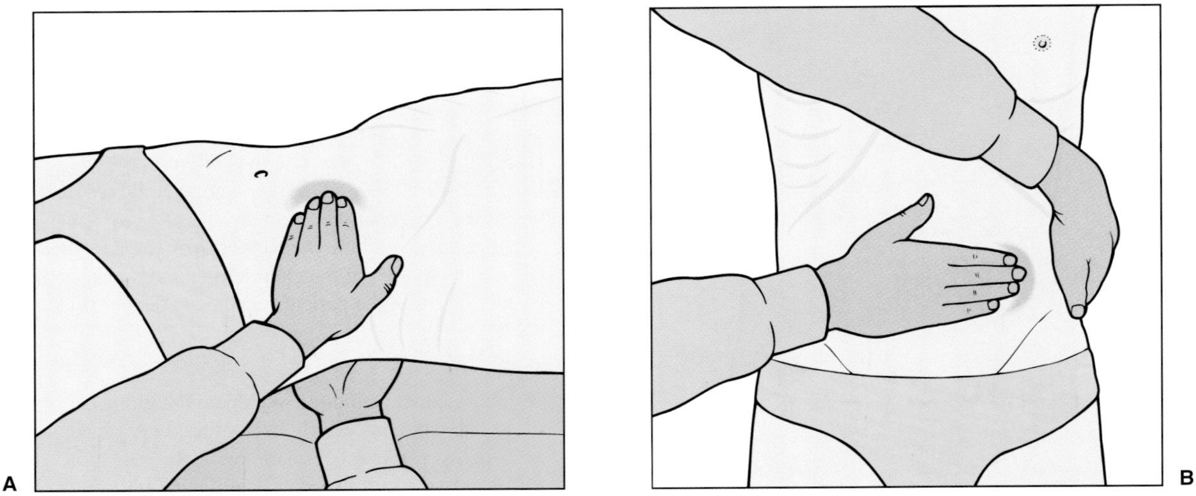

Fig. 5.13 Palpation of the left kidney. [A] From the same side and [B] from the opposite side.

TABLE 5.27 Important causes of palpable enlargement of the liver and/or spleen

Hepatomegaly	Splenomegaly	Hepatosplenomegaly
Congestive cardiac failure	Leukaemia	Infectious mononucleosis
Fatty infiltration, e.g. alcoholic liver disease	Haemolytic anaemia	Myelofibrosis
Congenital Riedel's lobe	Portal hypertension	Polycythaemia rubra vera
Viral hepatitis	Rheumatoid arthritis, systemic lupus erythematosus	Hepatic cirrhosis
Malignancy (primary or secondary)	Infections, e.g. malaria, subacute bacterial endocarditis	Lymphoma
		Amyloidosis, sarcoidosis

Gallstones are common with advancing years, especially in women and may result in acute cholecystitis, with tenderness overlying the gall bladder below the right costal margin in the mid-clavicular line. A palpable gall bladder is an abnormal finding and denotes enlargement. In the absence of jaundice, it is due to obstruction of the cystic duct leading to mucocele or empyema. Obstruction of the common bile duct produces jaundice; if the gall bladder is also enlarged, the obstruction is usually due to causes other than gallstones, such as carcinoma of the pancreas, since in cholelithiasis the gall bladder wall is diseased and thickened and cannot enlarge (*Courvoisier's law*).

A palpable spleen is always pathological and a spleen which remains palpable during expiration is grossly enlarged. Important causes of splenomegaly are shown in Table 5.27. Splenomegaly may be mistaken for an enlarged kidney; some features helpful in making this distinction are shown in Table 5.28.

Owing to the varying thickness of the abdomen, kidney enlargement is difficult for the inexperienced to assess unless there is gross enlargement. Irregularity of the surface or an abnormally hard consistency is more easily appreciated. When the liver is readily palpable, it may be difficult to decide whether the right kidney can also be felt, and the opposite is also the case. This is particularly true in polycystic disease of the kidneys especially in those patients who also have associated cystic disease of the liver.

Tenderness of the kidney is often greatest posteriorly and may be elicited by gently tapping the renal angle using a fist, with the patient sitting forward. Enlargement of one kidney is often the result of compensatory hypertrophy due to renal agenesis, hypoplasia or atrophy affecting the other kidney; alternatively, it may suggest the presence of a renal tumour or hydronephrosis. Enlargement of both kidneys may occur in polycystic disease and amyloidosis.

Rarely, the two kidneys are joined at their lower poles and may be palpable straddling the midline ('horseshoe kidney').

Other important causes of a palpable abdominal mass are given in Table 5.29.

Many patients with renal disease have small kidneys which are naturally non-palpable. Indeed, the possibility of chronic renal failure is more frequently suggested from the history than from the clinical examination as the signs are usually only present at an advanced stage (Fig. 5.15).

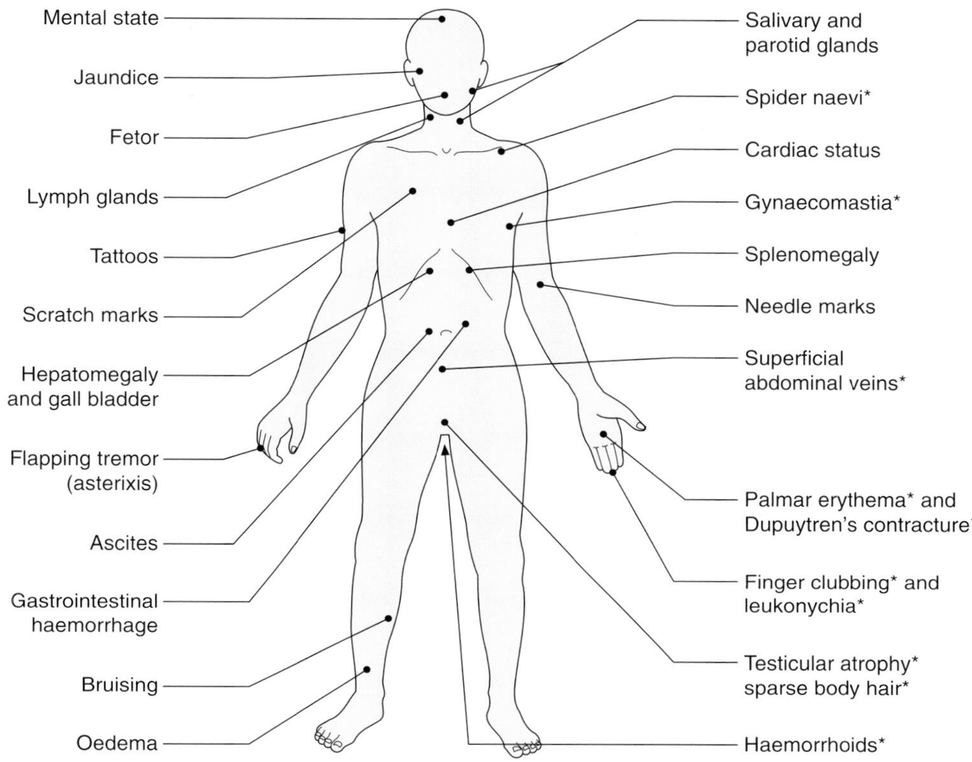

Fig. 5.14 Clinical features associated with advanced liver disease. Those features marked with an asterisk usually indicate the presence of chronic liver disease.

TABLE 5.28 Checklist to differentiate palpable spleen from left kidney

Distinguishing feature	Spleen	Kidney
Mass is smooth and regular in shape	More likely	Polycystic kidneys are bilateral, irregular masses
Mass descends in inspiration	Yes, moves superficially and diagonally	Yes, moves deeply and vertically
Able to feel deep to the mass	Yes	No
Able to insert fingers superficial to mass	No	Yes
Palpable notch on the medial surface	Yes, if very enlarged	No
Bilateral masses palpable	No	Sometimes (e.g. polycystic kidneys)
Percussion resonant over the mass	No	Sometimes
Mass extends beyond the midline	Sometimes	No (except with horseshoe kidney)

Percussion and auscultation

The principal value of abdominal percussion is to distinguish between distension due to gas, ascites, cystic or solid tumours. Normal peristaltic activity of the gut creates characteristic gurgling sounds which may be heard from time to time by the unaided ear (*borborygmi*). Through the stethoscope, they can be heard every 5–10 seconds, though the interval varies greatly and they occur more frequently after meals.

Examination sequence

General principles

- ☐ Percussion from resonance to dull.
- ☐ Place the percussing finger on the trunk parallel to the anticipated note change (Fig. 5.16A).
- ☐ Percuss lightly for superficial structures such as the lower border of the liver, more firmly for deeply placed structures such as the upper border of liver or the bladder.

TABLE 5.29 Important causes of palpable abdominal masses

Right iliac fossa masses	Appendix abscess Psoas abscess Carcinoma, e.g. colon, right ovary Transplanted kidney (note any overlying scar) Hard or impacted faeces (scybala) Crohn's disease (often adherent bowel loops) Ileocaecal TB
Midline masses	Aortic aneurysm Lymphoma (lymphadenopathy) Pancreatic pseudocyst Carcinoma, e.g. gastric, pancreatic, colonic Ovarian cysts or tumours (benign or malignant) Horseshoe kidney Bladder enlargement, e.g. retention of urine Uterine masses, e.g. pregnancy, fibroids, tumour
Left iliac fossa masses	Diverticular abscess Psoas abscess Hard or impacted faeces (scybala) Transplanted kidney (note any overlying scar) Carcinoma, e.g. colon, left ovary

- ☐ Examine the spleen with the patient holding the breath during full inspiration; percuss both below and then above the left costal margin.

Shifting dullness

- ☐ Examine the patient supine and percuss from the centre of the abdomen into the flank until a dull note is obtained (Fig. 5.16B).
- ☐ Mark the level or keep the finger in place as the patient rolls on to the other side.
- ☐ Pause for at least 10 seconds. Ascites is suggested if the note becomes resonant and confirmed by obtaining a dull note while percussing back towards the umbilicus (Fig. 5.16).
- ☐ To detect a fluid thrill, place a detecting hand on the patient's flank, flick the skin of the abdominal wall over the other flank using the thumb or forefinger.
- ☐ If a fluid thrill or impulse is felt, repeat the procedure with the patient's hand placed on the abdomen along the midline sagittal plane to dampen any possible thrill transmitted via the abdominal wall.

Auscultation

Examination sequence

- ☐ Auscultate for peristalsis bowel sounds for at least 3 minutes before deciding that they are absent.

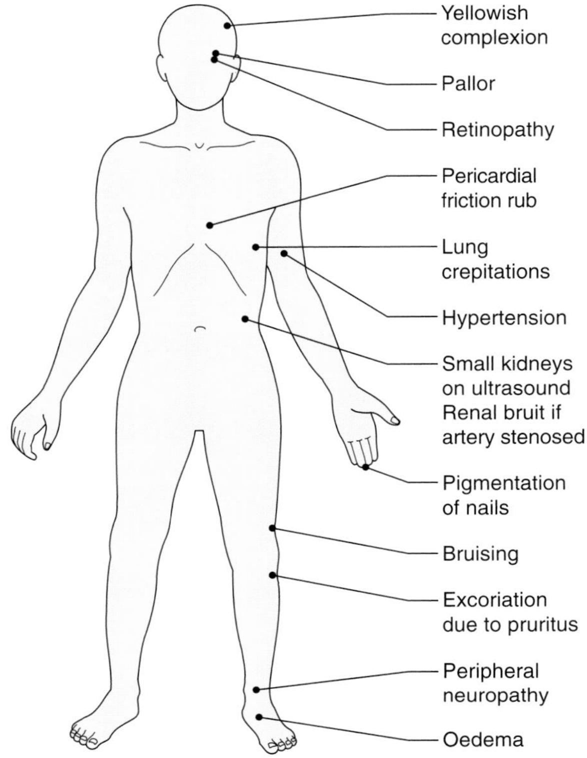

Fig. 5.15 Clinical features of advanced chronic renal failure.

- ☐ Auscultate over the aorta for a bruit.
- ☐ To elicit a succussion splash, place the hands over the lower ribs and shake the patient quickly and rhythmically from side to side.

Abnormal findings

Gaseous distension of the abdomen is resonant to percussion. The gravid uterus, bladder enlargement, ovarian cysts, and other solid pelvic masses extend out of the pelvis into the abdomen to produce central abdominal dullness with resonance of the flanks caused by gas in the surrounding displaced gut. In contrast, ascites is suggested by the presence of dullness in the flanks with central abdominal resonance. Ascites is often first suspected from the convexity of the abdomen and flanks on inspection, but is confirmed by percussion. In the presence of ascites, the gas-containing bowel floats uppermost. The liquid gravitates to the dependent part of the peritoneal cavity, namely the flanks and pelvis. Important causes of ascites are given in Table 5.30.

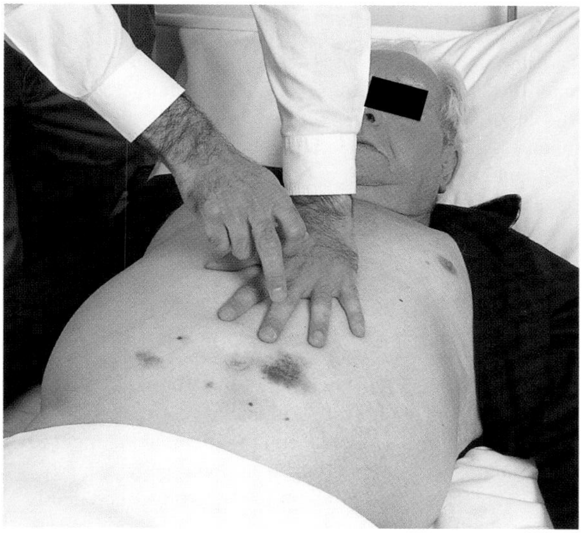

A

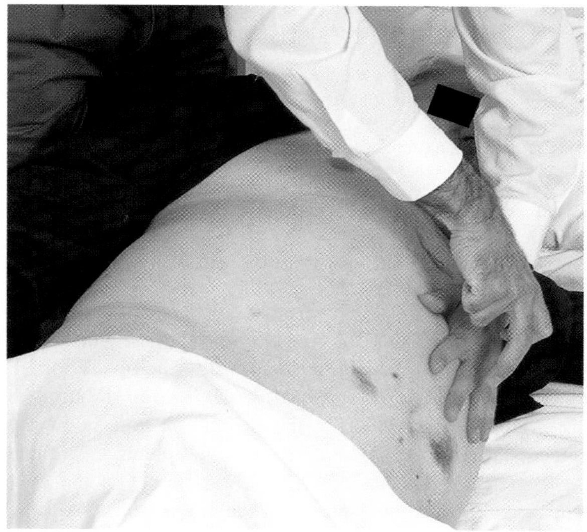

C

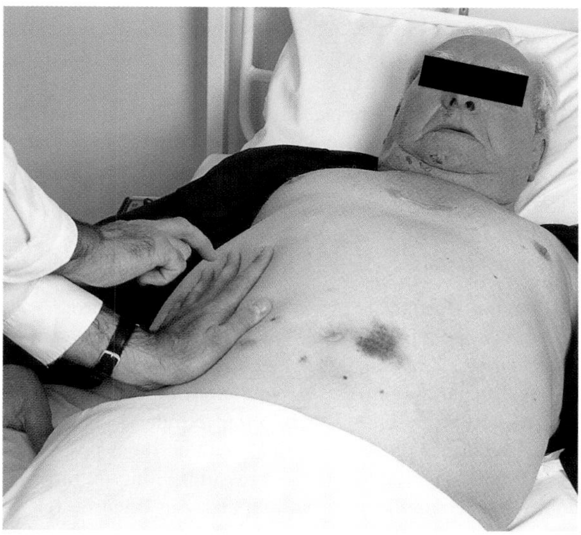

B

Fig. 5.16 Percussing for ascites. Percuss towards the flank from resonant [A] to dull [B], then ask the patient to roll on the other side. When ascites is present, the note has become resonant, percuss back towards the midline to detect the new level of dullness [C]. (Note the bruising caused by subcutaneous heparin injections.)

TABLE 5.30 Important causes of ascites

Exudate (> 30 g protein per litre)	Transudate (< 30 g protein per litre)
Carcinomatous infiltration of the peritoneum	Hepatic cirrhosis (portal hypertension)
Acute pancreatitis	Congestive cardiac failure
Infection (pneumococcal, TB, coliform)	Nephrotic syndrome
Inferior vena cava/hepatic vein obstruction (Budd–Chiari syndrome)	Ovarian tumour (Meig's syndrome)

TABLE 5.31 Causes of increased bowel sounds

Intestinal obstruction (with a high-pitched, tinkling quality)
Severe gastrointestinal bleeding
Small bowel malabsorption
Carcinoid syndrome (marked borborygmi)

The presence of small quantities of free fluid in the peritoneal cavity is not clinically detectable, since minor changes in percussion note may be due to gravitational shift of normal bowel. Minor degrees of ascites can only be detected by abdominal ultrasonography. Moderate ascites may be confirmed by demonstrating *shifting dullness* or eliciting a *fluid thrill*, but an enormous ovarian cyst may also produce a fluid thrill. It is rare for a fluid thrill to be present in the absence of shifting dullness.

Absent bowel sounds suggest cessation of bowel peristalsis, which is known as *ileus*. Ileus may be due to reduced nervous stimulation to the bowel, or to drugs – paralytic ileus – or may be a response to intra-abdominal inflammation or infection, such as bacterial peritonitis, or to long-standing bowel obstruction. Causes of increased bowel sounds are shown in Table 5.31.

The spleen. Percussion is of limited value in determining the size and position of the spleen as this can only be crudely assessed from the percussion note. However, dullness to percussion overlying a palpable mass in the left

TABLE 5.32 Causes of reduced liver dullness

Pulmonary hyperinflation, e.g. chronic obstructive airways disease
Small, shrunken liver, e.g. cirrhosis
Free air beneath the diaphragm, e.g. perforated hollow viscus
Interposition of the colon between the liver and the diaphragm (an unusual anatomical variant known as Chilaiditi's syndrome)

upper quadrant indicates that the mass is likely to be splenic in origin.

The liver. Percussion can give only a rough estimate of the size of the liver, particularly in regard to the upper border. Although this may be raised above the level of the fifth rib by a greatly enlarged liver, the percussion note is largely dependent upon the state of the lung and pleura (see Table 5.32). The apparent level of the lower border of the liver varies with the amount of gas in the colon, and a palpable lower border may be 3–4 cm below the edge detected by percussion. However, a positive finding on percussion implies that the borders of the liver extend at least as far as the extent of dullness.

Arterial bruits. Arterial bruits (harsh systolic murmurs) in the abdomen may arise from the aorta, or any other narrowed or partially occluded artery. Bruits due to stenosis of mesenteric or renal arteries may be difficult to hear owing to the distracting effects of bowel sounds, and a conscious effort should be made to listen for them. Renal artery bruits may be best heard posteriorly. Rarely, a systolic bruit may be heard over the liver in hepatoma.

Venous hum. A venous hum is occasionally audible between the xiphisternum and the umbilicus owing to turbulent blood flow in a well-developed collateral circulation from portal hypertension.

Friction sounds. Friction sounds resembling those of pleurisy may be present over an area of inflammation of the serosal surface of the spleen or liver (perisplenitis or perihepatitis).

Succussion splash. A sound like shaking a half-filled hot-water bottle is termed a succussion splash. This can be produced from a normal stomach up to 2 hours after food or drink. In other circumstances it is a feature of delayed gastric emptying, as seen in pyloric stenosis or diabetic autonomic neuropathy.

HERNIAL ORIFICES AND GENITALIA

The groins should be examined for hernias, femoral pulses (p. 106) and for lymph nodes (p. 59). In health, inguinal lymph nodes vary considerably in size and consistency.

Examination of the hernial orifices

The inguinal canal extends from the pubic tubercle to the anterior superior iliac spine and has an internal ring at the mid-inguinal point and an external ring at the pubic tubercle. The femoral canal lies below the inguinal ligament. Since hernias may reduce spontaneously as the patient lies supine, examination is better undertaken with the patient standing.

Examination sequence

- ☐ Ask the patient to stand, carefully inspect the inguinal and femoral canals and the scrotum for hernias; ask the patient to cough and observe any impulse over the femoral or inguinal canals and/or scrotum.
- ☐ Identify the anatomical relationships between the hernia, the pubic tubercle and the inguinal ligament to distinguish femoral hernias from inguinal hernias.
- ☐ Invaginate the scrotum with the little finger and gently palpate the external inguinal ring and posterior wall of the inguinal canal for possible muscle defects.
- ☐ Feel for any impulse as the patient coughs; if a hernia is present, reduce the hernia by massaging it towards the internal ring.
- ☐ Once the hernia is reduced, occlude the internal inguinal ring with finger pressure at the mid-inguinal point and check to see if the hernia reappears during coughing. Only a direct inguinal hernia should reappear.

Abnormal findings

Abdominal hernias are protrusions of a viscus through an abnormal opening. *External* hernias occur at the site of defects in the abdominal wall, e.g. operation scars and points of anatomical weakness. *Internal hernias* occur through defects of the mesentery or into the retroperitoneal space. External hernias of the abdominal wall are more prominent in the erect position, when the pressure within them rises, and during coughing when an impulse can often be felt in the hernia (*cough impulse*). After the identification of a hernia, an attempt should be made to replace the contents by the application of a gentle sustained pressure (*reduction*).

Hernias may be reducible or irreducible. Irreducible hernias may become *obstructed*, when the bowel lumen is occluded, and obstructed hernias may become *strangulated* when the vascular supply of the hernial contents is threatened. A strangulated hernia is tense and tender and shows no impulse on coughing; this is a surgical emergency if bowel infarction is to be avoided.

A *femoral hernia* is palpable below the inguinal ligament and lateral to the pubic tubercle. An *inguinal hernia* emerges from the abdominal wall through the external inguinal ring and is palpable above and medial to the pubic tubercle (Fig. 5.17). It is often difficult to accurately differentiate between direct and indirect inguinal hernias.

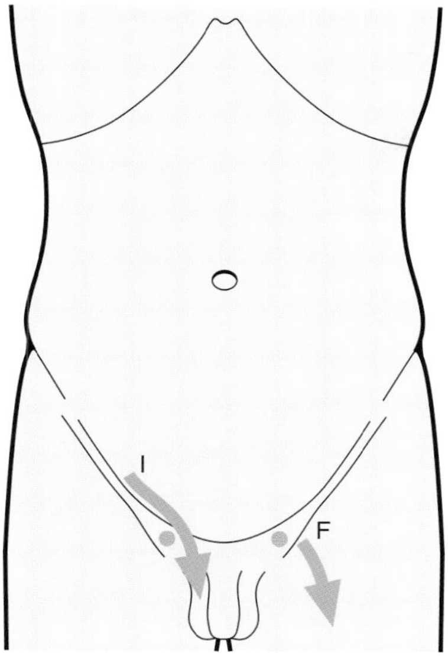

Fig. 5.17 Examining the hernial orifices. A femoral hernia lies below and lateral to the pubic tubercle. An inguinal hernia lies above and medial to the pubic tubercle.

An *indirect inguinal hernia* occurs into a persistent remnant of the processus vaginalis. It occurs in young men and may extend to the testes. Following reduction, control can be achieved by pressure over the internal inguinal ring, just above the midpoint of the inguinal ligament. A direct inguinal hernia occurs directly through the weakened posterior wall of the inguinal canal medial to the inferior epigastric artery and lateral to the rectus muscle. It is more common in older men and does not reach the testes. It will not be controlled by pressure over the internal inguinal ring.

Examination of the male genitalia

In the male, examination of the genitalia conveniently follows palpation of the groins. Some diseases of the external genitalia are both life-threatening and treatable, e.g. testicular carcinoma. It follows that serious consequences may ensue if the examination is omitted. In the scrotum, the main structures to be assessed are the testes, the epididymis and the spermatic cord. The contents of the male pelvis are shown in Figure 5.18.

Examination sequence

- ☐ Examine the penis and scrotum and carefully palpate the testes, epididymis and spermatic cords.
- ☐ Assess any scrotal swelling using the principles described on page 57.
- ☐ Confirm that any swelling originates in the scrotum and in the inguinal canal.

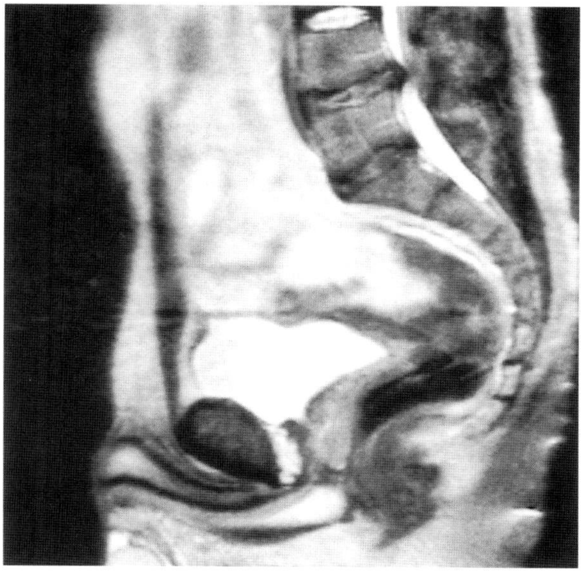

Fig. 5.18 MRI scan showing contents of the male pelvis. (Courtesy of Dr Andrew R. Wright.)

- ☐ Carefully palpate both testes to determine the exact site of any swelling.
- ☐ Use a small pen torch to transilluminate the scrotum to assess the nature of any swelling.

Abnormal findings

Hypospadias is a developmental abnormality of the penis in which there is incomplete development of the underside of the penis with an abnormal urethral orifice. Ulcerative mucosal lesions of the penis include herpes simplex, syphilis or squamous carcinoma. More rarely, they may be a feature of systemic disorders such as Reiter's syndrome or Behçet's syndrome. Non-ulcerating lesions include viral warts and infection of the prepuce (balanitis). Any evidence of urethral discharge should be noted and sampling performed for microscopy and culture.

Figure 5.19 shows some common abnormalities of the scrotum. A hydrocele is a relatively common swelling due to accumulation of fluid in the tunica vaginalis. It may be unilateral or bilateral. The fluid nature of the contents should be confirmed by *transillumination*. The possibility that a hydrocele may obscure a testicular tumour should not be overlooked and careful palpation of both testes is therefore necessary. Infections which affect the testis specifically (*orchitis*) are mumps and syphilis. The epididymis may contain a spermatocele or other cyst. It is prone to infection, often in association with urinary tract infection. This may be bacterial – usually due to coliform organisms – or tuberculosis, which produces a characteristic nodular change within the epididymis accompanied by thickening of the cord. Sometimes infection involves both the testes and the epididymis, and is known as *epididymo-orchitis*. Palpable varicosity of the spermatic vein (*varicocele*) can cause chronic local discomfort. Shortening of the spermatic cord is a characteristic of torsion of the testis.

Specific considerations

- The left testis usually lies lower than the right.
- Minor degrees of hypospadias are common (1 in 300 males).
- Bilateral testicular atrophy suggests hypogonadism, either congenital or acquired.
- Unilateral testicular atrophy may occur following mumps orchitis.
- Absence of one or both testes from the scrotum should lead to a search for incompletely descended testes in the inguinal canal or for ectopic testes in sites such as the groin.

Examination of the female genitalia

Vaginal examination is not routine. Its intimate nature raises medicolegal considerations necessitating both informed consent and the presence of a chaperone during the examination. The vaginal examination should be avoided if the hymen is intact, particularly as the information required can be obtained by digital examination of the rectum. Vaginal examination of a minor requires the consent of a parent or guardian. The contents of the female pelvis are illustrated in Figure 5.20.

Indications for a vaginal examination

- Surveillance for cervical carcinoma
- Vaginal discharge
- Postmenopausal bleeding
- Pelvic mass
- Symptoms of uterine prolapse
- Unexplained urinary tract obstruction
- Suspected tubal pregnancy

Examination sequence

- ☐ Ask the patient to empty the bladder.
- ☐ Position the patient comfortably either on her back or in the left lateral position with her head on a pillow, hips and knees flexed and thighs abducted.
- ☐ Use a lamp to illuminate the vulva adequately.
- ☐ Use suitable gloves and lubricate the examining fingers.
- ☐ Separate the labia minora with the forefinger and thumb of the left hand, bringing into view the clitoris anteriorly, then the urethra, the vagina and the anus posteriorly.

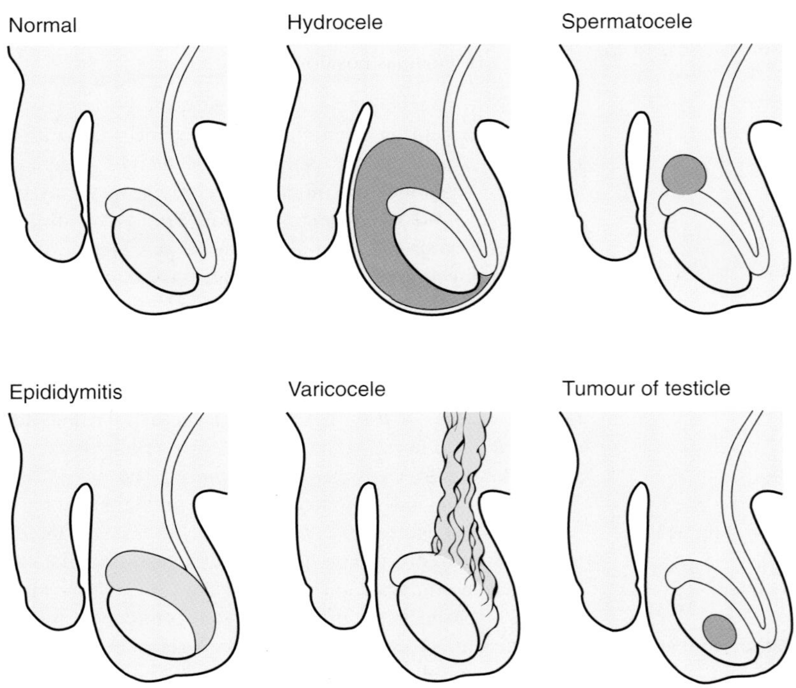

Fig. 5.19 Swellings of the scrotum.

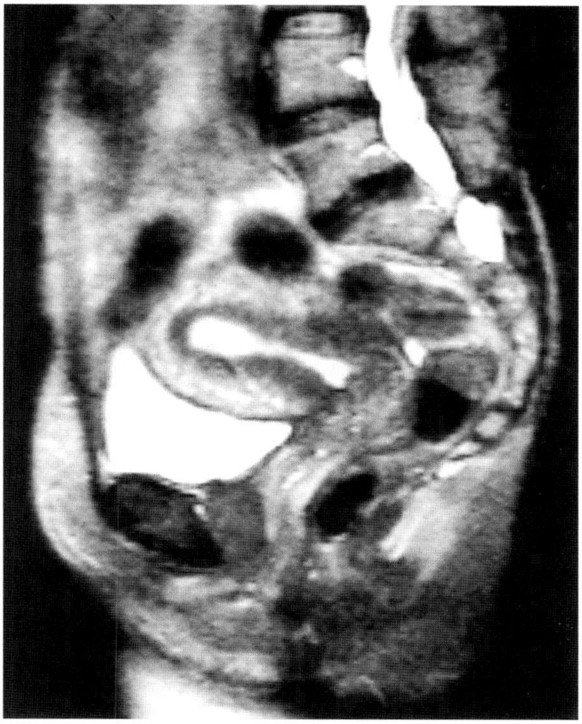

Fig. 5.20 MRI scan showing the contents of the female pelvis.
(Courtesy of Dr Andrew R. Wright.)

- ☐ Look for any evidence of discharge, ulceration or abnormalities of Bartholin's glands.
- ☐ Inspect the vaginal walls for prolapse by asking the patient to strain down and then to cough.
- ☐ Note the position and degree of any vaginal prolapse and the occurrence of any involuntary urinary incontinence on coughing.
- ☐ Insert the index and middle fingers of the right hand into the vagina and rotate palm-upwards (Fig. 5.21). Use only one finger if vaginismus (spasm of the vaginal muscles) or atrophic vaginitis makes examination painful.
- ☐ Palpate the cervix; the normal cervix points downwards and slightly backwards and feels like the tip of the nose.
- ☐ Note any tenderness on movement of the cervix (*cervical excitation*).
- ☐ Now perform bimanual palpation; with two fingers in the anterior fornix, place the left hand flat on the abdomen above the pubis.
- ☐ Identify the size, position and surface characteristics of the uterus between the hands.
- ☐ If the uterus is not palpable, palpate with the fingers in the posterior fornix as the uterus may be retroverted.

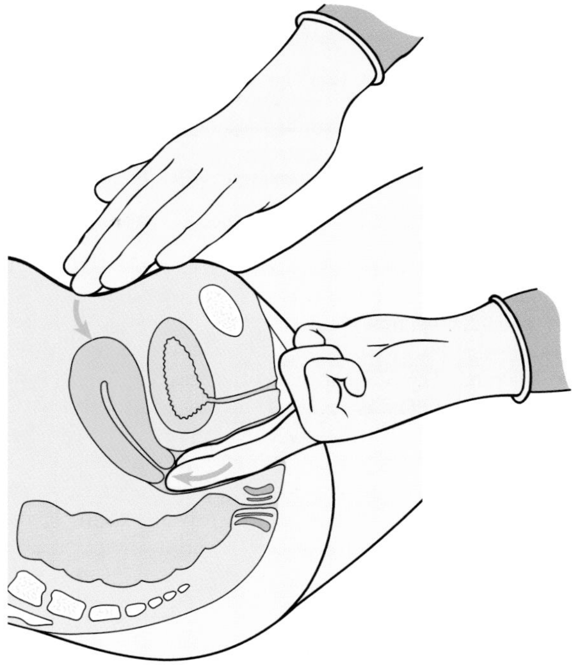

Fig. 5.21 Vaginal examination.

- ☐ Palpate each lateral fornix in turn bimanually.
- ☐ Note any tenderness or swelling of the Fallopian tubes or ovaries (adnexae), the bladder anteriorly and the pouch of Douglas posteriorly.
- ☐ Supplement digital examination by inspection of the vagina and uterine cervix using a vaginal speculum.

Using a vaginal speculum and taking a cervical smear

- ☐ Gently insert a lubricated, warmed speculum into the vagina; do not use a lubricant other than water if a cervical smear is being performed.
- ☐ Rotate the blades through 90 degrees pointing the handles anteriorly if the patient is supine and posteriorly if in the left lateral position.
- ☐ Gently open the blades and identify the cervix.
- ☐ Use the notched end of a spatula and rotate through 360 degrees to scrape off a cytological sample from the cervical os.
- ☐ Spread the sample thinly onto a labelled, cleaned glass slide and fix immediately with a 50/50 mixture of alcohol and ether.
- ☐ Swab any discharge from the urethra, vagina and cervix.
- ☐ Send one specimen for culture and smear another on to a glass slide for direct microscopy; unstained smears are helpful to confirm trichomonal infection and stained smears to confirm gonorrhoea or thrush.

EXAMINATION OF THE RECTUM

Digital rectal examination

Digital examination of the rectum is an important component of the clinical examination and the student should be familiar with the normal structures. Because this simple procedure is disagreeable to the patient, it is often inappropriately omitted.

The upper end of the anal canal is marked by the puborectalis muscle which is readily palpable and which contracts reflexly on coughing or conscious contraction by the patient. Beyond the anal canal, the rectum passes upwards and backwards along the curve of the coccyx and the sacrum. The normal rectum is usually empty and smooth-walled. The coccyx and sacrum lie posteriorly. In the male, anteriorly from below upwards, lie the membranous urethra, the prostate and base of the bladder. The normal prostate is smooth and has a firm consistency with lateral lobes and a median groove between them. In the female, the vagina and cervix lie anteriorly.

Indications for rectal examination

- *Alimentary problems.* All 'acute abdomens', suspected appendicitis, pelvic abscess, peritonitis and lower abdominal pain. Diarrhoea or constipation; mucus or blood in stools. Anal irritation or pain; tenesmus or rectal pain. Bimanual examination of a lower abdominal mass. In the search for tumours or transperitoneal metastases either diagnostically or in making a decision about treatment.
- *Genitourinary problems.* Assessment of the prostate in men with symptoms of prostatism (p. 155) or suspicion of prostatic carcinoma. Dysuria, frequency, haematuria. Epididymo–orchitis and in lieu of vaginal examination in patients where this would be inappropriate.
- *Miscellaneous problems.* Patients with unexplained backache, lumbosacral nerve root pain, unexplained bone pain or iron-deficiency anaemia. In all cases of pyrexia of unknown origin or unexplained weight loss.

Spasm of the external anal sphincter is commonly due to anxiety, but when associated with local pain, it is likely to be due to an anal fissure and a local anaesthetic suppository should be used before a satisfactory examination can be undertaken.

Examination sequence

- ☐ Position the patient in the left lateral position with the buttocks at the edge of the couch, the knees drawn up to the chest and the heels clear of the perineum.
- ☐ Reassure the patient and explain that the examination may be uncomfortable but should not be painful.
- ☐ Lubricate the examining index finger, protected by a suitable glove.
- ☐ Examine the perianal skin in a good light looking for evidence of skin lesions, external haemorrhoids or fistulae.
- ☐ Place the tip of the forefinger on the anal margin and with steady pressure on the sphincter pass the finger gently through the anal canal into the rectum (Fig. 5.22).
- ☐ If anal spasm is encountered, ask the patient to breathe out and relax. If anal spasm is present with anal pain, use local anaesthetic jelly before trying again. If pain persists, an examination under general anaesthesia may be necessary.
- ☐ Ask the patient to squeeze the examining forefinger with the anal sphincter, and note any weakness of sphincter contraction.
- ☐ Palpate around the entire rectum; note any abnormality and examine any mass systematically.
- ☐ Note the percentage of the rectal circumference involved by disease and its distance from the anus.
- ☐ Identify the uterine cervix in women and the prostate in men; assess size, shape, consistency, and note any tenderness elicited.
- ☐ Perform bimanual examination if necessary, using the other hand laid flat over the lower abdomen.
- ☐ Repeat the examination after the patient has defecated if in doubt about palpable masses.
- ☐ After withdrawal, examine the finger for stool colour and the presence of blood and mucus.
- ☐ Test the stool sample for blood using a 'Haemoccult' test card.

Abnormal findings

Haemorrhoids are not palpable unless thrombosed; similarly, normal seminal vesicles cannot be felt. In patients with chronic constipation the rectum is often loaded with faeces. Carcinoma of the lower rectum is palpable as a mucosal irregularity. An obstructing carcinoma of the upper rectum may produce ballooning of the empty rectal cavity below. Faecal masses are commonly palpable; they should be movable and can be indented. Metastases or colonic tumours within the pelvis may be mistaken for faeces and vice versa. Lateralised tenderness suggests pelvic peritonitis, e.g. right-sided tenderness in an appendix abscess.

In women, the normal cervix and the retroverted uterus are often palpable on the anterior wall; cervical carcinoma may be palpated. The presence of a vaginal tampon may confuse the inexperienced examiner. Acute salpingitis will cause lateralised tenderness. A 'frozen pelvis' from extensive peritoneal dissemination of tumour, e.g. ovarian cancer produces a hard, rigid feel to the pelvic organs.

In men, prostatic hyperplasia often produces a palpable symmetrical enlargement, but may not do so if the hyperplasia is confined to the median lobe. A hard, irregular gland suggests prostatic carcinoma. The median groove is often undetectable; in the presence of extracapsular spread

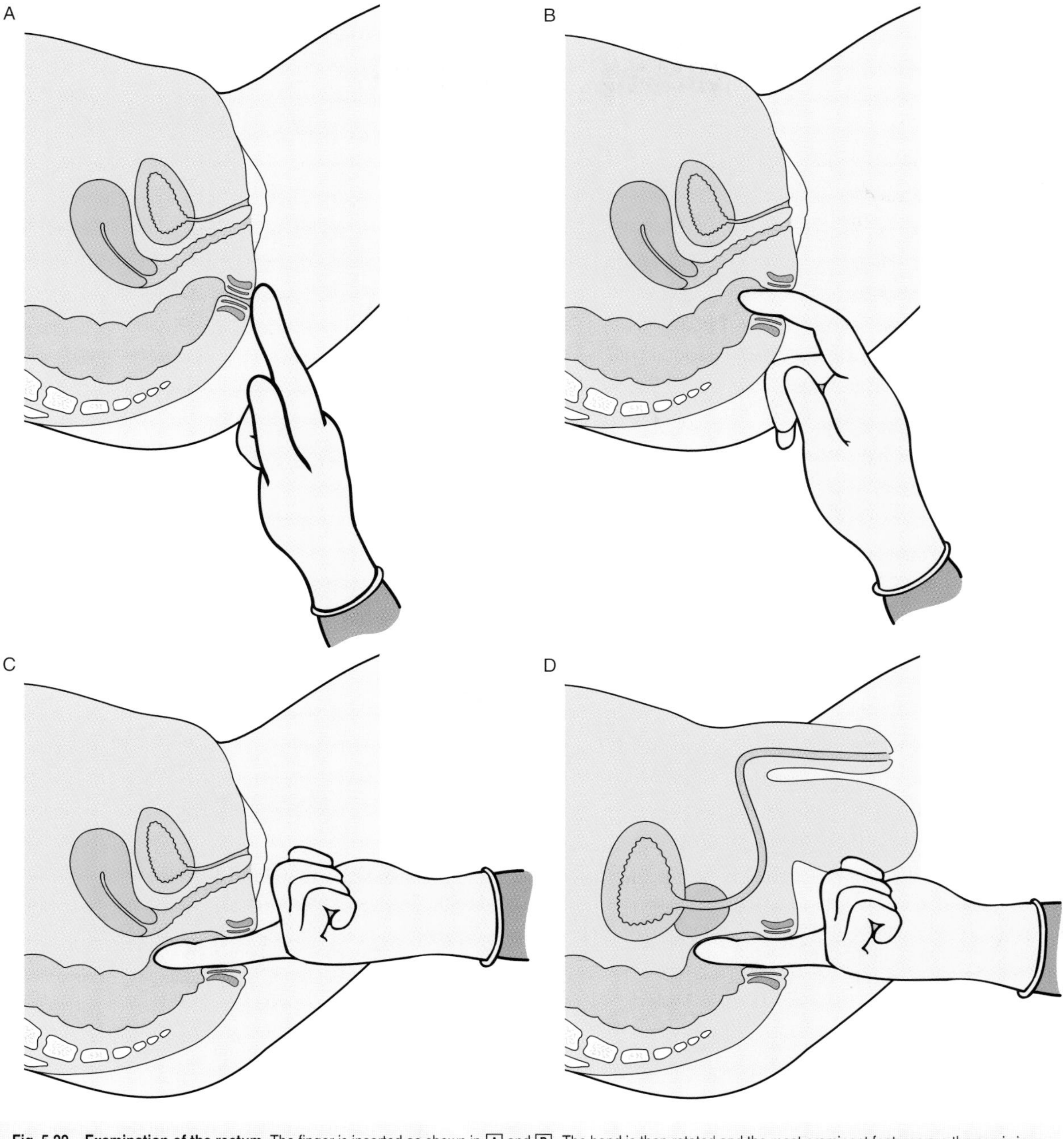

Fig. 5.22 Examination of the rectum. The finger is inserted as shown in [A] and [B]. The hand is then rotated and the most prominent features are the cervix in the female [C] and the prostate in the male [D].

there may be tethering of the rectal mucosa. The prostate is abnormally small in hypogonadism. Tenderness accompanied by a change in the consistency of the gland may be due to prostatitis or a prostatic abscess.

Proctoscopy

Visual examination of the rectum and anal canal complements digital examination but should always be preceded by digital examination. The appearance of normal rectal mucosa is similar to buccal mucosa apart from the presence of prominent submucosal veins.

Examination sequence

- ☐ Position the patient in the left lateral position with the buttocks at the edge of the couch, the knees drawn up to the chest and the heels clear of the perineum.
- ☐ Separate the buttocks with the forefinger and thumb of one hand and with the other hand gently insert a well-lubricated proctoscope with its obturator through the anal canal into the rectum in the direction of the umbilicus.
- ☐ Remove the obturator and examine the rectal mucosa carefully under good illumination, noting any abnormality seen.
- ☐ Ask the patient to strain down as the instrument is slowly withdrawn to detect any degree of rectal prolapse and the severity of any haemorrhoids.
- ☐ Carefully examine the anal canal for fissures, particularly if the patient has experienced pain during the procedure.

Abnormal findings

Only by proctoscopy can the anus and rectum be adequately examined for haemorrhoids, anal fissures (tears in the mucosa), rectal prolapse and mucosal disease. During straining, haemorrhoids distend with blood and may prolapse. Protrusion of more than 3–4 cm raises the possibility of a full-thickness rectal prolapse.

THE ACUTE ABDOMEN

Patients with acute upper GI haemorrhage are usually acutely ill and may require urgent management (Fig. 5.23). However, the term '*acute abdomen*' is generally applied to conditions in which the patient presents with acute distress related to an abdominal complaint. Usually the patient or relatives expect an immediate diagnosis and often a surgical cure. Many such situations are neither acute nor amenable to surgery and it is important not to perform a premature or unnecessary operation.

In some patients, clinical examination will reveal that the 'acute abdomen' has occurred in the context of pre-existing ill-health, in others underlying disease may be obscured by the acute complications. Corticosteroids, non-steroidal analgesics, alcohol abuse and previous surgery are examples of factors that may cause an 'acute abdomen' or modify the presentation.

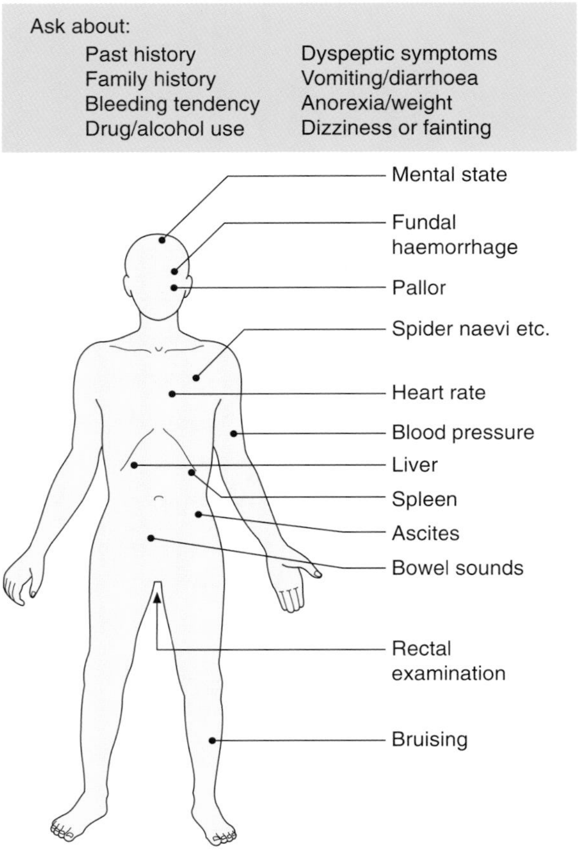

Fig. 5.23 Checklist in upper gastrointestinal tract haemorrhage.

The need to perform an appropriate history and examination are even more important than in non-acute situations when omissions or errors can be corrected at subsequent consultations. However, severe pain, shock and poor physical condition may make it difficult for a patient to concentrate and talk at length. Treatment may need to be commenced before a complete history and examination are possible. It is vital therefore to concentrate on the essential.

Important points in the history of a patient with an acute abdomen

- The patient's own history is the most valuable, and this should be obtained whenever possible.

- When patients are too ill to give their own account, the history should be obtained from observers.
- It is very important that the first history should be as accurate and as detailed as possible; ill patients may be disinclined to repeat their accounts of the illness.
- If, however, doubt remains as to the cause of the problem, the patient should be encouraged to recount the story again because histories relayed through other clinicians may be erroneous.
- Since abdominal pain may arise from disease outwith the alimentary tract, a thorough history is vital.
- The most recent and severe symptoms may occupy the patient's attention to such an extent that important but apparently unrelated details of the history are forgotten or omitted as being trivial.
- The history may appear to change as it is taken at different times by different clinicians; the patient's symptoms may also change as the disease progresses.
- Where appropriate, remember to pay specific attention to the:
  - reproductive, contraceptive and menstrual history
  - possibility of pregnancy and its complications
  - drug history, especially favoured remedies and alcohol consumption
  - past medical history and previous surgical operations.

Important points in the clinical examination of a patient with an acute abdomen

- The examination may begin with the abdomen but should then include the other systems since the disorder may be non-alimentary in origin.
- The hernial orifices, scrotal contents and rectum are important components of the examination.
- Rectal examination is uncomfortable. Repeated examination should be avoided. The examination is best performed by the clinician making the management decisions.
- Tenderness elicited by rectal and vaginal examination may be the sole sign of inflammation of the pelvic peritoneum in acute appendicitis and salpingitis respectively.
- Bimanual rectal and vaginal examination can be useful in assessing pelvic masses.
- Palpation of the abdominal wall overlying an inflamed organ may produce localised pain. In acute cholecystitis, Murphy's sign (p. 164) will be present.
- Localised peritonitis may be revealed by eliciting rebound tenderness on palpation.
- Attempts to elicit rebound tenderness are often both painful and unnecessary, and should not be made when evidence of peritonitis has already been established. Inflammation of the parietal peritoneum causes reflex contraction of the overlying abdominal muscles to produce guarding. Generalised peritonitis may produce 'board-like' rigidity when even light percussion may elicit pain.

Symptom patterns. In many abdominal disorders, there is a recognised typical pattern of specific features, although in many patients these are not all present. Such clusters of specific symptoms and signs can prove particularly useful diagnostic aids in patients with an 'acute abdomen'. These principles can be applied to a number of specific conditions (see Table 5.33 and Figs 5.24, 5.25 and 5.26).

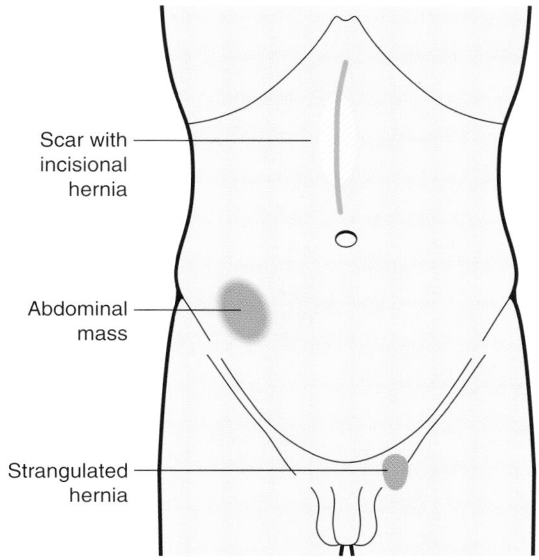

Fig. 5.24 Intestinal obstruction.

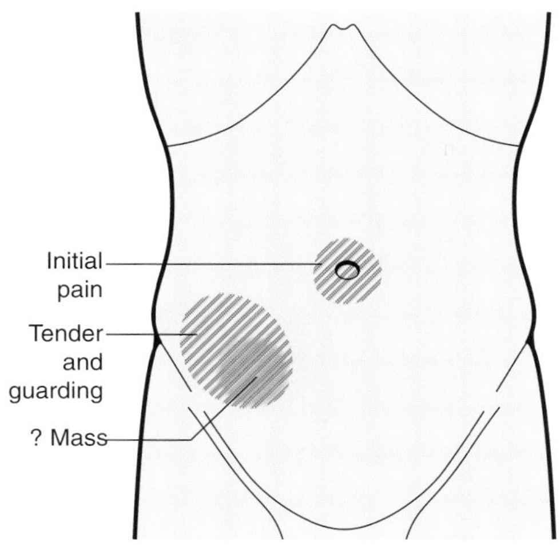

Fig. 5.25 Acute appendicitis.

TABLE 5.33 Some typical clinical features of the important causes of an 'acute abdomen'

Condition	History	Examination
Acute appendicitis	Nausea, vomiting, central abdominal pain which later shifts to the right iliac fossa (RIF)	Fever, tenderness and guarding in the RIF, palpable mass in the RIF, pelvic peritonitis on examination
Perforated peptic ulcer with acute peritonitis	Vomiting at onset associated with acute-onset severe abdominal pain, previous history of dyspepsia, ulcer disease, NSAID or corticosteroid therapy	Shallow breathing with minimal abdominal wall movement, abdominal tenderness and guarding, board-like rigidity, abdominal distension and absent bowel sounds
Acute pancreatitis	Anorexia, nausea, vomiting, constant severe epigastric pain, previous alcohol abuse/cholelithiasis	Fever, periumbilical bruising (Cullen's sign), bruising in the loin (Grey Turner's sign), epigastric tenderness, variable guarding, reduced or absent bowel sounds
Ruptured aortic aneurysm	Sudden onset of tearing, severe back/loin/abdominal pain, circulatory collapse, history of peripheral vascular disease and/or hypertension	Shock and hypotension, pulsatile, tender, central abdominal mass with an overlying bruit, asymmetrical femoral pulses Sometimes hypertension (renal artery involvement)
Acute mesenteric ischaemia	Anorexia, nausea, vomiting, bloody diarrhoea, constant, severe, sustained abdominal pain, previous history of cardiovascular disease	Atrial fibrillation, cardiac failure, asymmetrical peripheral pulses, absent bowel sounds, variable tenderness and guarding
Intestinal obstruction	Colicky central abdominal pain, nausea, vomiting and constipation	Surgical scars, hernias, abdominal mass, distension, visible peristalsis, increased tinkling bowel sounds
Ruptured ectopic pregnancy	Premenopausal; delayed/missed menstrual period, feeling faint, circulatory collapse, unilateral iliac fossa pain, pleuritic or shoulder-tip pain, vaginal discharge – 'late period', 'like prune juice'	Suprapubic tenderness, periumbilical bruising (Cullen's sign), pain/tenderness on vaginal examination (cervical excitation), swelling/fullness in the fornix on vaginal examination
Pelvic inflammatory disease (PID)	Sexually active female; previous history of STD/PID, recent gynaecological procedure, pregnancy or use of intrauterine contraceptive device. Irregular menstruation, dysuria, dyspareunia, lower or central abdominal pain, backache, pleuritic right upper quadrant abdominal pain (Fitz-Hugh–Curtis syndrome)	Fever, vaginal discharge, pelvic peritonitis causing tenderness on rectal examination, right upper quadrant tenderness (perihepatitis), pain/tenderness on vaginal examination (cervical excitation), swelling/fullness in the fornix on vaginal examination

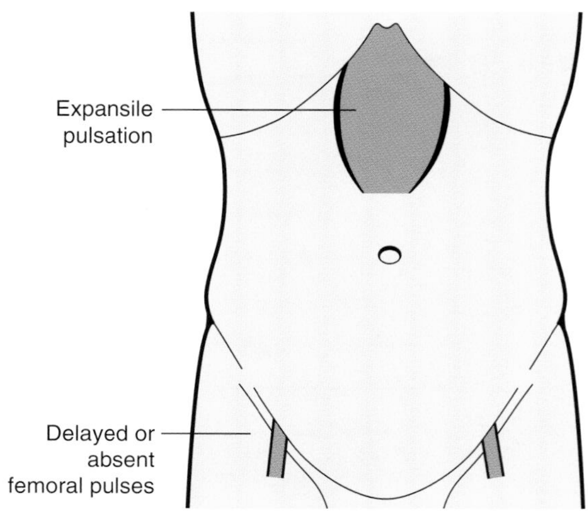

Fig. 5.26 Ruptured aortic aneurysm.

KEY POINTS

- A palpable spleen is always pathological.
- Pelvic peritonitis is often best elicited by rectal examination.
- A succussion splash is suggestive of gastric outlet obstruction only if it is elicited at least 2 hours after food or drink.
- Pancreatic carcinoma is the likely diagnosis in a jaundiced patient with a palpable gall bladder.
- Absence of one or both testes from the scrotum should promote a search for an incompletely descended or ectopic testis.
- Non-thrombosed haemorrhoids are not palpable on rectal examination.
- A hard craggy gland and loss of the median sulcus are features of carcinoma of the prostate.

EXAMINATION OF THE URINE

Useful diagnostic information can often be obtained from analysis of the urine. Indeed, significant kidney disease may develop without specific symptoms or signs, but is usually accompanied by urinary abnormalities. Urinalysis may also indicate disorders which do not primarily affect the kidneys, such as glycosuria in diabetes mellitus.

Urinalysis should therefore be performed on all new patients. It is particularly important in patients presenting with:

- symptoms of kidney or urinary tract disease
- thirst and/or polyuria
- weight loss
- abdominal pain
- jaundice
- hypertension
- pyrexia of uncertain origin (PUO).

Some of the clinical uses of urinalysis are shown in Table 5.34 and the main components of the examination are shown in Table 5.35. It is essential that microscopic and bacteriological examinations are performed on a freshly voided urine sample.

Macroscopic examination

Appearance. Normal fresh urine is clear, though its colour varies greatly. Cloudy urine is usually due to the presence of pus cells (*pyuria*), often with bacteria. Urine that is brownish and cloudy (*smoky urine*) may be due to the presence of blood, as in acute glomerulonephritis, or pigment, as in myoglobinuria. Other typical colour changes suggest the presence of blood, drugs or chemicals (Table 5.20, p. 155).

Odour. An unusually strong fishy smell suggests urinary infection, often with *Escherichia coli*. The typical ammoniacal smell of babies' nappies is due to bacterial decomposition. Some foods, such as asparagus, impart a characteristic smell to the urine.

Volume. Measurement of the urine volume during 24 hours is helpful in many clinical situations and may confirm oliguria or polyuria. In critically ill patients, hourly urine flow is usually measured, after bladder catheterisation, and can provide a useful dynamic indicator of 'core perfusion' in shock states.

Collecting a 24-hour urine sample:

- Ask the patient to empty the bladder on waking, e.g. 8 a.m., and to discard the urine.
- Collect all urine passed in the next 24 hours.
- Remind the patient to collect the final sample at 8 a.m. the following morning.

Biochemical examination

For most clinical purposes, use of a commercially available reagent strip test such as N-Multistix (Bayer Corporation) is sufficient to obtain the necessary diagnostic information. It is important to follow the instructions carefully, and to be alert to the causes of misleading results (see Tables 5.36, 5.37 and 5.38).

TABLE 5.34 Common uses of urinalysis

		Examples
Screening	Random	Diabetes mellitus Asymptomatic bacteriuria
	Selective	Antenatal care Hypertensive patients
Diagnosis	Primary renal disease Secondary renal disease Non-renal disorders	Glomerulonephritis Infective endocarditis Jaundice
Monitoring	Disease progression Drug toxicity	Diabetic nephropathy Gold therapy

TABLE 5.35 Checklist of urine tests

Macroscopic	Microscopic	Biochemical	Microbiological
Colour Clarity Odour Volume	RBCs, WBCs Bacteria Casts Crystals	Specific gravity, pH Blood, protein Glucose, ketones Bilirubin, urobilinogen	Culture and sensitivities

TABLE 5.36 Misleading reagent strip test results for proteinuria

False positive	Phenothiazine therapy Contamination with detergents, chlorhexidine Contamination with alkalis
False negative	Contamination with acid preservatives Bence Jones proteinuria

TABLE 5.37 Misleading reagent strip test results for haematuria

False positive	Non-urinary origin
Contamination with bleach (hypochlorite) Stale urine (bacterial peroxidases) Haemoglobinuria Myoglobinuria	Menstruation (common) Factitious (rare)

TABLE 5.38 Misleading urine reagent strip tests for bilirubin and urobilinogen

	Bilirubin	Urobilinogen
False positive	Phenothiazines Etodolac	Sulphonamides Salicylates
False negative	Vitamin C	Contamination with formalin

Urinary specific gravity. Urinary specific gravity, like osmolality, is an index of the concentration of solute in the urine. It varies in health between 1.002 and 1.035. Specific gravity depends upon the molecular weight of each solute present whereas the osmolality depends on the total solute concentration. In patients with unexplained polyuria, the concentrating ability of the kidneys can be assessed by an overnight fluid deprivation test. In healthy subjects, urinary specific gravity should rise above 1.022, corresponding to a urinary osmolality of greater than 800 mOsmol/kg, although this maximal value decreases with advancing age.

Urinary pH. Urinary pH varies in health between 8.0 and 4.5 and is usually lowest after an overnight fast. On a normal diet, a healthy subject excretes 40–80 mmol of acid, the majority of which is buffered by phosphates. In renal tubular acidosis, either congenital or acquired in origin, urinary acidification is impaired; urinary pH never falls below 5.3 even after an oral challenge with ammonium chloride.

Proteinuria. Urine testing for protein is best performed on fresh concentrated urine, and an early morning sample is therefore the most suitable. The lower limit of detection for urinary protein using reagent strips is 300 mg/l. Values in excess of this may occur transiently in the absence of renal disease (Table 5.39). Proteinuria of less than 1 g/l which disappears when lying supine (*orthostatic proteinuria*) is an occasional finding in healthy young subjects; protein will not be detected in the first urine passed after sleeping recumbent overnight, but will be present during the day.

Proteinuria may be due to increased leakage from the glomeruli, or may be due to tubular dysfunction. Even in health there is some filtration of proteins through the glomeruli, but most is reabsorbed and catabolised by the renal tubules. Proteinuria greater than 2 g per day suggests glomerular disease. Major renal disease may be present without significant proteinuria. This is common in polycystic kidney disease, renal scarring and obstructive uropathy. The proteinuria test strip is impregnated with tetrabromophenol blue, and false-positive and false-negative results may occur (Table 5.36). The test is relatively insensitive to Bence Jones proteins (immunoglobulin light chains, often found in the urine in myeloma), which should be sought by a specific laboratory test.

Urinary albumin excretion rates of as low as 30 mg/day can be detected using radioimmunoassay techniques. Excretion rates of 30–300 mg of albumin per day (*microalbuminuria*) occur in the early stages of diabetic nephropathy.

TABLE 5.39 Common causes of transient proteinuria

Cold exposure	Orthostatic proteinuria
Vigorous exercise	Abdominal surgery
Febrile illness	Congestive cardiac failure

Haematuria. Haematuria is detected by the peroxidase-like activity of the haem moiety oxidising chemicals in the reagent strip. A positive finding may occur as a result of conditions outwith the renal tract (see Table 5.37). The test is equally sensitive to haemoglobin and myoglobin, which can be measured with a specific laboratory test if indicated (e.g. in rhabdomyolysis). The presence of red blood cells in the urine should be confirmed by microscopy.

Urinary nitrite. Most Gram-negative bacteria convert urinary nitrate (derived from dietary nitrate) to nitrite, which can be detected by the reagent strip as an indicator of bacteriuria. A negative result does not exclude the presence of bacteria. Negative results are seen if the bacteria do not have the reductase which forms nitrite, if the urine has not been in the bladder for at least 4 hours (an early morning urine which has incubated within the bladder overnight is best), or if dietary nitrate is absent.

Microscopic examination

Urine microscopy is the most reliable way to establish the presence of erythrocytes, leucocytes, abnormal cells, casts or crystals. These structures disintegrate if urine is left standing, and a fresh sample is important. If present, bacteria can usually be discerned in an unstained wet film on low-power magnification. Higher-power magnification is necessary to distinguish erythrocytes from leucocytes, yeasts and small crystals. Phase contrast microscopy can be used to best identify casts and to assess red cell morphology. Polarised light can be used to best identify urinary crystals.

Urine microscopy

- Centrifuge 10 ml of fresh urine for 5 minutes at 3000 r.p.m.
- Remove the supernatant, leaving 0.5 ml of urine and the deposit.
- Mix the sediment gently and place one drop on a clean slide.
- Overlay a cover slip and examine under the microscope with low illumination and low-power magnification.
- Examine under high-power magnification if abnormalities seen require clarification.

Cells

Red blood cells can be recognised as small round cells without a nucleus. Those which have passed through the glomeruli are mostly dysmorphic (irregular in size and shape), whereas those from elsewhere in the urinary tract are of normal morphology. Phase contrast microscopy is the best way to assess urinary red cell morphology. It is however an operator-dependent process and should not form the sole basis of clinical decisions (e.g. renal biopsy or cystoscopy).

White blood cells have lobed nuclei and granular cytoplasm. White cells with no growth of bacteria on standard culture (sterile pyuria) may suggest renal tuberculosis, and indicate the need for mycobacterial cultures.

Epithelial cells Cells arising from the renal tubule are larger than white blood cells and have oval nuclei. They are present in urinary tract infection and to a lesser degree in inflammatory conditions such as tubulointerstitial nephritis and glomerulonephritis. Bladder epithelial cells are similar but even larger. Their presence is of no clinical significance.

Urinary casts

Casts are cylindrical structures which can be recognised as having formed in the renal tubules.

Hyaline casts are relatively clear and homogeneous cylindrical structures, which consist principally of Tamm–Horsfall mucoprotein secreted by tubular cells. It is unusual to see more than one per low-power field in health. An increase in their number is relatively non-specific and may be seen:

- after severe exercise
- in febrile illnesses
- in severe essential hypertension
- in chronic renal disease.

Granular casts are hyaline casts which in addition contain granules of albumin and immunoglobulins. They may also contain cellular debris to varying degrees (*granular and cellular casts*). They are pathological, and are typically found in disorders associated with significant proteinuria, such as:

- glomerulonephritis
- hypertension
- diabetic nephropathy.

Red cell casts are principally composed of well-defined erythrocytes, and are always accompanied by evidence of haematuria on urine testing (Fig. 5.27). They indicate haematuria of glomerular origin, and are most often seen in acute glomerular disease such as diffuse proliferative glomerulonephritis.

White cell casts suggest acute renal infection or inflammation, and are most often seen in acute pyelonephritis.

Crystals

These will form in any urine if left to stand for more than an hour. Crystals in fresh urine may indicate underlying disease, e.g. urate crystals in gout or urate nephropathy, oxalate crystals in hyperoxaluric stone disease, cystine crystals in cystinuria.

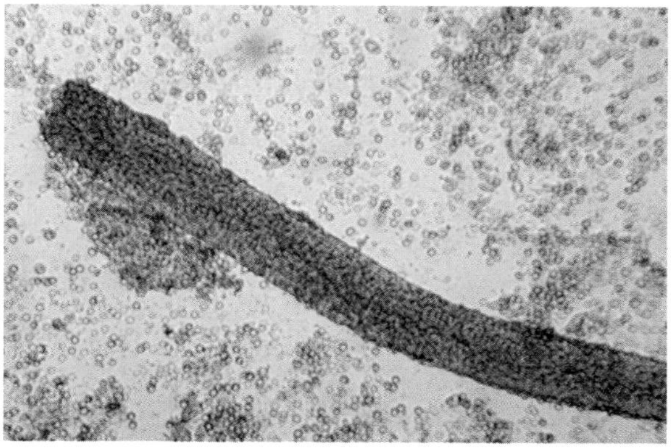

Fig. 5.27 Light microscopy of urinary sediment from a patient with acute glomerulonephritis, showing many red cells and a densely pigmented red cell cast.

Microbiological examination

For the detection of *Mycobacterium tuberculosis*, at least three early morning urine samples should be sent to the laboratory for specific TB culture. For all other suspected bacterial infections, a fresh, clean-voided, midstream urine sample is required.

Midstream urine sample

- Collect by placing the sterile container in the urine stream once micturition is well under way.
- Label the urine sample with the time, date and patient's name.
- Despatch to the laboratory without delay. If a delay is unavoidable, place the sample in an ordinary refrigerator (not freezer) until transport arrives.

KEY POINTS

- Microscopy provides the only reliable method of detecting cells and casts in the urine.
- Red cell casts are an indication of glomerular disease.
- Apparent haematuria due to menstrual contamination is a common finding.
- Transient minor proteinuria is non-specific and unlikely to be of clinical significance.
- Myoglobinuria is suggested by a positive result for blood without red cells on microscopy.
- Pyuria without obvious organisms suggests genitourinary tuberculosis.

FURTHER INVESTIGATIONS OF ALIMENTARY AND GENITOURINARY DISEASE

In most instances, the diagnosis can be made clinically, but requires confirmation by further investigation. When investigation involves any degree of hazard, including ionising irradiation, the risks and benefits require careful consideration.

Radiological investigations

The effects of ionising irradiation depend upon the dose rate, the tissue distribution and the type of radiation, i.e. photon (gamma-rays and X-rays) or particulate (alpha- and beta-particles). Since different types of radiation have different effects on different tissues, the effective dose equivalent, measured in sieverts (1 Sv = 100 rem), is used to express the equivalent dose of uniform whole-body

TABLE 5.40 Special investigations in gastrointestinal, hepatobiliary and genitourinary disorders (radiation dosage is shown in brackets (μSv))

Investigation	Diagnostic problem	Abnormal findings and comments
Chest X-ray (20 μSv)	Acute abdomen, perforated viscus, subphrenic abscess	Pneumonia, free air beneath diaphragm, pleural effusion, elevated diaphragm
Abdominal X-ray (500 μSv)	Intestinal obstruction, perforation, renal colic	Fluid levels, air above the liver, urinary tract calculi
Barium meal (2000 μSv)	Dysphagia, dyspepsia	Oesophageal obstruction/gastric pathology (endoscopy preferable if previous gastric surgery)
Small bowel barium enema (7000 μSv)	Malabsorption, subacute obstruction, unexplained GI bleeding	Duodenal diverticulosis, Crohn's disease, tumour
Large bowel barium enema (7000 μSv)	Altered bowel habit, iron-deficiency anaemia, rectal bleeding	Colonic carcinoma, colitis, diverticulitis
Upper abdominal ultrasound scan	Biliary colic, jaundice, pancreatitis, malignancy	Gallstones, liver metastases, cholestasis, pancreatic calcification, subphrenic abscess
Pelvic ultrasound scan	Pelvic masses, inflammatory diseases, ectopic pregnancy, polycystic ovarian disease	Pelvic structures and abnormalities Ascitic fluid
Urinary tract ultrasound scan	Haematuria, renal failure, hypertension, renal masses, prostatism, testicular/scrotal masses	Kidney size/shape; differentiate renal from post-renal disorders, cystic from solid lesions, post-micturition residual volume; guided biopsy
Intravenous urography (3000 μSv)	Haematuria, renal colic	Renal, ureteric or bladder stones, cysts, tumours, or other diseases
Renal angiography (6000 μSv)	Hypertension, renal failure (especially if kidney size unequal on ultrasound or vascular disease elsewhere)	Renal artery stenosis (unilateral or bilateral); possible angioplasty or stenting
Upper GI endoscopy	Dysphagia, dyspepsia, GI bleeding, gastric ulcer, malabsorption	Especially important in patients aged > 50 years even if barium meal is normal. Gastric and/or duodenal biopsies are useful
Lower GI endoscopy	Rectal bleeding, unexplained GI bleeding, colitis	Important even if the barium enema is normal. Biopsy confirmation of type of colitis
Endoscopic retrograde cholangiopancreatography (1500 μSv)	Obstructive jaundice, acute and chronic pancreatitis	Diagnostic and therapeutic role Stenting strictures
Abdominal CT scan (8000 μSv)	Suspected pancreatic or renal mass, tumour staging, abdominal aortic aneurysm	Useful to confirm or exclude metastatic disease and leaking from aortic aneurysm
Laparoscopy	Acute abdomen, chronic pelvic pain, suspected ovarian disease, peritoneal and liver disease	Appendicitis, hepatic cirrhosis, ectopic pregnancy, ovarian cysts, endometriosis, pelvic inflammatory disease
Aspiration cytology	Liver metastases, intra-abdominal or retroperitoneal tumours	Tissue biopsy guided by ultrasound scanning
Liver or renal biopsy	Parenchymal disease of liver or kidneys	Tissue biopsy guided by ultrasound scanning
Pancreatic function tests	Suspected pancreatic exocrine failure	Pancreolauryl test of exocrine function requires urine samples

irradiation. Irradiation of any area between the diaphragm and the knees should be avoided in pregnancy unless there are overriding clinical considerations. The normal annual UK background radiation is 2000 microsieverts (μSv). Typical radiation dosages are shown in Table 5.40 which gives the principal indications for performing various diagnostic procedures.

COMMON PITFALLS AND HOW TO AVOID THEM

- Oesophageal carcinoma may present with transient dysphagia. Even if the barium swallow is normal, patients with dysphagia require endoscopic examination to exclude malignancy.
- A common cause of iron-deficiency anaemia is gastrointestinal bleeding. Such patients require both upper and lower GI investigations.
- Rectal bleeding is often caused by haemorrhoids. However, haemorrhoids are so common that it is necessary to exclude alternative colorectal causes of bleeding, especially in patients with iron-deficiency anaemia.
- Acute pancreatitis can present as painless, paralytic ileus. Check the serum amylase concentration in all patients with an acute abdomen.
- Pelvic peritonitis may be present in the absence of abdominal tenderness. When this is a possibility, rectal examination should be performed to look for signs of tenderness.
- Ascites is often the result of portal hypertension and hepatic cirrhosis. However, the rapid development of ascites may be caused by intra-abdominal malignancy, peritoneal infection or cardiac failure. These possibilities should be excluded by clinical examination and paracentesis.
- Splenomegaly may be missed even by experienced clinicians; if doubt exists, perform abdominal ultrasonography.
- Sexually transmitted diseases affect all age groups irrespective of marital status or religion. When suspected, they should be positively excluded even if the patient is apparently not sexually active.
- Patients sometimes assume that 'cystitis' is normal, not worth mentioning to the doctor and not thought to be associated with urinary infection. Remember to ask about cystitis specifically.
- Haematuria with red cell casts indicates glomerular disease. Painless haematuria is a common presentation of bladder disease. Cystoscopy is necessary to exclude papilloma or carcinoma.
- Patients may present with renal failure having previously had persistent microscopic haematuria and/or proteinuria recorded but not investigated appropriately. Such abnormalities require explanation and investigation if necessary including renal biopsy.
- Advanced renal failure may present without any physical signs. Remember to undertake blood tests to exclude renal dysfunction in patients with non-specific symptoms, e.g. tiredness.
- Patients with metastatic bone disease commonly present with back pain; a rectal examination will help exclude prostatic carcinoma or intra-abdominal malignancy.
- Renal vascular disease is an important cause of hypertension and renal failure. Listen carefully for renal artery bruits and, if absent, look for bruits elsewhere, e.g. aortofemoral bruits.
- The oedema of the nephrotic syndrome is often misdiagnosed as cardiac failure. Remember to test the urine for protein; a 3-4+ positive test result will confirm the diagnosis.
- Weight loss may be the sole manifestation of diabetes mellitus; remember to test for glycosuria.

FURTHER READING

Davison A M, Cameron J S, Grunfeld J-P, Kerr D N S, Ritz E, Winearls C G 1998 Oxford textbook of clinical nephrology, 2nd edn. Oxford Medical Publications, Oxford
Gazzard B, Theodossi A (eds) 1985 Symptoms in gastroenterology. Clinics in gastroenterology. W B Saunders, London, vol 14:3
Haslett C, Chilvers E R, Hunter J A A, Boon N A 1999 Davidson's principles and practice of medicine, 18th edn. Churchill Livingstone, Edinburgh
Shearman D J C, Finlayson N D C, Camilleri M, Carter D C 1997 Diseases of the gastrointestinal tract and liver. Churchill Livingstone, Edinburgh
Thomson C R V, Plant W D 1997 Key topics in renal medicine. BIOS Scientific Publishers, Oxford

The nervous system

6

R. E. CULL • I. R. WHITTLE

THE HISTORY

Examination of the nervous system is founded on well-established principles of anatomy and physiology. In many instances, the taking of a detailed history and execution of a careful clinical examination will enable the clinician to localise the site of the neurological lesion and to establish a precise or differential diagnosis. When disease processes affect the *structure* of neural tissue (e.g. vascular disease, multiple sclerosis, tumours), significant changes are often found during clinical examination. Disorders of neural *function* (e.g. epilepsy, migraine) may produce no abnormal signs on examination, and the careful elicitation of the patient's history is of paramount importance.

A neurological examination requires to be systematic, irrespective of the order in which the different parts of the nervous system are examined. As experience is gained in clinical practice, aspects of the examination can be either abridged or focused depending upon the history, general observations of the patient's level of cognitive and sensorimotor function and preliminary examination findings.

The presenting symptoms of patients with neurological problems are very variable and largely dependent upon that part of the nervous system most affected. They may be very specific (e.g. sudden onset of headache or of double vision), or vague and diffuse (such as progressive forgetfulness or weakness). In many instances the diagnosis of a neurological illness can be based on details given from the patient's history. The general principles of history-taking apply as outlined in Chapter 1, but emphasis should be placed on the following special aspects relating to the nervous system:

Time relationships

- When did the symptoms start/stop?
- How long do they last?
- Do they occur at certain times of the day/week/month?
- Do symptoms evolve over seconds, hours, days, weeks or months?

Localisation

- Which part of the body is affected?
- Can the patient localise the problem to one limb or part of it?
- If more widespread, is the problem symmetrical?

Precipitating factors

- Are symptoms triggered by any specific activity, e.g. exercise, sleep, posture, reading, eating, coughing, micturition, sexual activity; or by external stimuli, e.g. light, sound, smell, heat or cold?

Associated symptoms

- Are the presenting symptoms accompanied by other features of neurological disease?
  - numbness, paraesthesiae, cold, warmth (sensory system)
  - weakness, clumsiness, stiffness, unsteady gait (motor system)
  - headache
  - nausea, vomiting
  - loss or alteration of consciousness
  - visual disturbances
  - psychological changes, e.g. depression or elation, weeping, agitation, sleep and appetite disturbance, change in energy and libido.

Past history

Some neurological disorders (e.g. epilepsy, hydrocephalus) may present many years after the causative event. It is therefore important to ask about:

- pregnancy (length of term; intrauterine problems)
- delivery (normal, assisted or operative)
- neonatal health (severe jaundice, respiratory difficulty, infections and convulsions)
- infancy (infections, convulsions, injuries)
- childhood and previous adult life (head and spinal injury, serious infections (particularly meningitis, encephalitis), surgical operations and drug therapy).

Family history

Many neurological disorders have a genetic component. Some may be strictly genetic disorders (e.g. muscular dystrophy, spinocerebellar degeneration, Huntington's chorea). In others, genetic factors appear to influence the development of the condition (e.g. epilepsy, migraine, multiple sclerosis, vascular disease).

Social history

The patient's *occupation* may be relevant in the causation or triggering of neurological disorders, e.g.:

- exposure to toxic chemicals (neuropathies and encephalopathy)
- recurrent overuse of certain joints predisposing to entrapment neuropathy (e.g. carpal tunnel syndrome)
- prolonged visual work, particularly with visual display units or under artificial light (tension headache and migraine).

Marital status and household dynamics and any change of lifestyle should be ascertained. Marriage, divorce, bereavement and change of occupation are important factors in

TABLE 6.1 Summary of neurological history-taking

Presenting complaint	Time relationships Localisation Trigger factors Associated features
Past medical history	Birth/pregnancy Head/spine injury Infections (meningitis/encephalitis) Surgical procedures Drug therapy
Family history	Epilepsy, migraine, multiple sclerosis, stroke, cerebral aneurysm, muscle disorders, dementia, spinocerebellar degenerations and neuropathies
Social history	Occupation Marital status Smoking habits Alcohol consumption Use of recreational drugs Sexual orientation and habits

emotionally based symptoms, particularly tension headache, migraine and depression, and may also trigger attacks of multiple sclerosis and epilepsy. Smoking habits both past and present should be elicited, as should the use and possible abuse of alcohol or other drugs. It may be appropriate to ask about the patient's sexual orientation and any possibility of exposure to sexually transmitted diseases including syphilis and HIV.

A summary of the information that should be obtained from patients presenting with neurological symptoms is given in Table 6.1.

Two of the commonest categories of symptom reported by patients seen in clinical neurology are:

- headaches
- attacks of altered consciousness – 'fits, faints and funny turns'.

HEADACHE

Headache is a very common symptom. A detailed history is frequently more important and more helpful than the physical examination. In the majority of patients, the diagnosis is tension-type headache; no underlying disease or abnormal physical signs are found and emotional factors often predominate. Headache is also a common non-specific feature of febrile illnesses and systemic diseases (see Table 6.2). The past medical history, family history, personal and social history and systemic enquiry together with details of current drug therapy are often relevant. Migraine is frequently a familial disorder. The assessment of headache should include its characterisation using the method described for pain (p. 7).

TABLE 6.2 Common causes of headache

Extracranial disorders	*Example*
Temporomandibular joint	Osteoarthritis
Cervical spine	Cervical spondylosis
Ophthalmological	Glaucoma
Teeth	Dental sepsis
Middle ear	Earache
Paranasal sinuses	Sinusitis
Arteries	Cranial arteritis
Intracranial disorders	
Migraine	
Meningitis	
Intracranial hypertension	
Tumour	
Subarachnoid bleed	
Psychosomatic disorders	
Tension headache	

Main site

Whether headache affects the entire head, half the head or a smaller area of the head, neck or face is often of paramount diagnostic significance. Examples of headaches and their relationship to the site are shown in Table 6.3.

Radiation

Unilateral pain radiating to the throat, ear, eye, nose, cheek or face is typical of the neuralgias. Facial pain extending beyond the territory of the trigeminal nerve and which may be bilateral or involve the tongue or mouth suggests a psychogenic cause. Pain radiating to the neck with tenderness of the neck muscles is typical of tension headache and cervicogenic headache.

TABLE 6.3 Relationship between the cause and site of headache

Disorder	Site
Subarachnoid haemorrhage	Bilateral, generalised or nuchal
Tension headache	Bilateral, generalised or nuchal
Migraine	Unilateral: different sides on separate occasions
Cluster headache	Unilateral: eye, nose, cheek
Cranial arteritis	Unilateral with scalp tenderness
Trigeminal neuralgia	Unilateral: maxillary or mandibular branches of the trigeminal nerve
Post-herpetic neuralgia	Unilateral: ophthalmic branch of the trigeminal nerve

Character

Pain likened to a tight band around the head or like a pressure over the head is characteristic of tension headache; in contrast, headaches that are described as sickening, dull aching or throbbing are usually migrainous in origin. Lancinating, paroxysmal pain like red-hot needles thrust through the face suggests trigeminal neuralgia.

Severity

The explosive onset of severe headache associated with neck stiffness is a common feature of subarachnoid haemorrhage, while a slowly progressive headache increasing in duration and severity is typical of raised intracranial pressure from a cerebral tumour. Severity is often also marked in migraine, cluster headache and trigeminal neuralgia; in the last, paroxysms of severe pain may cause the patient to wince and cry out momentarily.

Duration

The longer the history of headache without progression, the more likely that its cause is benign. Migraine attacks typically last 24–72 hours but occasionally last less than 6 hours. Episodes of cluster headache usually last less than an hour. In trigeminal neuralgia, each paroxysm lasts only seconds recurring over several minutes. The duration of tension-type headache is very variable, ranging from 15 minutes to many weeks or even months.

Frequency and periodicity

Attacks with a sudden or sub-acute onset occurring in repeated short bursts with pain-free intervals lasting weeks or months are characteristic of migraine, trigeminal neuralgia and cluster headache. Migraine attacks are often cyclical, occurring weekly or monthly, and are frequently perimenstrual in women. In between attacks, the migraine sufferer is usually well. Post-herpetic neuralgia and cranial arteritis have a subacute onset but are continuous, and meningitis and subarachnoid haemorrhage have an acute onset with rapid progression.

Special times of occurrence

Severe pain waking a patient from sleep in the early hours of the morning is typical of cluster headaches and raised intracranial pressure. Pain precipitated by facial movement such as eating, drinking, shaving or brushing the teeth suggests trigeminal or glossopharyngeal neuralgia. Jaw pain during chewing is typical of cranial arteritis. Headaches occurring at times of stress relief (e.g. weekend and holidays) are usually due to migraine.

Aggravating factors

Headache that is increased by bending, straining and coughing suggests raised intracranial pressure. Migraine may be precipitated by bright light, loud noise, strong odours, missed meals, intake of chocolate, cheese, alcohol and citrus fruits, changes in the weather, travel and by the contraceptive pill. Patients suffering from cluster headache are particularly sensitive to small amounts of alcohol and other vasodilators. The headache of benign intracranial hypertension is associated with weight gain and with the use of corticosteroids, tetracycline or contraceptive drug therapy.

Relieving factors

Migrainous attacks are characteristically less frequent and less severe during pregnancy. Acute attacks of migraine usually respond well to analgesic therapy or to more potent selective 5-HT_1 agonist agents such as sumatriptan. By contrast tension-type headache, especially when chronic, is often resistant to analgesics. A rapid and dramatic response in cranial arteritis to corticosteroid therapy is characteristic.

Associated phenomena

Nausea and vomiting typically accompany migraine; whereas raised intracranial pressure headache may be associated with vomiting, but often without nausea. Tension headache is not usually accompanied by any of these symptoms. Migraine is often accompanied by intolerance to light (photophobia) or noise (phonophobia), irritability, food cravings and hunger. In 15–20% of patients visual disturbances (teichopsia and fortification spectra) and/or peripheral and circumoral paraesthesiae occur, usually before the headache phase (migrainous aura). Patients with cluster headaches may experience watering of the eye or

CASE HISTORY

A 22-year-old undergraduate developed severe headache while attending a hockey team practice. She vomited and felt 'dazed'. She was driven to her flat by a friend and went to bed with a persistent headache. Her flat mate who was a student nurse returned home, and detected neck stiffness and took the patient to hospital. The patient was apyrexial and there were no focal neurological signs, but she had severe meningeal irritation. An urgent CT scan was arranged and confirmed the diagnosis of subarachnoid haemorrhage (Fig. 6.1).

Learning points

- Apparently healthy individuals may have life-threatening conditions.
- Because of the risk of potentially lethal rebleeding, the early diagnosis and treatment of subarachnoid haemorrhage is particularly important in patients who are conscious and neurologically intact.

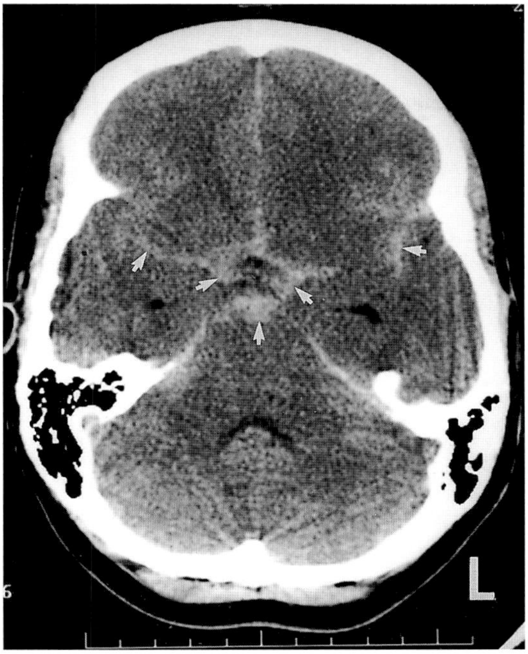

Fig. 6.1 CT scan of the brain showing subarachnoid blood in the suprasellar cistern and both sylvian fissures (arrowheads).

nose or even ptosis of an eyelid during attacks, and occasionally the ptosis may persist afterwards.

FITS, FAINTS AND FUNNY TURNS

The terms 'blackout', 'dizziness' and 'funny turn' are commonly used to describe the sudden onset of an altered state of consciousness. Such episodes may denote any of the following symptoms:

- *Vertigo*: a sensation of unsteadiness and loss of balance associated with a feeling of rotational movement due to dysfunction of the vestibular system of either a central or peripheral origin.
- *Syncope*: light-headedness or faintness associated with the feeling of impending and/or actual loss of consciousness due to a reduction in cerebral blood flow.
- *Epilepsy*: loss of consciousness associated with generalised or partial seizures due to paroxysmal excessive and hypersynchronous discharge of cerebral neurones.
- *Drop attack*: falls occurring without warning or loss of consciousness associated with sudden weakness of the legs.

Vertigo

The vestibular system includes the peripheral vestibular apparatus of the inner ear and vestibular nerve, the central connections of the vestibular nuclei within the brain stem and their cortical projections to the temporal lobes.

Any disorder which disrupts the balance of the two vestibular inputs may produce vertigo of varying severity from a 'swimming sensation' in the head to severe hallucinations of rotational movement with nausea and vomiting. A *peripheral disorder* producing vertigo is suggested by the association with cochlear symptoms, e.g. unilateral or bilateral *deafness* and *tinnitus* (abnormal noises in the ear). A *central disorder* producing vertigo is suggested by the association with neurological symptoms. It is important to establish the mode of onset: brief, acute episodes are usually due to a peripheral labyrinthine disorder, although acute brain stem ischaemia, temporal lobe epilepsy and Ménière's disease may also present in this way; chronic vertigo of gradual onset not associated with cochlear symptoms suggests a central lesion (see Table 6.4).

TABLE 6.4 Patterns of vertigo and their causes

Without deafness and tinnitus	With deafness and tinnitus
Acute	
Viral vestibular neuronitis	Skull fracture
Multiple sclerosis	Ménière's disease
Acute and recurrent	
Benign positional vertigo	Ménière's disease
Migraine	Chronic otitis media
Multiple sclerosis	Acoustic neuroma
Chronic and persistent	
Multiple sclerosis	Ototoxic drugs
Vertebrobasilar ischaemia	Acoustic neuroma

Syncope

Transient impairment of cerebral blood flow may result from a reduction in cardiac output, increased peripheral vasodilatation or a combination of the two (see Table 6.5).

TABLE 6.5 Causes of syncope

Vasovagal syncope
Postural syncope
Cough or micturition syncope
Vertebrobasilar arterial insufficiency
Carotid sinus hypersensitivity
Cardiogenic syncope
Arrhythmias
bradyarrhythmias (e.g. Stokes–Adams)
tachyarrhythmias
Outflow obstruction
aortic, pulmonary or mitral stenosis
hypertrophic, obstructive cardiomyopathy
atrial myxoma, constrictive pericarditis

Vasovagal syncope or simple faints usually occur in the standing position, or occasionally sitting. Apart from postural factors, attacks may be induced by pain or fear (e.g. of needles). Prodromal features include nausea, weakness and sensations of heat, tinnitus and dimming of vision. Bradycardia, peripheral vasodilatation and hypotension produce the transient loss of consciousness, which may be averted by lying down or putting the head well down. Sweating and skin pallor are often observed; urinary incontinence is unusual, but myoclonic jerks continuing for up to 10 seconds are relatively common and can cause confusion with epilepsy. Recovery from syncope is usually rapid.

Postural syncope occurs soon after standing upright or on prolonged standing and is common after periods of bed rest or following intense exertion. Its occurrence suggests impaired vasomotor reflexes due to autonomic neuropathy or vasodepressor drug treatment, or sodium and water depletion due to adrenal or renal insufficiency or to excessive intestinal or cutaneous losses.

Exertional syncope occurs during rather than following exertion and suggests impaired cardiac output due to pericardial, myocardial or valvular heart disease.

Syncope due to cardiac arrhythmias characteristically occurs suddenly and without warning; the patient may appear dead and be pale and pulseless as a result of either ventricular tachycardia or transient asystole ('Stokes–Adams attack'). Recovery is often rapid and accompanied by facial flushing.

Syncope associated with head movements suggests either carotid sinus hypersensitivity or vertebrobasilar arterial insufficiency; carotid sinus massage or extension of the cervical spine during upward gaze may precipitate further episodes.

Cough syncope characteristically follows a prolonged, purple-faced paroxysm of coughing in a patient with chronic obstructive airways disease.

Micturition syncope is uncommon and occurs usually in males, often with prostatism, who faint after emptying their bladder in the upright position after rising from sleep. The sudden relief of bladder wall pressure causes reflex vasodilatation and provokes the syncope.

Epilepsy

Not all epileptic discharges result in convulsions. Epileptic discharges may arise from one small area of the cerebral cortex and remain localised (*partial* or *focal seizures*) or may primarily involve or spread rapidly to both hemispheres (*generalised seizures*). Partial seizures may be *simple* and not impair consciousness, or *complex* and impair consciousness. The presentation will depend upon the area in the cortex from which the discharges arise. For example discharges in the temporal lobe may cause olfactory auras and the sensation of déjà vu. Both simple partial and complex partial seizures may progress to become generalised seizures (see Table 6.6).

TABLE 6.6 Classification of seizures

Generalised seizures
Absence attacks – petit mal (3 Hz spike and wave)
Myoclonic seizures – myoclonic jerks
Tonic – clonic seizures of grand mal or major fits
Tonic seizures
Atonic or akinetic seizures
Partial seizures
Simple partial seizures – no loss of consciousness
Complex partial seizures – loss of consciousness
Partial seizures evolving into generalised seizures
Generalised seizures with only EEG evidence of focal onset
Pseudo-seizures – non-epileptic attacks

TABLE 6.7 Aetiological clues in the history of epilepsy

Feature	Possible cause
Childhood onset	Idiopathic
Headaches	Intracerebral bleed or tumour
Focal symptoms	Intracerebral tumour
Nocturnal fits	Focal lesion Hypoglycaemia
Alcohol abuse	Alcohol withdrawal Subdural haematoma Hypoglycaemia
Sexual activity or drug abuse	HIV infection
Drug therapy	Iatrogenic
Pregnancy	Eclampsia
Hypertension/CVA	Cerebrovascular disease

The cause of epilepsy. Recognition that a patient's blackouts are epileptic in origin is the first stage in the diagnostic process. The underlying cause also requires to be determined (see Table 6.7). Epilepsy may be familial, congenital or acquired.

Differential diagnosis of syncope and epilepsy

Most blackouts are due to either syncope or epilepsy. Patients who fall to the ground may attribute the episode to a trip; those who are unable to recall hitting the ground have usually lost consciousness before falling. The diagnosis of blackouts is most readily made if a trained observer witnesses an episode. Every effort should be made to interview any available eyewitness.

Prodromal features. Nausea, visual dimming and a sense of impending loss of consciousness precipitated by prolonged standing, pain or intense emotional excitement favour syncope. Hyperventilation may be a prodromal feature to syncope, but may also produce epilepsy in susceptible patients. Episodes of sudden unconsciousness accompanied by abnormal movements, occurring while sleeping, soon after waking, or when watching television or stroboscopic discotheque lights suggest epilepsy.

Eyewitness account. A history of tonic or convulsive movements, facial grimacing, grunting, jaw clenching, tongue biting or irregular noisy breathing with cyanosis clearly suggests seizures. However, syncope may occasionally result in urinary incontinence, and patients with seizures may appear syncopal with pallor, sweating and limpness. Cardiac arrhythmias may result in a seizure due to cerebral hypoxia.

Falls and drop attacks

Changes in the erect posture and balance are normally monitored by visual, proprioceptive and vestibular receptors. Disorders of these systems may impair balance and are often first manifested by increased sway. Severe disorders of balance usually only ensue when more than one of the sensory systems are impaired. Proprioception is particularly important in maintaining static balance, while the vestibular system is more important in dynamic balance, e.g. walking on uneven pavements. In healthy elderly subjects, the shorter step length and increased sway alter the gait and the balance. The increased risk of falls in the elderly is particularly marked in those with dementia or cerebrovascular or locomotor disorders.

Accidental falls (trips or slips) should be distinguished from *spontaneous falls*. Occasionally patients may experience *drop attacks*, a sudden, unpredictable loss of power in the lower limbs causing the patient to crumple to the ground without dizziness or loss of consciousness. Characteristically, drop attacks patients are unable to stand upright for several minutes even with support (see Table 6.8).

TABLE 6.8 Checklist for the history of falls

Was it an accidental fall?
Recall of event
Trip or slip
Walking surface
Footware
Illumination
Visual acuity

Was it a spontaneous fall?
Preceding symptoms
Onset with head movement or standing upright
Associated symptoms of vertigo, deafness or tinnitus
Associated chest pain or palpitation
Awareness of hitting the ground
Eyewitness account
Resulting injuries or incontinence
Recall of events at the time
Ability to regain erect posture
Previous confusion, dementia or parkinsonism
Previous hypertension, blackouts or epilepsy
Drug therapy – antidepressants, hypnotics, hypotensive agents
Alcohol consumption

CASE HISTORY

For 12 months, a 60-year-old man had experienced episodes of auditory hallucinations and olfactory auras. On several occasions, he had been acutely confused. He presented with progressive headaches and left-sided weakness. The headaches were worse on waking in the morning. He was confused, particularly with regard to time, numbers and dates. He dragged the left foot and had some weakness in the left hand.

The MRI scan showed a large tumour involving the right temporal lobe with extensive oedema. There was effacement of the ipsilateral lateral ventricle, distortion of the third ventricle and displacement of the septum pellucidum across the midline to the left (Fig. 6.2).

Learning points

- Progression of symptoms usually indicates organic disease.
- Lesions which expand slowly may reach a considerable size before diagnosis.
- The site of the lesion explains the hallucinatory olfactory phenomena which were almost certainly epileptic in nature.

KEY POINTS

- Disorders of neural function may produce no abnormal signs. The diagnosis is often dependent on the history.
- Some neurological disorders may present many years after the causative event.
- Stress may induce neurological symptoms.

Headaches
- Tension headache is very common; most patients with headache do not have serious pathology.
- Headaches caused by organic disease are often progressive in nature and worse in the early morning and on bending.
- Subarachnoid haemorrhage should be considered in any patient with sudden-onset severe headache, radiating to the neck and accompanied by loss of consciousness or vomiting.

Altered consciousness
- Any eyewitness account of a 'blackout' is often the most critical part of the clinical examination.
- Patients who fall may attribute the episode to a trip. Those who lose consciousness before falling cannot recall hitting the ground.
- Epilepsy is not a diagnosis; it is always important to establish the underlying cause.

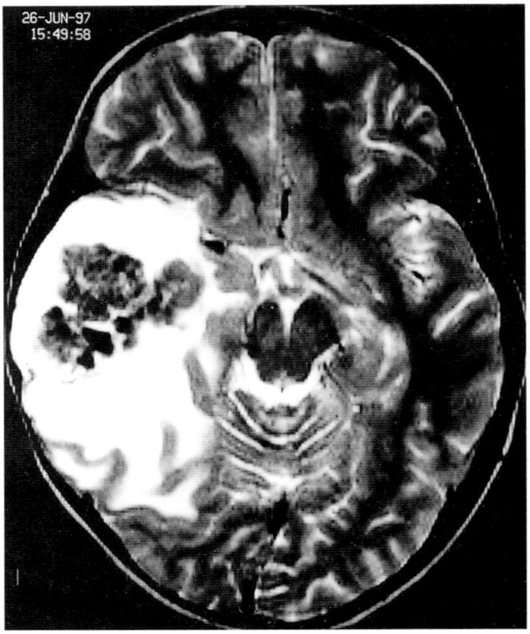

Fig. 6.2 T2-weighted axial MRI image showing large right temporal tumour with mass effect. Note the thinning of the right temporal skull vault which indicates that this lesion was very slow growing.

NEUROLOGICAL EXAMINATION

GENERAL OBSERVATION

Before starting the formal neurological examination it is often possible to obtain useful information by observing the patient (see Table 6.9). Thus the presence of involuntary movement is often detected during history-taking. The various types of involuntary movements are shown in Table 6.10. Additional information may be obtained during the general examination (Ch. 2). For example, the examination of the skin may provide important information (see Fig. 2.41, p. 58). Palpation for lymph nodes, cervical ribs or tenderness should be carried out in patients with arm and hand symptoms. Brachial plexus compression at the thoracic outlet is usually associated with tenderness, and sometimes sensory symptoms are evoked by firm pressure over the plexus. Likewise, scapular wasting may be observed after an episode of brachial neuritis (see Fig. 6.3). Vascular disease is the commonest cause of brain dysfunction in the middle-aged and elderly. Auscultation for cranial and cervical bruits (p. 193) should be included as part of the nervous system assessment. Evidence of stenoses in the carotid and vertebral systems may be found by listening for a systolic bruit over the affected vessel (Fig. 6.4), but the absence of a bruit does not exclude a significant stenotic lesion.

TABLE 6.9 The nervous system: general observations

- Gait
- Romberg's test
- Speech
- Handwriting
- Mental state
- Facial appearance
- Involuntary movements
- Movements of the neck and spine

Carotid artery stenosis occurs most often at its cervical bifurcation at the angle of the jaw, whereas bruits due to vertebral or subclavian artery stenosis are best heard at the supraclavicular fossa. It is best to also auscultate between the two sites for bruits arising from a common carotid lesion.

Bruits arising from cerebral arteriovenous malformations may be heard over the cranium, but because the orbit acts as an acoustic window, are better heard by listening with the stethoscope bell placed over a gently closed eyelid. The precordium should always be auscultated to ensure that

TABLE 6.10 Involuntary movements

Movement	Description	Sites affected
Tremor	Rhythmical oscillations 4–10/s	Hands, arms, legs, head/neck
Chorea	Jerky, rapid, semipurposive, changing in site and variable	Heads, arms, hands, legs, trunk
Athetosis	Slow, writhing, distal	Hands, feet
Dystonia	Slow, sustained, turning or postural	Head, neck, arms, legs, trunk
Myoclonus	Sudden shock-like non-purposive, affecting muscles, groups of muscles or whole body	Limbs, trunk, whole body
Hemiballismus	Proximal, flailing, continuous and of wide amplitude	Arm and leg on one side
Orofacial–lingual dyskinesias	Grimacing, chewing tongue, writhing	Face, mouth, tongue
Tics	Repetitive, purposive, stereotyped, jerky	Face, limbs, respiratory muscles, trunk, voice

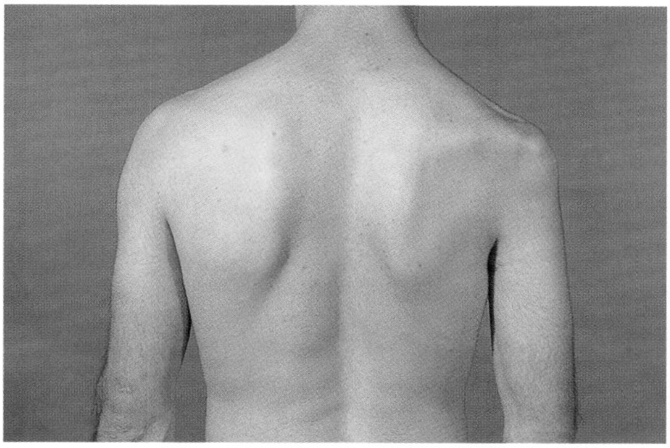

Fig. 6.3 Right scapular amyotrophy following brachial neuritis.

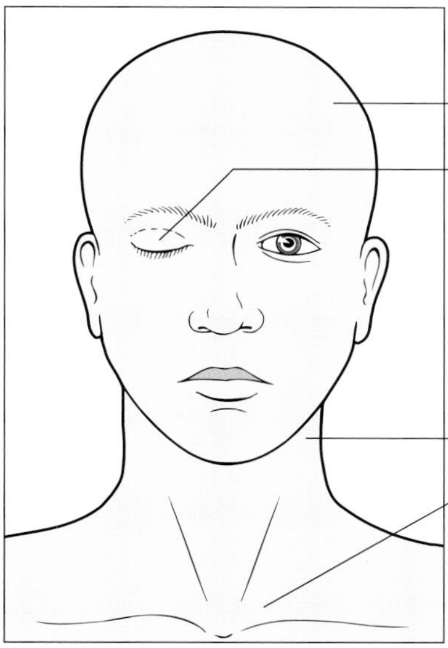

Fig. 6.4 Auscultation for cervical and cranial bruits. 1. Supraclavicular fossa. **2.** Carotid bifurcation. **3.** Over closed eyelid. **4.** Over cranium.

cardiac murmurs are not being transmitted to cranial vessels.

Gait

Ambulant patients should be observed walking and, if possible, patients in bed should be asked to walk to assess the gait (p. 214). Abnormalities such as hemiparesis and parkinsonism cause specific types of gait disturbance (see Table 6.11).

Balance mechanisms relying on cerebellar, vestibular and proprioceptive systems can be tested by heel–toe (tandem) walking and by carrying out *Romberg's test.*

CASE HISTORY

A 44-year-old Bangladeshi was visiting her sister, a resident in the United Kingdom. She awoke one morning with profound weakness of her left arm which felt heavy and awkward. Unsupported, she could only walk with difficulty and tended to bump into objects on the left side. On examination, she was normotensive, the pedal pulses were present and there were no vascular bruits. She was in atrial fibrillation with a ventricular rate of 160 per minute. The apex was tapping in nature and the auscultatory signs were consistent with pure mitral stenosis. She had an upper motor neurone paralysis of the left upper limb and face. There was minimal motor impairment of the left lower limb and the visual fields were intact. She exhibited left-sided visual inattention and sensory neglect. The MRI scan showed a wedge-shaped infarction in the territory of the right middle cerebral artery (Fig. 6.5). The echocardiogram confirmed mitral stenosis with clot in the left atrium as the source of the arterial (cerebral) embolism.

Learning points

- Strokes may be caused by primary cardiovascular disease.
- The anatomical site of the embolus accounts for the disability.
- Apparent disparity between functional disability and physical signs may sometimes be attributable to sensory and/or visual neglect.

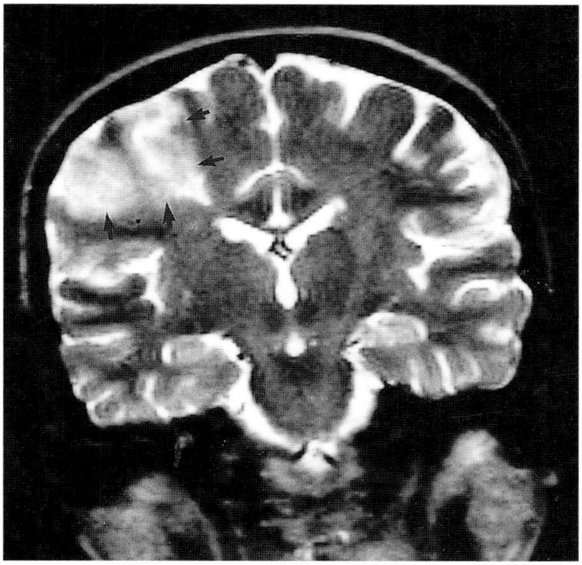

Fig. 6.5 T2-weighted coronal MRI scan showing a wedge-shaped area of signal change in the grey and white matter typical of a cortical cerebral infarct affecting a branch of the right middle cerebral artery (arrows).

Patients with cerebellar deficits will often have difficulty standing in this position even with the eyes open.

Examination sequence

- ☐ Ask the patient to stand with feet together and eyes open initially (Fig. 6.6A).
- ☐ Then ask the patient to close the eyes (Fig. 6.6B).

TABLE 6.11 Disorders of gait	
Hemiparesis	Patient drags affected leg stiffly, foot inverted, arm flexed at the side
Bilateral leg spasticity	Patient leans forward, legs adducted, and walks stiffly on toes (equinus)
Footdrop	Patient flexes the hip, lifting the foot off the ground. The foot slaps down noisily
Parkinsonism	Patient is slow to start walking and takes small strides. There is a tendency to walk faster or to suddenly freeze, failure to swing one or both arms and loss of postural reflexes if pushed from standing position
Cerebellar deficit (ataxia)	The gait is broad based. The patient may sway from side to side and may fall or have to hold on to furniture or walls
Apraxia (e.g. hydrocephalus or multi-infarct states)	Patient has a broad-based, small-stepping, unsteady gait and difficulty in turning

Where there is a proprioceptive or vestibular deficit, during Romberg's test, balance deteriorates when the eyes are closed, and the patient may fall if not caught.

Arm drift

A very useful but non-specific sign in clinical neurology is termed 'drift'. A positive sign suggests some underlying abnormality in nervous function and is an indication for performing a more detailed neurological examination.

Examination sequence

- ☐ Ask the patient to close the eyes and outstretch the limbs, placing palms uppermost and the fingers extended and adducted, and then to maintain this position.

Normally the limbs do not drift with eyes closed. Abnormality may involve a subtle change in finger position (e.g. a slow flexion) or a more gross drift downwards or pronation of the whole arm.

Speech

Much may be learned about the patient's speech and language function during history-taking (p. 17). Speech disorders may be divided into two main groups:

1. Disorders of articulation (*dysarthria*) and phonation (*dysphonia*).

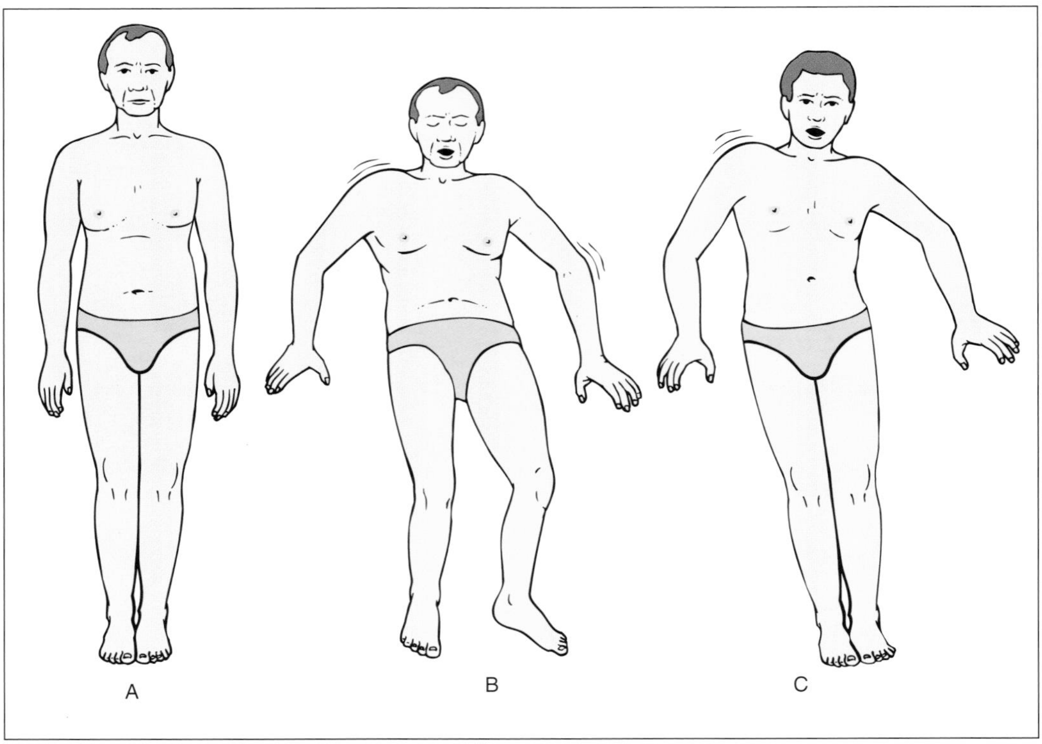

Fig. 6.6 Romberg's test for position sense. The patient can stand with feet together and eyes open [A] but falls with eyes closed [B]. In contrast, the patient with a cerebellar lesion cannot stand with feet together and eyes open [C].

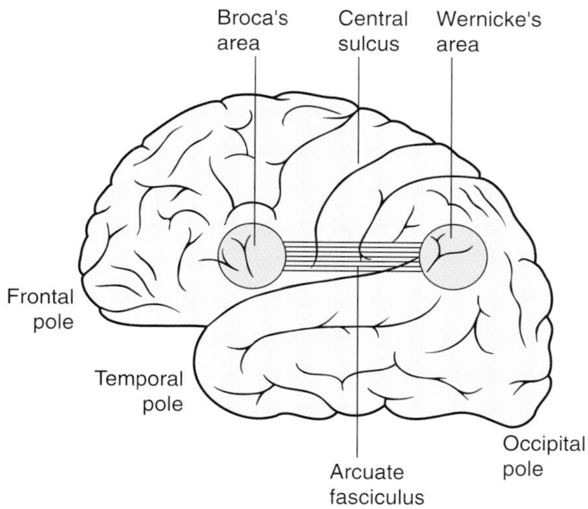

Fig. 6.7 The main language areas.

2. Disorders of language areas in the dominant hemisphere (*dysphasia*).

If a deficit of speech is evident a more thorough examination should be undertaken. By careful examination of speech and language it is often possible to localise the causative lesion.

Anatomy

The language areas are situated in the dominant cerebral hemisphere. In the vast majority of right-handed people the left hemisphere is dominant. About a third of left-handers have a dominant right hemisphere; the others have either left-sided or bilateral language localisation. The main language areas are shown in Figure 6.7.

Broca's area (the inferior frontal region) is concerned with the generation of motor programmes for the production of words or parts of words (phonemes).

Wernicke's area lies in the posterior temporal lobe and the adjoining parietal region and is concerned with the comprehension of language and the selection of words to convey meaning.

Examination sequence (Table 6.12)

- ☐ *Spontaneous speech*: Assess the output of spontaneous speech, fluency and use of inappropriate words (paraphasias and neologisms) during conversation. If dysarthria is suspected, ask the patient to repeat a phrase which requires precise articulation (e.g. 'West Register Street').
- ☐ *Naming of objects*: Ask the patient to name a shown object (e.g. a comb or a pen). The test can be made more difficult by asking the patient to name an object or a concept that is described but not shown.
- ☐ *Comprehension of spoken speech*: Assess comprehension of spoken speech by asking the patient to carry out commands. Staged commands (e.g. 'pick up the blue card, fold it in half and put it under the white card') help bring out subtle defects. A collection of coins can provide suitable objects for similar arrangement tasks. It is important to avoid giving visual clues.
- ☐ Ask the patient to say simple sentences such as 'Today is Tuesday'. This is often sufficient to detect repetition failure due to conduction dysphasia.
- ☐ Ask the patient to read aloud from a book or paper. This may reveal an associated dyslexia.
- ☐ Examine the patient's handwriting. This cannot be assessed if there is a motor deficit affecting the writing hand. Errors of form, grammar and syntax may be found in association with dysphasia, indicating a disorder not only of speech but more globally affecting language function.

TABLE 6.12 Examination of speech and language

Spontaneous speech	Naming objects, concepts
Articulation	Comprehension of spoken commands
Fluency	Repetition of spoken phrases
Paraphasias	Reading aloud
Grammar	Handwriting
Syntax	

Common abnormalities

Dysarthria. Dysarthria may be caused by purely mechanical factors such as ill-fitting dentures, but it is usually due to weakness or impaired coordination of the orolingual muscles concerned with the production of consonants (see Table 6.13). Dysarthric speech is indistinct and difficult for the listener to discern. However, its grammatical construction is normal, and the patient's comprehension of spoken

TABLE 6.13 Causes of dysarthria and dysphonia

Mechanism	Example
Weakness of facial and tongue muscles	Myasthenia gravis
Lesions of lower brain stem (bulbar palsy)	Motor neurone disease
Bilateral corticospinal tract lesions above the pons	Multiple lacunar infarcts
Impaired control of phonation and articulation	Parkinsonism
Imprecise motor control systems	Cerebellar lesions
Impaired larynx function	Recurrent laryngeal nerve palsy

and written language is retained. With cerebellar deficits the dysarthria has a slurred quality with imprecise control of word length and tonal inflection, giving it a drawling, 'sing-song' quality. Dysarthria is often evident during conversation with the patient while the history is being taken.

Elevation of the soft palate is used to close off the nasopharynx for the production of explosive consonants ('b' and 'g'). Palatal weakness or anatomical defects in the palate cause 'nasal' speech with failure to produce these sounds correctly. For example, when such a patient tries to say the word 'egg' it is pronounced as 'eng'.

Dysphonia. The production of tones in speech is achieved by movement of expired air through the larynx. Vibration of the vocal cords produces the frequency changes used in speech and singing. Poor respiratory function may cause dysphonia, but more typically it is the result of laryngeal problems, causing hoarseness of the voice, often with reduced speech volume.

Dysphasia. Difficulty with language function is called dysphasia. Damage to *Broca's area* causes:

- reduced number of words used
- poorly articulated and non-fluent speech
- errors of grammar and syntax.

Such speech has a clipped, telegrammatic quality, but if the lesion is relatively localised, comprehension of spoken and written language is usually preserved.

With dysfunction in *Wernicke's area*, the output of spontaneous speech may be normal or increased, the speech fluent and the articulation of phonemes is usually intact. However, the speech may contain:

- incorrect words (verbal paraphasias)
- incorrect letters (literal paraphasias)
- nonsense words (neologisms).

Conduction dysphasia. In this disorder the patient is unable to repeat phrases or words spoken by the examiner. The causative lesion lies in the perisylvian area with damage to the arcuate fasciculus of fibres.

Global dysphasia. In this condition there are elements of both anterior (Broca) and posterior (Wernicke) dysphasias. This results from large lesions in the middle cerebral artery territory. It may be so marked as to abolish speech completely (aphasia).

The neck and cervical spine

Various aspects of the examination of the neck are described in Chapter 2 (cervical lymph glands, p. 58; thyroid gland, p. 62), Chapter 3 (carotid pulse, p. 83 and jugular venous pulse, p. 88) and Chapter 8 (neck movements p. 268). In particular, a neurological assessment may be incomplete without testing active and passive movements of the cervical spine, especially side rotation and flexion for obvious reasons.

Degenerative arthrosis of the cervical spine is common, especially in the middle-aged and elderly. Such patients may develop neck pain, long tract features or radicular symptoms.

- Flexion of the neck sometimes evokes electric shock-like sensations which shoot into the limbs, when the cervical spinal cord sensory tracts are diseased (*Lhermitte's sign*). This phenomenon is particularly common in multiple sclerosis but is also seen in syringomyelia, cervical cord tumours and spondylotic myelopathy.
- Neck movements are restricted by meningeal irritation.

Meningeal irritation. Inflammation of the meninges due to infection or blood evokes reflex spasm in the paravertebral muscles. This results in neck stiffness in the cervical area. In the lumbar area muscle spasm may produce a positive Kernig's sign.

Evidence of meningeal irritation should be looked for in any patient in whom meningitis or subarachnoid haemorrhage is a possibility. The signs, however, may be absent in the early evolution of a subarachnoid haemorrhage or in the deeply comatose patient.

Examination sequence

Neck stiffness

- ☐ Ask the patient to lie supine and to relax the head onto a single pillow.
- ☐ Support the occiput with both hands and gently flex the neck until the chin touches the chest – *Kernig's sign.*
- ☐ Ask the patient to lie supine with both legs exposed and fully extended.
- ☐ Passively flex one leg at the hip and the knee.
- ☐ Then extend the knee while maintaining the hip in flexion and observe the other limb for reflex flexion at the hip – *Kernig's test.*

If neck stiffness is present it is not possible to passively flex the neck sufficiently for the chin to reach the chest. Indeed, attempted neck flexion may cause the trunk to rise from the bed (Fig. 6.8A). When Kernig's test is positive, attempts to extend the knee joint when the hip joint is flexed are resisted by hamstring muscle spasm and the other limb may flex at the hip (Fig. 6.8B).

EXAMINATION OF THE CRANIAL NERVES

An understanding of the applied anatomy is essential for correct interpretation of clinical findings. This involves being familiar with the functions, locations and major connections of the cranial nerve nuclei.

The olfactory (I) nerve

Anatomy

The olfactory nerve subserves the sense of smell. Smell

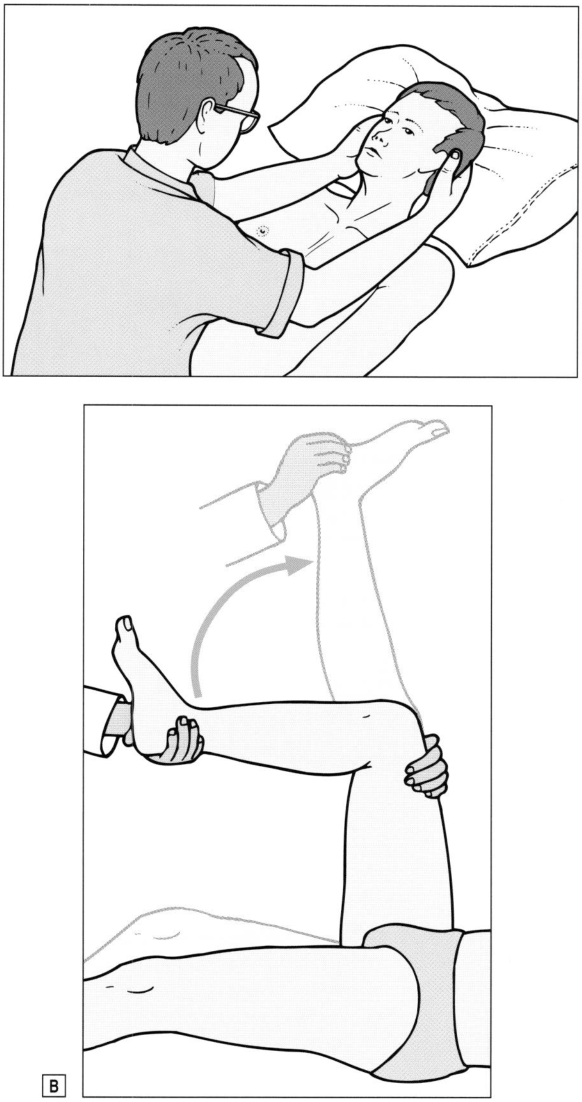

Fig. 6.8 **Testing for meningeal irritation.** A Neck rigidity B Kernig's test.

receptors are situated high in the nasal cavity, and these bipolar olfactory cells project axons through the cribriform plate of the ethmoid bone to the olfactory bulb. Second-order neurones (mitral cells) then project centrally together with the pyramidal cells of the olfactory nucleus down the olfactory tracts and stria to the primary olfactory cortex (medial temporal lobe) and the ipsilateral amygdaloid body, the anterior perforated substance and the septal area. The primary olfactory cortex has numerous connections with the hypothalamus, reticular system and the limbic lobe.

Testing the sense of smell

Commonly used test substances include vials of peppermint, vanilla, coffee, almond oil or even stronger odours such as whisky or isopropyl alcohol used for skin cleaning.

Examination sequence

☐ Check that the nasal passages are clear.
☐ Test the sense of smell for each nostril separately.
☐ Occlude one nostril by digital pressure.
☐ Ask the patient, with eyes closed, to sniff and identify in turn the test substances.

Common abnormalities

The commonest cause of anosmia is obstruction of the nasal passages. The commonest neurological cause of anosmia is a previous head injury causing shearing damage to the olfactory filaments as they pass through the cribriform plate to the olfactory bulbs. Nasofrontal tumours such as olfactory groove meningiomas and carcinomas arising from the paranasal air sinus are less common causes.

Perversion of smell (parosmia) is sometimes of psychological origin but may occur following partial recovery of the olfactory nerves after trauma. Certain drugs and sinus infection also cause this phenomenon. Olfactory hallucinations, usually of an unpleasant nature, are a characteristic of seizures arising from the temporal lobe. These olfactory hallucinations are often associated with smacking movements of the lips and unusual feelings in the epigastrium.

The optic (II) nerve

Examination of the optic nerve involves testing:

- visual acuity (see p. 244)
- pupillary reflexes
- visual fields
- colour vision (see p. 245)
- fundoscopy (see p. 251).

Much of the examination of the optic nerve is described in Chapter 7. This section deals with the pupillary reflexes and with the visual fields.

Anatomy

The optic nerve transmits the axons of the retinal ganglion cells. It begins at the back of the globe and passes through the optic canal of the sphenoid bone into the cranium, where it joins with the contralateral nerve to form the optic chiasma. The optic tract then passes posteriorly to the lateral geniculate bodies of the thalamus and then to the primary visual cortex (area 17) in the occipital lobe. This tract is termed the geniculocalcarine tract or the optic radiation. The visual association cortex and areas 18 and 19 are in close proximity in the occipital lobe.

The afferent limb of the pupillary reflex involves the retina, optic nerve, chiasma and tract. These fibres terminate in both sides of the midbrain pretectum. The axons then pass to the accessory oculomotor nuclei of Edinger–Westphal. The efferent limbs of the reflex arc are preganglionic parasympathetic fibres in the III nerve, the ciliary ganglion and post-ganglionic fibres that innervate the constrictor muscle of the iris.

The normal visual field extends 160° horizontally and 130° vertically, with the physiological blind spot 15° from fixation in the temporal field. The field for red colour vision is much smaller than that for monochrome.

Pupillary reflexes

If a light is directed at one eye, both pupils will normally constrict. The reaction of the pupil on the side stimulated is called the *direct light reflex*, and the constriction of the other pupil the *consensual light reflex*.

When a near object (e.g. at 10 cm) is viewed, convergence of the eyes is accompanied by bilateral pupillary constriction referred to as the *accommodation reflex*.

Examination sequence

- ☐ Examine the pupils in a dimly lit room for size and symmetry.
- ☐ Check the direct and consensual reflex in each eye in turn by shining a bright pen torch from the side and from below with the patient looking into the distance in order to avoid an accommodation response.
- ☐ To test the reaction to accommodation ask the patient first to look into the distance and then at an object held close to the face; observe any change in the pupil size.

Common abnormalities

Abnormal pupillary reflexes. Impairment or absence of the pupillary reaction to light may be due to damage to either the afferent or efferent sides of the reflex arc. Since both pupils constrict in response to light directed into one eye, afferent lesions can easily be distinguished from damage to the efferent pathway.

With afferent pupillary defect, the dysfunction is on the afferent limb of the reflex arc (retina or optic nerve). The pupil does not have a direct light reflex but constricts when light is shone into the opposite eye (i.e. the consensual reflex is preserved).

With efferent pupillary defect, the lesion is on the efferent limb of the unreactive eye (oculomotor nerve, ciliary ganglion). One pupil is fixed and dilated and does not respond to light directly, but the contralateral pupil responds consensually.

TABLE 6.14 Drugs affecting the pupil

Dilated (mydriasis)	*Mode of action*
Atropine/homatropine	Anticholinergic
Amphetamine and derivatives	Sympathomimetic
Constricted (miosis)	
Neostigmine, morphine and derivatives	Parasympathomimetic

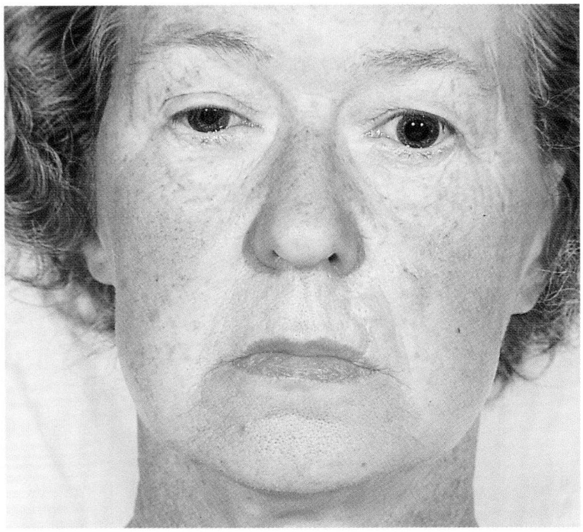

Fig. 6.9 Right Horner's syndrome in a patient with bronchogenic carcinoma. Note the ptosis and enophthalmos. (Courtesy of Dr D.H.A. Boyd).

Other abnormalities of pupillary reflexes include the Parinaud syndrome (p. 202), oculomotor paresis (see p. 202) and following structural damage to the iris. In the Holmes–Adie syndrome absence of ankle jerks and other deep tendon reflexes is seen in association with myotonic pupils. (See Table 7.2, p. 249.)

Abnormalities of pupillary size Some abnormalities in pupil size are shown in Table 7.2. Symmetrically small or dilated pupils are commonly drug induced (see Table 6.14).

Pontine haemorrhage causes bilateral pupil constriction, and in anxiety the pupils are symmetrically dilated.

In Horner's syndrome (Fig. 6.9) unilateral miosis is associated with ptosis, impaired sweating and enophthalmos (recession of the globe in the orbital fossa). Paresis of the light reflex and accommodation as a result of a lesion in the ciliary ganglion is termed an internal ophthalmoplegia.

Visual fields

Testing fields assesses the function of the peripheral and central retina, the optic pathways and the cortex. Since colour vision tends to fail early in many disorders of the retina and optic nerve, a red hat-pin is a particularly useful test object for detecting scotomas. Visual fields can be estimated quickly by the method of confrontation or measured accurately using perimeters. Both methods require a cooperative patient.

If a patient is unable to cooperate (because of an impaired conscious state or dysphasia) a crude test of visual field integrity can be made by moving the hand quickly towards the patient's face. This menacing stimulus will usually evoke reflex blinking if the incoming stimulus is detected.

Examination sequence

- ☐ Sit directly opposite and facing the patient.
- ☐ Examine each eye separately first.
- ☐ Ask the patient to cover one eye and look at the examiner's opposing eye (Fig. 6.10).
- ☐ Examine the outer aspects of the visual fields with a waggling finger or preferably a fine probe with a large red or white head (e.g. a hat-pin).
- ☐ Bring the test object into the field of vision in a curve, not a straight line. Approach from the periphery at several points on the circumference of the upper and lower, nasal and temporal quadrants of the visual fields.
- ☐ Ask the patient to respond as soon as the movement of the test object is observed.
- ☐ Map out central field defects by moving the test object across the visual field (Fig. 6.11).
- ☐ When using a red test object instruct the patient to report as soon as the colour is perceived.

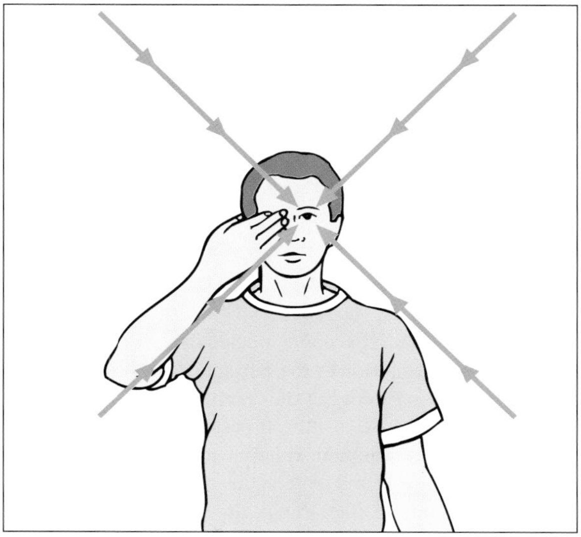

Fig. 6.10 Testing the visual fields.

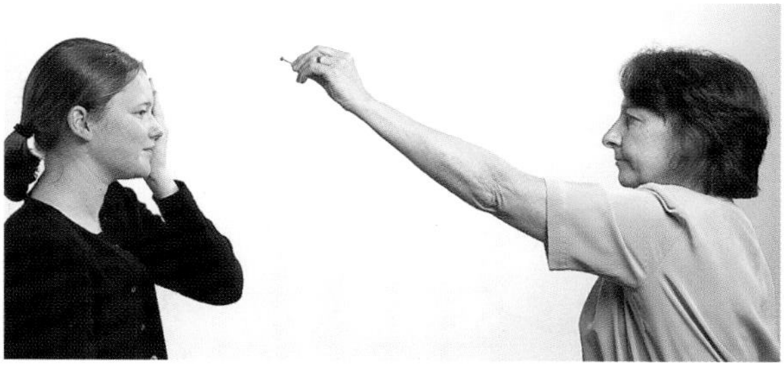

Fig. 6.11 Testing for a central field defect using a red hat-pin.

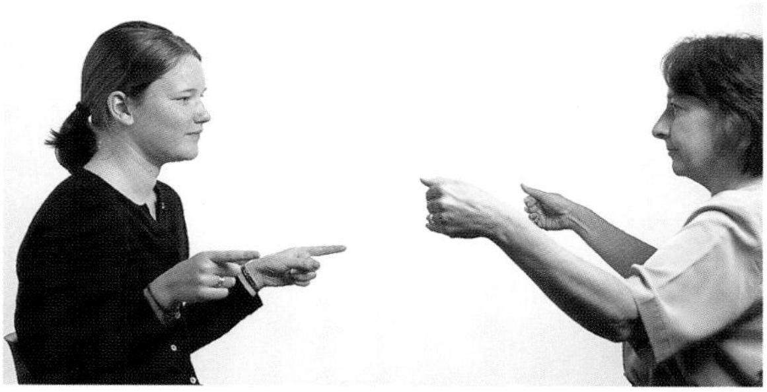

Fig. 6.12 Testing for visual inattention.

- ☐ Test for visual inattention by asking the patient to report when the fingertip is moved on one or both sides simultaneously (Fig. 6.12).

Common abnormalities

Impaired visual acuity can be due to lesions of the cornea, lens, vitreous, retina or optic nerve and the more distal visual pathway. Characteristics of optic nerve lesions are shown in Table 6.15.

The common patterns of visual defect are illustrated in Figure 6.13. Lesions proximal to the optic chiasma cause monocular dysfunction. Lesions of the optic chiasma and distal visual pathways will produce binocular visual field defects. Lesions of the optic tract and lateral geniculate body (LGB) region are frequently vascular in origin.

TABLE 6.15 Common features in optic nerve lesions

Abnormalities	*Common causes to consider*
Abnormal pupillary response	Multiple sclerosis, optic neuritis
Enlargement of blind spot	Vascular disease
Scotomas	Retrobulbar and parasellar neoplasms (e.g. pituitary adenomas, craniopharyngioma and meningioma)
Impaired visual acuity	
Impaired colour vision	
Abnormal fundoscopy	

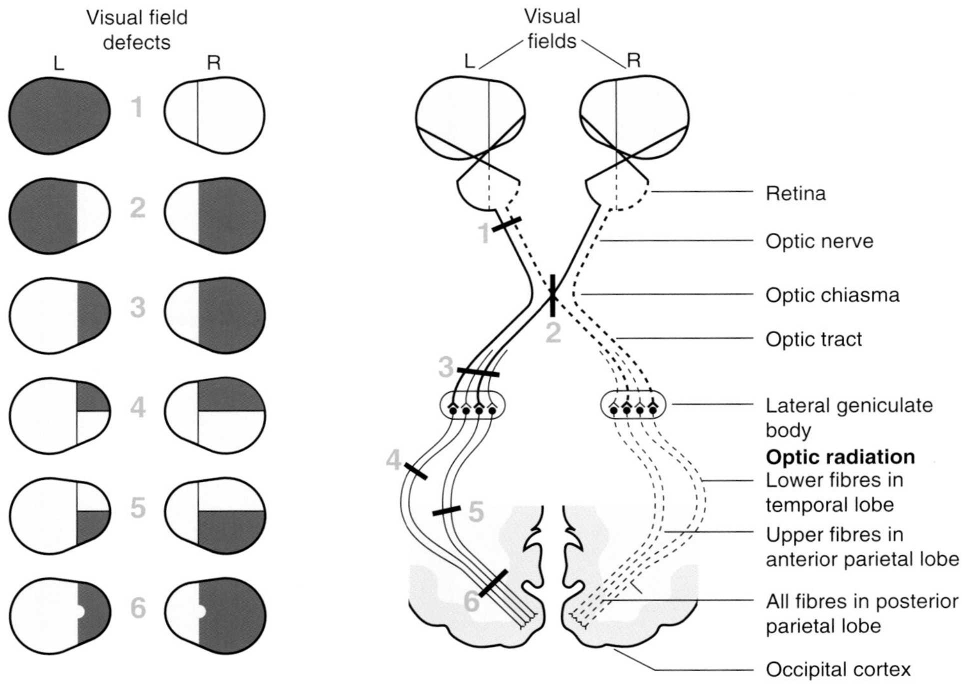

Fig. 6.13 Visual field defects. 1. Total loss of vision in one eye because of a lesion of the optic nerve. **2.** Bitemporal hemianopia due to compression of the optic nerve. **3.** Right homonymous hemianopia from a lesion of the optic tract. **4.** Upper right quadrant hemianopia from a lesion of the lower fibres of the optic radiation in the temporal lobe. **5.** Less commonly a lower quadrantic hemianopia occurs from a lesion of the upper fibres of the optic radiation in the anterior part of the parietal lobe. **6.** Right homonymous hemianopia with sparing of the macula due to lesion of the optic radiation in the posterior part of the parietal lobe.

Common lesions in the optic radiation and occipital cortex are vascular (e.g. posterior cerebral artery infarction), inflammatory (e.g. multiple sclerosis) or neoplastic (e.g. glioma, metastatic neoplasia).

Visual field defects are termed homonymous if the same part of the visual field is affected in each eye. Homonymous defects are due to lesions distal to the optic chiasma (see Fig. 6.13). The field defect may be hemianopic (i.e. half of the visual field is lost) or quadrantinopic (i.e. one-quarter of the visual field is lost). Such a defect will be either upper or lower depending upon which part of the visual field is affected. If the visual field loss is not identical in both eyes it is termed incongruous; this type of defect is seen in lesions of the optic tract. Homonymous hemianopia due to occipital cortical lesions tends not to involve the central part of vision (macular sparing). When inattention is present the patient will be able to detect single targets on both sides, but will ignore objects on one side when two fields are stimulated simultaneously.

The oculomotor, trochlear and abducent (III, IV and VI) nerves

These three cranial nerves innervate the muscles controlling eye movement and pupillary size. Although the nerves subserve discrete actions they are examined together because of their close functional interrelationships.

Anatomy

- The oculomotor (III) nerve nucleus lies in the ventral midbrain just anterior to the periaqueductal grey matter. The nerve passes between the cerebral peduncles into the interpeduncular CSF cistern. It passes just below the free edge of the tentorium in relation to the posterior communicating artery and enters the dura surrounding the cavernous sinus. It then enters the orbital fossa through the superior oblique fissure, where it subdivides into its terminal branches. The nerve innervates the superior (SR), medial (MR) and inferior (IR) recti, the inferior oblique (IO) and levator palpebrae superioris (LPS) muscles. These muscles open the upper lid (LPS) and move the globe upwards (SR, IO), downwards (IR) and medially (MR). Through the parasympathetic fibres arising from the Edinger–Westphal nerves, the nerve also indirectly supplies the sphincter muscles of the iris, which cause constriction of the pupil, and the ciliary muscle, which is responsible for focusing the lens for near vision.

- The trochlear (IV) nerve arises from a nucleus in the caudal midbrain. The fibres decussate before leaving the midbrain just below the inferior colliculus. The nerve then passes forward and laterally in relation to the rostral pons and the free edge of the tentorium. It pierces the dura of the tentorial edge and passes through the cavernous sinus and superior orbital fissure. In the orbit it innervates the superior oblique (SO) muscle, contraction of which causes downward movement of the globe when the eye is adducted.
- The abducent (VI) nerve originates from a nucleus located near the midline of the caudal pons, where it forms part of the facial colliculus. The nerve emerges from the ventral pontomedullary junction just lateral to the pyramid, passes through the prepontine CSF cistern and pierces the basal dura to enter Dorello's canal and then traverse the cavernous sinus. Here the nerve is in direct relation to the internal carotid artery before it passes through the superior orbital fissure to the lateral rectus (LR) muscle. Contraction of the LR causes abduction of the eye.

Ocular motility is dependent not only on the integrity of the III, IV and VI nerves but also on a central brain stem tract, the medial longitudinal fasciculus (MLF), which interconnects the nuclei. The MLF also receives direct and indirect input from the vestibular nuclei, cerebellar flocculus and the para-abducens nucleus, also called the nucleus of the paramedian pontine reticular formation (PPRF). This is important for lateral gaze. The MLF provides a mechanism by which the optical axes remain parallel or conjugate when the eyes are turned to one side or when there is movement of the head. There are also supranuclear connections. There is also a centre for vertical gaze at the mesodiencephalic junction with medial and lateral neuronal pools subserving downgaze and upgaze respectively. Sympathetic fibres dilate the pupil and also innervate part of the LPS. The preganglionic sympathetic fibres arise in the posterior hypothalamus to emerge through the ventral roots of the first two or three segments of the thoracic spinal cord and ascend through the sympathetic chain to the superior cervical ganglion. Postganglionic fibres ascend in the carotid neural plexus and into the orbit with the ophthalmic artery to terminate in the radial muscle of the iris (dilator of the pupil). In area 8 of the frontal lobe there is the frontal eye field (FEF). When this area is stimulated the eyes turn conjugately away from the side of stimulation.

Eye movements

The six external ocular muscles move the eyeball in the directions shown in Figure 6.14.

While the MR and LR subserve horizontal eye movements, vertical eye movement is more complex and mediated both by the IO and SR (upgaze) and the SO and IR (downgaze). Because of the different long axes of the various ocular muscles, the superior oblique is mainly responsible for downgaze and the inferior oblique mainly responsible for upgaze in the adducted eye. The appropriate recti are responsible for vertical gaze in the abducted eye (see Fig. 6.14 and Fig. 7.9, p. 250).

The assessment of eye movements is conveniently combined with looking for nystagmus. Minor degrees of nystagmus occur in normal subjects at extremes of lateral gaze, particularly if maintained for more than 10 seconds.

Examination sequence

- ☐ Inspect the eyes for any abnormality.
- ☐ With both eyes open, test for ocular movements with the patient's head in the neutral position and, if necessary, held there by one of the examiner's hands on the crown of the head.
- ☐ Examine carefully for any squint (strabismus) or other abnormality, including nystagmus.
- ☐ First ask the patient to look up and down, and to the right and the left.
- ☐ Then ask the patient to fix the gaze on the examiner's finger and to report if double vision occurs while following the movement of the finger held about 60 cm away.

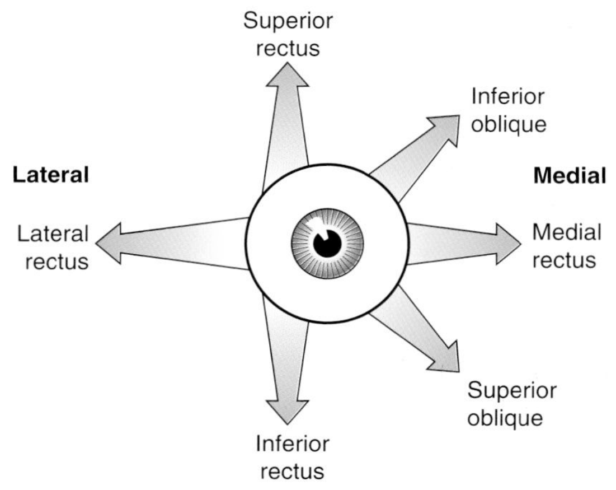

Fig. 6.14 External ocular muscle function.

- ☐ Move the finger up and down, then to the right and up and down, and then to the left and up and down. If necessary, repeat the examination, one eye at a time, to distinguish muscle and gaze palsies.
- ☐ Record the direction in which double vision is present and where maximal separation of the images occurs.
- ☐ If diplopia is reported ask the patient to close one eye at a time to identify which eye is producing the false image.
- ☐ To test convergence, ask the patient to focus on the finger as it is brought from a distance towards the tip of the nose.
- ☐ Look for nystagmus while examining eye movements.
- ☐ Record the presence of vertical, horizontal or rotatory nystagmus and the direction of gaze in which it is most marked.
- ☐ Note the direction of the fast component of nystagmus, whether it changes direction with the direction of gaze and whether the degree of nystagmus is different in each eye.

Common abnormalities

The palpebral fissures are normally symmetrical. Abnormalities that may be present on inspection include ptosis (drooping of an eyelid), widening of the palpebral fissures, inequality in pupillary size (anisocoria), abnormal eye movements at rest (nystagmus, opsoclonus and square wave jerks), asymmetrical blinking, conjunctival injection and orbital pulsation. A lesion of the sympathetic pathway gives rise to Horner's syndrome (Fig. 6.9).

Disorders of ocular movements

There are many non-neurological causes of disordered eye movements. These include disorders of the ocular muscles (myopathies) and the neuromuscular junction (e.g. myasthenia gravis) and metabolic encephalopathy (e.g. toxic levels of phenytoin, carbamazepine).

Cranial neuropathies that involve III, IV and VI cause characteristic patterns of eye movement disorders with diplopia (double vision).

Oculomotor nerve (III). A complete unilateral lesion of III causes ptosis, weakness of superior, medial and inferior eye movements, pupillary dilatation and an absent direct reflex. Common causes of an isolated III palsy are diabetic mononeuropathy, carotid-posterior communicating artery aneurysms, pituitary or other tumours, trauma and vascular disease. The III palsy associated with a contralateral hemiplegia (Weber syndrome) is due to a midbrain stroke. III nerve lesions may be incomplete depending on the location and type of lesion. Lesions due to diabetes or vascular disease tend not to involve the pupil, in contrast with compressive lesions (e.g. aneurysm).

Trochlear nerve (IV). Isolated lesions are not common. The patient usually complains of diplopia, particularly bad when looking down and reading. The patient will often adopt a compensatory head tilt. Causes of an isolated IV lesion are ischaemic mononeuropathy (diabetes, hypertension) and head trauma, in which the associated intracranial damage to the IV nerve is sometimes bilateral. Damage to the trochlear itself, through which the superior-oblique tendon passes, may be responsible for the IV palsy after head injury, ENT surgery and in patients with rheumatoid arthritis.

Abducent nerve (VI). Isolated lesions are common. In many cases, particularly following head injury and in patients with raised intracranial pressure, it is a 'false localising' sign (i.e. the VI nerve is affected by intracranial pathology elsewhere). The patient experiences diplopia worse looking towards the side of the paretic LR. The paralysis may be complete or partial. Abducent paresis may be associated with diabetes and with suppurative otitis media (Gradenigo's syndrome). Lesions of the cavernous sinus (aneurysms, pituitary adenoma, meningioma) quite commonly cause VI nerve paresis. However, cavernous sinus lesions usually produce a constellation of cranial neuropathies. Lesions of the VI nerve are occasionally found in conjunction with ipsilateral V and VII paresis and contralateral hemiplegia in unilateral pontine stroke.

Other lesions affecting eye movement

Paresis of conjugate upgaze and downgaze may be seen in space-occupying lesions around the pineal gland and tectal region and in patients with aqueductal stenosis and hydrocephalus. Failure of upgaze, together with loss of the pupillary light response but preservation of miosis on accommodation, is termed Parinaud's syndrome or the pretectal syndrome. This is usually due to a lesion of the pineal gland and ventral midbrain.

Lateral gaze paresis may be due to a lesion in the frontal eye field (FEF). If the lesion is destructive (e.g. intracerebral haemorrhage), the eyes are deviated towards the side of the damaged frontal lobe. In most cases the paresis lasts only a few days and eye movements return to normal. If the FEF lesion is irritative (e.g. epileptic) the eyes and head may be deviated to the side opposite the lesion. If there is a lesion in the paramedian pontine reticular formation (PPRF) the eyes are deviated away from the side of the lesion. This is most commonly caused by a pontine stroke and therefore associated with a plethora of other brain stem signs. Resolution of the paresis in such cases is much slower than that following damage to the FEF.

Internuclear ophthalmoplegia (INO) occurs when there is a lesion of the MLF. The ipsilateral eye is unable to adduct and there is nystagmus in the contralateral abducting eye.

INO is most commonly seen in multiple sclerosis but can also occur with vascular disorders and neoplasms of the brain stem. Supranuclear ophthalmoplegia occurs when the corticonuclear fibres are damaged. Spontaneous eye movements and doll's eye elicitation of ocular movements are preserved, but there is paresis of voluntary eye movements (usually downgaze and sometimes upgaze). They may be associated with parkinsonian and dystonic clinical signs in the Steele–Richardson–Olzewski syndrome.

Nystagmus. *Pendular nystagmus* occurs when the amplitude of the two phases of movement are equal and is often due to poor vision. It is thought to be an exaggeration of the normal tiny movements made by the eye to prevent fatigue of the retinal photoreceptors. Congenital blindness and ocular albinism are often associated with coarse pendular nystagmus.

Horizontal phasic (jerk) nystagmus is usually due to labyrinthine, cerebellar or brain stem dysfunction. The direction of horizontal nystagmus is determined by the direction of the fast phase. The amplitude is usually increased by gaze to that side. It is termed first degree if present only on looking in that direction, second degree if present when looking straight ahead, and third degree if still present on gaze in the opposite direction.

- Nystagmus due to lesions of the brain stem is usually multidirectional. Common causes are Wernicke's encephalopathy, multiple sclerosis, anticonvulsant toxicity and brain stem ischaemia.
- Labyrinthine nystagmus is horizontal or rotary.
- Lesions of the cerebellar hemisphere cause horizontal nystagmus to the side of the diseased hemisphere. *Downbeat nystagmus* (usually due to a lesion of the cervicomedullary junction), *see-saw nystagmus* (due to parasellar lesions) and *convergence-retraction* nystagmus (due to lesions of the tectal and pineal region) are rare forms of disturbance.

Other jerky abnormalities of eye movement which mimic nystagmus are *ocular bobbing* (usually due to a pontine haemorrhage), which is characterised by spontaneous downward jerks of both eyes followed by a slow return to rest position, and *opsoclonus*. The latter is characterised by chaotic rapid eye movements and is seen in children with metastatic neuroblastoma or adults with bronchogenic carcinoma.

The trigeminal (V) nerve

The trigeminal nerve has both sensory and motor functions. It transmits sensation from the face, mouth, lips, eyes, forehead and anterior part of the scalp as well as the dura of the anterior cranial and middle fossae. The motor function involves supplying the muscles responsible for various movements of the jaw, initiation and coordination of swallowing and dampening the amplitude of vibration of the tympanic membrane.

Anatomy

Sensory function. Sensation is provided through three major branches which join together to form the Gasserian ganglion which sits in Meckel's cave in the petrous temporal dura.

- *The ophthalmic branch (V_1).* This supplies sensation to the skin of the upper nose and eyelid, forehead and scalp (see Fig. 6.15) as well as the cornea, conjunctiva, intraocular structures, parts of the mucosa of the frontal, sphenoidal and ethmoidal sinuses and the upper part of the nasal cavity. The ophthalmic branch passes through the superior orbital fissure and then reaches the Gasserian ganglion via the wall of the cavernous sinus.
- *The maxillary nerve (V_2).* It innervates the lower eyelids, skin of the temple, upper check and adjacent areas of nose and upper lip, the mucous membranes of the upper mouth, nose, roof of the pharynx and parts of the maxillary, ethmoid and sphenoidal sinuses as well as the gums, teeth and palate of the upper jaw (see Fig. 6.16). The maxillary nerve enters the base of the skull through the foramen rotundum to reach the Gasserian ganglion.
- *The mandibular division (V_3)* supplies the teeth and gums of the lower jaw, mucosa of the cheek and floor of the mouth, the epithelium of the anterior two-thirds of the tongue, the temporomandibular joint, external and internal

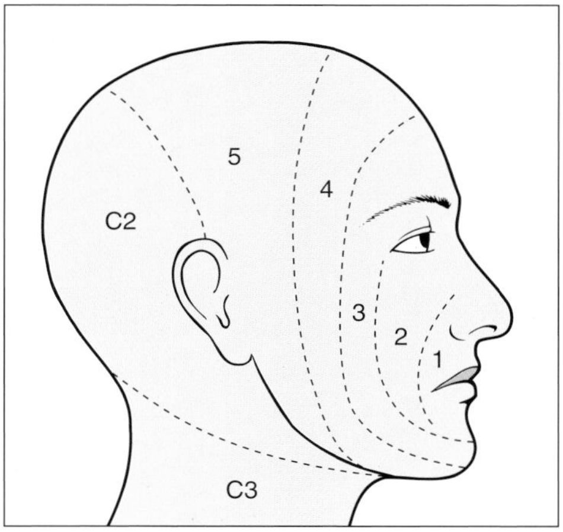

Fig. 6.15 Pain fibres to the head. Areas marked 1 to 5 indicate the central distribution within the spinal tract of the V cranial nerve. 1 is represented in the pons, 2 the pontomedullary region, 3 the lower medulla, 4 and 5 the upper cervical cord. The areas labelled C2 and C3 derive from the spinal segments directly.

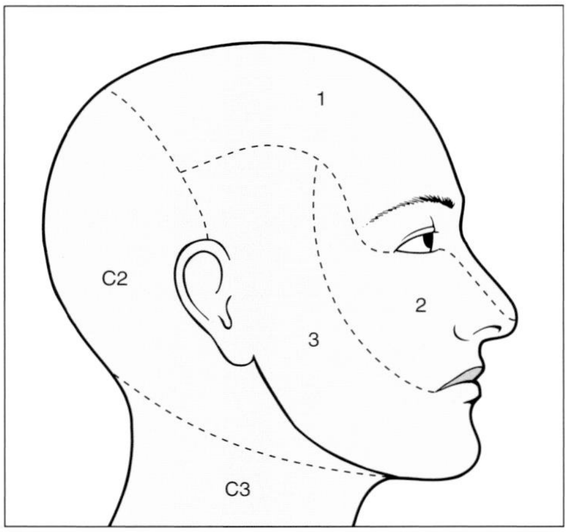

Fig. 6.16 Cutaneous distribution of the trigeminal nerve. 1. Ophthalmic division. **2.** Maxillary division. **3.** Mandibular division. **C2.** Second cervical root. **C3.** Third cervical root.

ear and the skin of the lower lip and jaw region. The nerve passes through the infratemporal fossa, entering the skull through the foramen ovale to reach the Gasserian ganglion. It is joined by its lingular branch which receives parasympathetic ganglion fibres from the chorda tympani of the VII nerve which control saliva excretion.

The trigeminal nerve also innervates the dura mater of the anterior and middle cranial fossae.

From the Gasserian ganglion, nerve rootlets traverse the prepontine CSF system to pass into the pons at the anterolateral surface to enter three sensory nuclei. These are:

- the principal nucleus of the trigeminal nerve (touch, joint position sense and two-point discrimination)
- the mesencephalic nucleus (unconscious proprioceptive information from periodontal membrane, palate, masticatory muscles and the temporomandibular joint)
- the spinal trigeminal nucleus (pain and temperature). This nucleus extends from the pons to the C2 segment of the spinal cord. Owing to inversion of the fibres going into this nucleus, the upper part of the face is represented in the caudal part of the spinal trigeminal nucleus (see Fig. 6.15).

The sensory nuclei have multiple connections to the thalamus, particularly the activating system and limbic nuclei.

Motor functions. The motor branch of V is conveyed in V_3 and innervates muscle of mastication (the masseters, temporalis, medial and lateral pterygoids, the anterior belly of the digastric). It also supplies the mylohyoid, tensor veli palatini and tensor tympani muscles.

Examination

In addition to testing the sensory and motor function, examination of the V nerve includes testing two reflexes.

The corneal reflex. Touching the cornea, which is very sensitive, evokes a brisk contraction of the orbicularis oculi (i.e. blinking). Because of the presence of interneurones, a unilateral corneal stimulus produces a bilateral reflex blink, i.e. the reflex has direct and consensual responses. The afferent part of the corneal reflex is the nasociliary branch of V_1 and the efferent limb is the facial nerve.

The jaw jerk. This is analogous to the tendon reflexes in the limbs. The afferent and efferent pathways are subserved by the V cranial nerve. The reflex response is a brisk contraction of the jaw muscles, producing closure of the jaw. This is often not visible in young people but is commonly present above the age of 50.

Examination sequence

Sensory

- ☐ Test light touch and pain sensation in the territory of the three sensory regions using cotton wool and pin prick respectively. (Temperature sensation may also be tested.)
- ☐ Test two-point discrimination (pp. 229) on the upper and lower lips using calipers. Normally a separation of 3–4 mm can be detected.
- ☐ Check sensation in each division of the trigeminal nerve independently, comparing the right with the left.

Motor

- ☐ Inspect the muscles of mastication for wasting, most easily seen in the temporalis muscle above the zygomatic arch.
- ☐ Ask the patient to open the jaw against resistance (pterygoids, mylohyoid, anterior belly of the digastric).
- ☐ Palpate the masseters and estimate their bulk and symmetry as the patient clenches the teeth.

Corneal reflex

- ☐ Approach from the side as the patient looks in the opposite direction, very lightly touch the cornea, not the conjunctiva, with a wisp of damp cotton wool (Fig. 6.17).
- ☐ Observe the presence of both direct and consensual corneal reflexes.

Jaw jerk

- ☐ Place the thumb or forefinger in the midline over the tip of the patient's mandible, with the mouth slightly open.
- ☐ Tap the examiner's finger downwards with a tendon hammer (see Fig. 6.18).

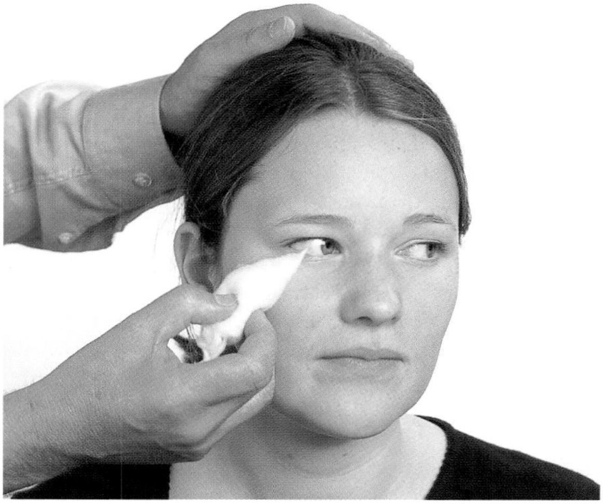

Fig. 6.17 Testing the corneal reflex.

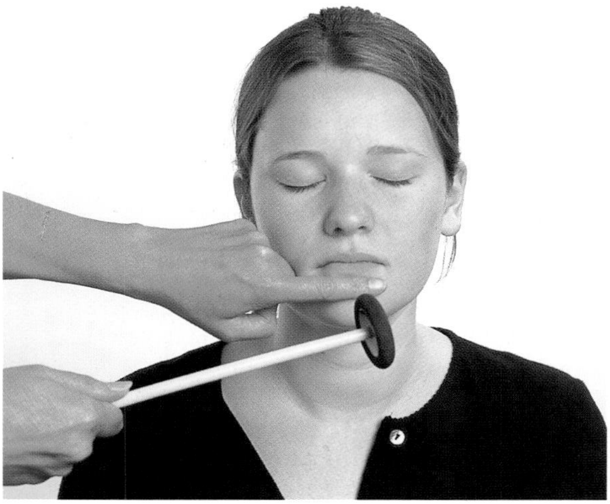

Fig. 6.18 Eliciting the jaw jerk.

Common abnormalities

Unilateral loss of sensory modalities from the distribution of one or more of the branches of the trigeminal nerve is an important finding.

- Lesions within the cavernous sinus commonly cause loss or reduction in corneal reflex as well as diminished forehead sensation (V_1 lesion). This is frequently associated with dysfunction in III, IV or VI.
- Neoplasms of the base of middle cranial fossa (e.g. meningioma, squamous carcinoma from the air sinuses, nasopharyngeal carcinoma, trigeminal neuroma) will lead to sensory impairment in one or more branches of the V nerve.
- Patchy sensory loss such as on the cheek, certain teeth or forehead may result from direct injury or laceration to peripheral branches of the V (e.g. infraorbital nerve damage with fractures of the zygoma, alveolar nerve damage with fractures of the mandible or maxilla and supraorbital or supratrochlear nerve damage with eyebrow lacerations).
- Large tumours in the cerebellopontine angle region (e.g. acoustic neuroma, petrous meningioma, epidermoid) also may impair V function, as well as VII and VIII.
- Unilateral pterygoid weakness causes the jaw to deviate to the weak side when the mouth is opened. When the patient tries to move the jaw from side to side there is difficulty in moving it to the contralateral side. Facial asymmetry resulting from a VII nerve lesion may give rise to an apparent deviation of the jaw.

Detection of bilateral paresis or atrophy in the muscles of mastication is very difficult, even when there are obvious signs of sensory V nerve dysfunction. The muscles may be involved in various myopathies, myasthenia gravis or progressive bulbar palsy.

A brisk jaw jerk occurs in bilateral diseases of the upper motor neurone above the level of the pons (e.g. multiple sclerosis or motor neurone disease). Determination of whether a jaw jerk is pathologically brisk can be difficult because hyperreflexia is common in the anxious.

The facial (VII) nerve

This nerve has various functions:

- It innervates the muscles of facial expression.
- It is the efferent limb of the corneal reflex (see p. 204) and also the palmomental reflex (a contraction of the ipsilateral mentalis muscle in response to scratching the thenar eminence), the pout or snout reflex (a bilateral pursing of the lips following a brisk tap on the lips), the nasopalpebral reflex (glabellar tap) and the efferent limb of the stapedius reflex.
- Through the nervus intermedius (sensory and parasympathetic fibres) it supplies parasympathetic secretomotor fibres to the lacrimal gland (producing tears) and submandibular gland (producing saliva).
- It supplies taste sensation to the anterior two-thirds of the tongue through the chorda tympani branch.

Anatomy

The motor nucleus of VII lies in the lower pons and its fibres initially pass posteriorly and medially to loop around the VI nucleus before turning forwards and emerging from the lateral pontomedullary junction (see Fig. 6.19).

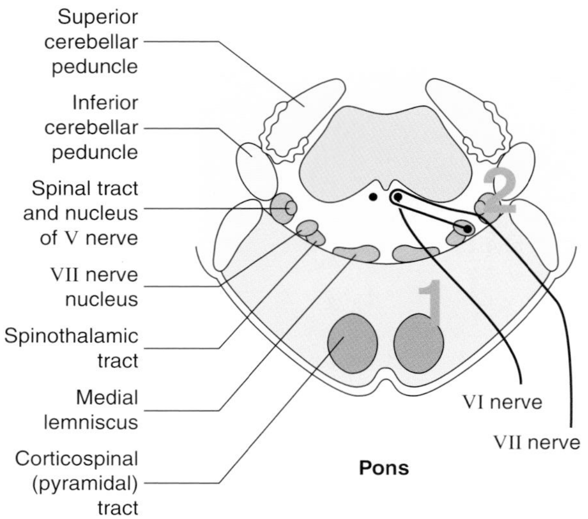

Fig. 6.19 Lesions of the pons. Lesions at **1.** (e.g. haemorrhage) cause ipsilateral VI and/or VII nerve palsies and contralateral pyramidal signs. Lesions at **2.** (e.g. basilar thrombosis) cause ataxia on the side of the lesion (damage to the cerebellar peduncles). There may also be impaired sensation on the ipsilateral side of the face (spinal tract and nucleus of V nerve) and on the contralateral side of the body (spinothalamic tract) and occasionally a VII nerve lesion. Lesions in the pons often cause internuclear ophthalmoplegia (p. 202) and ataxic nystagmus.

The nervus intermedius contains parasympathetic fibres from the superior salivatory nucleus and taste fibres, which have their cell bodies in the geniculate ganglion and synapse centrally in the gustatory nucleus or nucleus solitarius. It emerges from the pons in close proximity to VII, and the two nerves pass through the pontomedullary CSF cistern in close relationship to the vestibular and cochlear (VIII) nerves. All these nerves enter the internal acoustic meatus. The facial nerve and the nervus intermedius then pass through the facial canal of the temporal bone. The facial nerve emerges from the stylomastoid foramen, passes through the parotid gland and subdivides into several branches which innervate the muscles of the face, the corneal reflex and the other reflexes. Within the temporal bone and distal to the geniculate ganglion the facial nerve has branches to the stapedius muscle (which dampens down tympanic vibrations), to the pterygopalatine ganglion (from which arises the greater petrosal nerve, which is secretomotor to the lacrimal gland) and to the tongue (chorda tympani which conveys taste).

Examination

Examination of the VII nerve depends largely on inspection to assess facial asymmetry.

Taste sensation is rarely tested in clinical practice; electrical stimulation of the tongue with a small current is more reliable and practical (electrogustometry). Secretomotor function of the lacrimal gland is usually only tested by ophthalmologists doing a Schirmer test.

Testing for decreased saliva production owing to denervation of the submandibular gland is not performed in clinical practice.

Examination sequence

Inspection

- ☐ Observe the face for any asymmetry which may be related to paresis of the facial muscles.
- ☐ Observe the symmetry of blinking and eye closure and the presence of any tics or spasms of the facial musculature.
- ☐ Observe spontaneous movement of the face, particularly the upper and lower facial musculature during such actions as smiling.

Motor function

- ☐ Test the facial muscles by asking the patient to raise the eyebrows, wrinkle the forehead (this can be achieved by asking the patient to look upwards at the examiner's hand), close the eyes as strongly as possible, to show the teeth (even if these are false), to blow out the cheeks against the closed mouth, to purse the mouth and to whistle (Fig. 6.20A–D).
- ☐ Check the strength of eye closure for paresis or asymmetry.

Taste sensation

- ☐ Instruct the patient not to speak during the test because this will cause the tongue to retract and dissipate the substance into the contralateral side of the tongue as well as its posterior one-third.
- ☐ Gently hold the protruded tongue with a swab.
- ☐ Place a test substance (e.g. sweet, salt, bitter or sour substances) on the anterior two-thirds of each side of the tongue in turn.
- ☐ Ask the patient to identify the substance by pointing to the appropriate word written on a card.

Schirmer's test

- ☐ Put a piece of special blotting paper under the lower eyelid and remove it after 5 minutes. Normally at least 10 mm of the blotting paper will be dampened by evoked tear secretion.

Common abnormalities

Upper motor neurone lesions affecting the corticonuclear fibres will cause facial paresis that is worse in the lower facial muscles with relative sparing of the upper face (because of bilateral cortical innervation of the upper facial

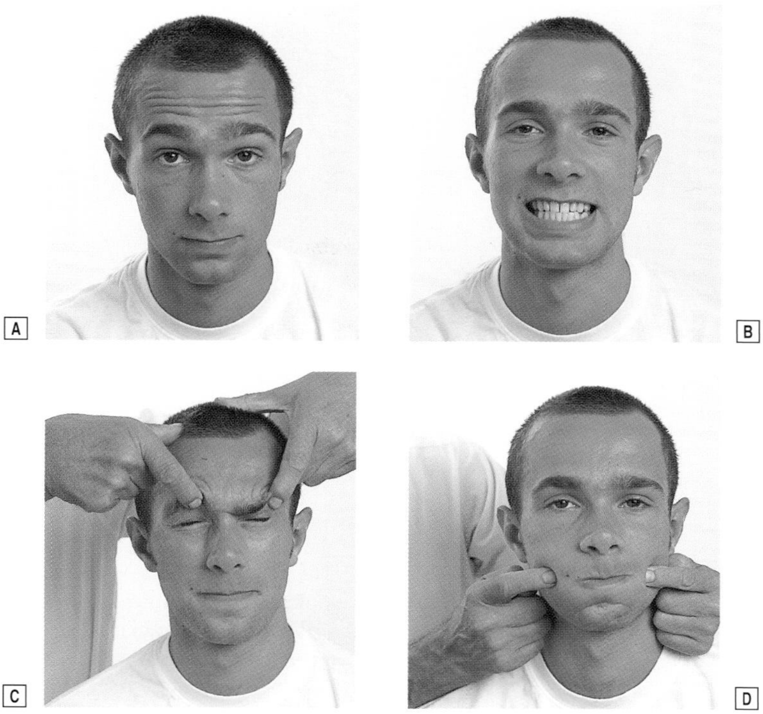

Fig. 6.20 Testing the motor function of the facial nerve. Ask the patient to [A] raise the eyebrows, [B] show the teeth, [C] close the eyes against resistance and [D] blow out the cheeks.

muscles). The corner of the mouth will droop and saliva may dribble, the nasolabial fold will be flattened, but eye closure, although paretic, is usually well preserved. Smiling may also be preserved because emotional facial movements employ additional neural pathways. Taste is normal. The commonest cause of this type of unilateral facial dysfunction is a vascular lesion involving the contralateral rolandic cortex or its subcortical pathways. Usually there will also be weakness of the ipsilateral upper limb (faciobrachial paresis).

With lower motor neurone lesions affecting the facial nucleus or its nerve, there is unilateral paresis of both upper and lower facial muscles with inability to close the eye and impaired blinking, loss of the nasolabial fold and forehead wrinkles (Fig. 6.21). Taste to the anterior two-thirds of the tongue is impaired if the chorda tympani is also damaged. The commonest cause is idiopathic Bell's palsy (see Table 6.16). A frequent feature in such patients is Bell's phenomenon. This is an upward rotation of the eye on trying to contract the paretic orbicularis oculi.

The location of the VII lesion can be deduced from the clinical findings. Taste and lacrimation will be preserved in those lesions distal to the stylomastoid foramen. A lesion involving the nerve to the stapedius will cause hyperacusis (e.g. sounds appearing louder than normal). A lesion involving the greater petrosal nerve will cause a dry eye.

Bilateral facial weakness can be due to the upper or lower motor neurone lesions as well as disorders of the muscles and neuromuscular junctions. Progressive supranuclear paresis will cause a bilateral facial paresis associated with a lability of emotional expression and a disassociation between emotional (well preserved) and voluntary (poorly preserved) movement. Such patients may exhibit an obvious snout reflex. Causes of bilateral lower motor neurone facial type paresis (Table 6.16) are relatively uncommon and may be difficult to detect.

The vestibulocochlear (VIII) nerve

The VIII cranial nerve has two functional parts, the vestibular and the cochlear components.

Anatomy

The cochlear branch subserves hearing. The fibres arise from the end organs in the inner ear. They pass centrally along the internal acoustic meatus and cross the cerebellopontine CSF cistern to enter the lateral brain stem at the

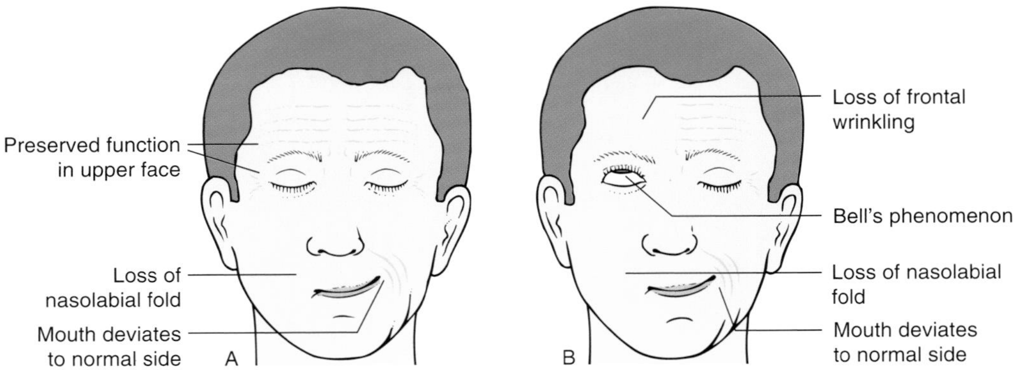

Fig. 6.21 Types of facial weakness. Caused in A by lesion of precentral area or pyramidal tract (upper motor neurone); B by lesion of facial nerve or nucleus (lower motor neurone), also showing Bell's phenomenon.

TABLE 6.16 Common causes of VII nerve palsies

Unilateral	Bilateral
Upper motor neurone type weakness	
Usually vascular	Often vascular
Cerebral tumour	Consider motor neurone disease
Multiple sclerosis	
Lower motor neurone type weakness	
Usually Bell's palsy	Neurosarcoidosis
Consider parotid tumour, head injuries, skull base tumours	Myasthenia gravis
	Generalised polyneuropathies (Guillain–Barré syndrome)
	Some myopathies (e.g. myotonic dystrophy)

pontomedullary junction. The fibres then synapse in the cochlear (dorsal, ventral) and vestibular (inferior, superior, lateral and medial) nuclear complexes. From the cochlear nucleus second-order fibres ascend to the superior olivary and trapezoid nuclei. Central fibres then ascend up the lateral lemniscus, and synapse in the inferior colliculus and medial geniculate body (MGB) before entering the primary auditory cortex in the superior temporal gyrus (areas 41 and 42). The ascending auditory pathways decussate at several levels so that each cortical region receives impulses from both ears.

The inferior and superior vestibular branches and the associated vestibular pathways are very important in the maintenance of correct posture, eye coordination and movement.

The vestibular part of the VIII is also the afferent limb of both the oculocephalic (doll's eye reflex) and oculovestibular (caloric) reflexes. The oculocephalic reflex involves conjugate movements of the eyes in response to changes in head position. The oculovestibular reflex involves elicitation of eye movements following irrigation of the external ear canal by either cold or warm water.

The central connections of the four vestibular nuclei are complex. Through fibres in the MLF they interconnect with the III, IV and VI cranial nuclei. Other fibres project to the cerebellar vermis and flocculus, while others descend in the vestibulospinal tracts. Ascending fibres relay through the medial geniculate body (MGB) to the posterior temporal lobe.

Examination

In clinical practice deafness or impaired hearing is best studied using audiometry and brain-stem evoked potentials to determine their precise aetiology. 'Bed-side' tests are relatively crude but should give some indication as to whether hearing is normal, abnormal or asymmetrical.

Whispering numbers or words tests hearing for higher frequencies in particular. Rinne's test determines whether air conduction is better than bone conduction. Normally the air-conducted sound is perceived as louder. Weber's lateralising test provides supplementary information about the nature of any hearing impairment. Normally, the sound appears to arise in the midline (Fig. 6.22).

Vestibular function can be assessed clinically by testing the oculocephalic reflex, or doll's eye manoeuvre, and by induction of positional nystagmus. In the former, the normal response is for the patient's eyes to deviate to the left as the patient's head is turned to the right and vice versa on contralateral head turning. If the patient's head is briskly extended the patient's eyes should move downwards. In the doll's eye manoeuvre, the normal response to unilateral irrigation with cool water is for the patient to develop nystagmus towards the contralateral side. If the ear is irrigated with warm water the patient will have nystagmus towards the side of the irrigated ear.

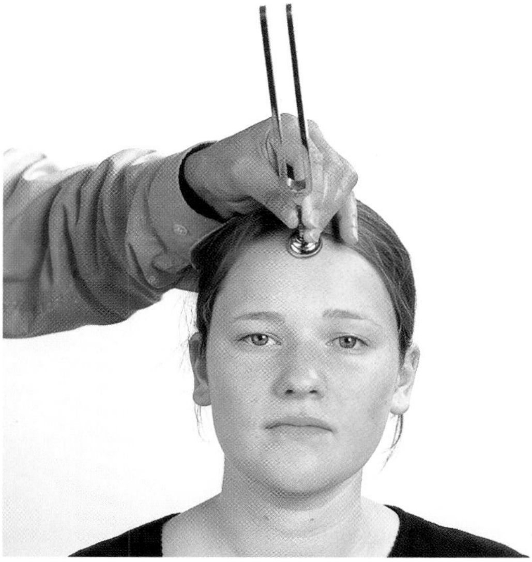

Fig. 6.22 Weber's test.

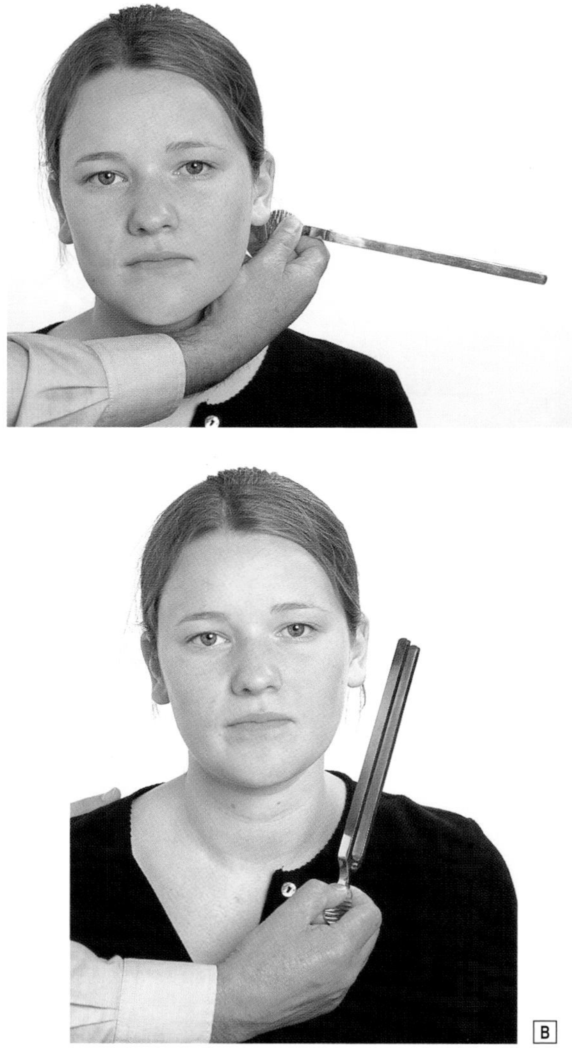

A

B

Fig. 6.23 Rinne's test. A Testing bone conduction. B Testing air conduction.

Usually caloric vestibular tests are carried out in a special laboratory set up to record eye movement electronically.

Examination sequence

Hearing

- ☐ Mask hearing in the non-tested ear by either rubbing the forefinger and thumb together over the external acoustic meatus or gently massaging the patient's external acoustic meatus with the examiner's forefinger.
- ☐ Test hearing in each ear by asking the patient to repeat whispered numbers or words.
- ☐ Perform Rinne's test by placing a vibrating tuning fork (256 or 512 Hz) on the mastoid process (to assess bone conduction of sound) then just lateral to the external ear (Fig. 6.23).
- ☐ Ask the patient which of the two sounds appears louder.
- ☐ Perform Weber's test by placing the strongly vibrating tuning fork to the middle of the forehead. Ask the patient where the sound is heard loudest (in the midline or preferentially to one side).
- ☐ Examine the external acoustic canal using an auroscope. Visualise the tympanic membranes and note any abnormal vascularity of the membrane or retrotympanic fluid level (p. 50).

Induction of positional nystagmus (Hallpike's test)

- ☐ Support the patient's head, with eyes open, and lower it briskly below the horizontal plane of the couch, turning the head to one side (Fig. 6.24).
- ☐ Sit the patient up again, and repeat the test, turning the head to the other side.
- ☐ Note the response of the eyes to head movement.

Oculovestibular reflex

- ☐ Inspect the canal to ensure that the tympanic membranes are visualised.
- ☐ If necessary, remove any impacted wax.
- ☐ Gently irrigate the canal with patient's eyes open using water at either 30°C or 44°C and observe the response.

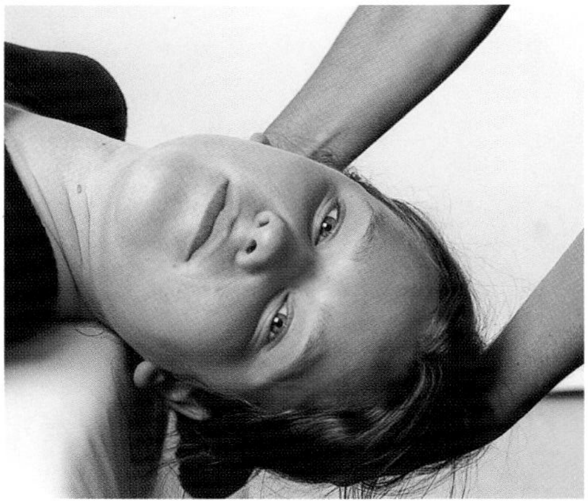

Fig. 6.24 Testing for positional nystagmus.

Oculocephalic reflex

- ☐ Perform the test with the patient lying down.
- ☐ Stand above and behind the patient at the head of the bed.
- ☐ Slightly flex and support the patient's head.
- ☐ Briskly rotate the head from one side to the other and note lateral movements of the eyes.

Common abnormalities

If impaired hearing is unilateral it should be determined whether it is either conductive (i.e. due to disease of the tympanic membrane or ossicular chain) or sensorineural (e.g. involving the organ of Corti or the cochlear nerve) in origin. If bone conduction is better than air conduction in Rinne's test this indicates a conductive defect. In Weber's test, a patient with sensorineural deafness will perceive the sound as arising from the better ear. In conduction deafness, however, the sound appears to arise from the deaf side; this is because of the improved efficiency of bone conduction in the presence of middle ear damage.

Common causes of deafness are shown in Table 6.17.

Acute abnormalities of the vestibular nerves and labyrinth will usually evoke phasic nystagmus (p. 203), positional nystagmus or impairment of the caloric response.

There are two main types of positional nystagmus and vertigo:

1. Peripheral lesions (usually calcific deposits in the otolith organ) cause vertigo and nystagmus after a latent period of a few seconds; the nystagmus declines if the position is maintained.
2. Nystagmus due to rare 'central'-type lesions has no latency, does not show fatigue and is less likely to cause vertigo.

TABLE 6.17 Common causes of deafness

Conduction deafness	*Effect*
Wax in the external canal Damage to tympanic membranes Fluid in inner ear Ossicular chain disruption (head injury) Otosclerosis (degenerative)	Diminished hearing on affected side Rinne's test: bone conduction louder Weber's test: to affected side
Sensorineural deafness	*Effect*
Damage to cochlear nerve and organ of Corti Acoustic neuroma Transverse fracture of petrous temporal bone Bilaterally in the elderly (degenerative)	Diminished hearing on affected side Rinne's test: air conduction louder Weber's test: to unaffected side

- Following acute labyrinthine damage or vestibular nerve lesions (fractured petrous temporal bone after head injury, acute vestibular neuronitis, etc.) the patient will complain of severe nausea, vertigo or dizziness and disturbance of balance. These symptoms are all aggravated by head movements. In such cases there is frequently phasic nystagmus with the fast phase towards the side of the lesion.
- Positional nystagmus will not be elicited in normal subjects. However, where there is a disorder of the labyrinth or its vestibular connection, the patient may complain of vertigo and develop nystagmus within 10 seconds of head movement.
- The oculocephalic reflex is primarily of value in testing for brain stem death (p. 234). If the patient is unconscious there will be no nystagmus but on irrigation of one ear with cool water the eyes deviate to the irrigated side. Conversely, if the ear of the unconscious patient is irrigated with warm water, the eyes will deviate to the contralateral side. Bilateral irrigation with either cool or warm water induces vertical eye movements. The reflex is absent in brain stem death.
- Chronic lesions of the vestibular nerve (e.g. acoustic neuroma) are not normally accompanied by vertigo or nystagmus.

Many patients who complain of vertigo and *tinnitus* (a subjective awareness of noise such as hissing in the ear) may have entirely normal clinical examinations, and require detailed audiometry and vestibular tests for diagnosis.

The glossopharyngeal (IX) and vagus (X) nerves

These nerves are considered together, being related anatomically, functionally and in terms of clinical examination.

Anatomy

Both nerves arise as a series of rootlets from the post-olivary sulcus of the lateral medulla. They pass antero-laterally across the cerebellomedullary CSF cistern and exit the skull through the jugular foramen. They traverse the CSF cistern in close relationship to the vertebral artery and posterior inferior cerebellar artery. The motor component of both of these nerves arises from the nucleus ambiguus in the medulla.

Glossopharyngeal nerve:

- The motor component is small and innervates the stylopharyngeus muscles. It sometimes contributes to the innervation of the palatal and upper pharyngeal muscles.
- The large sensory component innervates the mucosa of the pharynx and tonsillar region, conveys taste for the posterior third of the tongue and sensation for part of the lining of the tympanic cavity and Eustachian tube.
- Secretomotor parasympathetic fibres supply the parotid gland.

Vagus nerve:

- It innervates the muscles of the upper pharynx and soft palate, as well as the intrinsic muscles of the larynx and the cricothyroid.
- It conveys sensory sensation from the dura mater of the posterior cranial fossa and from part of the skin of the external auditory meatus.
- It has extensive afferent and efferent connections with the heart, lungs and intestines.

The IX and X are also involved in several reflexes:

- The gag reflex involves constriction and elevation of the pharynx and palate (X efferent limb) in response to tactile stimulation of the upper pharynx and tonsils (IX afferent limb).
- The oculocardiac reflex (slowing of the heart rate after orbital compression).
- The carotid sinus reflex.

Examination sequence

- ☐ Observe movements of the palate and uvula by asking the patient to say 'aah'.
- ☐ Assess tonsillar, palatal and upper pharyngeal tactile sensation using a dampened swab stick and tongue depressor.
- ☐ The gag reflex may be elicited by touching either the tonsil or pharynx. Test each side separately. Testing for the gag reflex is unpleasant. It should be performed only if there is other evidence of nerve paresis.
- ☐ Assess the volume and quality of the patient's speech, noting if the voice is hoarse or has a nasal quality.
- ☐ Ask the patient to cough to determine whether this is more nasal or bovine than normal.
- ☐ Ask the patient to puff out the cheeks, to test palatal closure of the nasopharynx.

Common abnormalities

- Lesions of IX and X cause *dysphagia* (difficulty in swallowing due to palatal and pharyngeal paresis), loss of the gag reflex and *dysphonia* (altered voice quality, usually hoarseness, resulting from weakness of the muscles moving the vocal cords and palate).
- IX nerve dysfunction is usually seen with other signs of cranial nerve or brain stem dysfunction. An isolated IX nerve lesion is very unusual. It is suggested by unilateral loss of palatal, tonsillar or pharyngeal sensation, together with an absent or depressed gag reflex.
- Disorders of the X nerve will cause asymmetrical elevation of the soft palate with deviation of the uvula away from the side of the lesion (Fig. 6.25). The voice may have a nasal quality.
- With lesions to the recurrent laryngeal branch of the vagus nerve, the voice will sound hoarse and the cough 'bovine'.

Some clinical conditions causing IX and X nerve lesions are shown in Table 6.18.

Normally both sides of the palate elevate in a symmetrical fashion and the uvula remains in the midline. In order to puff out the cheeks the palate must elevate and occlude the nasopharynx. If palatal movement is weak, air will escape audibly through the nose. The gag reflex produces elevation of the palate and the pharynx, very similar to the motions seen at the beginning of vomiting.

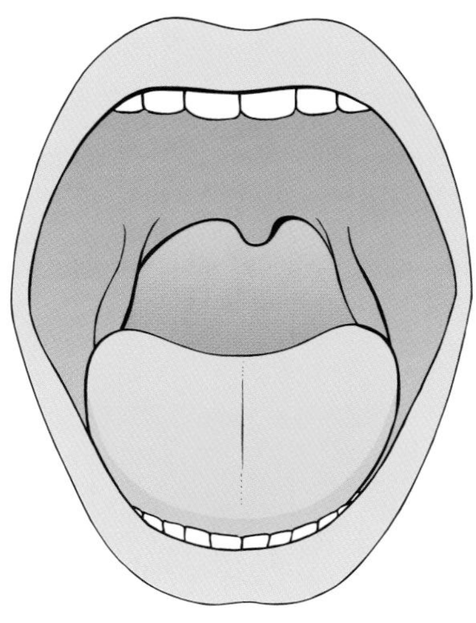

Fig. 6.25 Right X nerve palsy; note the uvula is pulled over to the left side.

TABLE 6.18 Common causes of IX and X nerve lesions

Unilateral of IX and X
Skull base neoplasms (including meningioma)
Skull base fracture
Recurrent laryngeal
Bronchial carcinoma
Mediastinal lymphoma
Aortic arch aneurysms
Bilateral X
Progressive bulbar palsy (motor neurone disease)
Bilateral supranuclear lesions (pseudobulbar palsy)
Cerebrovascular disease
Multiple sclerosis

Neither the oculocardiac or carotid reflexes nor taste in the posterior one-third of the tongue are routinely tested in clinical practice.

The accessory (XI) nerve

Anatomy

This motor cranial nerve has two nuclei, one of which is intimately related to that of X in the caudal part of the nucleus ambiguus (innervates the intrinsic muscles of the larynx). The much larger spinal element is derived from segments C1–C5. This arises as an extensive series of rootlets from the lateral medulla and spinal cord. Its fibres ascend through the foramen magnum then merge to exit the skull base through the jugular foramen, where the bulbar component rejoins the vagus nerve (see X). The spinal component descends to supply the sternomastoid and the upper half of the trapezius muscle.

Examination sequence

- ☐ Inspect the trapezius muscle from behind.
- ☐ Ask the patient to shrug the shoulders and maintain them in elevation, then apply downward pressure to the shoulders to check for paresis of the trapezius muscle (Fig. 6.26A).
- ☐ Inspect the sternomastoids for hypertrophy or atrophy and palpate to assess tone and bulk.
- ☐ Test the left sternomastoid by asking the patient to rotate the head to the right side with a hand placed against the right side of the chin in an effort to stop this rotatory movement (Fig. 6.26B).
- ☐ Examine the right sternomastoid during rotation to the left.

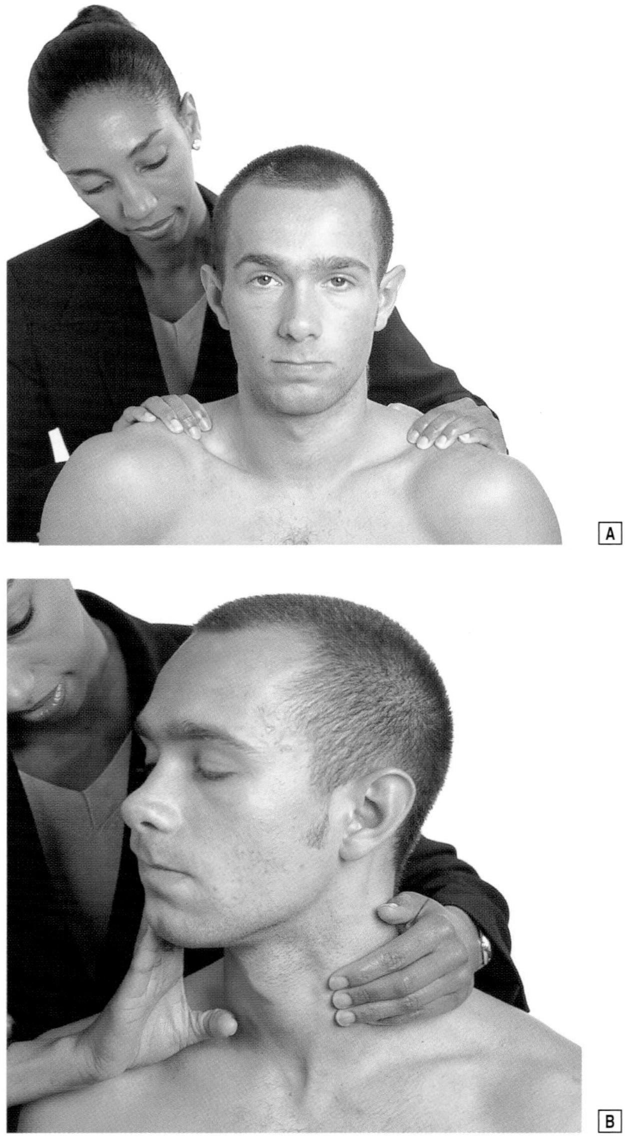

Fig. 6.26 Testing A the trapezius muscle and B the left sternomastoid.

Common abnormalities

- Wasting or weakness of the trapezius muscle will produce a flaring of the vertebral border of the scapula, which will be displaced away from the spine in its upper part and rotated towards the spine at its lower end. The point of the shoulder will appear dropped and the arm will appear lower.
- Isolated XI lesions are unusual.
- Isolated paresis of the trapezius can occur if branches of the spinal accessory nerve are cut during surgery in the posterior triangle of the neck.

- The nerve may be involved with other lower cranial nerves in basal skull tumours or following penetrating injury.
- Upper motor neurone lesions involving the spinal accessory nerve or damage to corticobulbar fibres may produce little in the way of clinical signs.
- Lower motor neurone lesions may occur as part of a progressive bulbar palsy.
- Paresis of the sternomastoid muscle occurs in a range of myopathic disorders, especially dystrophia myotonica.

Involuntary turning movements of the head that involve the sternomastoid and other neck muscles are a feature of spasmodic torticollis and other dystonic conditions. If dystonia is long-standing the sternomastoid may be hypertrophic and the mobility of the neck very restricted.

The hypoglossal (XII) nerve

Anatomy

The XII nerve arises from a motor nucleus located beneath the floor of the fourth ventricle. Its rootlets arise from the pre-olivary sulcus and pass anterolaterally in front of the vertebral and posterior inferior cerebellar arteries. It exits the skull base through the hypoglossal canal in the occipital bone. It then passes to the root of the tongue, where it divides into branches that innervate the tongue muscles. Normal tongue movement is essential for articulation, adequate chewing and the onset of swallowing.

Examination sequence

- ☐ Ask the patient to protrude the tongue; observe the symmetry of movement, bulk and look for wasting and fasciculation.
- ☐ Assess movements of the tongue from side to side.
- ☐ Ask the patient to press the tongue against the cheek and feel the strength of contraction and assess muscle bulk.
- ☐ Assess hypokinesis of tongue movements by asking the patient to say ‘lah lah lah’ as quickly as possible, and to make rapid in-and-out and side-to-side movements of the tongue.

Common abnormalities

- With unilateral atrophy the tongue becomes wrinkled and thinner on the affected side and deviates towards that side on protrusion.
- Spontaneous contraction (fasciculation) of small parts of the muscles may be apparent and more easily seen when the tongue is protruded.
- Unilateral XII nerve lesions are usually seen with other cranial neuropathies, and the causes may be neoplastic (skull base tumour), vascular (medullary infarct, vertebral artery aneurysm) or traumatic.
- Bilateral lower motor neurone lesions may be seen as part of a wider clinical syndrome (e.g. motor neurone disease or syringobulbia) and are often components of bulbar palsy.
- Myopathic disorders involving the tongue will generally be part of a more widespread syndrome (e.g. myasthenia gravis). Such lesions cause dysarthria, dysphagia and dysphonia.
- Unilateral upper motor neurone lesions may produce deviation of the protruded tongue which is not associated with fasciculation or wasting. This is most typically seen immediately after an acute cerebrovascular event; the asymmetry of tongue protrusion tends to resolve after several days.
- With bilateral upper motor neurone lesions, voluntary movements of the tongue are hypokinetic (slow) and the tongue appears small and tends to assume a more conical form. There tends to be dysarthria and dysphagia. Such dysfunction (pseudobulbar palsy) may occur in

KEY POINTS

- The commonest cause of anosmia is obstruction of the nasal passages.
- The field for red colour vision is much smaller than that for monochrome.
- If a lesion occurs distal to the optic chiasma, the same side of each visual field will be affected in each eye and the defect is termed homonymous.
- The superior oblique muscle is supplied by the IV cranial nerve and is responsible for downward movement of the adducted eye.
- Conjugate ocular motility is dependent not only on the integrity of the cranial nerves but also on a central brain stem tract, the medial longitudinal fasciculation (MLF).
- Parasympathetic fibres constrict and sympathetic fibres dilate the pupil.
- In many cases a VI cranial nerve palsy is a ‘false localising’ sign caused by raised intracranial pressure.
- Minor degrees of nystagmus are seen in normal patients at extremes of lateral gaze, particularly if maintained for more than 10 seconds.
- Pendular nystagmus is often due to long-standing poor vision.
- Unilateral loss of sensation in one or more branches of the trigeminal nerve is an important finding.
- A pathologically brisk jaw jerk occurs in patients with bilateral upper motor neurone lesions above the level of the pons.
- An upper motor neurone lesion affecting one corticobulbar (facial) tract results in relative sparing of the upper face because of bilateral innervation of those muscles.
- In clinical practice deafness is often best studied using audiometry.
- Many patients with vertigo and tinnitus have no detectable abnormality on clinical examination.
- IX cranial nerve dysfunction is usually seen with other signs of cranial nerve or brain stem dysfunction.
- With lesions of the recurrent laryngeal branch of the vagus nerve, the voice will sound hoarse and the cough bovine.
- Inspect the trapezius muscle from behind.
- Orofacial dyskinesias are usually drug induced.

supranuclear or suprabulbar disorders, which may be vascular (e.g. bilateral insular infarction) or inflammatory (e.g. multiple sclerosis) in origin.

- Orofacial dyspraxias involve inability to move the tongue and parts of the face on command and are usually seen after parietal lobe lesions.
- Involuntary movements of the tongue (and usually parts of the facial musculature as well) may occur in a group of disorders called orofacial dyskinesias. These are most often drug induced (e.g. major tranquillisers, anti-parkinsonian drugs) and may persist, or even worsen, after drug withdrawal. They may be choreiform in type or tremulous in some patients.
- Lesions of the cranial nerves IX, X, XI and XII may be simultaneously affected, usually by diffuse disorders – typically motor neurone disease. The condition is known as *bulbar palsy* with clinical features of dysphonia, dysarthria and dysphagia.

Where there are bilateral supranuclear lesions of IX–XII due to vascular disease, motor neurone disease or demyelination, there is loss of voluntary palatal and pharyngeal movements, but with an intact gag reflex (*pseudobulbar palsy*).

THE MOTOR SYSTEM

It is convenient to consider motor and sensory function separately, although precise movements require sensory and cerebellar input. In the dyspraxias the organised sequence of complex motor activation is impaired although there is no deficit of spontaneous movement or pathways to individual muscles.

The examination of the motor system normally incorporates:

- inspection and palpation of muscle groups (wasting, hypertrophy, and fasciculation)
- assessment of tone
- testing of power
- elicitation of deep tendon reflexes and plantar responses
- testing of coordination.

Anatomy

The corticospinal motor pathways are outlined in Figure 6.27. This primary motor pathway is modulated by sub-cortical (basal ganglia), cerebellar and vestibular input. Patterns of motor dysfunction, therefore, may be determined by both focal and systematic neuropathology (Table 6.19).

TABLE 6.19 Patterns of motor dysfunction
Paralysis or weakness
Impairment of coordination
Changes in tone and posture (dystonia)
Involuntary movements (dyskinesia)
Changes in the rate at which movements are performed (hypokinesis and bradykinesis)
Loss of learned movement patterns (dyspraxia)

Inspection and palpation

The patient should be examined in underwear in order to observe the limbs and muscles clearly. There is considerable variety between normal subjects in muscle bulk and power. It is important to take this into consideration along with factors such as age and occupation when assessing 'normality'. In health, lower limb musculature is usually symmetrical. In the upper limbs, the musculature in the dominant side is often more developed; as in the racquet arm of a professional tennis player.

Common abnormalities

Muscle wasting can have a multiplicity of different causes (see Table 6.20). In order to determine the anatomical cause of atrophy, it is necessary to assess its distribution; whether it is focal or diffuse, primarily proximal or distal or whether or not the atrophy involves a peripheral nerve or a spinal segment. Conversely, muscle hypertrophy may be occupational or a manifestation of certain rare forms of muscular dystrophy (e.g. Duchenne).

Fasciculations appear as subcutaneous twitches overlying muscle bellies when the muscles are at rest. They result from disease of lower motor neurones that innervate that particular muscle and are caused by brief contraction of single motor units. They may be coarse or fine in amplitude and are most commonly found in wasted muscles. They can occur in normal people after vigorous exercise. A similar usually benign phenomenon, myokymia, involves fasciculations of the orbicularis oculi. This condition is commonly caused by anxiety and tiredness.

Myoclonus is a sudden shock-like muscle contraction which involves one or more muscles of a whole limb. Myoclonic jerks may be focal or diffuse and may occur singly or repetitively. They may occur in normal people, particularly when falling asleep. Some patients with primary generalised epilepsy experience myoclonic jerks, especially after waking. Less common causes of myoclonic jerks are rare diseases such as Creutzfeld–Jakob disease, subacute sclerosing panencephalitis, familial myoclonic epilepsies, and anoxic cerebral damage.

Choreiform movements are irregular, jerky, semipurposeful and ill sustained. They tend to be multifocal and are classically seen in Huntington's chorea.

Tics or habit spasms are much more stereotyped and localised than choreiform movements, and sometimes can be temporarily resisted at will by the patient.

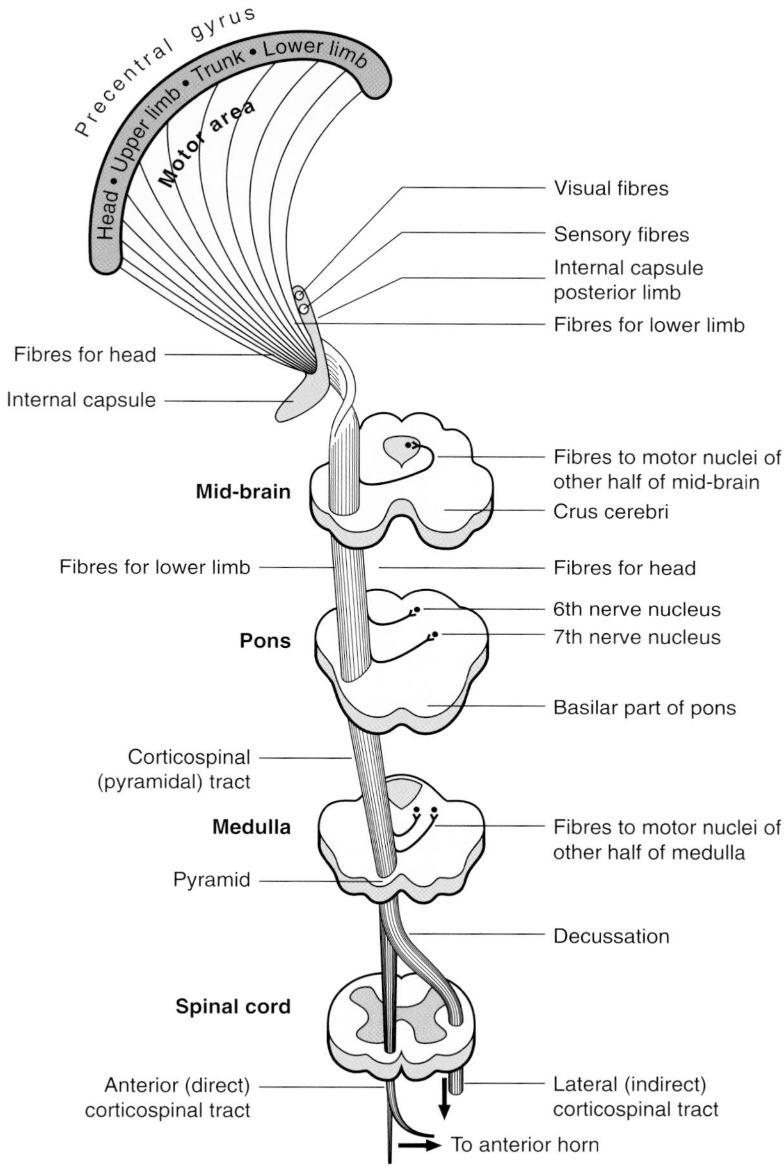

Fig. 6.27 The motor pathways.

Tremor is defined as rhythmic movement resulting from alternating contraction and relaxation of groups of muscles (see Table 6.21). Tremors produce oscillations about a joint or group of joints. The pattern of tremor most frequently seen is rapid and fine in amplitude and is an exaggeration of physiological tremor. It is prominent in patients with hyperthyroidism and some patients who indulge excessively in alcohol, coffee or other drugs. A distal upper limb tremor is a cardinal feature of parkinsonism and characteristically involves a beating of the thumb towards the index finger. In its fully developed form, it is of 'pill rolling' type with the thumb moving across the tips of all fingers. Parkinsonian tremor is maximal at rest and reduced by voluntary movement. Intention tremor is absent at rest, present on actively maintaining a position and exacerbated by movement. It is due principally to disorders of the cerebellum or its connections. Much coarser and often more violent tremors usually involving the upper limb are induced by

TABLE 6.20 Causes of muscle weakness

Anatomical aetiology	Associated features	Common causes
Lower motor neurone	Muscle atrophy Fasciculation Reflexes absent or diminished Hypotonia	Peripheral neuropathies Radiculopathies Anterior horn cell damage (e.g. poliomyelitis) Motor neurone disease
Upper motor neurone	'Patterned' weakness Little or no muscle wasting Hyperreflexia Hypertonia Hypokinesia of movement	Cerebrovascular disease (e.g. hemiplegia) Spinal injury or disease (e.g. paraplegia) Multiple sclerosis
Myopathies	Muscle wasting (usually proximal) Hypotonia Tenderness (myositis)	Hereditary conditions (e.g. muscular dystrophy) Alcohol and other toxins
Psychological	Inconsistent weakness No associated features	Stress Anxiety Compensation claims

TABLE 6.21 Types of tremor

Name	Frequency (Hz)	Examples	Rest	Posture	Movement
Action (or postural)	10	Hyperthyroidism Anxiety and fatigue	–	+	+
Intention	5	Cerebellar	–	+	++
Resting	5	Parkinsonism	++	±	±

active movements (action or kinetic tremors) and abolished by rest in patients with multiple sclerosis, cerebrovascular disease involving the midbrain red nucleus (and thus termed 'rubral'-type tremor) or subthalamic nucleus. The last classically causes hemiballismus, in which there are violent throwing movements of the limbs on one side.

Dystonic movements are slow and writhing and often lead to sustained abnormal contracture and limb posturing. These are often called torsion spasms and are most commonly seen in spasmodic torticollis, following infantile hemiplegia and in dystonia musculorum deformans. Athetosis describes slow writhing movements of distal parts, usually fingers and toes. Dystonia is typically due to extrapyramidal dysfunction, usually involving the basal ganglia.

Palpation is of limited value. Abnormalities include:

- tenderness in inflammatory conditions (myositis)
- 'doughy' in Duchenne's dystrophy as a result of fatty infiltration of the pseudohypertrophied muscles
- 'woody' in some forms of acute muscle necrosis (e.g. alcoholic rhabdomyolysis).

Percussion of muscle bellies may enhance the production of fasciculations, or occasionally elicit sustained contraction in myotonic disorders (percussion myotonia).

Tone

There are also considerable individual variations in muscle tone which may be defined as the resistance felt when a joint is moved passively through its range of movement. In normal people who are relaxed the manipulation of a joint evokes slight 'elastic' type of resistance from the adjacent muscles. The normal degree of this tension can be gauged only by repeated examination of healthy people.

Examination sequence

- ☐ Note any involuntary movement or abnormalities of posture or gait.
- ☐ Inspect the muscles for symmetry and for fasciculation, noting the nature and anatomical distribution of any abnormality.
- ☐ Palpate and/or percuss muscle groups to elicit tenderness or other features.

Tone

- ☐ Ask the patient to relax and 'go floppy'.
- ☐ Passively flex and extend each joint in turn; do this slowly at first and then more rapidly to get a feel of muscle tension (Fig. 6.28A).
- ☐ In the upper limbs test muscle tone at the shoulder, elbow joint and wrist joint.

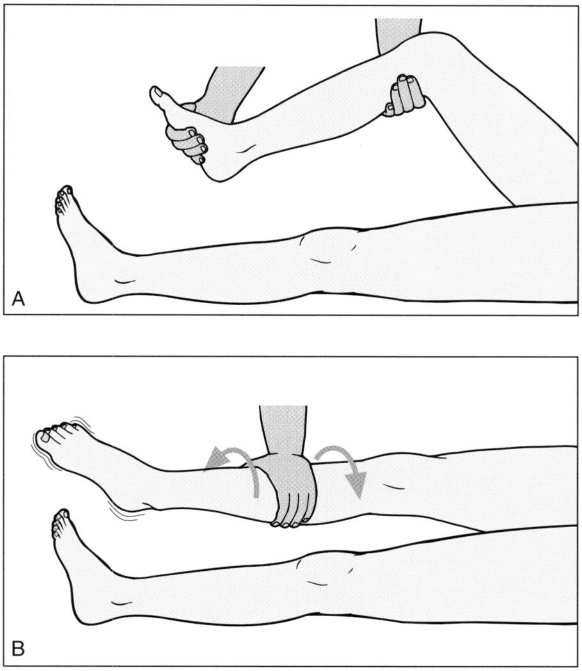

Fig. 6.28 Testing for tone. A Check the full range of movement at the knee. B Rock the relaxed leg to and fro.

- ☐ In the lower limbs test tone by internally and externally rotating the resting leg (Fig. 6.28B) and by briskly raising the patient's knee off the bed and observing whether the ankle is also raised off the bed.

Knee clonus

- ☐ Sharply push the patella towards the foot while the patient lies supine and relaxed with the knee extended.
- ☐ Following the initial jerk, exert sustained pressure with the thumb and index finger in a downwards direction on the patella.

Ankle clonus

- ☐ Support the flexed knee with one hand in the popliteal fossa so that the ankle rests gently on the bed.
- ☐ Using the other hand briskly dorsiflex the foot and sustain the pressure (Fig. 6.29).

Abnormal findings

Abnormalities in tone should be interpreted in the light of other clinical findings.

Hypertonia may be manifest as either spasticity or rigidity. Spasticity is characterised by rapid build-up of resistance during the first few degrees of passive movement and then as the movement continues there is sudden lessening of resistance. *Hypertonia* is a feature of upper motor neurone pathology. It is usually associated with increased deep tendon reflexes, clonus, an extensor plantar reflex and typical patterns of weakness. It is a common finding in cerebrovascular disease, multiple sclerosis, traumatic spinal injury and degenerative spondylotic myelopathy. Spasticity in the upper limb is frequently more obvious in attempted extension, whereas in the lower limb it is more obvious with attempted flexion. Rigidity is a term used to describe sustained resistance to passive movement. *Rigidity* is most frequently encountered in patients with Parkinson's disease (who will often have the other manifestations of this disease such as bradykinesia, tremor, gait and postural abnormalities). The rigidity may be sustained throughout the range of movement or may have a phasic component giving it a jerky feel (cogwheel rigidity), as in parkinsonism.

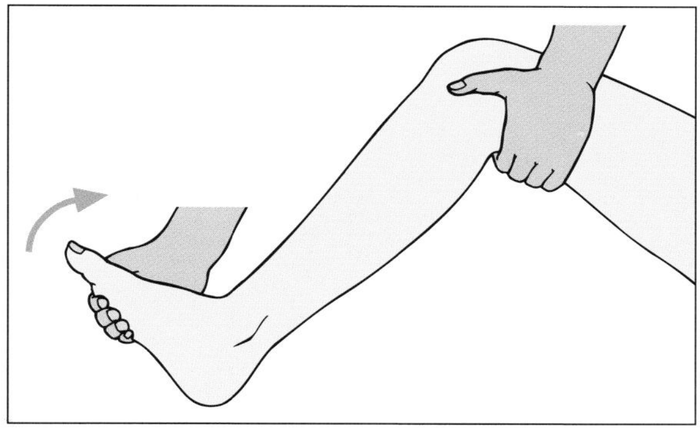

Fig. 6.29 Testing for ankle clonus.

Hypotonia may be very difficult to discern in a relaxed patient. In the upper limb, hypotonia may be evident from the posture of the outstretched hands, which show flexion at the wrist and extension of the fingers (dinner fork deformity). *Hypotonia* is encountered in lower motor neurone and cerebellar disorders and in chorea. It is often associated with hyporeflexia, muscle wasting and paresis. Hypotonia is also seen transiently in the early phase following capsular cerebrovascular accident in which the plegic limb is atonic prior to becoming spastic and hyperreflexic. Cerebellar hypotonia is subtle and often difficult to detect but may be evident if knee reflexes are pendular (see below).

Clonus is a term applied to a rhythmic series of involuntary muscle contractions evoked by sudden stretch of the muscles. If knee clonus is present, the patella will jerk up and down following a solitary jerk stimulus. If sustained ankle clonus is present there will be a rhythmical beating (alternating plantar and dorsiflexion) of the foot for as long as the pressure is maintained.

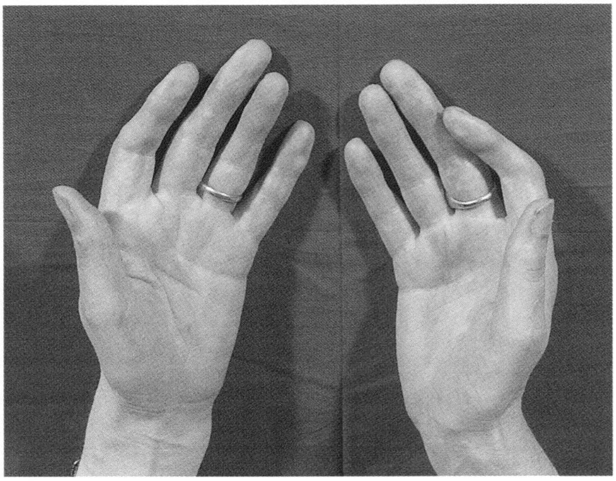

Fig. 6.30 Muscle wasting in patient with dystrophia myotonica.

Although a few beats of clonus are present in some normal people, sustained clonus indicates damage to the upper motor neurones and is a 'hard' neurological sign.

In dystrophia myotonica, there is muscle wasting (Fig. 6.30) and the delay in muscle relaxation time gives an impression of abnormal tone.

Power

When evaluating muscle power it is important to relate the strength of the muscles to the patient being tested. For example, a labourer may complain of weakness in an arm which to the examiner is extremely strong, while an elderly patient may have no symptoms despite being generally paretic.

There are two methods by which muscle power can be determined, isometric and isotonic. Isometric testing is more sensitive in detecting subtle degrees of weakness. Muscle power is usually determined using the gradient recommended by the Medical Research Council (UK) (see Table 6.22). Using this system, in most clinical situations, paresis occurs within the grade 4 range; this can be subdivided into 4^+ and 4^- to give greater precision. One system of testing is shown in Table 6.23.

TABLE 6.22 MRC scale for muscle power

0	No muscle contraction visible
1	Muscle contraction visible, but no movement of joint
2	Joint movement when effect of gravity eliminated
3	Movement sufficient to overcome effect of gravity
4	Movement overcomes gravity plus added resistance
5	Normal power

TABLE 6.23 One method of testing the motor system

Test in a proximo-distal direction

In the upper limbs examine for:
- Abduction and adduction of the shoulder
- Flexion and extension of the shoulder
- Flexion and extension of the elbow
- Flexion and extension of the wrist
- Supination and pronation of the forearm
- Extension of the fingers at both the metacarpophalangeal and interphalangeal joints
- Finger and thumb flexion, extension, adduction and abduction

Test the abdominal muscles by asking the supine patient to flex the neck or sit forward.

In the lower limbs examine for:
- Hip flexion and extension, adduction and abduction
- Knee flexion and extension
- Foot dorsiflexion, plantar flexion, inversion and eversion, toe plantar flexion and dorsiflexion

Examination sequence

- ☐ Examine individual muscle groups in both limbs alternately, or in some instances simultaneously, so that strength of the right and left can be directly compared.
- ☐ Either ask the patient to contract a group of muscles as powerfully as possible and then to maintain that position while the examiner tries to overpower the muscle group being tested (*isometric testing*).
- ☐ Or ask the patient to put the joint through a range of movement while attempting to halt movement progression (*isotonic testing*).

Common abnormalities

When considered with other clinical features, a weakness in a particular muscle or limb will identify the category of the underlying disease (Table 6.20). If such a weakness is found, a more detailed examination of muscles innervated by the same peripheral nerve or spinal segment should be undertaken (see Ch. 8).

Deep tendon reflexes

Anatomy

A neurological reflex depends on an arc which consists of an afferent pathway, which is activated by a specific receptor, an efferent system, which activates a stereotyped response, and a simple or complex pathway that interconnects the afferent and efferent systems. Since the reflex response to an appropriate stimulus is involuntary, disturbances of reflexes afford objective signs of neural dysfunction. The deep tendon reflexes of the limbs provide essential information about the status of the central and peripheral nervous systems. They are phasic stretch reflexes which involve only two neurones. Being monosynaptic the deep tendon reflexes are subserved by a particular spinal cord segment. However, suprasegmental influences modify activity of the reflex arc. Reflexes are evoked by sudden stretch of a muscle. This activates the muscle spindles, which produce an afferent volley that travels up 1A fibres, which enter the dorsal horn of the spinal cord and synapse on an μ-motor neurone in the ventral horn of the cord. Excitation of the neurone leads to direct activation and contraction of the muscle.

Examination

It is important to strike the tendon since mechanical stimulation of a muscle belly may produce contraction of that muscle which is not dependent on the reflex arc. The important deep tendon reflexes are the biceps jerk (BJ), the supinator jerk (SJ), the triceps jerk (TJ) and the knee jerk (KJ) and ankle jerk (AJ). These reflexes are illustrated with their segmental innervation in Figures 6.31–6.36. The ankle jerk is usually elicited in the position shown in Figure 6.35. However, if the patient has difficulty in relaxing, the position shown in Figure 6.36 is particularly useful.

Other deep tendon reflexes which may be useful occasionally include the deltoid reflex (C5), the pectoral reflex (C7), the finger flexion jerk, the Hoffmann reflex (C7,C8,T1), and the hamstring jerk (L5,S1).

Deep tendon reflexes are classified as hyperactive (+++), normal (++), sluggish (+) or absent (–). If a reflex is present only with reinforcement it may be annotated as ±. It is only from examination of a large number of patients that the clinician will get a feel for the normal spectrum.

Examination sequence

Tendon reflexes

- ☐ Place the patient in a comfortable relaxed position which allows the examiner to reach the limbs easily.

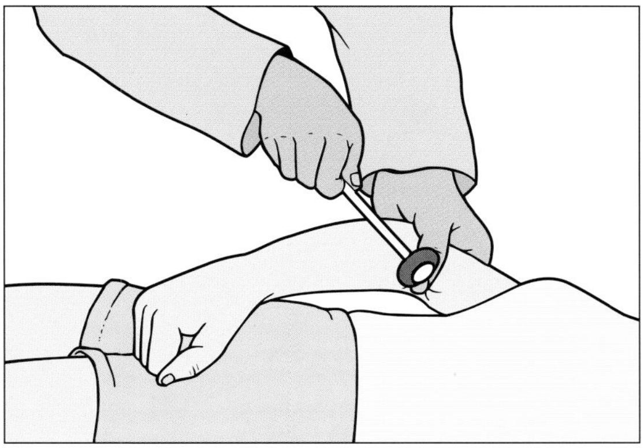

Fig. 6.31 Eliciting the biceps jerk, C5 (C6).

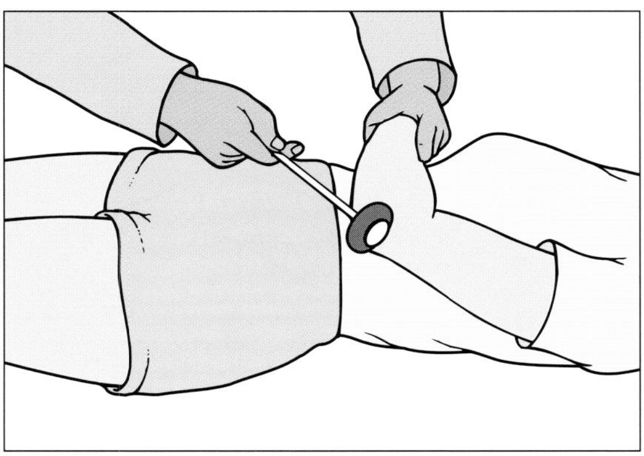

Fig. 6.32 Eliciting the triceps jerk, C6, C7.

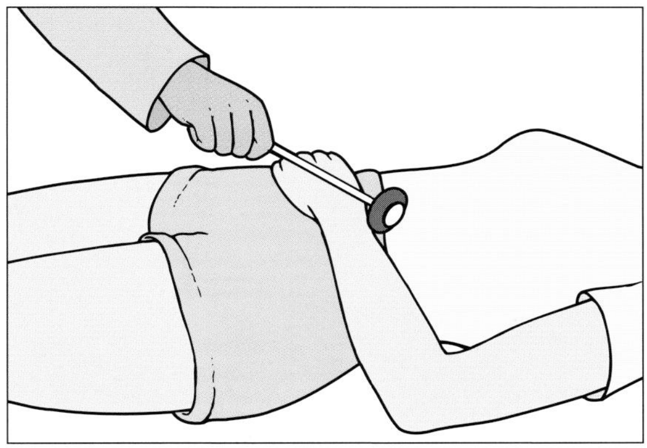

Fig. 6.33 Eliciting the supinator jerk (C5), C6.

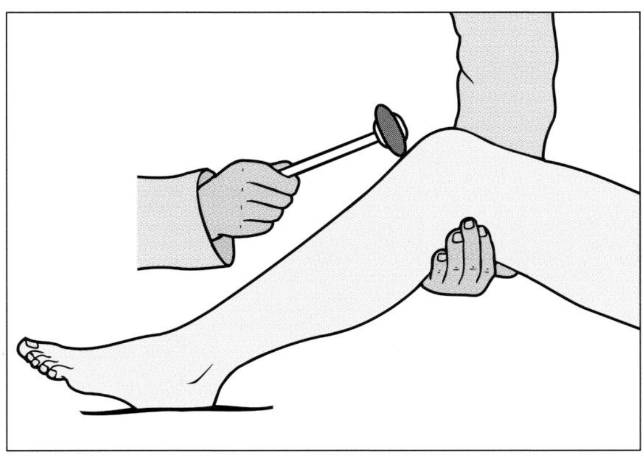

Fig. 6.34 Eliciting the knee jerk (note that the legs must not be in contact with each other), L3, L4.

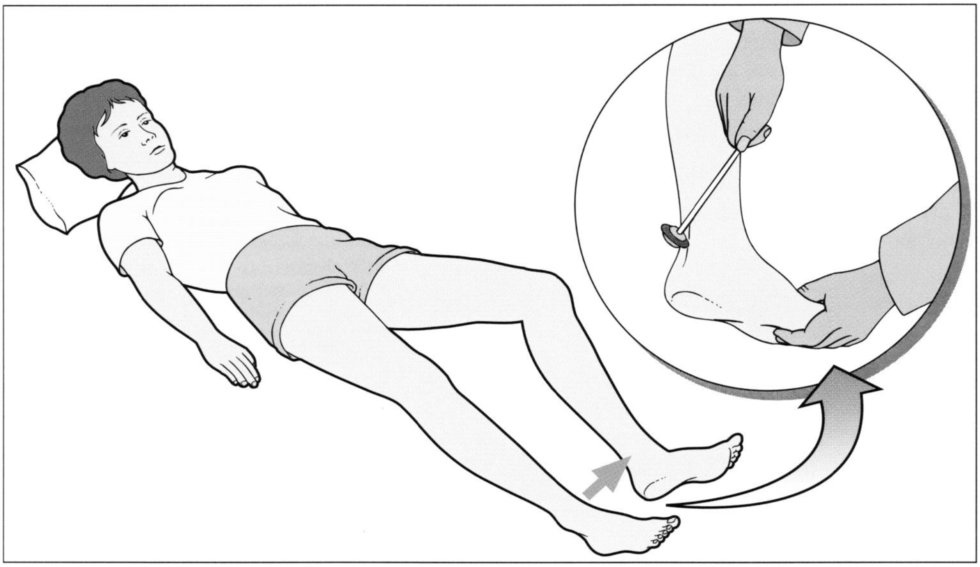

Fig. 6.35 Eliciting the ankle jerk of recumbent patient, S1.

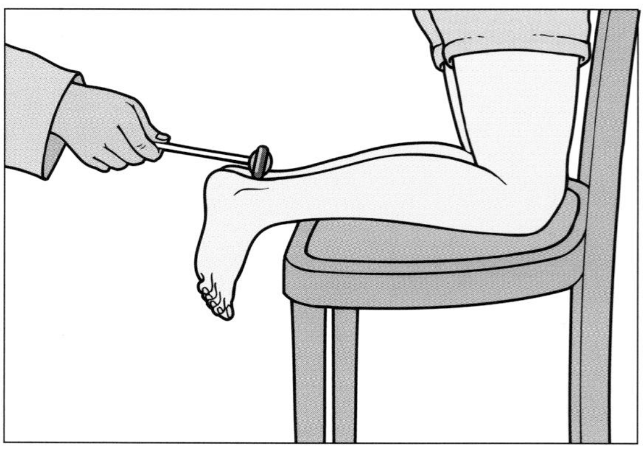

Fig. 6.36 Eliciting the ankle jerk of kneeling patient, S1.

- ☐ Ensure that the muscle being tested is visible.
- ☐ Strike the tendon, not the muscle belly, with a sharp tap from a tendon hammer.
- ☐ Observe the muscle contraction.
- ☐ Test the symmetry of the reflex by comparing the amplitude of movement on one side with the other.
- ☐ In those patients in whom reflexes are difficult to elicit or appear to be absent, use the technique of reinforcement: for lower limb reflexes ask the patient to interlock the flexed fingers (Fig. 6.37). Then ask the patient to 'tighten' immediately before striking the tendon and to relax thereafter.
- ☐ When reinforcing upper limb reflexes, ask the patient to clench the teeth or squeeze the knees together whilst the tendon reflexes are being elicited, and to relax immediately thereafter.

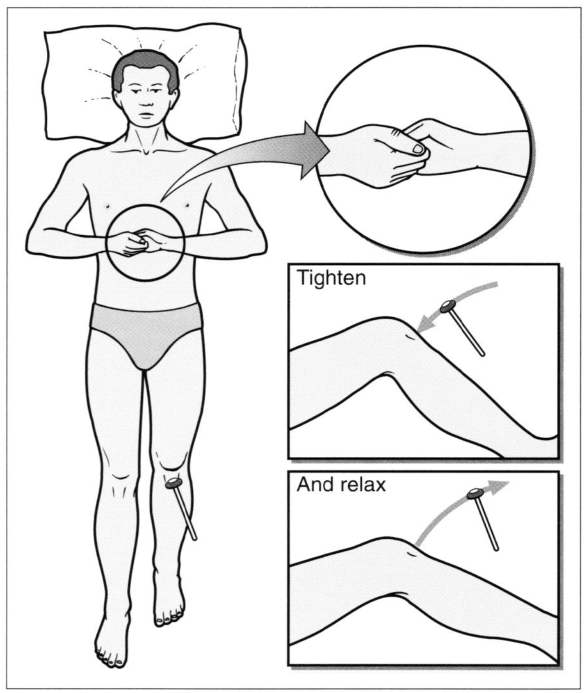

Fig. 6.37 Reinforcement in eliciting the knee jerk.

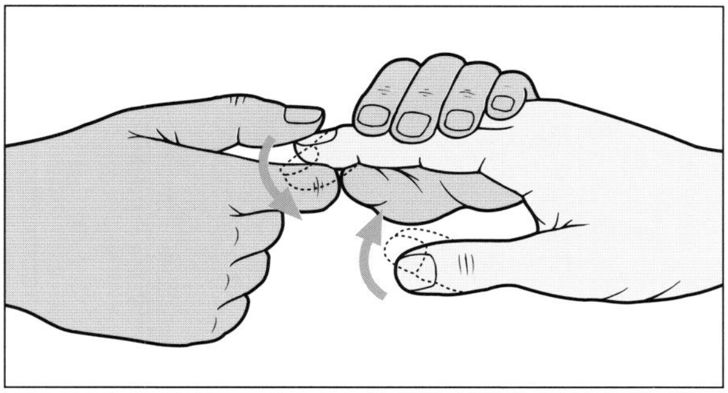

Fig. 6.38 Hoffmann's sign.

The finger jerk

- ☐ Place the tips of the examiner's middle and index fingers across the palmar surface of the proximal phalanges of the patient's relaxed fingers.
- ☐ Tap the examiner's fingers lightly with a tendon hammer. The normal response is slight flexion of the patient's fingers. This becomes exaggerated if there is hyperreflexia.

The Hoffmann reflex

- ☐ Place the examining right index finger under the distal interphalangeal joint of the patient's middle finger.
- ☐ Briskly flick down the patient's fingertip with the examining right thumb tip, and allow it to spring back to the normal position while observing the patient's thumb for any movement (Fig. 6.38). Reflex flexion of the thumb is exaggerated in hyperreflexion.

Pectoral reflex

- ☐ Place the examiner's extended index and middle fingers on the lateral border of the pectoralis muscle.
- ☐ Tap them with the tendon hammer.

Deltoid reflex

- ☐ Place the examiner's index finger across the tip of the shoulder (on the deltoid muscle belly).
- ☐ Tap the examiner's finger with a tendon hammer.

Common abnormalities

Deciding whether deep tendon reflexes are pathologically brisk or a variant of normal can be very difficult. Ancillary clinical findings such as muscle tone, pattern of paresis, the presence of clonus and extensor plantar response should clarify the significance of deep tendon hyperreflexia.

- Pathological hyperreflexia is a sign of upper motor neurone disease.
- Diminished or absent tendon reflexes are in general caused by diseases of the lower motor neurone. Diseases of the neuromuscular junction and myopathies may also produce hyporeflexia, but this tends to occur late in the disease process.
- Diminution or loss of ankle jerks may be present in some healthy elderly people.
- In some patients who have myotonic pupils (see p. 249) some of the deep tendon reflexes may be absent (Holmes–Adie syndrome).
- Isolated loss of a reflex may suggest a radiculopathy affecting that segment (e.g. loss of biceps jerk with C5–6 disc prolapse, loss of triceps jerk with C6–7 prolapse, loss of ankle jerk with lumbosacral (S1) disc prolapse).
- Symmetrical loss of reflexes may reflect an isolated or generalised peripheral neuropathy.
- Lesions involving the anterior horn cell (poliomyelitis, motor neurone disease) will also lead to depressed or absent deep tendon reflexes.
- A normal reflex contraction followed by delay in the relaxation time is a feature of hypothyroidism (Fig. 2.47, p. 63).
- During Hoffmann's test the thumb flexes excessively when there is hyperreflexia
- 'Inversion' of deep tendon reflexes may be seen with combined spinal cord and root pathology (myeloradiculopathy), most commonly associated with cervical spondylosis. The term refers to an absent or minimal response in the reflex arc being tested but with a much more obvious reflex response from muscles innervated from an adjoining spinal segment. This is most commonly seen when attempts to elicit the biceps or triceps jerk evoke strong finger flexion or, less often, a triceps reflex.
- Crossed reflex induction may also occur in spinal cord lessions. For example, elicitation of the knee jerk on one side may produce a reflex response on the contralateral side.
- Cerebellar lesion may be associated with hypotonica and hyporeflexia, the reflexes being pendular in character.

Superficial reflexes

This group of reflexes includes the plantar response, the superficial abdominal reflex and cremasteric reflex. These are polysynaptic reflexes, which are evoked by cutaneous stimulation.

Plantar response

Following strong tactile stimulation of the lateral border of the sole of the foot, the normal plantar reflex is plantar flexion of the hallux with flexion and adduction of the other toes (S1,S2) (Fig. 6.39).

Superficial abdominal reflex

This involves reflex contraction of the anterior abdominal

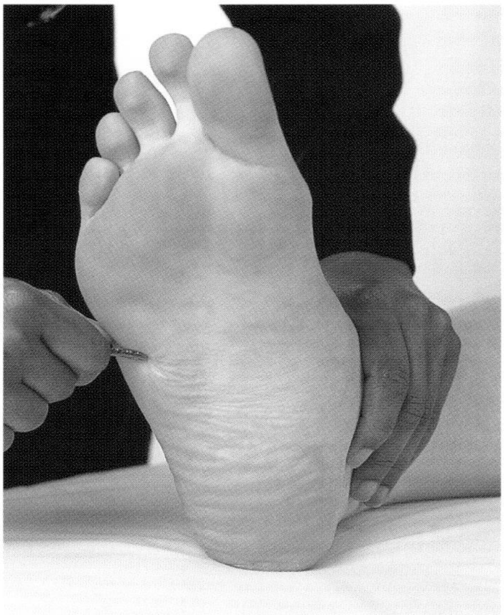

Fig. 6.39 Eliciting the plantar reflex.

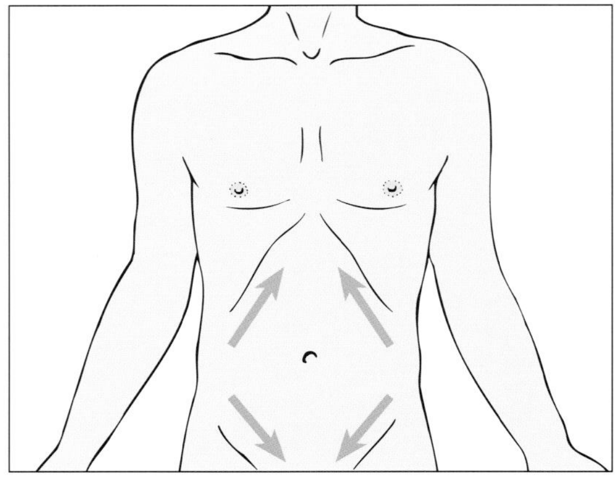

Fig. 6.40 Abdominal reflexes. Site of stimuli for their elicitation.

wall in response to light tactile stimulation. The segmental innervation of the reflex arc ranges from approximately T8 to T12.

The normal response is for the umbilicus to either elevate or depress and move laterally towards the quadrant of stimulation.

This reflex can be elicited easily in children and young adults but becomes much more sluggish in the elderly, the obese and after childbirth.

Cremasteric reflex

This involves brisk elevation of one testicle following ipsilateral stimulation of the inner thigh. This reflex is subserved by the genitofemoral nerve (L1,L2).

Examination sequence

Plantar response

- ☐ Place the patient supine with the legs extended.
- ☐ Slowly rake a blunted point, such as the end of a car key or the examiner's thumbnail along the lateral border of the foot from heel towards the little toe.
- ☐ Stop as soon as the first movement of the big toe occurs.

Superficial abdominal reflex

- ☐ Position the relaxed patient supine.
- ☐ Stroke the upper and lower quadrants of the abdominal wall on each side swiftly but lightly with an orange stick (Fig. 6.40).
- ☐ Observe any muscle contraction.

Cremasteric reflex

- ☐ Position the patient with the thigh externally rotated and abducted.
- ☐ Stroke the skin of the upper thigh using an orange stick.
- ☐ Observe the response of the ipsilateral testicle.

Common abnormalities

An abnormal or extensor plantar response (Babinski response) occurs when the hallux dorsiflexes and the other toes fan (abduct) and dorsiflex. An extensor plantar response is an unequivocal sign of upper motor neurone lesion. It will often be associated with hyperreflexia, hypertonicity and clonus. In many people elicitation and interpretation of the reflex can be difficult because of either poor response or excessive ticklishness. In some instances, it is necessary to record the response as equivocal.

The superficial abdominal reflex is lost in upper and lower motor neurone lesions. However, because it is difficult to elicit in many subjects it is at best only a useful ancillary sign.

The cremasteric reflex may be lost with either upper motor neurone disease or damage to the L1,2 spinal segment. In some normal patients, particularly the elderly, it may be difficult to elicit. Clinically it is only of relevance when assessing patients with spinal injury or other evidence of myelopathy.

Coordination: cerebellar function

Anatomy

The cerebellum plays an important role in the coordination of voluntary, automatic and reflex movement. The anatomical subdivision of the cerebellum into the midline vermis and the lateral cerebellar hemispheres is useful in clinical practice.

- The *nucleus of the vermis* has multiple interconnections with the vestibular nuclei and is important in the maintenance of body posture and equilibrium.
- The *cerebellar cortex* and subcortical nuclei are important in smoothing and synchronising the timing of muscle contraction and relaxation when the limbs are moved. One lateral cerebellar hemisphere controls limb movement on its own side.

The cerebellum also receives information from the spinal cord (spinocerebellar tracts), motor cortex (via the pontocerebellar fibres) and brain stem (red nucleus, reticular nuclei and the inferior olivary nuclear complex).

Clinical testing

Clinical tests of cerebellar function use movements of varying complexity to demonstrate the precision of motor function of both limb and postural musculature. In the upper limbs, the commonly used tests are:

- The *finger–nose test*. This involves observing the speed, smoothness and accuracy of the movement and whether any tremor occurs.
- *Rapid alternating movement* of supination and pronation of the forearm. This test is usually performed more quickly on the dominant side.

In the lower limbs, tests include the *heel–shin test* and the *heel–toe test of gait*. Additional tests that provide complementary information about the cerebellar function involve testing for truncal ataxia, assessing speech for dysarthria (p. 195), checking for nystagmus (p. 203), hypotonia (p. 217) and the presence of pendular reflexes (p. 221).

Examination sequence

The finger–nose test

- ☐ Ask the patient to hold one arm outstretched and then, with the tip of the index finger, to alternately touch the tip of the nose and then the examiner's fingertip as accurately as possible (Fig. 6.41).
- ☐ Perform the test with the patient's eyes open and test each arm in turn.

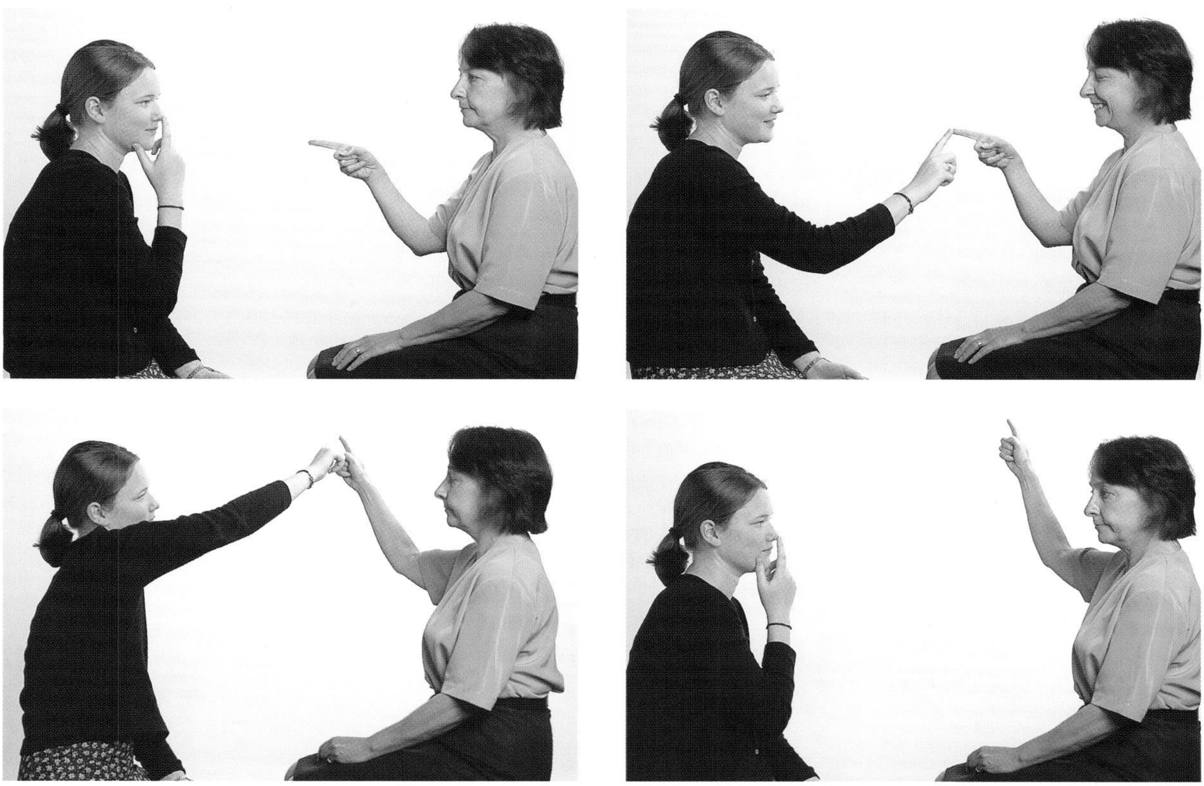

A B C D

Fig. 6.41 The finger–nose test. Ask the patient to touch the tip of the nose [A] and the examiner's finger [B], moving the finger from one position to another backwards and forwards as well as side to side ([C], [D]).

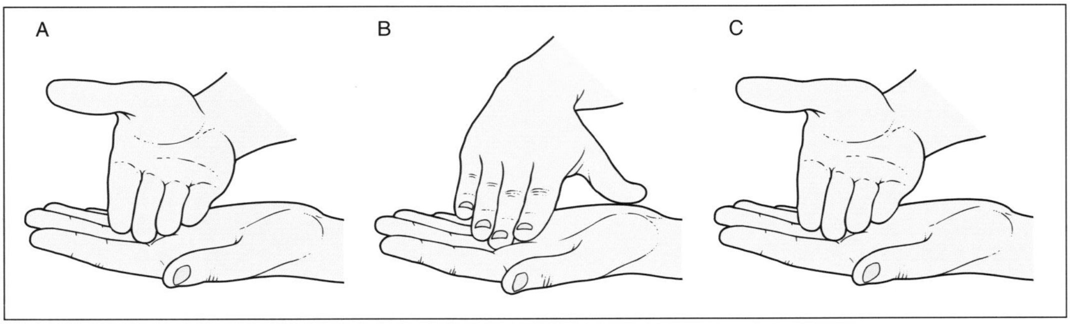

Fig. 6.42 Testing rapid alternating movement.

- ☐ Make the test more discerning by moving the target fingertip so that the patient has to readjust 'aim'.
- ☐ To test for ataxia due to proprioceptive deficit (sensory ataxia), now ask the patient to bring the outstretched fingertip to touch the tip of the nose with the eyes closed.

Rapid alternating movement

- ☐ Ask the patient to place one palm upwards and then alternately hit the upfacing palm with the palmar and then dorsal aspects of the fingertips of the other hand as quickly as possible (Fig. 6.42).

The heel–shin test

- ☐ Ask the patient to raise one leg at the hip and then place the heel of the flexed leg on the contralateral knee and to then run the heel down the surface of the tibial shaft towards the ankle and then back again (Fig. 6.43A and B).
- ☐ To render the test more complex ask the patient first to raise the leg and touch the examiner's finger held in a suitable position with the big toe before placing the heel on the knee.

The heel–toe test of gait

- ☐ Perform this test with the patient either barefoot or wearing flat shoes.
- ☐ Ask the patient to walk along a straight line so that, in turn, the heel of one foot comes directly in contact with the toes of the other foot.
- ☐ Observe the gait in general, and in particular note any tendency to stagger and the side to which the patient preferentially falls.

Common abnormalities

Lesions of the cerebellar vermis. These cause truncal and gait ataxia.

- In severe lesions the patient may have difficulty maintaining balance when sitting, and unassisted walking may be impossible.
- The gait may be wide based (i.e. the legs are held further apart than normal), and there may be unsteadiness of both gait and standing posture.

A

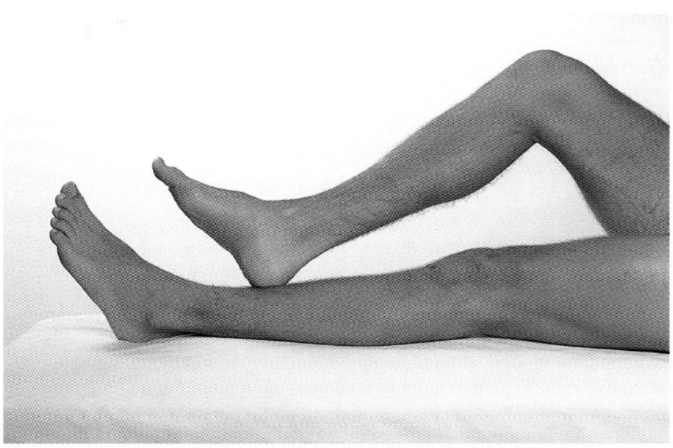

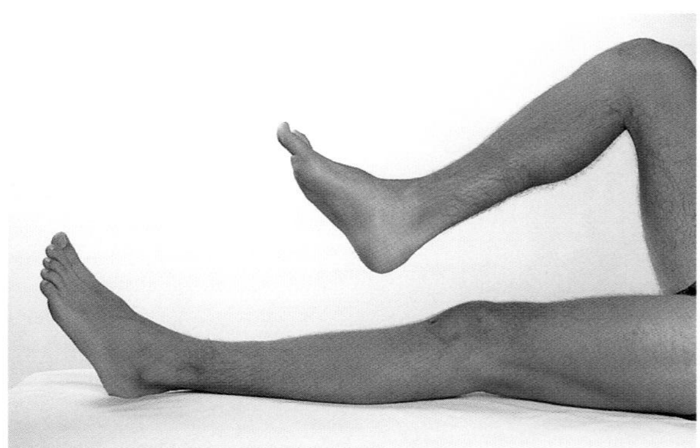

B

Fig. 6.43 The heel-shin test.

- The patient may fall when attempting to do a heel-toe test.

Such features are most commonly seen in patients with alcoholic cerebellar degeneration and neoplasms of the vermis. If the patient is examined only lying in bed, such signs may be missed.

Disease of the cerebellar hemisphere. There may be:

- abnormalities in the finger–nose test ipsilateral to the lesion, impaired rapid alternating movement and heel–shin test
- horizontal phasic nystagmus towards the side of the lesion
- an intention tremor when performing the finger–nose test with past pointing or *dysmetria* (i.e. the patient under- or overshoots the examiner's finger)
- generalised incoordination and clumsiness of the movement (*dyssynergia*)
- slowness and incoordination when performing rapid alternating movement (*dysdiadochokinesis*).

Cerebellar signs in adults are often due to cerebrovascular disease or multiple sclerosis involving the cerebellum or its brain stem connections. Specific syndromes due to occlusion of certain branches of the vertebrobasilar system are recognised by specific constellations of symptoms. Spontaneous intracerebellar haemorrhage, usually of hypertensive origin, is also a relatively common cause of acute-onset cerebellar signs in adults. Although cerebellar neoplasms are common in children, the predominant signs often tend to be those of intracranial hypertension with signs of cerebellar dysfunction occurring later. Metabolic intoxications (alcohol, phenytoin, carbamazepine) also frequently cause generalised cerebellar dysfunction. Generalised and progressive failure of cerebellar functions is seen in degenerative disorders with a genetic basis (the spinocerebellar degenerations) and as a non-metastatic effect of some malignancies, especially lung cancer.

THE SENSORY SYSTEM

Anatomy

Each of the modalities of light touch, pain, temperature, proprioception (joint position sense) and vibration have specific receptor systems and afferent pathways. Sensations of touch, pressure and position sense are carried in the peripheral nerves in relatively large fast-conducting fibres, while pain and temperature modalities are subserved principally by smaller, slower-conducting fibres. The cells of origin of peripheral sensory fibres lie in the dorsal root ganglia. The central processes of those ganglion cells subserving pain, temperature and some light touch synapse in the laminae of the dorsal horn of the spinal cord then decussate (cross over the midline) into tracts in the contralateral spinal cord (anterior and lateral spinothalamic tracts). These fibres ascend to either the ventral posterior thalamic nuclei (25%) or the reticular nuclei of the brain stem and thalamus. Those ganglion cells subserving proprioception, discriminative light touch and vibration sense synapse in the gracile and cuneate nuclei in the caudal medulla. The latter fibres ascend in the dorsal columns (cuneate and gracile fasciculi) of the spinal cord (Fig. 6.44A).

Symptoms

The most common symptoms related to the sensory system include the following.

Hypoaesthesia (decreased sensation). This may be an awareness that the sensations of temperature, pain or light touch are diminished when compared with normal limbs. A patient may inadvertently burn the fingers if pain and temperature modalities are disturbed (as, for example, in cervical syringomyelia).

Altered sensations. These may be spontaneous (*paraesthesiae*) or elicited by touch or other stimuli (*dysaesthesiae*). They

KEY POINTS

- Abnormalities of tone need to be interpreted in the light of other clinical findings.
- Although a few beats of clonus are present in some normal people, sustained clonus indicates upper motor neurone damage and is a hard clinical sign.
- The pattern of weakness and associated clinical features will indicate which anatomical category of disease underlies a paresis.
- Disturbances in deep tendon reflexes afford objective signs of neural dysfunction.
- It is important to strike the tendon, not the muscle, when eliciting a tendon reflex.
- Deciding whether or not a deep tendon reflex is pathologically brisk can be difficult.
- Diminished or absent tendon reflexes are usually caused by diseases of lower motor neurones.
- An extensor plantar response is an unequivocal sign of a pyramidal tract lesion.
- Rapid alternating movements in the upper limbs are normally performed more quickly on the dominant side.
- Lesions of the cerebellar vermis causing truncal and gait ataxia may be missed if the patient is examined only lying in bed.

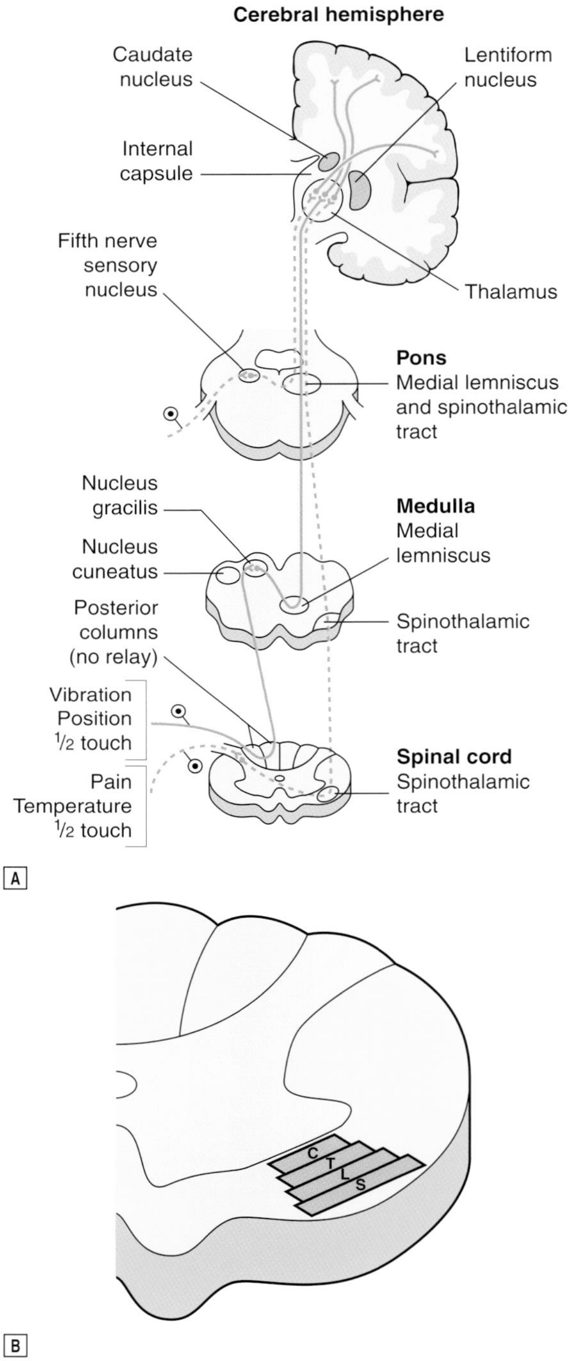

Fig. 6.44 A **The main sensory pathways.** B **Spinothalamic tract.** To show layering of the spinothalamic tract in the cervical region: C represents fibres from cervical segments which lie centrally; fibres from thoracic lumbar and sacral segments (labelled T, L and S respectively) lie progressively more laterally.

may be pins and needles, tightness or constriction or feelings of warmth or coldness.

Pain. Pain is an extremely common symptom. In some diseases, such as trigeminal neuralgia (V nerve distribution), glossopharyngeal neuralgia (IX nerve distribution), post-herpetic neuralgia and discogenic radiculopathies, the description of distribution of pain and its type may be diagnostic. In most cases, however, symptoms of pain do not conform to standard dermatomal or peripheral nerve distribution (Figs 6.45 and 6.46), and often pain may be perceived inappropriately (e.g. touch felt as pain); this phenomenon is termed hyperpathia or allodynia.

Numbness. Caution should be exercised when a patient describes a limb as 'numb' since this means weakness or heaviness to some people rather than loss of feeling.

The sensory modalities

From the clinical viewpoint, the important sensory modalities are joint position sense (proprioception), light touch, pin prick, vibration, temperature and two-point discrimination. Other sensory functions are important but will be covered under the section on the cortical examination (see Table 6.24). It is unusual for a patient to experience only one sensory symptom.

The aims of sensory testing are:

- to determine if any modalities are impaired
- to determine the site of any lesion from the topographic pattern of dysfunction (e.g. dermatomal distribution, peripheral nerve distribution).

When performing these tests it is important to avoid inflicting unnecessary discomfort upon the patient and to explain what is being performed. If physical signs are present, the examination should also cover a search for the underlying cause (see Fig. 6.47).

TABLE 6.24 Tests of sensation

Modality	Pathway
Light touch Proprioception Vibration Two-point discrimination	Large fast-conducting axons Dorsal columns Medial lemniscus
Pinprick (superficial pain) Deep pain Temperature	Smaller slower-conducting axons Spinothalamic tracts
Stereognosis Graphaesthesia Two-point discrimination	Parietal cortex (only valid if peripheral sensory function intact)

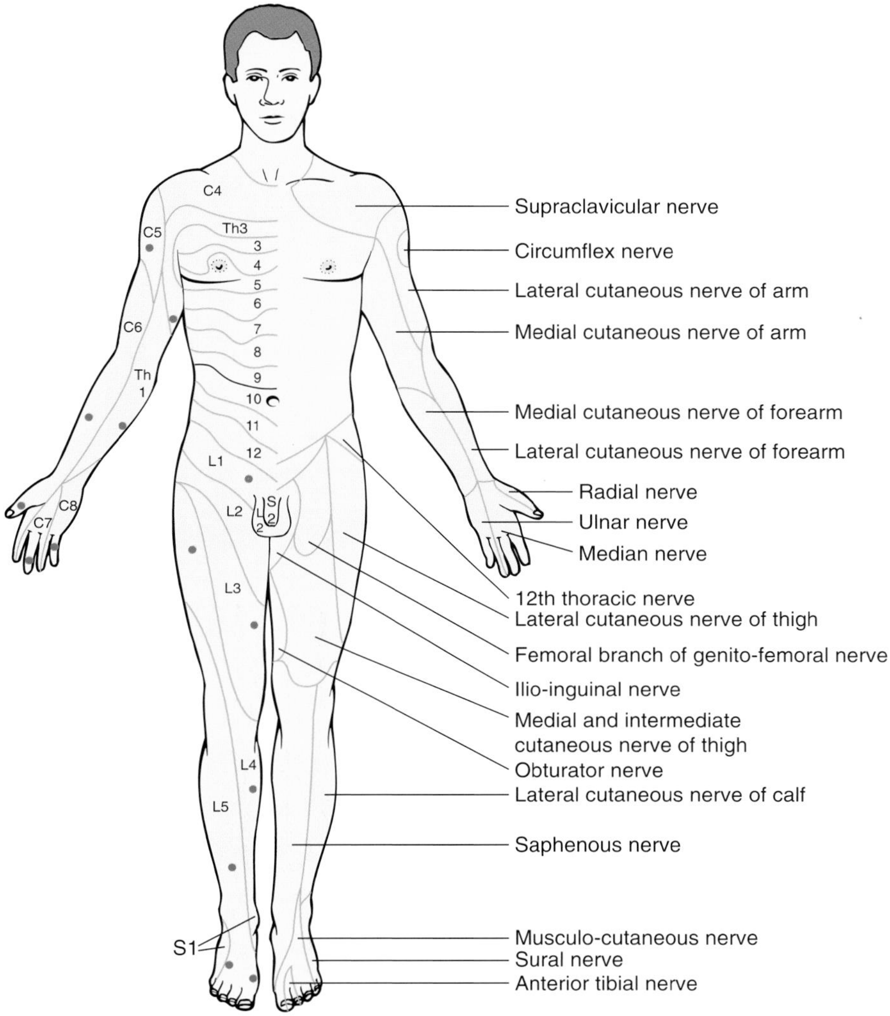

Fig. 6.45 Segmental and peripheral nerve innervation and points for testing anterior cutaneous sensation of limbs. By applying stimuli at the points marked, both the dermatomal and main peripheral nerve distribution are tested simultaneously.

Examination sequence

Touch

- ☐ Ask the patient to close the eyes and to respond verbally to each touch.
- ☐ Touch the skin with a small piece of cotton wool; tissue paper and light digital touch are alternative stimuli.
- ☐ Avoid regularly timed stimuli so that the patient does not anticipate the test.
- ☐ Examine the spinal segments sequentially (e.g. in the upper limb start on the outer border of the arm (C5), then proceed downwards to the lateral border of the forearm and thumb (C6), index finger (C7), etc.).
- ☐ Compare sensation on each limb for symmetry.
- ☐ Outline the borders of any abnormal area of sensation by testing from the hypoaesthetic area towards normal.
- ☐ If the patient complains of dysaesthesia (an uncomfortable or abnormal feeling) map from the normal to the abnormal area.

Pain

- ☐ Because of the risk of transmitted hepatitis and HIV, use a new dressmaking pin or a dedicated disposable pin. Avoid using a hypodermic needle, which is too sharp.
- ☐ Establish a baseline for sharpness (e.g. sternal area) before examining the limb.

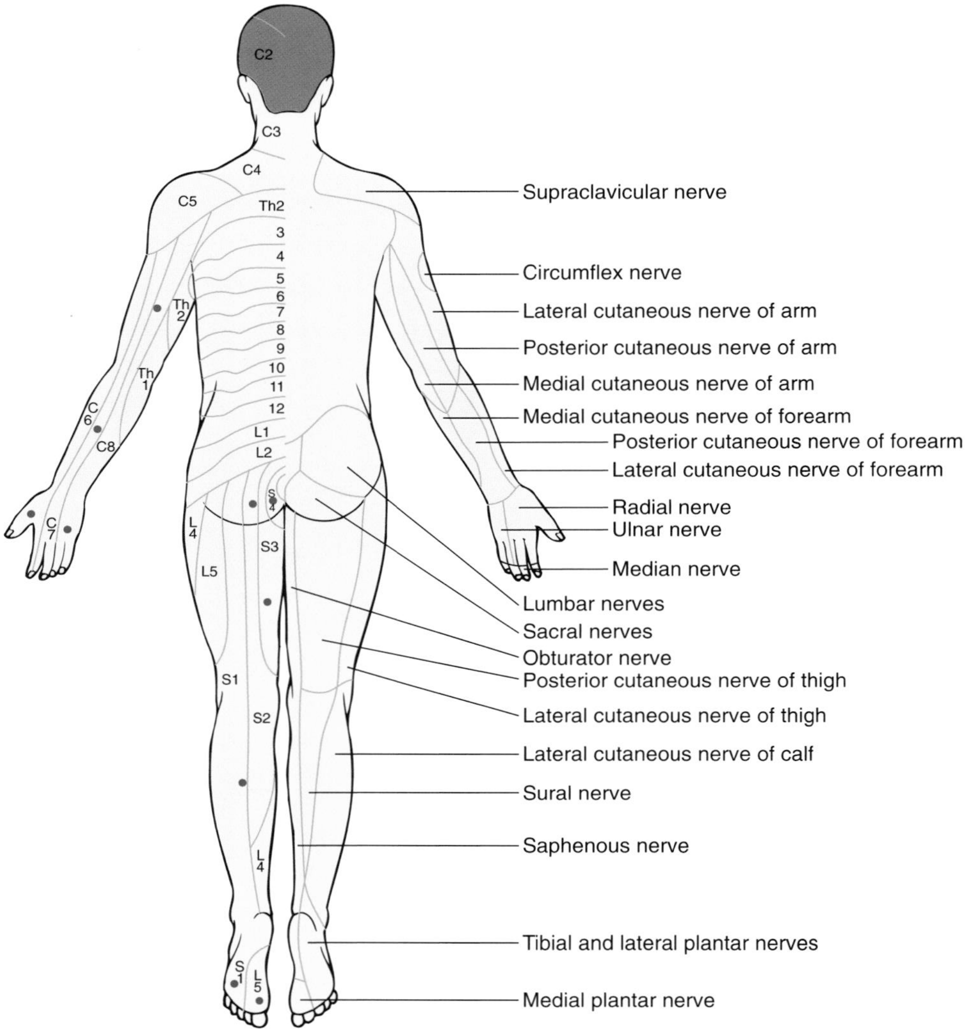

Fig. 6.46 Segmental and peripheral nerve innervation and points for testing posterior cutaneous sensation of limbs. By applying stimuli at the points marked, both the dermatomal and main peripheral nerve distribution are tested simultaneously.

- ☐ Test pin prick sensation down each limb and over the trunk.
- ☐ Ask the patient to report if the quality of sensation changes, either becoming blunter (hypoaesthesia) or feeling sharper or more painful (hyperaesthesia).
- ☐ Test each dermatome in turn, but also bear in mind peripheral nerve distributions.
- ☐ Map out the boundaries of any abnormal area as described for light touch.

Deep pain

- ☐ Squeeze muscle bellies (e.g. calf, biceps or triceps) or apply firm compression over the patient's fingernail and toenail beds.
- ☐ Ask the patient to report as soon as the sensation becomes painful.

Temperature

- ☐ Touch the patient with a cold object (e.g. a tuning fork) and ask the patient about the quality of the temperature sensation. This can be performed on face, forearms, hands, trunk and legs.
- ☐ For improved discrimination fill two plastic containers (e.g. serum bottles) one with warm and the other with

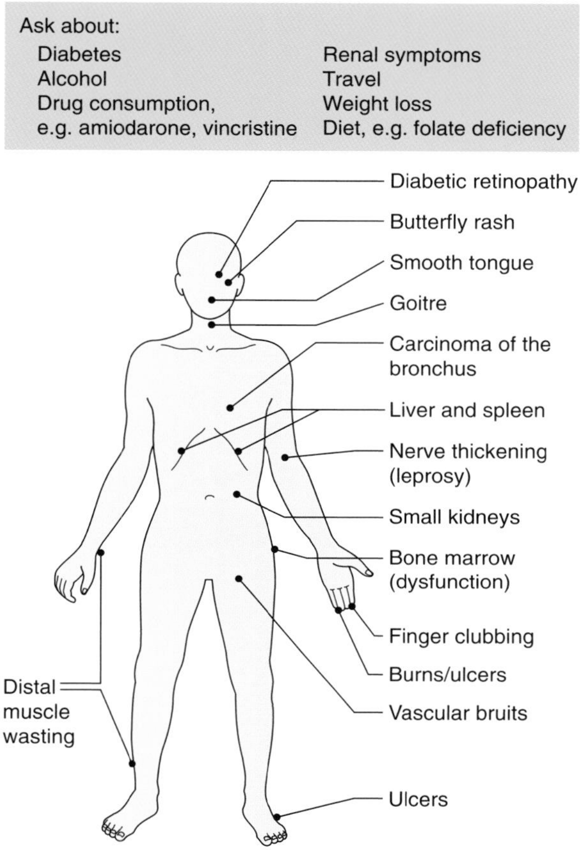

Fig. 6.47 General assessment of a peripheral neuropathy.

cool water. Ask the patient to close the eyes and to distinguish between warm and cool while applying the containers to the skin in a random sequence.

Joint position sense (JPS)

☐ Test this sensation initially at the most distal part of the limb. In the upper limb, first test at the distal interphalangeal joint of the index finger.
☐ Show the patient the intended movements of the joint and name them (e.g. 'that's up' and 'that's down').
☐ Ask the patient to close the eyes and to avoid guessing.
☐ Grasp the proximal phalanx of a finger with one hand while holding the medial and lateral borders of the distal phalanx of the same finger with the other thumb and finger.
☐ Move the patient's distal phalanx up and down.
☐ Ask the patient to identify the direction of movement during a random sequence of small movements (e.g. up, down, down, up).
☐ Then test the contralateral limb.
☐ If there is any abnormality of JPS at the distal interphalangeal joint, test at the proximal interphalangeal joint and, if necessary, at the metacarpophalangeal joint, progressing to the wrist and elbow if JPS remains impaired.

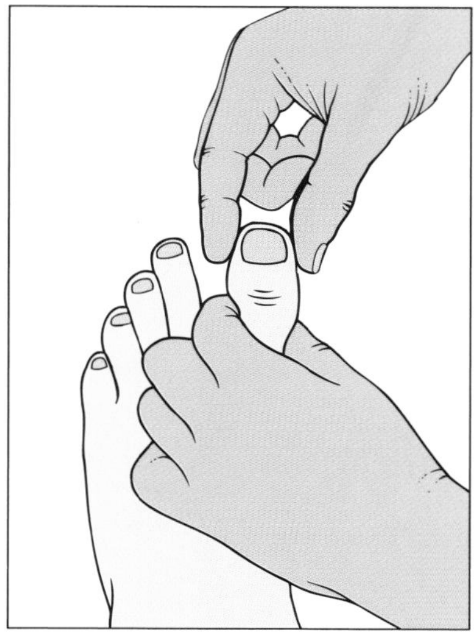

Fig. 6.48 Testing for position sense in the big toe.

☐ In the lower limb start at the interphalangeal joint of the big toe, holding the proximal phalanx in the other hand (Fig. 6.48).
☐ Take care to ensure that the examiner's fingers do not rub against the patient's other toes.
☐ If there is impairment proceed to examine the metatarsophalangeal joint and, if necessary, the ankle and knee.

Vibration sense

☐ Examine the patient with his or her eyes closed.
☐ First hold the vibrating tuning fork (128 Hz) over the sternum so that the patient identifies the sensation.
☐ In the lower limbs test the big toe (Fig. 6.49A). If necessary, next move proximally in turn to the ankle (Fig. 6.49B), tibial shaft and tuberosity and the anterior iliac crest.
☐ In the upper limbs test the interphalangeal joint of the forefinger; if impaired, proceed to the metacarpophalangeal joint and then more proximal bony prominences.
☐ If in doubt, ask the patient to identify as soon as the tuning fork stops vibrating when 'stopped' by the examining fingers.

Two-point discrimination

☐ Use a two-point discriminator if one is available, or an opened-out paper clip.
☐ Perform the test with the patient's eyes closed.

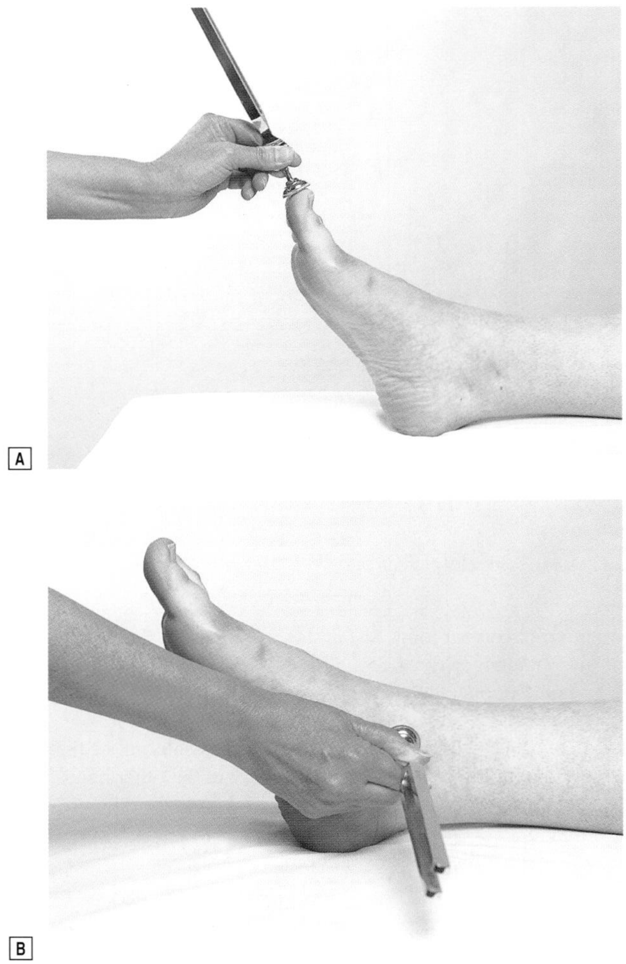

Fig. 6.49 Testing vibration sensation at [A] the big toe and [B] the ankle.

- ☐ Hold the patient's index finger and apply either one or two of the test object points to the finger pulp.
- ☐ Ask the patient to determine if one or two stimuli were applied.
- ☐ Then determine the minimum distance at which two points are felt to be separate.
- ☐ Perform the test on the pulp of both index fingers and thumbs.
- ☐ Repeat the test several times during the course of the clinical examination to determine variation in two-point discriminatory distance.

Common abnormalities

It may be difficult to decide if an apparent sensory loss is significant. Some patients may be vague in their perception of the sensory stimulus, while others may be obsessive and comment on minor variations in the intensity of the stimulus applied. Organic alterations of sensation are usually consistent and reproducible in their nature, degree and extent.

In the normal person two separate stimuli can be discriminated when they are applied as close together as 3–5 mm on the pulps of the index finger. On the soles of the feet, the distinguishing distance may be anything up to 10 times greater. It is one of the few objective parameters of sensory function. Its documentation prior to surgery or any other therapy is a useful way of gauging clinical response to treatment. Patients who have considerable alteration of superficial sensation will volunteer sensory symptoms. The finding of extensive or apparently severe sensory loss in the absence of symptoms should be assessed with caution.

Peripheral nerve damage. Impaired vibration sense over bony prominences occurs with age and is often lost at the ankles over the age of 70. However, loss of vibration sense is seen in patients at an earlier stage than impairment of JPS. For example, it is an early feature in diabetic peripheral neuropathy.

Joint position sense impairment is also first detected distally. Joint position is most commonly impaired in patients with large-fibre peripheral neuropathies and spinal cord disorders (myelopathies) affecting the dorsal columns. Disturbances of JPS may occur without paresis. In such patients the following findings may be noted:

- impaired fine-finger function and alterations of gait as a result of loss of feedback concerning muscle activity and joint position
- sensory ataxia when the finger–nose test is carried out with the eyes closed
- positive Romberg's test
- walking in the dark their gait becomes unsteady or they may fall when performing movements that require complex postural adjustments
- with the hands outstretched and eyes closed, the fingers may make small slow movements (pseudoathetosis).

Two-point discrimination in the fingers is impaired in many peripheral neuropathies, particularly those involving large sensory fibres, and in cervical myeloradiculopathies. In these conditions its loss is associated with other abnormal clinical findings suggestive of dorsal column dysfunction (light touch, JPS, vibration).

Disorders of touch, pain and temperature perception (hypoaesthesia, dysaesthesia and hyperaesthesia), JPS and two-point discrimination are common in peripheral neuropathies and nerve injuries, discogenic radiculopathies and spinal injuries.

Lesions of individual peripheral nerves or sensory nerve roots commonly give rise to subjective feeling of numbness and diminution of all sensory modalities in their areas of distribution (Figs 6.45 and 6.46). Less commonly, partial lesions of the peripheral nerve give rise to pain of a burning, unpleasant quality, as in causalgia, a condition occurring infrequently after injury to either the median or sciatic nerve. In polyneuropathies the numbness or paraesthesia and objective sensory features affect the distal parts of the limbs and often involve the legs before the arms. Superficial sensory loss in a polyneuropathy is found over the distal parts of the extremities and extends up the limbs to a level which may be relatively uniform around their whole circumference as a 'stocking and glove'-type sensory disturbance.

Spinal cord lesions. There may be a disassociated sensory loss (i.e. not all modalities are affected equally). Most commonly pain and temperature sensations are lost while touch, vibration and JPS are intact. This pattern results from lesions which damage the lateral spinothalamic pathways but not the dorsal columns. Disassociated sensory loss is classically found in patients with cervical syringomyelia but may arise from other intramedullary and brain stem pathology. Other characteristic patterns of sensory (and motor) loss occur in the anterior spinal artery syndrome (preservation of dorsal column function, with loss of motor function and spinothalamic modalities) and in the Brown–Séquard syndrome (ipsilateral loss of motor function, vibration and JPS with contralateral loss of spinothalamic sensations). Lesions of the conus medullaris and cauda equina (central disc prolapse, neurofibroma, ependymoma, primary and metastatic neoplasia) cause sensory loss from the feet, up the back of the legs, to the buttocks, perineum and genitalia.

Intracranial lesions are frequently vascular in origin. Various patterns of sensory abnormalities may be found:

- Unilateral lesions of the lower brain stem may cause impairment of pain and temperature perception on the ipsilateral side of the face (as a result of V nerve nucleus involvement) and on the contralateral side of the body below the neck (sometimes called alternating analgesia). Spinothalamic tract lesions above the mid-pontine level may damage both the spinothalamic tract and the medial lemniscus, which lie close together. This will cause sensory impairment of all modalities on the contralateral face and body.
- Lesions of the thalamus may give rise to spontaneous, intense, burning pain on the contralateral side associated with diminution of touch over the same area. The pain is poorly localised and has a particularly unpleasant quality.
- Damage to the sensory cortex may not impair perception of pain, temperature and touch but causes alterations in the qualitative, affective and discriminatory aspects of sensory appreciation and is usually accompanied by loss of two-point discrimination or astereognosis.

Parietal lobe lesions may cause marked loss of two-point discrimination in the absence of other modality changes.

Cortical function

Tests that examine sensory cortical function depend on the integrity of the peripheral sensory pathways. If these are impaired, testing of cortical sensory function is pointless. This section deals with aspects of cortical function which have localised anatomical substrates. When damaged these give rise to discrete patterns of clinical abnormality. The range of skills which can be tested include:

- calculating ability, body awareness, right and left orientation and integrative perception of sensory information (stereognosis)
- cortical vision (p. 200)
- speech and other language functions (e.g. reading, writing, verbal comprehension) (p. 195)
- ability to carry out skilled movements. *Apraxia* is the inability to carry out skilled movements despite satisfactory understanding of the task and normal motor power, cerebellar and sensory functions.

If language functions are impaired many of the tests cannot be performed.

Examination sequence

Point localisation

☐ Ask the patient with the eyes closed to localise tactile stimuli applied to various parts of the body, e.g. hands, fingers, different parts of the face.
☐ In addition, ask the patient to discriminate the right side from left, and to name individual fingers, when these are touched by the examiner.

Stereognosis

☐ Ensure that the patient's eyes are closed.
☐ Place various identifiable objects in the palm of the patient's hands (e.g. pen top, coin, key, matchstick, piece of cotton wool).
☐ Ask the patient to identify the object by feel alone.

Graphaesthesia

☐ Perform the test with the patient's eyes closed.
☐ Using a suitable object, such as the blunt end of a pencil, trace digits or letters on the patient's palm.
☐ Ask the patient to identify each symbol in turn.
☐ Repeat the test in the lower limb over the shin, if appropriate.

Sensory inattention

☐ Perform the test with the patient's eyes closed and arms outstretched.
☐ Confirm that the patient can feel a stimulus on either side when tested separately.

☐ Touch both hands simultaneously and ask the patient to report if the stimulus was applied to the left, right or both sides.

Calculating skills

☐ Ask the patient to perform subtraction sums. Alternatively, ask how much change would be expected from, say £10, if goods were bought costing a specific price.

Constructional and dressing apraxia

☐ Assess the ability of the patient to copy geometrical patterns (constructional apraxia) and see if there is any difficulty in dressing, e.g. putting an arm into a pyjama sleeve (dressing apraxia).

Common abnormalities

- The inability to localise tactile discrimination in the various parts of the body occurs with lesions in the posterior inferior parietal cortex. *Finger agnosia* is a particular type of this deficit.
- The inability to recognise objects by touch alone (*astereognosis*) suggests an abnormality of the angular and supramarginal gyra in the parietal lobe.
- An inability to recognise symbols written on the palm of the hand (*dysgraphaesthesia*) also suggests an abnormality of the parietal sensory association cortex.
- Sensory inattention arises from lesions in a similar location and is often found with visual inattention (p. 199). The normal subject is aware when both sides are touched. Abnormality can only be assessed if the peripheral sensory system is intact on both sides.
- An inability to perform simple calculations (*dyscalculia*) suggests a lesion in the dominant inferior parieto-temporal region.
- The association of right/left disorientation, finger agnosia, dyslexia and dyscalculia is termed Gerstmann's syndrome and occurs in lesions of the dominant angular gyral region.

Primitive reflexes

Primitive reflexes are normally present in neonates and young children but are lost with maturation of the central nervous system. Many of these reflexes return with generalised structural or functional diseases of the adult central nervous system (or with ageing); and indeed some remain present in a proportion of normal people. The commonly performed reflexes are the *pout* and *snout* reflex, the *grasp* reflex and the *palmomental* reflex (see below).

Examination sequence

Pout reflex

☐ With the patient's eyes closed, gently tap over the upper lip with the index finger.

Grasp reflex

☐ Create a distraction, e.g. by asking the patient to count backwards slowly from 10, then gently run the examiner's index and middle fingers across the patient's palm.

Common abnormalities

The pout reflex is part of the suckling reflex. It involves the lips pursing forwards. The grasp reflex will produce involuntary gripping by the patient. When present, they have minimal localising value, but in patients with neurological dysfunction, their presence suggests a diffuse, usually cortical, neuropathological process.

KEY POINTS

- Caution should be exercised when a patient describes a limb as 'numb' since this means weakness or heaviness rather than loss of feeling to some people.
- When performing sensory tests it is important to explain what is being performed and to avoid unnecessary discomfort.
- Organic alterations of sensation are consistent and reproducible in nature, degree and extent.
- Parietal lobe lesions may cause marked loss of two-point discrimination and stereognosis in the absence of other sensory changes.
- Sensory cortical function cannot be evaluated if peripheral sensory pathways are impaired.
- Primitive reflexes have minimal localising value but suggest a diffuse neuropathological process affecting the cerebral hemispheres.

EXAMINATION OF THE UNCONSCIOUS PATIENT

By definition patients are in coma if they do not open their eyes, utter sounds or obey commands in response to verbal or other stimuli. Wherever possible an account of events preceding coma should be obtained directly from friends or relatives and supplemented by any further information, e.g. from ambulance personnel. It is useful to establish when the patient was last seen alert and conscious because the possible diagnoses are influenced by the rate of onset of coma. Thus cerebrovascular episodes, drug abuse, hypoglycaemia, a fulminating infection or a post-ictal condition may all develop suddenly whereas coma associated with ketoacidosis, chronic renal failure or hepatic dysfunction is usually more insidious in onset. The causes of coma in young patients are usually different from those in the elderly (see Fig. 6.50).

Initial examination involves an assessment of the cardiac and respiratory status. Blood pressure, pulse rate and rhythm and respiratory rate, rhythm and volume may suggest or establish the aetiology of the coma. Profound

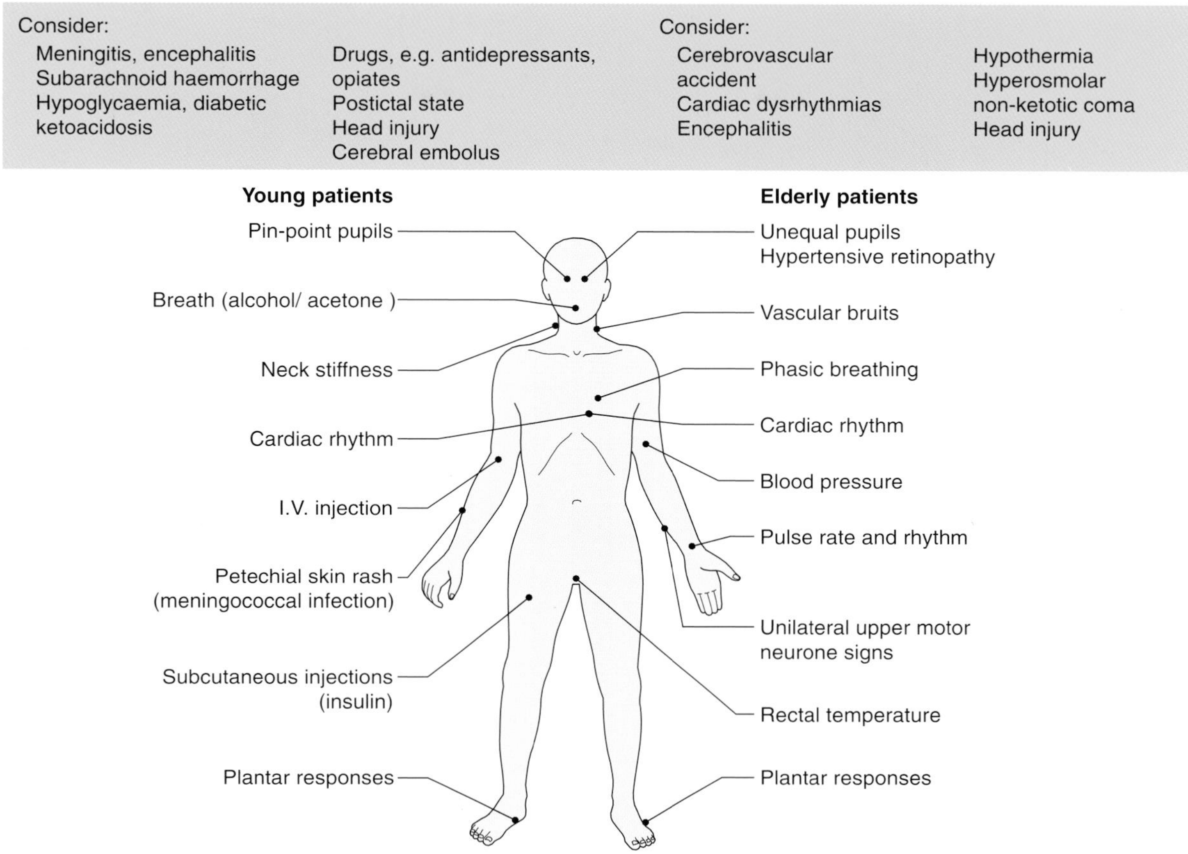

Fig. 6.50 Causes of coma.

abnormalities may require immediate treatment. Only once the airway is established and the cardiac output is satisfactory, should further examination be undertaken to look for an underlying cause. These include signs of trauma, acute or chronic medical disease, drug intake (needle marks or breath smelling of alcohol) or acute infection (pyrexia, nuchal rigidity). If the patient is diabetic, a rapid estimation of blood glucose should be performed and intravenous glucose administered while awaiting the result. If there is evidence of head injury, particular care should be taken since the cervical spine may also be injured.

Examination of the head should include a search for lacerations (? underlying depressed skull fracture), bruising over the mastoid process (Battle's sign indicative of a middle fossa fracture) and CSF or bloody discharge from the ears or nose. An anterior cranial fossa or nasal fracture may be associated with bilateral periorbital haematomas (racoon eyes). Palpation of the orbital margins may reveal a zygomatic or malar fracture. The severity of facial injuries can be gauged by checking the stability of the alveolar process of the mandible (grasp the upper jaw with a gloved hand and see if the alveolar process is stable).

The degree of coma can be assessed by the Glasgow Coma Scale (GCS) (see Table 6.25). The response to pain is best tested by digital pressure on the supraorbital ridge because if pressure is applied to a limb, there may be no response in the presence of spinal cord or peripheral nerve damage. In recording the various aspects of the GCS, the best response obtained is scored if there is asymmetry.

The temptation to dilate the pupils with mydriatics in order to obtain a better view of the fundus should be resisted because of the importance of assessing the size of the pupils and the response to the light reflex.

- *Bilaterally fixed dilated pupils* can occur with bilateral nerve III paresis (owing to massive brain swelling and tentorial herniation or midbrain damage) and following

TABLE 6.25 The Glasgow Coma Scale

Motor response (score range 1–6)	
Obeys commands	6
Localises to pain	5
Flexion withdrawal to pain	4
Abnormal flexion	3
Extension	2
No response	1
Eye opening (score range 1–4)	
Spontaneous eye opening	4
Eye opening to voice	3
Eye opening to pain	2
No eye opening	1
Verbal response (score range 1–5)	
Normal speech, orientated	5
Normal speech, disorientated	4
Abnormal speech	3
Incomprehensible sounds	2
No verbal response	1

When assessing the patient's GCS the *best* scores from verbal, eye and motor assessments are used and added. The GCS will therefore range from 3 to 15. This scale gives an indication of the patient's conscious state and is not a substitute for neurological examination. For example, a patient may have had nondominant hemispheric stroke causing a dense hemiplegia yet still have a normal GCS.

ingestion of anticholinergic drugs (e.g. magic mushrooms, tricyclic antidepressants).

- A *unilateral fixed dilated pupil* suggests an ipsilateral intracranial mass lesion (e.g. spontaneous intracerebral haemorrhage, traumatic haematoma) causing a III nerve palsy.
- *Pin-point pupils* occur following pontine vascular lesions and after narcotic overdose
- *In metabolic coma* the pupils are normally reactive to light.

Unconscious patients are unable to fixate and will therefore have 'roving' eye movements. Not infrequently the ocular axes will not be conjugate.

In patients with severe raised intracranial pressure and signs of cerebral herniation the blood pressure will be high and the pulse slow (Cushing's response).

Assessment of asymmetry on the motor aspects of the GCS will give supportive evidence concerning unilateral intracranial pathology (e.g. with a right fixed dilated pupil, if the motor response is worse on the left side than the right, this further supports a diagnosis of an acute intracranial mass lesion).

Assessment of the corneal, oculocephalic, oculovestibular and gag reflexes will provide additional information about the integrity of brain stem function.

Examination of limb tone and reflexes will provide information about the presence of spinal cord injury. Rectal examination may reveal poor anal tone in cauda equina damage. With cervical spinal cord injury there is usually associated hypotension (due to loss of sympathetic vascular tone) and bradycardia due to unopposed vagal activity to the heart.

KEY POINTS

- It is essential that the airway is protected and both ventilation and cardiac output are satisfactory before further detailed physical and neurological examination is undertaken.

BRAIN DEATH TESTING

The clinical diagnosis of brain death is now an inevitable aspect of practice in intensive care units on patients receiving ventilatory support. Prior to testing for brain death, it is necessary that the cause of the irreversible brain damage has been established (e.g. intracerebral haemorrhage, encephalitis) and that reversible conditions such as hypothermia, drug intoxication and metabolic defects have been excluded. In patients who have been previously neuromuscularly paralysed, restoration of normal neuromuscular function requires to be tested electrically or by elicitation of the deep tendon jerks. Brain death can only be diagnosed in the absence of the following functions:

- pupil reflex to light
- corneal reflex
- oculovestibular reflex using iced-water irrigation of the external ear canal
- gag reflex
- cough reflex
- spontaneous respiration when the $Pa\text{CO}_2 > 6.6$ kPa or > 50 mmHg
- response to painful stimuli, within the cranial nerve territories.

Spinal reflex activity in response to peripheral stimulus (e.g. pressing the toenail bed) is usually absent but may be preserved in the brain-dead. EEG testing is not necessary to diagnose brain death but usually shows a flat, isoelectric trace.

The 'brain death tests' should be performed by two experienced clinicians either together or separately. The tests are then repeated, after an interval, prior to the declaration of brain death.

THE DIAGNOSTIC PROCESS

Following the neurological examination, the diagnostic formulation normally comprises:

- an assessment of the nature of the patient's dysfunction
- the definition of the distribution of lesions
- an assessment of the most likely pathological diagnosis. In other words, what is disturbed, where and why?

DISTURBANCE OF FUNCTION

The first step involves determining from the physical signs which parts and paths of the nervous system may have been disturbed (Table 6.26).

The full combination of signs is not to be expected in every case and the clinician has to deduce which part of the nervous system has been damaged when incomplete patterns of signs have been demonstrated.

DISTRIBUTION OF LESIONS

The clinical recognition of neural dysfunction is followed by the identification of the site or sites of their involvement. All the observed signs may be due to a single localised lesion affecting adjacent structures or may be the consequence of more widespread damage.

Single lesions

The extent and nature of the dysfunction will often enable the location of a lesion to be deduced fairly precisely.

Cerebral cortex. Although the cerebral cortex functions in an integrated manner, certain cortical areas are associated with specific functions. The effects of lesions at different sites in the parietal, frontal, occipital and temporal lobes are summarised in Figure 6.51. Impairment of specialised functions results in dementia, dysphasia, apraxia, astereognosis and other forms of agnosia, often associated with lesions in the visual pathway. Cortical motor neurones are spread over a wide area and lesions typically affect function in only part of the opposite side of the body. Thus, unless the lesion is very large, paresis confined to one limb (monoplegia) or to one side of the face is more likely than a hemiplegia.

In contrast, a profound hemiplegia involving face, arm and leg, associated with loss of sensation of all modalities on the paralysed side, suggests a lesion affecting the *internal capsule*, where the upper motor neurone and sensory pathways are packed closely together.

Brain stem. Lesions are characterised by ipsilateral impairment of one or more cranial nerves with concurrent contralateral dysfunction in one or more long tracts. The cranial nerve dysfunction will depend on the part of the brain stem affected. A midbrain lesion is suggested by a III nerve palsy; pontine damage by VI and VII nerve signs accompanied by contralateral upper motor neurone signs. Occasionally other tracts such as the spinothalamic or sympathetic pathways are interrupted. Examples of lesions involving the midbrain, pons and medulla are given in Figures 6.52 and 6.53 (see also Fig. 6.19).

TABLE 6.26 Signs attributable to lesions in different parts and paths of the nervous system

Upper motor neurone (pyramidal tract) lesions
Weakness or paralysis of movement
Increase in tone of 'clasp-knife' type
Increased amplitude of tendon reflexes
An extensor plantar response
Lower motor neurone lesions
Weakness or paralysis of muscles
Wasting of muscles with fasciculation
Reduction in tone
Diminution or loss of tendon reflexes
Extrapyrimidal lesions
Resting tremor (especially 'pill-rolling')
Rigidity, cogwheel or 'lead pipe'
Bradykinesia, expressionless face, festinant gait
Cerebellar lesions
Ataxia of gait
Intention tremor of limbs
Jerking nystagmus
Dysarthria of staccato or scanning type
Dysmetria and past-pointing
Hypotonia and pendular tendon reflexes
Smooth movements may be replaced with jerking movements
Generalised neuropathies
Diminution of superficial sensation affecting the distal aspect of limbs with 'stocking' and 'glove' distributions
Wasting and weakness of distal limb musculature
Early loss of tendon reflexes
Sensory tracts
Dorsal columns:
Ataxia of gait and limb movements aggravated by eye closure (positive Romberg's test)
Impaired position sense
Diminished appreciation of vibration
Lateral spinothalamic tracts:
Impairment of pain and temperature sensation
Muscles
Wasting and weakness, usually proximal
Reduction in reflexes when muscle wasting is marked
Cerebral cortex dysfunction
Dysphasia and dyscalculia
Right and left disorientation
Astereognosis, sensory inattention
Apraxia
Amnesia and cognitive disorders
Visual field homonymous defects
Hemiparesis, monoparesis

Stroke disease. Cerebrovascular accidents (strokes), due to either cerebral infarction or haemorrhage comprise the

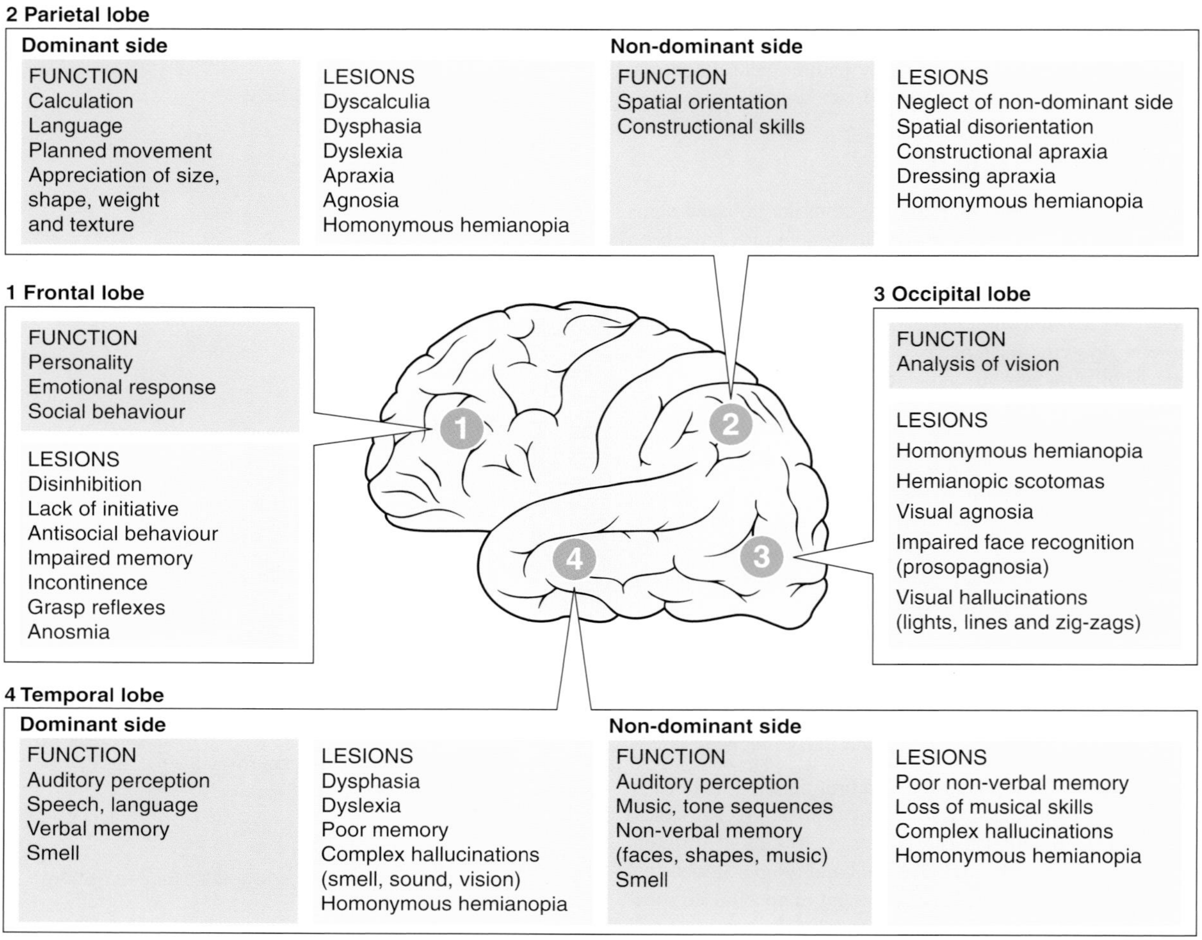

Fig. 6.51 Features of localised cerebral lesions.

commonest neurological abnormality seen in medical wards. Strokes may affect the cerebral cortex or the brain stem. Table 6.27 shows the clinical features of stroke in different arterial territories subserved by either the internal carotid or vertebral arteries.

Spinal cord. Damage is localised by correlating motor, sensory and reflex changes. Upper motor neurone signs arising from cord lesions are often, but not always, bilateral. Their presence helps to locate the site of lesion very roughly. If they are present in the arms the lesion lies above the fifth cervical segment; if the abdominal reflexes are pathologically absent, a segment above the eighth thoracic is implicated. Pyramidal tract signs in the legs indicate a lesion above the conus medullaris.

The site of spinal damage is localised more precisely if the lesion also involves the anterior horn cells or motor roots, thereby causing lower motor neurone signs, with weakness and wasting in a segmental distribution. Sensory signs often help to delineate the position of cord lesions. Impairment of sensation over a segmental dermatome will indicate the level of a lesion. Interruption of sensory tracts may give rise to an upper level of sensory loss which roughly corresponds to the site of the spinal lesion but which is often at a more caudal level. Spinal cord lesions which disrupt reflex arcs with loss of tendon reflexes indicate the segments which have been damaged.

Often the segmental level and the cross-sectional areas of a spinal cord lesion may be gauged (Fig. 6.54). Below a hemisection of the cord on the ipsilateral side there will be found (1) upper motor neurone signs, (2) impaired joint position and vibration senses and sometimes (3) signs of

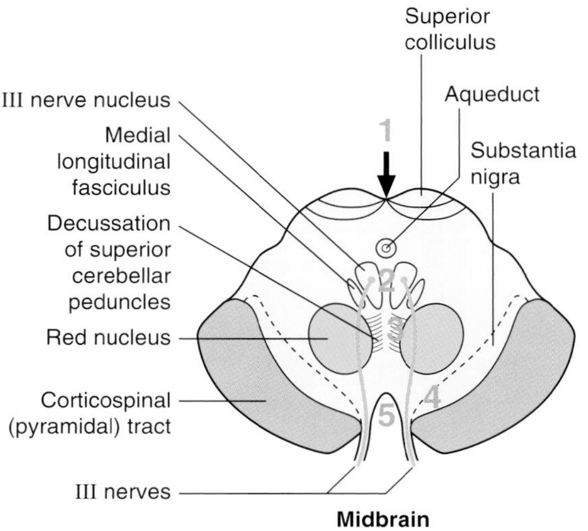

Fig. 6.52 Lesions of midbrain. Lesions at **1.** (e.g. pressure from a pineal tumour) cause weakness of upward gaze which may first be manifest as nystagmus in a vertical plane. Lesions at **2.** produce bilateral, partial lesions of the III nerve and anterior internuclear ophthalmoplegia (p. 202, damage to medial longitudinal fasciculus). Lesions at **3.** cause ipsilateral III nerve palsy and contralateral cerebellar signs (damage to decussating cerebellar peduncles) and/or tremors and athetoid movements (damage to red nucleus). Lesions at **4.** cause ipsilateral III nerve signs and contralateral pyramidal involvement. Lesions at **5.** cause bilateral pyramidal signs. Lesions which affect the midbrain immediately below this level also implicate the IV nerve.

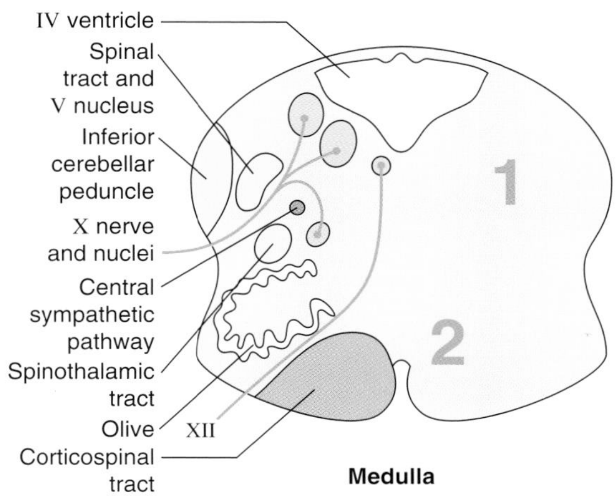

Fig. 6.53 Lesions of the medulla. Lesions affecting the lateral medulla **1.** (e.g. thrombosis of the posterior inferior cerebellar artery) cause ataxia and intention tremor on the ipsilateral side; jerking nystagmus on turning the eyes to the side of the lesion (damage to the spinocerebellar tract in the inferior cerebellar peduncle); analgesia on the ipsilateral side of the face and contralateral limbs (affection of spinal tract of V nerve and the lateral spinothalamic tract); Horner's syndrome (involvement of the central sympathetic pathway); dysphonia, dysphagia and weakness of soft palate and paralysis of the vocal cords on the side of the lesion (damage to the X nerve). Lesions affecting the paramedian area **2.** (e.g. infarction) cause a crossed paralysis – wasting and fasciculation of ipsilateral side of tongue (damage to XII nerve) and contralateral pyramidal signs.

vasomotor disturbance. On the contralateral side there will be reduced sensation to pain and temperature. This composite picture is called the *Brown–Séquard syndrome*.

Peripheral nerve. The most common causes of damage to a single peripheral nerve (mononeuropathy) are entrapment especially in fibro-osseous tunnels (e.g. carpal tunnel syndrome), trauma (e.g. radial nerve palsy), diabetes mellitus (e.g. femoral nerve palsy) or in obesity (e.g. meralgia paraesthetica). Symptoms and signs of some common entrapment neuropathies are summarised in Table 6.28.

Multiple lesions

Discrete lesions. An analysis of a patient's signs may show that they cannot be explained by a single lesion. Two or more discrete lesions may be required, as in multiple sclerosis, in which optic nerve and spinal dysfunction may be found concurrently.

TABLE 6.27 Features of stroke in different arterial territories

Main artery	Branch	Clinical features	Side
Internal carotid	Middle cerebral	Hemiparesis (face and arm > leg), hemianaesthesia Dysphasia, dysarthria, dyspraxia, hemianopia	Opposite side to lesion
	Anterior cerebral	Hemiparesis (leg > arm and face), incontinence	
Vertebral	Posterior cerebral	Hemianopia, cortical blindness, amnesia Thalamic pain	Nuclear symptoms ipsilateral to lesion; contralateral sensory and pyramidal signs
	Cerebellar basilar	Ataxia, diplopia, nystagmus, dysarthria, dysphagia, facial weakness/numbness, bilateral sensory symptoms, loss of consciousness	

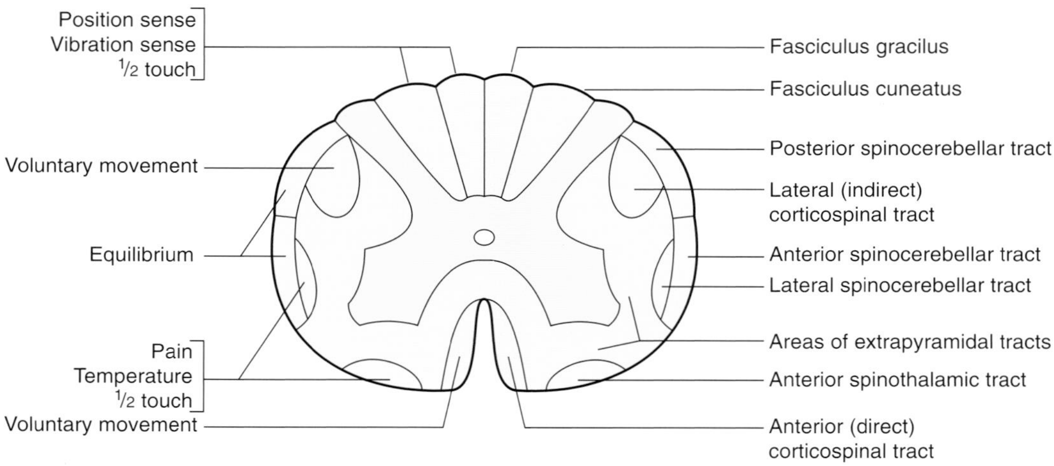

Fig. 6.54 Transverse section of the spinal cord.

TABLE 6.28 Symptoms and signs in entrapment neuropathy (from Haslett et al 1999)

Nerve	Symptoms	Muscle weakness/wasting	Area of sensory loss
Median (at wrist) (carpal tunnel syndrome)	Pain and paraesthesia on palmar aspect of hands and fingers, waking the patient from sleep. Pain may extend to arm and shoulder	Abductor pollicis brevis	Lateral palm and thumb, index, middle and half ring finger
Ulnar (at elbow)	Paraesthesia on medial border of hand, wasting and weakness of hand muscles	All small hand muscles, excluding abductor pollicis brevis	Medial palm and little finger, and half ring finger
Radial	Weakness of extension of wrist and fingers, often precipitated by sleeping in abnormal posture, e.g. arm over back of chair	Wrist and finger extensors Supinator	Base of dorsum of thumb
Peroneal	Foot drop, trauma to head of fibula	Dorsiflexion and eversion of foot	Nil or dorsum of foot
Meralgia paraesthetica	Tingling and dysaesthesia on lateral border of the thigh (lateral cutaneous nerve of the thigh)	Nil	Lateral border of thigh

Selective damage. Some neuropathological lesions afflict specific tracts in different parts of the nervous system. A polyneuropathy may be widespread, symmetrical or asymmetrical depending on aetiology (see Fig. 6.47). Involvement of motor or sensory fibres may predominate. Damage may be confined to upper and lower motor neurones, as in motor neurone disease, or to dorsal root ganglion cells, as in some forms of carcinomatous neuropathy. Spinal tracts may be selectively damaged, singly or in combination, as when dorsal and lateral columns are disrupted by vitamin B_{12} deficiency (subacute combined degeneration).

Diffuse damage. Diffuse damage may be demonstrated when disorders affect wide areas of grey and white matter and traverse structural and functional boundaries. Thus alcohol abuse may cause generalised cortical neuronal loss, cerebellar degeneration, selective damage to the limbic circuitry and midbrain (as in Wernicke's encephalopathy) and peripheral neuropathy. All of these disturbances may not be present. However, combinations of several lesions are commonly found in the same patient. Repetitive head injuries may also cause randomised, diffuse cerebral atrophy resulting in the dementia of the 'punch-drunk' state, in which parkinsonism is also typical.

PATHOLOGICAL DIAGNOSIS

Specific clues to aetiology may be contained in the history. The story of an antecedent head injury in an elderly patient with a progressive intracranial lesion may suggest a chronic subdural haematoma. A family history of epilepsy, muscle disease or ataxia may clarify the nature of a patient's illness.

The general medical examination may suggest that the neural lesion is due to a process which involves other systems. Evidence of peripheral vascular disease or a cardiac arrhythmia might imply that a cerebral lesion was vascular in nature. Anaemia and a smooth tongue could implicate vitamin B_{12} deficiency as the cause of a myelopathy. Features of hepatic cirrhosis may suggest an alcohol-related problem or Wilson's disease.

The nature and distribution of the neurological signs suggest some conditions and help to exclude others. Signs of focal brain dysfunction together with papilloedema suggest a space-occupying lesion, such as a tumour. Patients with multiple but transient neurological abnormalities, particularly drowsiness and nystagmus, may be suffering from alcohol intoxication or drug overdosage.

With this approach, it is often possible to make a firm diagnosis on clinical grounds alone. On other occasions the probable causes should be considered and a rational scheme of investigation designed.

FURTHER INVESTIGATIONS

The general investigation of a patient with a neurological complaint is important. Examples include assessing haematological parameters, renal and hepatic function, checking for electrolyte abnormalities, testing for HIV status, checking for vitamin B_{12} deficiency and taking chest radiographs.

Some neurological investigations cause discomfort and may be hazardous. It is wise to start with those clinically appropriate investigations which are least disturbing and only proceed to invasive tests if these become essential. Sometimes, however, the clinical urgency is such that the definitive investigation needs to be performed immediately.

COMMON PITFALLS AND HOW TO AVOID THEM

- Neurological symptoms and signs can change rapidly. In patients under observation, up-date the history and repeat the physical examination at appropriate intervals.
- Unexplained symptoms may be the result of psychological illness. Anxiety may trigger somatic symptoms via several mechanisms, e.g. hyperventilation. Remember to examine the mental state tactfully and with sensitivity.
- In patients with a headache of sudden onset, lack of a neurological deficit does not exclude subarachnoid haemorrhage nor does a normal CT brain scan. Lumbar puncture should be performed to exclude the diagnosis.
- The symptoms and signs of atypical meningitis can be subtle. Where there is doubt, if the CT scan is normal, lumbar puncture should be undertaken without delay.
- Nerve root pain is a common early feature of spinal cord compression. In order to avoid overlooking this possibility, examine the patient regularly for evidence of a progressive neurological deficit.
- The lower limit of the spinal cord involvement is reflected by the pattern of neurological signs. In contrast, the upper limit may be difficult to define clinically. This may require spinal MRI of the entire spinal cord up to the foramen magnum.
- In patients with an intramedullary cord lesion, the diagnosis may be concealed. However, the presence of a dissociated sensory loss and preservation of sacral sensation strongly suggest the possibility.
- Somatic neurological symptoms, especially headache, are frequent in patients suffering from depressive illness. Specific enquiry about life events, sleep disturbance, appetite and libido may be useful in making a positive diagnosis.
- Patients with neurological symptoms suggesting a functional disorder may need 'permission to get better'. Recovery is more likely to occur if the clinician makes allowance for this by admitting ignorance of the cause of such a disability rather than adopting a confrontational approach.
- 'Stroke' is a clinical diagnosis. The appropriate management of the patient with a stroke requires making a pathological diagnosis and, for this, a CT brain scan is necessary, e.g. to distinguish between haemorrhage and thrombosis.
- Dysphasic syndromes may present as apparent confusional states. Remember to look carefully for evidence of receptive dysphasia in patients with confusion.
- Following stroke, neurological damage may be increased if the early management is suboptimal. It is important to look for and correct such remediable factors as hypoxia, anaemia, severe hypertension and cardiac failure.
- Failure to obtain an eyewitness account in a patient with unexplained blackouts can lead to delayed diagnosis and inappropriate investigations. The telephone can be a more useful tool than the CT scanner in such patients.
- Presentation with apparent status epilepticus is common in patients with pseudoseizures. Ask relatives and/or carers about previous unexplained or inconsistent blackouts or funny turns. 'Funny turns' which only occur in the presence of witnesses are usually not seizures.
- When doubt exists about whether blackouts are epileptic or cardiovascular in origin, accurate recall of events immediately preceding the blackout, absence of headache or other symptoms after the event and the rapid and complete recovery all strongly favour a non-epileptic origin. Ask specifically about these features to aid the diagnosis.

- Benign intracranial hypertension signifies the absence of cerebral tumour. Papilloedema is always a serious sign and requires urgent investigation. Remember that patients may lose their sight permanently if the condition is not promptly treated irrespective of its cause.
- When a patient has difficulty in walking ('off legs') do not forget to check for features of spinal cord compression: spastic paraplegia (upper motor neurone signs in lower limbs), a 'sensory level', e.g. sensory loss up to T10 dermatome, with an atonic bladder which can be palpated on abdominal examination.

FURTHER READING

Haslett C, Chilvers E R, Hunter J A A, Boon N A 1999 Davidson's principles and practice of medicine, 18th edn. Churchill Livingstone, Edinburgh

The examination of the eye

7

M. J. MACDONALD

THE HISTORY

An accurate history is essential. As vision is the most important sense in man, fear of blindness makes patients especially anxious about eye problems. This should be appreciated while taking the history.

Symptoms fall into three main categories:

- abnormal appearance
- pain
- disturbance of vision.

Abnormal appearance

Abnormal appearance may be a presenting symptom, or may be noted as a sign during examination. It is important to establish whether the abnormality is congenital or acquired, its speed of onset and whether there are any associated features. In conditions causing severe pain the eye is often very red. Table 7.1 gives a few examples of conditions which may present with an abnormal appearance of the head, face or eyes.

Pain

The character of pain in eye disease falls into four main categories:

- foreign body sensation
- deep severe pain
- eye strain
- headache unrelated to the eye but with visual symptoms.

Foreign body sensation. This is associated with disorders of the conjunctiva and cornea, the external coats of the eye. It ranges from a feeling of mild discomfort and grittiness usually associated with conjunctival inflammation to a severe burning sensation with photophobia (light sensitivity) characteristic of corneal epithelial damage. There may, for example, be a history of rheumatoid disease (Sjögren's dry eye syndrome), cold sores (herpes simplex corneal ulcers) or of using ultraviolet light (welder's flash burns). In external disorders, the eye is usually pink and there may be a sticky or watery discharge.

Deep severe pain. Severe eye pain is distressing and often associated with nausea and vomiting. It is vaguely localised to the eye and brow. It is characteristic of intraocular inflammatory disease (uveitis, scleritis and endophthalmitis) and of high intraocular pressure (acute glaucoma). The eye is usually very red. Similar pain occurs in herpes zoster ophthalmicus (shingles affecting the first division of the V nerve) and intracranial aneurysms pressing on the V nerve.

Eye strain. This symptom is generally vague. The eyes feel tired and aching, often with frontal headache. The most usual cause is tension headache or fatigue. Occasionally it is caused by uncorrected optical errors or problems with binocular vision and requires an optician's advice.

Headache. Pain in the head is often associated with visual symptoms. A migraine attack classically begins with the flashing or zigzag lights of a visual aura but may also be associated with a hemianopia. Visual obscurations (temporary visual loss when bending) occur with headache in chronic raised intracranial pressure.

CASE HISTORY

A 70-year-old woman presented complaining of attacks of blurred vision in one eye.

On questioning she admitted to feeling 'done'. Examination of the eye was normal. Her hair was untidy as combing had been uncomfortable due to tender spots on the head. The ESR was markedly raised at 100 mm in the first hour. High-dose systemic steroids were prescribed with an immediate improvement in the tiredness and scalp tenderness.

Learning points

- Giant cell arteritis commonly causes prodromal attacks of blurred vision.
- The most common associated features are tiredness and headache which may be accepted as normal in an elderly person.
- Untreated, the arteritis will cause irreversible and often bilateral visual loss due to ischaemic optic neuropathy.
- A normal eye examination does not exclude serious pathology. In this case the history suggested the diagnosis which was established by the high ESR.

Disturbance of vision

When taking the history it is important to establish time sequences, associated features and whether the disturbance

TABLE 7.1 Examples of abnormal appearance of head, face and eyes

Site	Appearance	Associated features	Cause
Head	Abnormal head posture	Squint and diplopia on straightening head	Vertical muscle palsy
Face	Asymmetry and fullness of supraorbital ridge	Cranial nerve palsies	Sphenoidal ridge meningioma
Eyes	Proptosis	Lid lag and lid retraction	Dysthyroid eye disease
Lids	Xanthelasma	Corneal arcus	Hypercholesterolaemia

is unilateral or bilateral. Apparent sudden loss of vision may have only been noticed suddenly when the normal eye was covered. The main disturbances of vision are:

- blurred vision
- loss of vision
- double vision (diplopia)
- flashing lights (photopsia) and haloes
- floaters.

Blurred vision. Blurring is usually due to an ocular problem. When the media (cornea, lens, aqueous or vitreous) are hazy, vision blurs and there is often dazzle in bright light. Cataracts cause such symptoms. The blur caused by refractive errors is cured by spectacles.

Loss of vision. Sudden visual loss suggests a vascular aetiology. The nature of the loss may help localise the lesion. Loss of vision in one eye indicates that the problem is anterior to the chiasm; hemianopic field defects in both eyes that it is post chiasmal (Fig. 6.13, p. 200). Patients often state that they cannot see out of the right eye when they cannot see the right side of the visual field (right hemianopia), and likewise those with a left hemianopia may equate this with loss of vision in the left eye. Scotomas or blind spots are often observed accurately by the patient, who will describe the defect in the field of vision.

DISORDERS
Causes of reduced visual acuity
• Uncorrected refractive errors
• Hazy media
• Retinal disease
• Optic nerve disease
• Psychological.

Diplopia. Patients may complain of double vision when they mean blurred vision. True double vision becomes single when one eye is covered. Sudden onset of double vision usually indicates a neurological problem (p. 202).

DISORDERS
Causes of diplopia
• Neurological disorders, e.g. disseminated sclerosis
• Muscle and neuromuscular junction disorders, e.g. myasthenia gravis
• Decompensating long-standing squint
• Refractive errors
• Incorrect spectacles
• Media opacities
• Macular disease.

Photopsia and haloes. Seeing flashes and zigzags of light is called photopsia. It occurs when the retina is stimulated by the vitreous tugging on it. Very similar sensations are noted in both eyes in migraine. Haloes are due to prismatic effects, usually water drops in the cornea or lens in corneal oedema or cataract.

Floaters. Seeing occasional small 'floaters' is physiological, but patients may be alarmed when they are first noticed. A sudden rush of many floaters or large black 'tadpoles' suggest a vitreous haemorrhage.

KEY POINTS

- Patients with eye and visual disorders are often very anxious.
- Sudden loss of vision is usually vascular.
- Sudden onset of diplopia is often neurological.
- Patients may mistake hemianopia for loss of vision in one eye.

THE EXAMINATION

The examination of the eye is an intrinsic component of every clinical consultation. The willingness of the patient to establish and maintain eye-to-eye contact may provide valuable information regarding the patient's personality. It may also indicate whether or not the clinician has achieved satisfactory rapport with the patient.

It is necessary to develop a routine for examining the eye. This chapter describes an effective sequence:

- *General inspection* to overview the external appearance and observe any behavioural characteristics.
- *Visual function*. Measurement of visual acuity and visual field and colour vision testing are best performed before dazzling the eye with lights.
- *Detailed inspection* of eyes using torch or slit lamp.
- *Pupil reactions*. These can be observed during the inspection.
- *Ocular movements*. This involves checking eye movements binocularly and uniocularly in all positions of gaze and carrying out cover/uncover test.
- *Ophthalmoscopy*. This includes dilated ophthalmoscopy if indicated.

Common abnormal findings are given in the Disorders box.

GENERAL INSPECTION

It is important to take time to overview the appearance of the face and head before making a detailed inspection of the eyes. An abnormal head posture suggests problems with ocular motility, asymmetry of the face or head or facial

DISORDERS
Common abnormal findings in eye disease
• Reduced visual acuity
• Abnormal visual field
• Red eyes
• Hazy media
• Squints
• Diplopia
• Abnormal pupil reactions
• Retinal haemorrhages and exudates
• Optic atrophy
• Papilloedema

dysmorphia can indicate developmental abnormalities, eczema can suggest the likelihood of associated allergic eye disease.

Observation of behaviour may suggest the clinical problem. Patients with severe eye pain often wear dark glasses or screen themselves from light. People with double vision may close one eye. People with restricted peripheral visual fields often have great difficulty going into a strange room and if there is a hemianopia may bump into objects on the blind side. When central vision is lost people may not make eye contact but look to one side of the person they are addressing.

VISUAL FUNCTION TESTS

All tests of visual function are best performed before any detailed eye examination.

Visual acuity

Visual acuity (VA) is measured by testing the ability of the retinal cones to distinguish test objects, most commonly letters. It should be assessed at the beginning of an eye examination for several reasons. It ensures that the test is not forgotten, a common omission of potential medicolegal significance. As patients occasionally attribute visual loss to the eye examination itself, it is best to measure and record it at the start. The bright light of the ophthalmoscope and other optical instruments may dazzle the patient if it is used before testing vision.

Testing visual acuity

Distance visual acuity should be measured using distance spectacles if worn, with a Snellen chart at 6 metres (Fig. 7.1). Distance VA is recorded as two numbers written one over the other. The number on top is the distance between the patient and the test chart. This is usually 6 metres but may be 3 metres or less when vision is poor. The number below records the smallest line of letters read. Each line of letters on the Snellen chart is marked with a number – 60, 36, 24, 18, 12, 9 and 6. This represents the distance in metres at which a normally sighted person could read that line. Normal VA is written as 6/6, subnormal 6/9, etc. Vision of 6/9-6/12 is needed for driving. Vision of less than 3/60 is legal blindness. This figure indicates that the individual can not see the line at 3 metres which a normally sighted person could read at 60 metres.

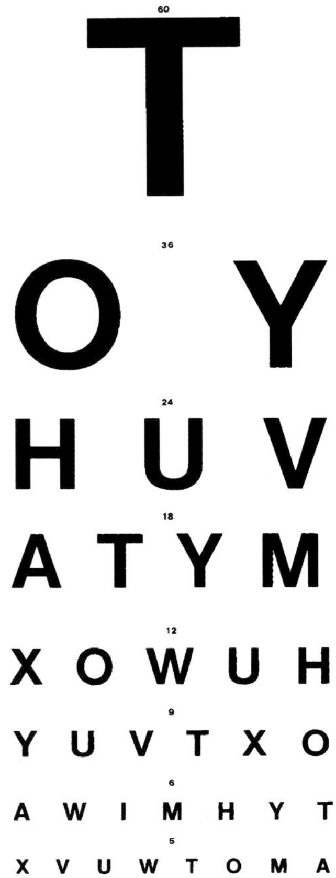

Fig. 7.1 Snellen test.

Other methods of testing VA are available for children and people who cannot read. Near vision is measured using standard near charts with the patient wearing reading glasses.

Examination sequence

- ☐ Test each eye separately, with patients wearing their distance glasses, and while ensuring that the other eye is totally occluded.

- ☐ If possible, use a line rather than single letters and use different letters for each eye, as patients, especially children, memorise quickly.
- ☐ If the vision is abnormal, check it again using a pinhole which partially corrects optic errors, though children and the elderly often find this difficult to use.
- ☐ If VA is less than 6/60 repeat the test with the chart 3 metres away as 3/60, etc.
- ☐ If the vision is less than 3/60, ask the patient to count fingers held 1 metre from the face, to detect a moving hand or perceive light.
- ☐ Measure near vision in each eye using reading glasses and standard reading charts.
- ☐ If no near charts are available, use a newspaper and record the smallest print seen.

Colour vision

Tests of colour vision assess the function of the retinal cones and optic nerve. Ishihara plates are the most commonly used test. They consist of a series of plates in which coloured spots contain shapes which the patient is asked to pick out. Errors are made when colour vision is defective. Colour vision tends to fail early in a number of conditions. Abnormalities are found in:

- congenital red/green colour blindness, which is carried on the X chromosome and affects 7% of males
- age-related macular disease
- optic nerve disease.

Visual fields

Testing fields assesses the function of the peripheral and central retina, the optic pathways and the cortex. The normal field extends 160° horizontally and 130° vertically with a blind spot 15° from fixation in the temporal field.

Defects in fields are described as central or peripheral. A scotoma is a field defect surrounded by a seeing area. Lesions anterior to the chiasm cause binocular field defects only if both eyes or optic nerves are affected.

DISORDERS
Causes of abnormal visual fields
• Glaucoma
• Retinitis pigmentosa
• Age-related macular disease
• Cerebrovascular disease
• Carotid vascular disease
• Brain tumours
• Trauma

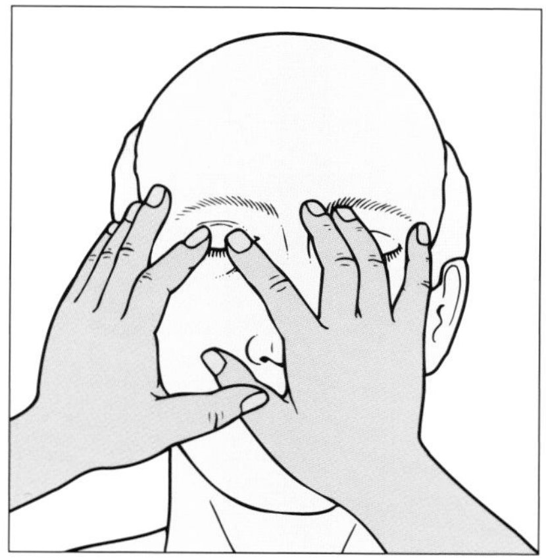

Fig. 7.2 Testing intraocular tension.

Central scotomas involve fixation and are characteristic of diseases affecting the macula and the axons leading from it.

Centrocaecal scotomas lie between fixation and the physiological blind spot and occur in toxic optic neuropathy. *Ring scotomas* forming a circular defect around fixation are typical of retinitis pigmentosa; *arcuate scotomas* are characteristic of glaucoma. Both may progress to 'tunnel vision' with extensive loss of visual field almost to fixation.

Altitudinal hemianopia is loss of the upper or lower field in one eye, common in vascular disease of the optic nerve.

Posterior to the chiasm, lesions result in binocular field defects and are discussed in Chapter 6 (p. 200).

Examination of visual fields can be carried out at the bedside by confrontation (Fig. 6.10). The technique is described on page 199. An accurate and permanent record of visual fields can be made using a perimeter. Patients unable to cooperate with confrontation testing are not suitable for perimetry.

DETAILED INSPECTION

Examination sequence

- ☐ Observe any behavioural characteristics
- ☐ Stand back a little to overview the head, face and eyes, inspecting them from the front, side and above.
- ☐ Note abnormal head postures, asymmetry, prominent or squinting eyes, bony abnormalities – anything which looks out of the ordinary.
- ☐ Inspect the eyes closely using a pen torch.
- ☐ Assess the pupillary reactions to light and accommodation.
- ☐ Evert both lids to examine the palpebral conjunctiva and the fornix.
  - Pull down the lower lid while the patient looks up.

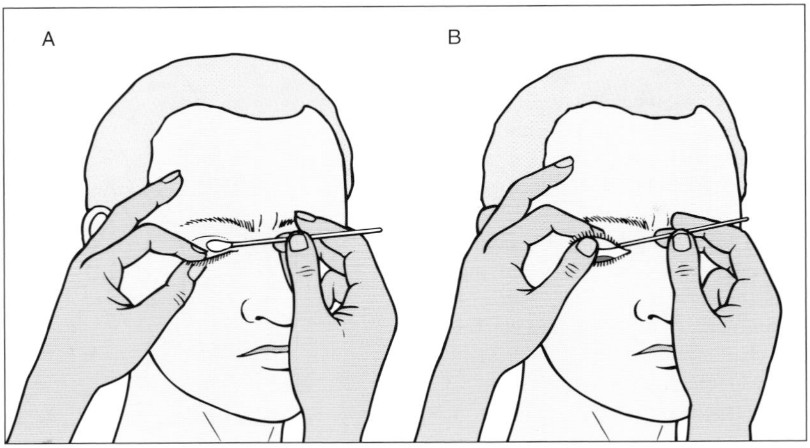

Fig. 7.3 Everting the upper lid.

- To evert the upper lid ask the patient to look down, grasp the lashes, press gently on the upper border of the tarsal plate with a cotton tip and swing the lashes up (Fig. 7.3).

☐ Make a rough estimation of intraocular pressure by fluctuating the eye gently with the index finger (Fig. 7.2). Accurate measurements are made with a tonometer.

☐ Use slit lamp microscopy for detailed inspection of the eye.

COMMON ABNORMALITIES

Eyelids

The lids normally cover the upper and lower margins of the iris. The palpebral fissures should be symmetrical. The palpebral aperture is narrowed in blepharospasm (spasm of the eyelids) and photophobia (light sensitivity), which are often associated with painful eye conditions. Photophobia also occurs in migraine and in association with meningeal irritation.

Ptosis (upper lid drooping) can be due to congenital or acquired levator palpebrae paresis (third nerve palsy), or to sympathetic paresis (Horner's syndrome, Fig. 6.9, p. 198).

Lid retraction, with widening of the palpable aperture, is obvious when sclera is visible above and below the iris (Fig. 7.4). It occurs in hyperthyroidism, usually with a lag of the upper lid on looking down (lid-lag) and when the eye is pushed forward (proptosed) by retrobulbar tumours or inflammation. Proptosis is also called exophthalmos. It is common in auto-immune thyroid disease. The periorbital tissues are loose and the lids swell easily. Periorbital oedema occurs commonly in congestive heart failure, glomerulonephritis, hypersensitivity reactions and thyroid

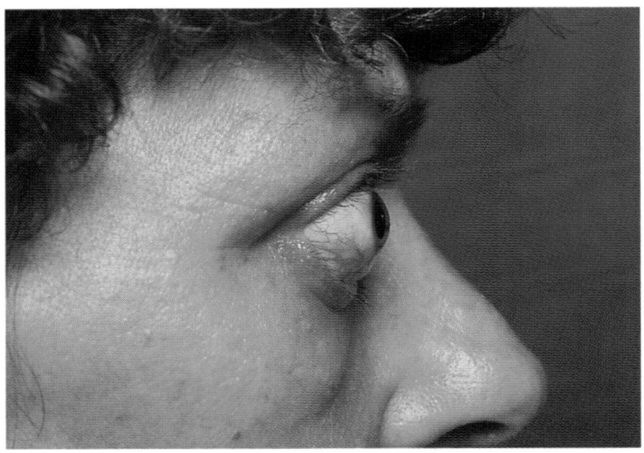

Fig. 7.4 Proptosis and lower lid retraction in dysthyroid eye disease.

disease. There may be associated conjunctival oedema (chemosis).

The lids may turn in (*entropion*) (Fig. 7.5), causing corneal damage, or out (*ectropion*), causing watering. Both malpositions occur in the lax tissues of the elderly but can also result from conjunctival or skin scarring respectively.

Common lumps on the lids include styes (microabscesses of lash follicles), tarsal cysts (pea-like swellings of the tarsal glands) and rodent ulcers (basal cell carcinoma).

Lacrimal apparatus

The lacrimal gland secretes tears. It is situated under the lateral part of the upper lid and is visible on lid eversion. The tears drain away through the lacrimal puncta and canaliculi in the medial edge of both eyelids. The lacrimal

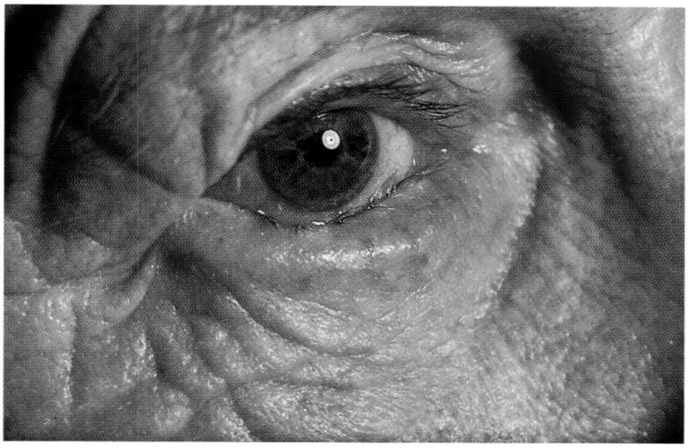

Fig. 7.5 Senile entropion of the lower lid.

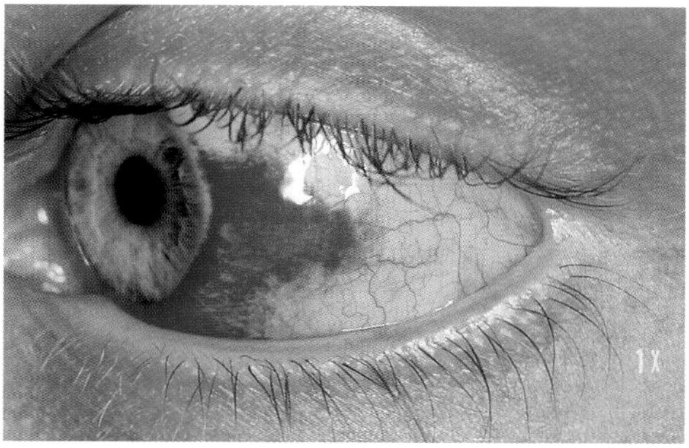

Fig. 7.6 Subconjunctival haemorrhage.

sac lies between the medial canthus and the nose. It may enlarge in viral infections such as mumps, granulomatous conditions like sarcoidosis or malignancy such as lymphoma or carcinoma. Damage to the secretomotor part of the lacrimal nerve or to the gland itself causes a dry eye with associated corneal problems. Blockage of the nasolacrimal duct causes watering, sticky discharge and may result in acute dacryocystitis with abscess formation in the lacrimal sac. Blocked tear ducts are most common in infants and in the elderly.

Conjunctiva

Conjunctival inflammation (conjunctivitis) is common and causes a red eye with the injection maximal towards the fornix (the fold between globe and lid). Other causes of a red eye are shown in the Disorders box. Conjunctivitis is often accompanied by photophobia and excessive lacrimation. Infective causes are associated with a sticky yellow discharge which glues the lashes together. Lymph follicles may be seen as sago-like lumps on the tarsal conjunctiva and are particularly characteristic of chlamydial conjunctivitis. Allergic inflammation is characterised by itch, a white discharge and conjunctival oedema (*chemosis*). Other causes of chemosis include alcoholism, chronic respiratory failure and superior vena cava obstruction.

Subconjunctival haemorrhage (Fig. 7.6) causes an alarming bright-red splash of blood which usually occurs spontaneously but may appear in whooping cough or labour or as a result of local trauma or bleeding disorders. *Pingueculae* are triangular yellow deposits beneath the conjunctiva between the canthus and the edge of the cornea. They develop with advancing years and are of no clinical significance. *Pterygium* is a triangular fold of conjunctiva in the same area which may encroach upon the cornea, particularly in tropical countries. Foreign bodies stuck under the upper lid cause severe irritation and photophobia. They are easily removed on everting the lid.

Sclera

Normal sclera is white, often with small brown spots of pigmentation marking perforating blood vessels in the elderly. The sclera are yellow in jaundice (Fig. 2.3B, p. 26). In osteogenesis imperfecta and severe iron deficiency anaemia the sclera are thin and appear blue (Fig. 2.1A, p. 25). Inflammation (*scleritis*) causes a dusky red colour, severe eye pain and tenderness. It is often a feature of connective tissue disease. The condition scleromalacia may also be found in rheumatoid arthritis and may rarely progress to perforation (scleromalacia perforans).

Cornea

Normal cornea is transparent with blood vessels only at the limbus, the junction between cornea and conjunctiva. General loss of transparency and lustre occurs in corneal oedema and extensive epithelial damage. Acute glaucoma characteristically causes corneal oedema. Extensive damage to the

DISORDERS
Causes of red eyes
• Trauma
• Subconjunctival haemorrhage
• Conjunctivitis
• Keratitis
• Acute glaucoma
• Uveitis.

corneal epithelium occurs in advanced exophthalmos, chemical corneal injuries, vitamin A deficiency and severe dry eye syndrome, which may be associated with connective tissue disease (Sjögren's syndrome), or occur as part of the sicca syndrome. More localised corneal haze is often caused by trauma with foreign bodies or ulcers due to infection, the herpes simplex virus being a common cause. Damage to the epithelium may be difficult to see but can be detected by instilling yellow fluorescein drops, which stain the affected area.

The blood vessels around the limbus dilate in response to corneal disease or injury (an appearance known as ciliary flush). They may also invade the cornea when they are visible as a little leash growing from the limbus with surrounding haze.

Corneal arcus is a white ring near the outer margin of the cornea. In elderly subjects it is common and of no clinical significance. In younger patients it may indicate hypercholesterolaemia.

A *Kayser-Fleischer* ring is a yellow or brown deposit of copper at the periphery of the cornea found in Wilson's disease (hepatolenticular degeneration). *Corneal calcification* at the medial and lateral aspects of the corneoscleral junction suggests long-standing hypercalcaemia.

Loss of corneal sensation is associated with V nerve lesions (p. 204). An insensitive cornea (Fig. 7.7) is very vulnerable to trauma and infection and may need to be protected with a shield or by a tarsorrhaphy (artificial closure of the lids).

Iris

Heterochromia (different colours of the irides) may indicate intraocular disease. In inflammation (*iritis*) the iris looks muddy with a small pupil and there is ciliary flush. Iritis may be a manifestation of systemic disease.

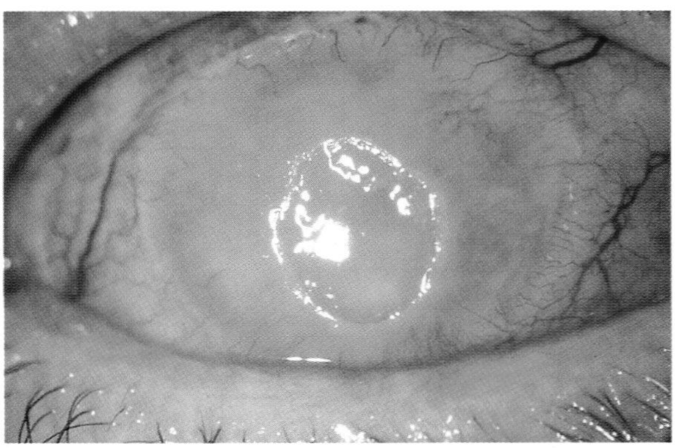

Fig. 7.7 Loss of transparency, ulceration and vascularisation in an insensitive cornea.

Lens

The normal lens is not visible on inspection. Advanced cataracts can be seen as a milky whiteness in the pupil.

Intraocular pressure

This is low in dehydration and high in glaucoma.

PUPIL REACTIONS

Normal pupils are round, regular and nearly equal in size. They are miotic (constricted) in infancy, old age, bright light, sleep and convergence. They are mydriatic (dilated) in excitement and in the dark. When light is directed at one pupil, it constricts (direct light reflex), as does the other pupil (consensual light reflex). When the eyes converge both pupils constrict (accommodative reflex). A detailed description of the pupillary reflexes and their examination is given in Chapter 6. Normal pupils are often described as PERLA in case notes (pupils equal and reactive to light and accommodation). Table 7.2 lists some examples of pupil abnormalities.

Ocular movements

The eyes are normally parallel in all positions of gaze except convergence. When they are not, a squint is present. Squints may be associated with paresis of one of the extraocular muscles (paralytic or inconcomitant squint) or with defective binocular vision (non-paralytic or concomitant squints).

Acquired paralytic squints cause diplopia, the images being maximally separated and squint greatest in the direction of action of the paretic muscle. Congenital and long-standing paralytic squints often result in abnormal head postures with the head turned or tilted to minimise the diplopia.

Concomitant squints are the same in all positions of gaze. They usually become manifest in childhood (Fig. 7.8) when they are not associated with diplopia, as this symptom is suppressed centrally in young children. Central suppression causes amblyopia (lazy eye).

Eye movements should be examined by:

- Testing movements in all positions of gaze (pp. 201–2). Both eyes should move symmetrically with no diplopia. If diplopia is present, the most peripheral double image is the one from the paretic eye (Fig. 7.9).
- *The cover test.* The cover/uncover test is particularly helpful in detecting small concomitant squints in children.

Examination sequence

☐ Ask the patient to look at a distant object.
☐ Cover one eye.

TABLE 7.2 Pupil abnormalities

Cause	Appearance	Reaction
Retinal/optic nerve disease	Abnormal > normal side	*Afferent pupil defect* Poor direct light reaction, normal consensual reaction and normal accommodative reaction on affected side Reduced consensual reaction on normal side
Neurosyphilis causing pretectal lesion	Small, irregular, unequal	*Argyll Robertson pupils* No reaction to light Normal reaction to accommodation
III nerve palsy Parasympathetic blocking drops	Abnormal > normal side	*Efferent pupil defect* No reaction to light or accommodation Normal side reacts consensually
Ciliary ganglion lesion	Abnormal > normal side	*Holmes–Adie (myotonic) pupil* No reaction to light Slow, sustained reaction to accommodation
Sympathetic lesion	Abnormal < normal side	*Horner's* Reacts to light/accommodation Does not dilate with cocaine drops
Inflammation of iris	Abnormal < normal side Festooned	Poor/absent reaction to light/accommodation Other pupil reacts consensually
Iris ischaemia in acute glaucoma	Abnormal > normal side	No reaction to light/accommodation Other pupil may not react consensually

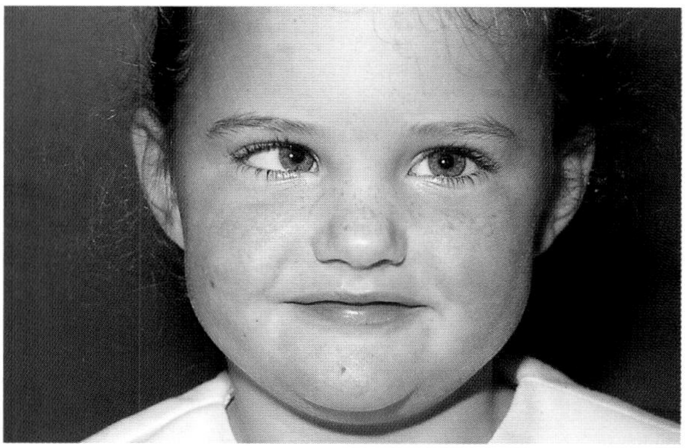

Fig. 7.8 Concomitant right convergent squint in a child.

☐ Closely observe the uncovered eye for any movements. If it moves to take up fixation, that eye was squinting.
☐ Repeat the sequence for the other eye.

OPHTHALMOSCOPY

Ophthalmoscopy can be used to:

- detect opacities in the media
- estimate optical errors
- examine the fundus (the back) of the eye.

Technique

The direct ophthalmoscope is the most commonly used instrument. It provides a 15× magnified upright image of the retina. A beam of light from the instrument is deflected by a mirror into the patient's eye, illuminating the retina, which the clinician observes through a hole in the mirror. Lenses can be rotated into place to compensate for short sight (myopia) or long sight (hypermetropia) in examiner and/or patient (Figs 7.10 and 7.11).

Learning to use the ophthalmoscope successfully takes a lot of practice. Rough handling, prolonged dazzling, poking the eye with the ophthalmoscope and garlicky breath do not help patient cooperation! The key points are summarised in Table 7.3 and the techniques illustrated in Figures 7.12 and 7.13.

Ophthalmoscopy is much easier through a dilated pupil. Dilatation is essential in infants and children and for accurate examination of the periphery and macula and is

TABLE 7.3 Keys points for successful ophthalmoscopy

- Practice
- Dark room
- Bright opththalmoscope light
- Correct position of patient
- Correct position of examiner
- Correct use of eye and hand
- Dilating drops if possible

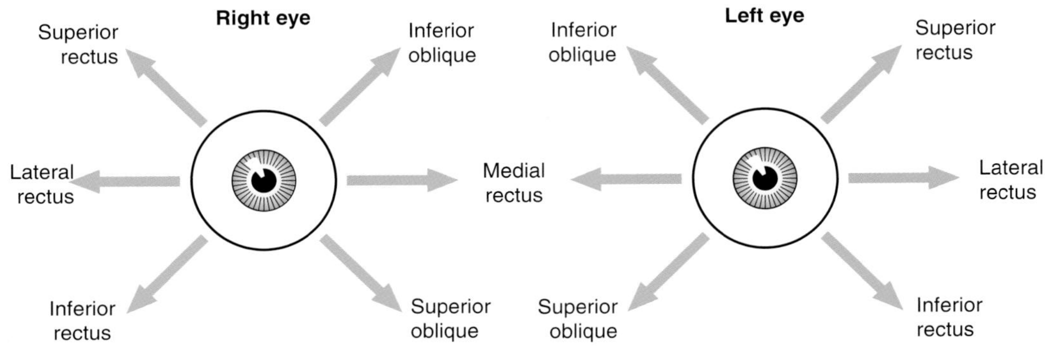

Fig. 7.9 Fields of actions of pairs of extraocular muscles. This diagram will help to work out which eye muscle is paretic. For example, a patient whose diplopia is maximum on looking down and to the right has either a weak right inferior rectus or a weak left superior oblique. Cover one of the patient's eyes and ask which image disappears – the most peripheral image comes from the affected eye.

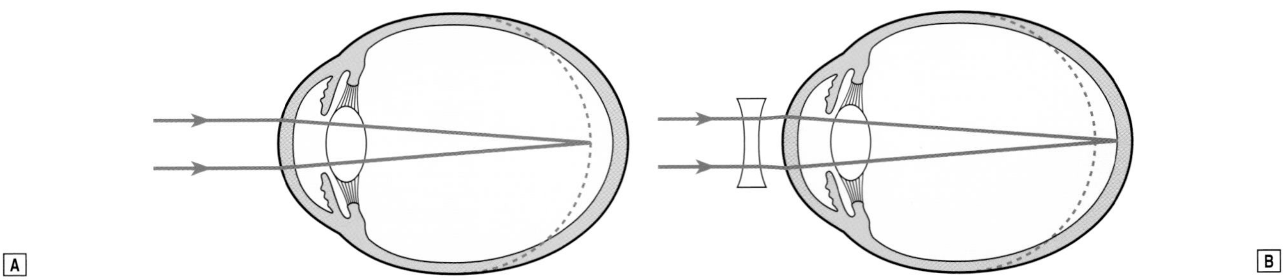

Fig. 7.10 The myopic (short-sighted) eye. A The eye is too long and the retina is not in focus when no lens is used. B The use of a concave (minus) lens brings the retina into focus.

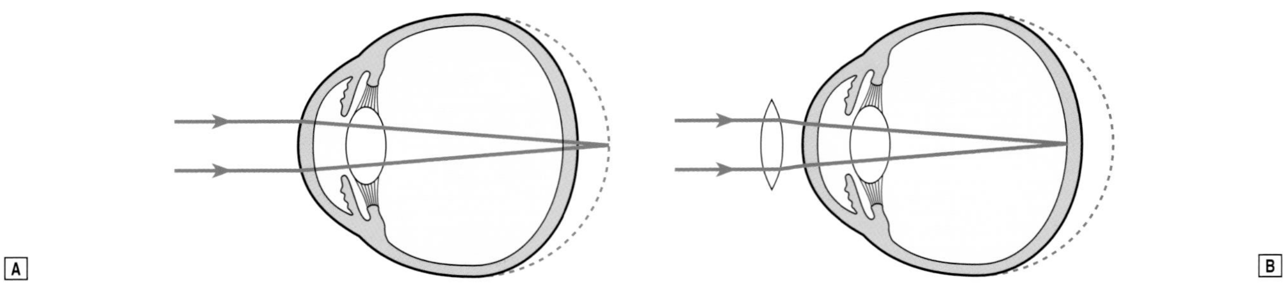

Fig. 7.11 The hypermetropic (long-sighted) eye. A The eye is too short and the retina is not in focus when no lens is used. B The use of a convex (plus) lens brings the retina into focus.

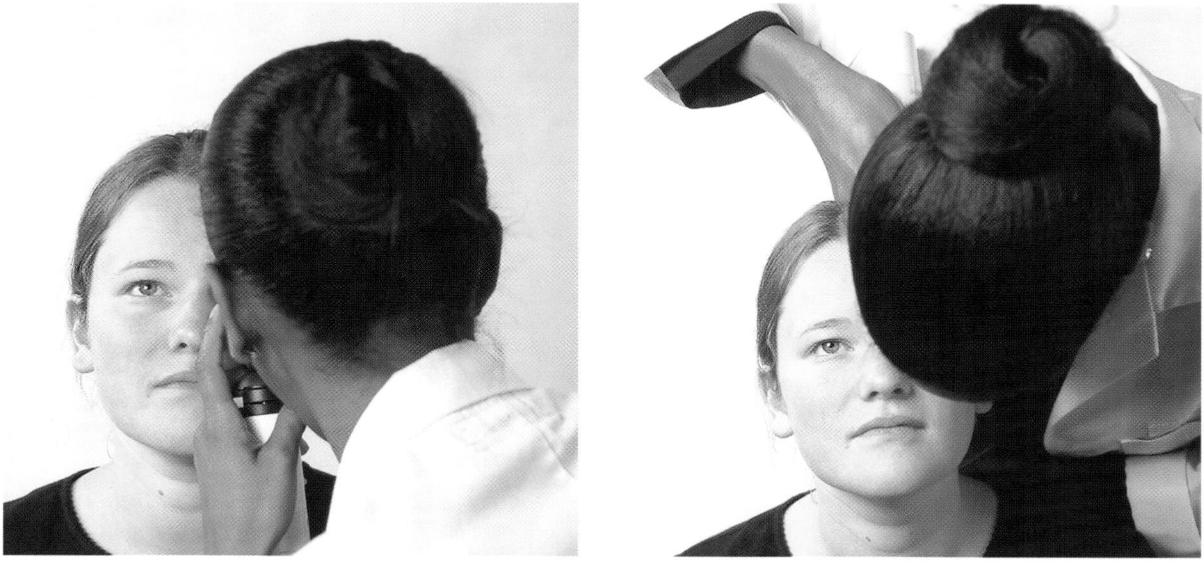

A B

Fig. 7.12 Ophthalmoscopy: correct methods. [A] The patient's gaze can be fixed on a distant point. [B] Using the right (dominant) eye to inspect the patient's left eye from above by an examiner who has difficulty in using the left eye. The patient's gaze is not obstructed.

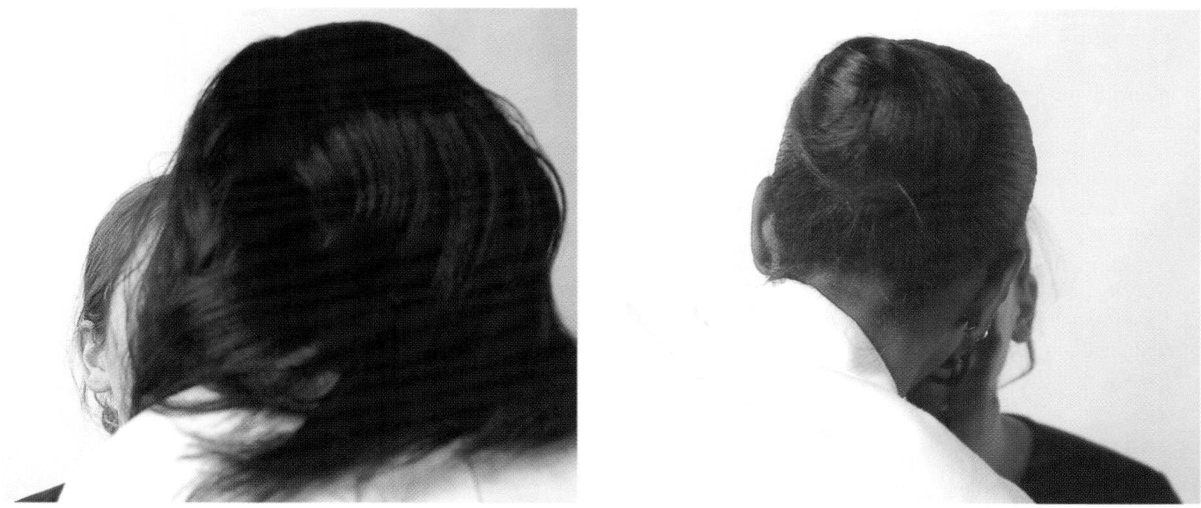

A B

Fig. 7.13 Ophthalmoscopy: incorrect methods. [A] The clinician is using her right eye to examine the patient's left eye but the view is obstructed by hair. [B] The clinician is using her right eye to examine the patient's left eye, thereby obscuring the patient's view.

advised when screening for diabetic retinopathy. The pupils should not be dilated when intracranial pathology requires pupillary monitoring. There is a very small risk of precipitating angle closure glaucoma by dilating eyes with shallow anterior chambers. Patients should be warned that after dilatation vision will be slightly blurred and easily dazzled, that driving and reading may be affected and that medical advice is required should prolonged blur, haloes or eye pain occur. Tropicamide 0.5% drops are recommended as they work in 20 minutes and wear off in 8 hours. Pilocarpine drops should not be used to constrict the pupil after the examination; they cause eyeache, blurring and do not protect against glaucoma. It is important to record pupil reactions before instilling drops and to note the drops used.

Examination sequence for ophthalmoscopy

- ☐ Use a dark room and effective ophthalmoscope batteries.
- ☐ Ask the patient to look at a distant object and blink and breathe normally.
- ☐ Stand or sit on the side to be examined an arm's length from the patient and with eyes level with the patient's.
- ☐ To look at the right eye, hold the ophthalmoscope with the lenses at zero in the right hand.
- ☐ Use the right eye to examine the patient's right eye (and use the left eye while examining the patient's left eye).
- ☐ If the examiner has difficulty using the non-dominant eye, examine the patient from above to permit the patient to continue to fix on a distant object (Fig. 7.12B).
- ☐ Switch on the instrument and shine it at the pupil, angling it slightly towards the nose.
- ☐ If the eye closes, open it gently.
- ☐ Demonstrate the red reflex and note the nature of any opacities in the media, which will be outlined black against the glow.
- ☐ Keeping the beam pointing in the same slightly nasal direction and the red reflex in view, move close to the patient, stopping just clear of the lashes.
- ☐ Steady the instrument by resting the middle and ring fingers of the right hand against the patient's cheek.
- ☐ The optic nerve (disc) should now be in view because of the angle of approach. If, instead of the disc, retinal blood vessels are seen, the 'arrow' made at bifurcations points to the disc.
- ☐ If the image is out of focus, use the index finger of the right hand to rotate the lens wheel until the view is clear.
- ☐ Examine the fundus systematically.
- ☐ Note any abnormality as though the fundus were a clock with the disc at the centre. The disc diameter (1.5 mm) is used as the unit of measurement, e.g. 'haemorrhage at 6 o'clock two disc diameters from disc'.
- ☐ Examine the macula last; it is difficult to see through an undilated pupil. Use a narrow beam and ask the patient to look straight at the light.

Opacities in the media

The ocular media (cornea, aqueous, lens and vitreous) are normally clear. Any opacities are noted when observing the red reflex. Dense opacities completely obscure the reflex – an example is advanced cataract. The depth of the opacity can be determined by moving the ophthalmoscope. Corneal opacities move in the opposite direction, lens opacities stay still and vitreous opacities move in the same direction.

Refractive errors

Providing the examiner does not have an uncorrected refractive error, the lenses required to focus on the patient's retina give an indication of any optical abnormality.

DISORDERS
Causes of hazy media
• Corneal dryness
• Corneal scarring
• Cataract
• Vitreous haemorrhage
• Uveitis.

Myopia. Minus (concave) lenses are required. In high myopia it may not be possible to focus on the retina unless patients wear their glasses. The optic disc often looks abnormal in high myopia, appearing very large and pale with surrounding chorioretinal atrophy (Fig. 7.14).

Hypermetropia. Plus (convex) lenses are required. The discs may look pink and slightly swollen (pseudopapilloedema).

Astigmatism. When severe, the refractive error cannot be fully corrected with the ophthalmoscope. The disc may look distorted.

The normal fundus

Retina

The colour of the retina varies considerably according to skin pigmentation, from reddish black in those with black skin to pale pink in albinos (Fig. 7.15). Retinal pigment is often clumped, giving a tigroid appearance. Large choroidal vessels are visible if pigment is very sparse. The normal macula lies temporal to the disc within the vascular arcades,

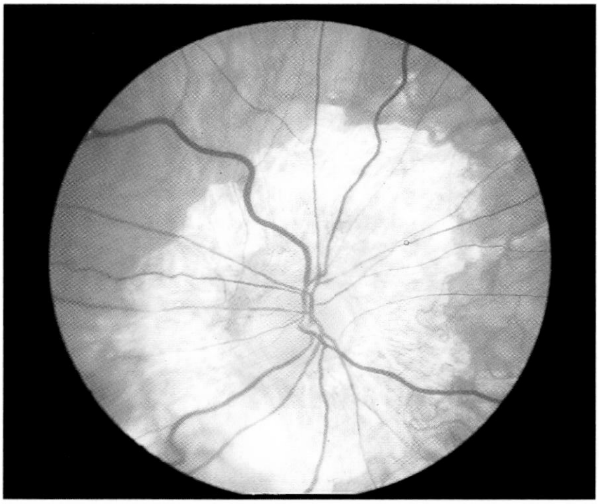

Fig. 7.14 Highly myopic disc.

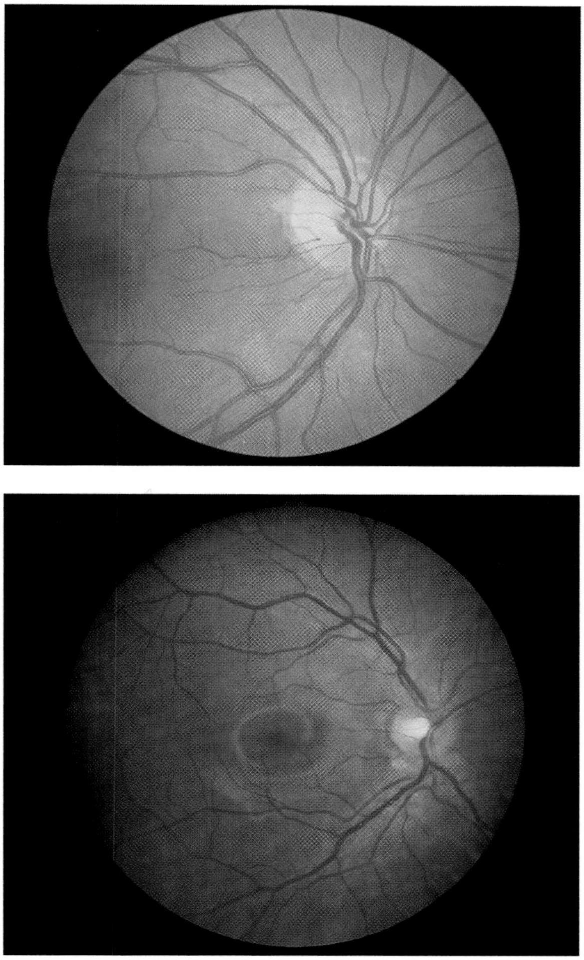

Fig. 7.15 Normal fundus. A Caucasian; B Asian.

is darker than the rest of the retina and has a shiny central (foveal) reflex. There are normally no deposits in the retina.

Optic disc

The optic disc is pink with slight temporal pallor. The margin is well demarcated except nasally. Quite commonly there is a surrounding pigment rim or partial white crescent of exposed sclera. The optic cup is paler than the rest of the disc and varies in depth and size but the diameter should not exceed more than 50% of the disc.

Blood vessels. The bifurcation of the central artery and vein are visible at the disc. A transmitted physiological pulsation of the vein may be present; arterial pulsation is abnormal. The upper and lower branches of the artery divide into nasal and temporal arterioles (lacking internal

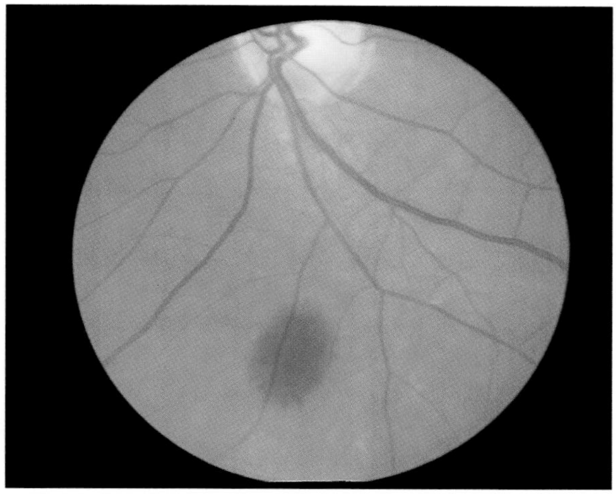

Fig. 7.16 Benign melanoma at 6 o'clock two disc diameters from the disc.

elastic lamina) with corresponding venous tributaries. The arterioles have a smaller calibre than the veins and are a brighter red. Healthy vessel walls are invisible.

The abnormal fundus

Retinal atrophy

Old injuries and inflammation result in atrophic scars. The white sclera is exposed and there is often surrounding hyperpigmentation. White patches of atrophic retina also occur in congenital coloboma, high myopia and retinal degeneration.

Abnormal pigmentation

The commonest pigmentary abnormality is that associated with age-related macular degeneration in which retinal pigment epithelial changes cause hypopigmentation and pigment clumping at the macula. Central vision is poor.

Benign choroidal melanomas are flat dark lesions (Fig. 7.16). Malignant melanomas are raised, enlarge progressively and often metastasise.

Retinitis pigmentosa is associated with pigment deposits shaped like bone spicules.

Abnormal deposits

Hard exudates. These are well-defined, yellowish-white deposits in the retina, often arranged in rings. They are caused by lipoproteins leaking out of an abnormally permeable blood vessel, which may be visible in the centre of the ring. At the macula they tend to accumulate in a star

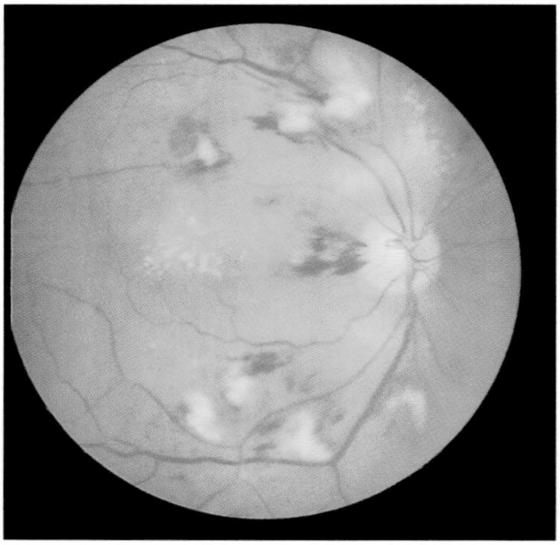

Fig. 7.17 Retinal soft exudates, flame haemorrhages and early macular star of hard exudate in hypertensive diabetic patient.

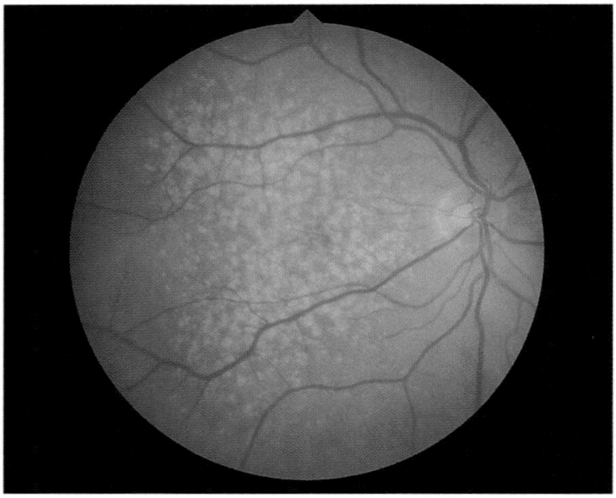

Fig. 7.18 Colloid bodies at the macula.

shape because of the unique horizontal arrangement of the deep retinal layers around the fovea (Fig. 7.17). They are commonly seen in hypertension, diabetes and following retinal vascular occlusions.

Soft exudates. These look like deposits of cotton wool in the superficial retina. They occur around areas of infarcted retina and may be associated with other features of retinal ischaemia (venous dilatation, haemorrhages and new blood vessels). They are due to swelling of the nerve fibre layer axons (Fig. 7.17).

Colloid bodies. These may be mistaken for hard exudates. They are small, round yellow deposits in the deepest retinal layer appearing most commonly in the elderly and around the macula (Fig. 7.18).

Other abnormal deposits include foci of active chorioretinal inflammation, metastatic infections (e.g. CMV, miliary tuberculosis) and carcinomas.

Congenital abnormalities of the optic nerve

Examples include myelinated nerve fibres (Fig. 7.19) and persistent hyaloid artery remnants. The appearance in refractive errors has already been mentioned.

Glaucoma

A larger and deeper than normal cup suggests glaucoma (Fig. 7.20). Such a finding is an indication for measuring intraocular pressure by tonometry.

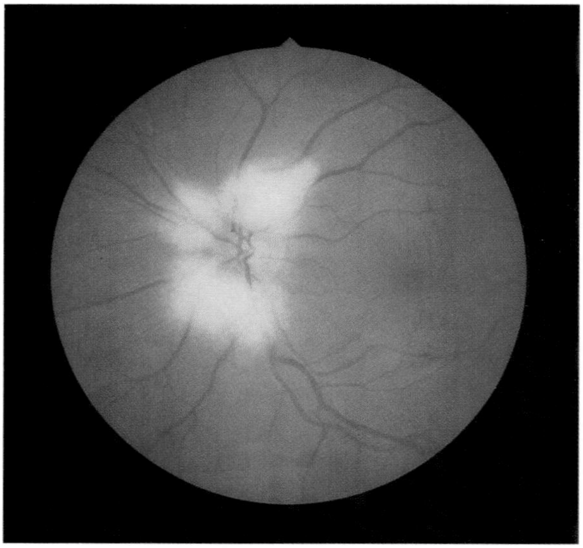

Fig. 7.19 Myelinated nerve fibres.

Optic atrophy

An atrophic optic disc is pale. Subtle changes are hard to interpret – it is helpful to compare the two discs, as marked asymmetry in colour is significant. The terms primary, secondary and consecutive optic atrophy are confusing and are best avoided. Optic atrophy is usually associated with decreased vision and afferent pupillary defects. It is not a diagnosis but a sign. Glaucomatous optic atrophy is illustrated in Fig. 7.20. The Disorders box lists the causes.

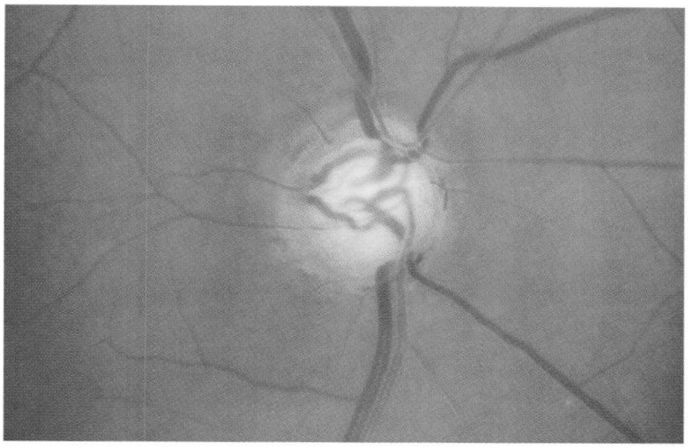

Fig. 7.20 Optic disc atrophy and cupping in glaucoma.

DISORDERS
Causes of optic atrophy
• Inherited, e.g. Leber's optic atrophy
• Toxic, e.g. methanol poisoning
• Glaucoma
• Extensive retinal disease
• Ischaemic optic neuropathy
• Demyelinating disease
• Trauma, e.g. avulsion of optic nerve
• Tumours, e.g. pituitary adenoma, craniopharyngioma.

Papilloedema

Swelling of the disc is called papilloedema. The swollen disc is pink with congested veins and surrounding small haemorrhages, the margins are blurred and the cup is lost (Fig. 7.21). It can be due to inflammation of the optic nerve head (papillitis) or to increased intracranial pressure or cerebral oedema (see Disorders box). In papillitis there is associated marked visual loss, an afferent pupil defect and the papilloedema is most likely to be unilateral. In increased intracranial pressure the vision is normal at first, papilloedema is most likely to be bilateral and there are other characteristic features such as headache and vomiting. In accelerated hypertension cerebral oedema and papilloedema are features.

DISORDERS
Causes of papilloedema
• Increased intracranial pressure
• Cerebral oedema
• Accelerated/malignant hypertension
• Optic nerve tumours
• Papillitis
• Pseudopapilloedema.

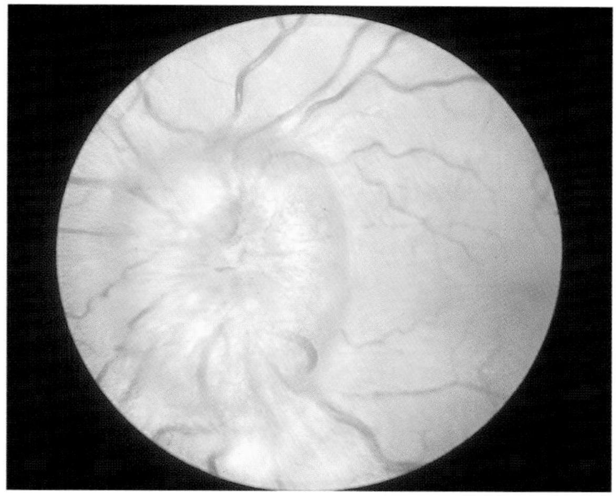

Fig. 7.21 Papilloedema.

Retinal vascular abnormalities

Haemorrhages. *Superficial retinal haemorrhages* are flame shaped because of tracking of blood along the horizontally arranged nerve fibres. They occur in hypertension (Fig. 7.17).

Deep haemorrhages are dark-red blots contained by the vertically arranged deep retinal layers. Microaneurysms look very similar. Both occur in the dots and blots of diabetic retinopathy (Fig. 7.22).

Preretinal haemorrhages obscure the underlying retina. Initially round, they form a flat-topped fluid level and may burst into the vitreous (Fig. 7.23). They may occur following subarachnoid haemorrhage or follow bleeding from retinal new vessels.

In *vitreous haemorrhage* the fundus view is hazy or absent and the red reflex abnormal. The blood may be distributed diffusely through the vitreous gel or form clots which cause tadpole-like floaters.

Choroidal haemorrhages are very dark red and often large with wavy margins. They occur in trauma and age-related choroidal vascular disease.

Retinal artery occlusion. Obstruction of the central retinal artery results in sudden, and often total, loss of vision. The retina is pale and swollen and the macula stands out a bright cherry red. In branch artery occlusion the affected

DISORDERS
Causes of retinal haemorrhages
• Diabetes
• Hypertension
• Trauma
• Retinal breaks
• Subarachnoid haemorrhage
• Retinal vein occlusions
• Sickle cell disease
• Anticoagulants
• Age-related macular disease.

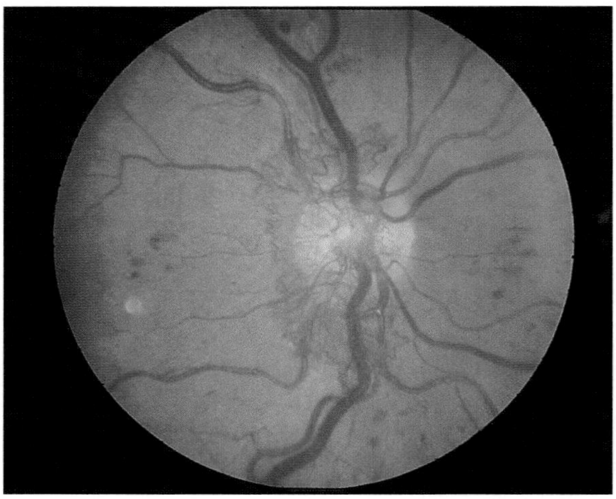

Fig. 7.22 Dots, blots and optic disc new vessels in proliferative diabetic retinopathy.

arteriole is attenuated and the corresponding retinal segment pale (Fig. 7.24). Emboli may be visible in the arterioles as shiny (cholesterol) or white (platelet) plaques. They may cause transient loss of vision (amaurosis fugax) as well as arterial occlusions.

Retinal vein occlusion. In central vein occlusion a little vision is retained. The ophthalmoscopic picture is a dramatic 'stormy sunset' with large flame haemorrhages and cotton wool spots splashed over the fundus (Fig. 7.25). In branch vein occlusion the same picture is confined to the affected segment and marked nipping often marks the site of the occluded vein.

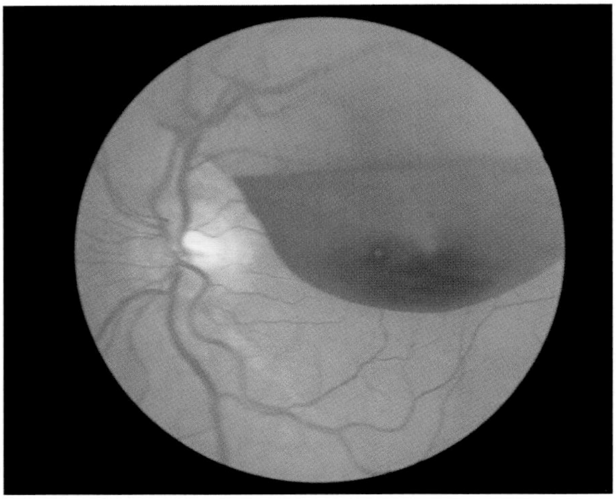

Fig. 7.23 Preretinal haemorrhage.

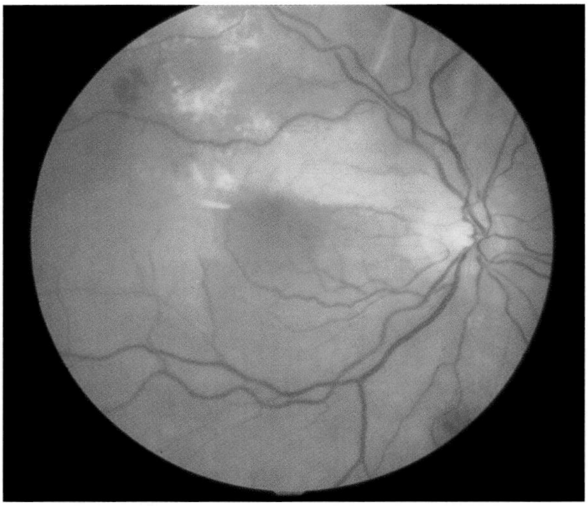

Fig. 7.24 Branch retinal artery occlusion showing retinal oedema above the macula and a cherry red spot.

Ischaemic optic neuropathy. Occlusion of the blood supply to the optic nerve head results in pale papilloedema. There is irreversible loss of sight. Giant cell arteritis is a common cause of ischaemic optic neuropathy.

Hypertension. Chronic hypertension leads to diffuse or segmental narrowing of the arteriolar blood column as the vessel walls thicken. In extreme sclerosis the sheathing of the vessel walls is visible. The thick-walled arterioles compress the veins at crossings, causing venous nipping.

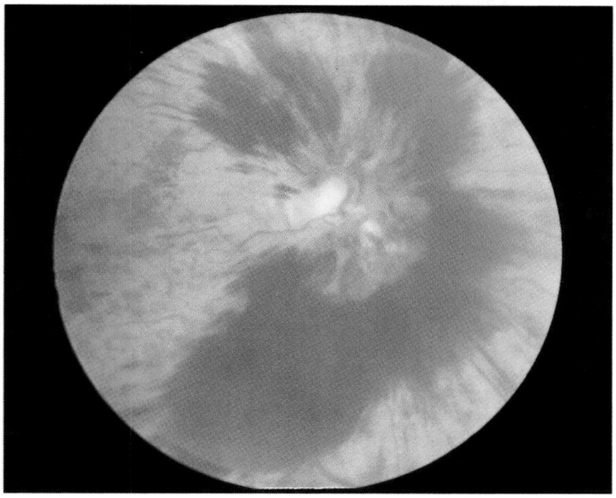

Fig. 7.25 Central retinal vein occlusion.

Flame haemorrhages, hard exudates and papilloedema are features of accelerated hypertension. Hypertension seldom affects vision.

Diabetic retinopathy. Microangiopathy affects the retinal capillaries in diabetes, leading to widespread capillary non-perfusion. Early (background) disease is characterised by dot and blot haemorrhages and microaneurysms; as capillary non-perfusion increases, signs of retinal ischaemia appear. These are cotton wool spots, venous dilatation and intra-retinal new vessels. Neovascularisation sprouting from the optic nerve and surface of the retina characterises proliferative retinopathy (Fig. 7.22). Blindness often follows.

CASE HISTORY

A 10-year-old boy hit his head in a fall from his bicycle. He did not lose consciousness but was thought to be concussed. A few days later he complained of double vision when trying to read.

On examination, he had adopted an abnormal head posture with a depressed chin and head tilt. Ocular movements showed defective depression of the left eye in adduction indicating a IV nerve palsy causing paresis of the superior oblique muscle. The visual acuity was normal but he had bilateral papilloedema which settled after a few days. A CAT scan excluded a subdural haematoma. The double vision did not improve, he was unable to ride his bike and could not see to read without prismatic lenses. Corrective squint surgery was required 18 months later.

Learning points

- Concussional head injury without loss of consciousness can cause serious contusional brain damage as shown in this case by papilloedema and the left IV nerve palsy.
- The diplopia on looking down associated with IV paresis is often not evident until some time after head injury when the patient is well enough to concentrate on reading and to get up and about.
- Apparently minor head injury can be associated with serious and long-term visual problems.

EXAMINATION OF INJURED EYES

It may be very difficult to inspect a painful or injured eye without an anaesthetic. Avoid forcing open an injured eye as pressure on an eye with an open wound may cause further damage. Local anaesthetic drops may relieve pain enough to allow the eye to open itself. In small children an examination under a general anaesthetic may be required.

EXAMINATION CHECKLIST

A normal eye examination can be carried out quickly using simple equipment and should conclude that:

- External inspection is normal.
- Vision in each eye is normal.
- Confrontation visual fields are full.
- Ocular movements are normal.
- Pupil reactions are normal.
- Optic discs are flat and of normal colour.
- Retinal vessels are normal.

KEY POINTS

- General observation and inspection should precede detailed eye examination.
- Visual acuity should always be measured.
- Ophthalmoscopy is easier through a dilated pupil.
- Pupil dilatation is contraindicated if neurological observations are required.

COMMON PITFALLS AND HOW TO AVOID THEM

- Listening to patients give their story in their own words is vital. Rushing into the examination without taking a careful history may be misleading. In many conditions affecting vision – for example, migraine and giant cell arteritis – the diagnosis is suggested by the history, and examination may be normal.
- It is common to focus too quickly on the details of the eye examination and neglect to make general observations about the patient's general behaviour and appearance, which can be very helpful.
- Visual function should always be checked. If the appropriate test charts are not available, distance vision in the eyes can be compared using print on notice boards, and a newspaper used to assess near vision.
- Very poor vision in one eye with no abnormal examination findings is often due to amblyopia, suggested by a previous

history of a squint, wearing patches or having a lazy eye at school.

- Serious eye disease, like diabetic retinopathy and glaucoma, can be asymptomatic until the sudden onset of blindness. All diabetic patients should be advised to have an eye examination annually and everyone over 40 should have an examination for glaucoma every 2 years.

FURTHER READING

Firth P, Gray R, Maclennan S, Ambler P 1994 The eye in clinical practice. Blackwell, Oxford

Huber M, Reacher M 1990 Clinical tests in ophthalmology. Wolfe, London

Kanski J 1994 Ophthalmology. Churchill Livingstone, Edinburgh

Khaw P T, Elkington A R 1994 ABC of eyes, 2nd edn. British Medical Journal, London

Murray P, Fielder A 1997 Pocket book of ophthalmology. Butterworth-Heinemann, Oxford

The locomotor system

8

P. J. ABERNETHY • N. P. HURST

THE HISTORY OF RHEUMATIC DISORDERS

The diagnostic process is partly intuitive and partly follows a simple algorithmic process. From an initial impression of the patient and the patient's story, the clinician starts to form a list of possible diagnoses. This is modified, revised or reinforced as the history (Table 8.1) and examination proceed. For the inexperienced diagnostician, following a simple routine provides a sound framework and reduces the apparent complexity of musculoskeletal symptoms, but with experience this will be modified and become increasingly efficient.

The principal clinical features of rheumatic disease are joint pain, stiffness and swelling, bone pain and muscle weakness. Since many rheumatic diseases follow an easily recognisable pattern, important information leading to a preliminary differential diagnosis, can be obtained by identifying the following:

- the joints which have been affected, whether monoarticular (single joint), oligoarticular (a few joints), or polyarticular (many joints) (Table 8.2)
- mode of onset and duration, i.e. acute, chronic, episodic or migratory
- day-to-day behaviour of symptoms, such as the presence or absence of morning stiffness and the response to physical activity
- whether the involvement is symmetrical or asymmetrical
- the presence of extra-articular inflammatory features, particularly in the skin and eyes.

Rheumatic symptoms may be the presenting complaint of systemic disorders, thus the patient's age, sex, general medical history and the immediate clinical context such as obvious ill health, may provide additional vital clues.

Pain

The patient may have difficulty localising the pain because musculoskeletal pain is often referred to sites well away from the site of pathology (somatic referral) (Table 8.3). The severity, type of onset (acute or insidious), diurnal variation and relation to physical activity should be assessed (Table 8.4). The severity of pain may be judged by the presence of night pain and sleep disturbance, but it is important to establish whether it is pain which is actually waking the patient or whether the patient is waking for some other reason. Persistent pain is also frequently associated with anxiety or lowered mood which may cause 'pain amplification'; allowance must therefore be made for this when interpreting the story.

TABLE 8.1 The history summarised

- Pattern of joint involvement
- Mode of onset
- Character of pain – relieving and exacerbating factors
- Stiffness – early morning and after immobility
- Extra-articular features
- Family history
- Social history
- General medical history
- Past medical history

TABLE 8.2 Some common anatomical patterns of rheumatic disease

Inflammatory disorders (synovitis)	
Polyarticular	
MCP, PIP and MTP joints*	RA,† SLE,† psoriasis
DIP joints	Psoriasis
Girdle joints	Polymyalgia rheumatica, RA
Oligoarticular	
Asymmetrical large joints or dactylitis (sausage digit)	Reactive arthritis, Reiter's syndrome, psoriasis or AS†
Monoarticular	
Acute	Gout, pseudogout, infection, psoriasis
Chronic	Psoriasis, RA, AS, chronic infection (e.g. TB)
Axial, sacroiliac and girdle joints	AS
Degenerative disorders (bony swelling ± synovitis)	
Polyarticular	
DIP or PIP joints and/or first CMC joint*	Nodal OA†
Monoarticular	
Chronic	OA
Axial joints	Lumbar or cervical spondylosis

* MCP, metacarpophalangeal; PIP, proximal interphalangeal; DIP, distal interphalangeal; MTP, metatarsophalangeal; CMC, carpometacarpal
† RA, rheumatoid arthritis; SLE, systemic lupus erythematosus; OA, osteoarthritis; AS ankylosing spondylitis

TABLE 8.3 Sites of somatic referral of joint pain

Cervical spine	to	Head or over shoulders
Lumbar spine	to	Buttocks/posterior thigh
Shoulder	to	Lateral aspect of upper arm
Elbow	to	Forearm
Hip	to	Anterior thigh or knee or both

TABLE 8.4 Assessing joint pain

- Mode of onset
- Variation with time
- Effect of activity
- Site and distribution
- Night pain
- Mood disturbance

Stiffness

This occurs with inflammatory and degenerative lesions but in inflammatory joint disease it is more marked and often shows a characteristic diurnal variation. It is worse after rising from bed for at least 30 minutes and may return at the end of the day. In severe cases the stiffness can persist throughout the day. Such patients also describe immobility stiffness or 'gelling' after periods of inactivity.

Swelling

A history of swelling should be sought but interpreted with caution. Swelling in the absence of trauma is suggestive, but not pathognomonic of inflammation. It is necessary to define the site of the swelling, and whether it is local or diffuse. Furthermore it is important to be aware that pain or sensory disturbance may give rise to the sensation of swelling (i.e. altered body image) without actual swelling being present. This may also be a feature of psychological disorders.

Weakness

This may occur as a result of joint disease but where weakness is the dominant presenting symptom it is highly suggestive of a myopathy.

Extra-articular or systemic features

Extra-articular features are often crucial in making a correct diagnosis of inflammatory joint disease and should be carefully sought in the history and examination (Fig. 8.1). The pattern of joint involvement, (e.g. polyarticular, oligoarticular, etc.) will usually suggest which extra-articular features should be sought (Table 8.5).

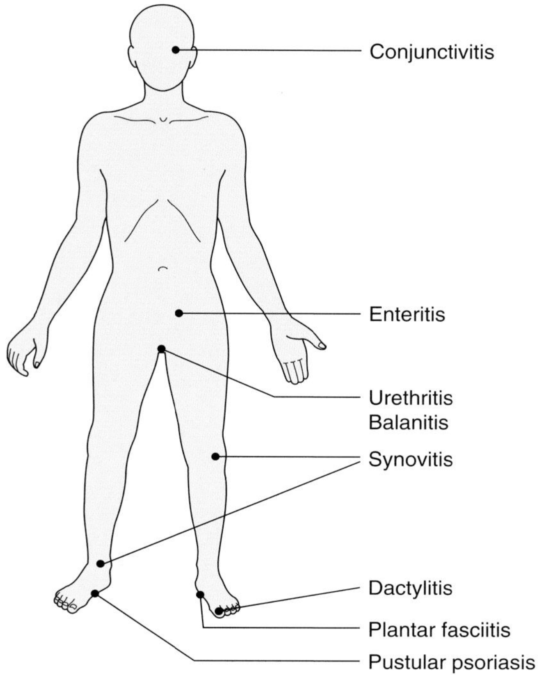

Fig. 8.1 Clinical features of reactive arthritis.

TABLE 8.5 Examples of extra-articular features associated with rheumatic disease

Disease	Non-articular features
Symmetrical polyarthritis	
RA	Subcutaneous nodules, Raynaud's phenomenon, sicca syndrome, pleurisy, episcleritis
SLE	Raynaud's phenomenon, serositis, alopecia, photosensitivity, rash, fever, episcleritis
Asymmetrical oligoarthritis	
Psoriatic arthritis	Psoriasis, nail dystrophy
Reactive arthritis (including Reiter's syndrome)	Urethritis, conjunctivitis, fever, penile ulcers, psoriasiform rash, iritis, mouth ulcers, diarrhoea, enthesitis (e.g. Achilles tendonitis, plantar fasciitis)
Ankylosing spondylitis	Iritis, enthesitis
Sarcoidosis	Erythema nodosum and hilar adenopathy
Monoarthritis	
Gout	Tophi, obesity, renal impairment
Septic arthritis	Fever, malaise, source (usually skin), throat

GUIDE TO THE FEATURES OF PAIN AND STIFFNESS ENCOUNTERED IN SPECIFIC CONDITIONS

Inflammatory arthritis

In acute lesions, such as osteomyelitis, septic arthritis or gout, the pain is severe and throbbing, disturbs sleep and prevents use of the limb or affected joint. When a joint is infected, any attempt at movement causes severe pain. In chronic inflammatory lesions, such as rheumatoid arthritis, there is diurnal variation of stiffness and pain.

Degenerative arthritis

The patient with peripheral or axial joint osteoarthritis will usually give a history of gradually increasing pain over months or years, with loss of movement of the joint. Early morning stiffness and pain is usually minimal but when present will usually settle with gentle use of the joint over approximately 15–30 minutes, but may return as the day progresses, with impairment of activities. In more severe cases, rest pain and night pain occur.

Psychogenic symptoms

The complaint of chronic polyarthralgia or myalgia, which is constant day and night and does not conform to any clear pattern, should raise the suspicion that this may be a somatic presentation of an underlying psychological or psychosocial problem, for which an explanation should be sought. Other clues include lack of objective abnormal clinical findings, such as reduced movement or joint swelling, and the prominence of features such as tiredness, lack of energy, change in mood, sleep patterns or appetite although such features may be the consequence of chronic pain.

Traumatic lesions

A sprained ligament is one which has been partially torn in response to trauma. Immediately after a sprain the pain may be severe and constant. Subsequently, pain only occurs with movement that stretches the damaged ligament and is relieved when the ligament is relaxed. A complete ligament tear may produce an unstable joint which becomes increasingly painful as the day progresses when the supporting muscles tire and the related ligaments stretch. At times there is a characteristic pattern of instability, e.g. following lateral ligament rupture of the ankle the hindfoot is subject to recurrent episodes of inversion.

GENERAL MEDICAL BACKGROUND, FAMILY AND SOCIAL HISTORY

The medical background may be important and a careful enquiry into past illnesses and medication often brings to light diagnostic clues, e.g. diuretics may precipitate gout. The family history may also be helpful (Table 8.6). The patient's domestic or working environment may be relevant to the patient's symptoms. Inability to hold a pen or tools, to kneel, stand for long periods or to use ladders may have profound social and economic consequences, particularly for those in manual or unskilled jobs.

TABLE 8.6 Conditions in which the family history may be diagnostically helpful

Diseases linked to the HLA-B27 tissue type – ankylosing spondylitis, iritis, reactive arthritis, weaker association with psoriasis, inflammatory bowel disease
Psoriasis – psoriatic genes may be expressed in either skin, joints or both in any order and at any time
Hypermobile joints – Marfan's syndrome, Ehlers–Danlos syndrome, benign familial hypermobility, floppy (prolapsing) mitral valve
Gout

Any patient with a significant rheumatic disorder should be assessed for the ability to perform the activities of daily living, i.e. ability to dress, wash, use a lavatory, walk, climb steps and do daily chores. Simple self-assessed questionnaires are available for this purpose (e.g. the Stanford Health Assessment Questionnaire).

CASE HISTORY

A 40-year-old female developed painful polyarthralgia involving the metacarpophalangeal (MCP) and proximal interphalangeal (PIP) joints of the fingers, the knees and forefeet. She felt unwell. On wakening in the morning she was stiff and took an hour to get dressed but her joint stiffness improved with gentle activity. As the day progressed her weight-bearing joints became more swollen. At night her sleep was disrupted by joint pain and she was often awakened in the early hours with numbness and diffuse pain in her hands, which only improved when she got out of bed. On questioning, there were no other extra-articular features such as Raynaud's phenomenon or rash. There was diffuse but mild periarticular swelling and she had reduced grip strength because of pain and stiffness.

Her age, and sex, and the polyarthralgia and stiffness associated with a systemic upset suggested the diagnosis of symmetrical inflammatory arthropathy such as rheumatoid arthritis or systemic lupus erythematosus. The additional symptoms are highly suggestive of carpal tunnel syndrome, probably secondary to wrist synovitis. Subsequent investigations confirmed the diagnosis of rheumatoid arthritis.

Learning point

- Polyarthralgia and diurnal stiffness with systemic symptoms suggest inflammatory arthropathy.

KEY POINTS

- Listen to the patient's story, and assess the impact of symptoms on the patient's normal function.
- Establish the precise site and distribution of pain and pattern of joints involved.
- Establish the variation of symptoms over time.
- Enquire about extra-articular features and family history if inflammatory joint disease is suspected.
- Remember that joint disease may be a manifestation of a general medical problem.

PHYSICAL EXAMINATION OF THE LOCOMOTOR SYSTEM

General inspection

The examination begins on first meeting the patient, with observation of the patient's overall posture, gait, ease of movement and demeanour. Guided by the history, a search for relevant non-articular features of joint disease and significant general medical abnormalities should be made.

TABLE 8.7 Physical examination – the principles

Anatomy	Bony, articular, ligamentous, tendinous, muscular or neurological
Inflammation	Tenderness, erythema, warmth, synovitis, effusion
Function	Range of movement and specific functions (e.g. walking, rising, power grip)
Complications	Deformity, instability, muscle wasting, calluses, extra-articular features

Aims of examination

The locomotor examination is aimed at identifying the site and type of pathology, loss of function and associated complications (Table 8.7). This is achieved by inspecting the joints, palpating them, observing their movement and performing specific manoeuvres to test the integrity and function of supporting structures.

Basic techniques

Inspection

In certain joints, such as the hip and shoulder, deformities may not be evident and have to be 'unmasked' during formal examination. The term valgus is used to describe deviation of the limb distal to the joint away from the midline (e.g. knock knee) and varus to describe deviation towards the midline (e.g. bow-leg).

Palpation

Joint line tenderness is present in articular disorders. Disorders of tendon, bursae, ligaments and their attachments (entheses) are associated with tenderness localised to the site of pathology.

Movement

Some joints, such as the subtalar joint of the hindfoot, which have limited movement, are most easily examined passively. Relatively immobile joints, including sternoclavicular, acromioclavicular, manubriosternal, costochondral and sacroiliac joints, have to be examined by palpation or stressing manoeuvres to elicit pain.

The neutral zero method of recording movement is recommended. All joints are considered to be in the neutral position when the body is in the classical anatomical position, with two exceptions, namely the hands are flat against the thighs in the sagittal plane and the feet are at right angles to the leg (Fig. 8.2).

A goniometer (Fig. 8.3) is helpful to assess joint movement or deformity and its response to therapy, particularly in the knee, hip and elbow. Quite wide individual variations in the normal range of movement are found with age.

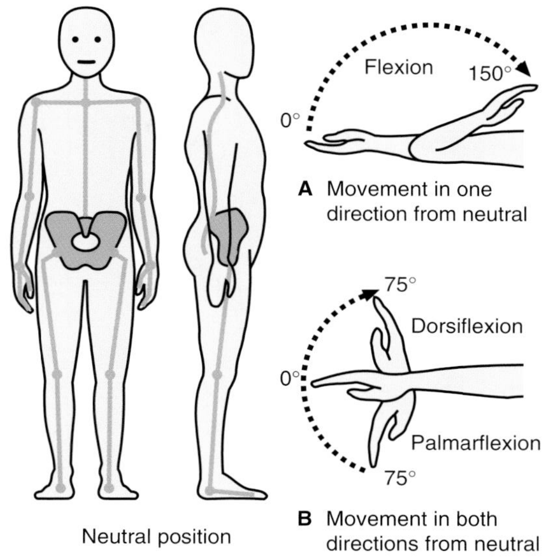

Fig. 8.2 Measuring movements of joints.

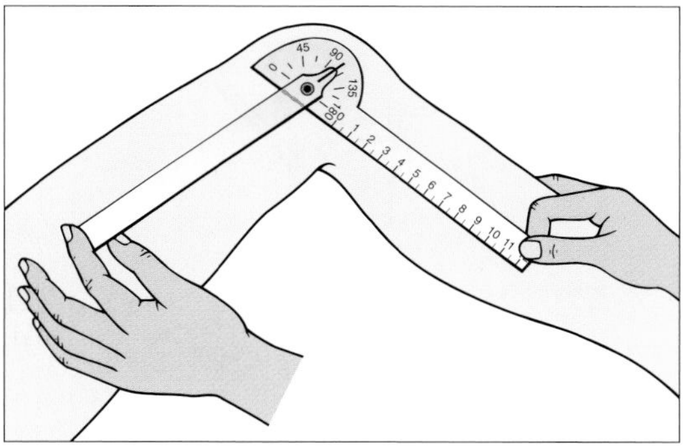

Fig. 8.3 Goniometer.

Examination sequence

- ☐ Inspect for swelling, local muscle wasting, skin changes and joint deformities.
- ☐ Palpate the joint to identify sites of warmth and tenderness and distinguish fluid and soft tissue swelling from bony swelling.
- ☐ Use one hand to feel for crepitus or clicks during active movement of the joint.
- ☐ Whenever possible, compare the affected joint with the patient's other limb acting as a 'normal control'.
- ☐ Measure any restriction of movement.
- ☐ Assess the patient's gait and if abnormal determine whether it is painful (antalgic) or painless.

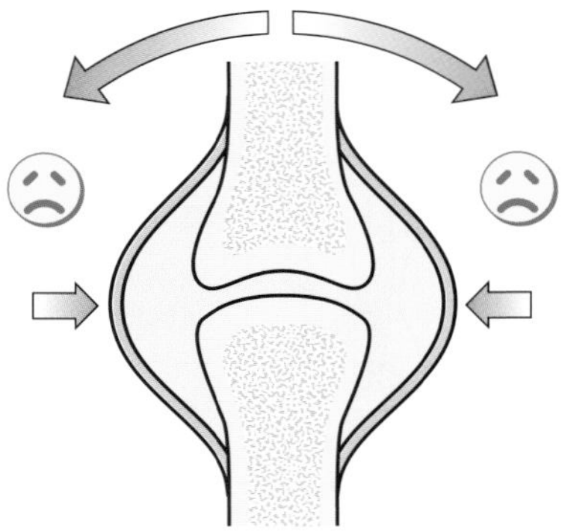

Fig. 8.4 Inflammation of a joint.

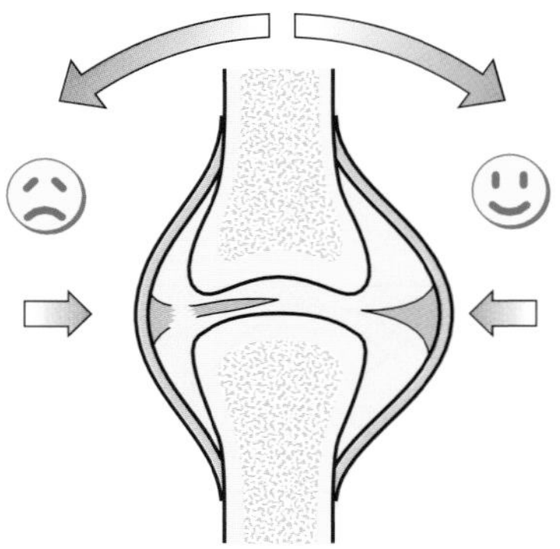

Fig. 8.5 Rupture of a semilunar cartilage.

Basic abnormal signs

Pain, swelling, stiffness or laxity may be due to pathology in the joint or an adjacent structure.

Intra-articular structures

Articular disorders are characterised by pain, restriction of movement, joint line tenderness on palpation, swelling and sometimes crepitus arising from soft tissues or cartilage erosion. Precise localisation of tenderness is important in determining the site of the pathology. In acute lesions, the whole joint may be tender to palpation (Fig. 8.4). Palpation or manoeuvres that increase pressure on a damaged structure, such as a torn semilunar cartilage, will elicit pain (Fig. 8.5). Synovitis feels rubbery and warm and is usually associated with a fluctuant effusion.

Complete lack of movement, accompanied by severe pain, is due to acute inflammation or recent trauma. Complete lack of movement without pain indicates spontaneous fusion (ankylosis) or surgical fusion (arthrodesis) of the joint.

Joint capsule or ligament

An incomplete tear of a joint capsule or ligament (sprain) is painful when stretched by active or passive movements and such movements are restricted by protective muscle spasm. Movement which eases tension on the structure relieves the pain (Fig. 8.6A). Tenderness is localised to the damaged area. An effusion may be present if the capsule remains intact; otherwise it leaks out.

A completely ruptured ligament will give rise to gross instability and swelling over the ligament, rather than within the joint, owing to the escape of joint fluid through the ruptured capsule. Passive movement of the joint is painful and demonstrates an excessive degree of mobility.

Muscles and tendons

Damage to, or inflammation arising in, a muscle tendon unit or the tendon attachment to bone (enthesis) is associated with local tenderness. Inflammation of the tendon sheath (tenosynovitis) results in swelling, sometimes accompanied by tenderness and crepitus along the line of the sheath. Any

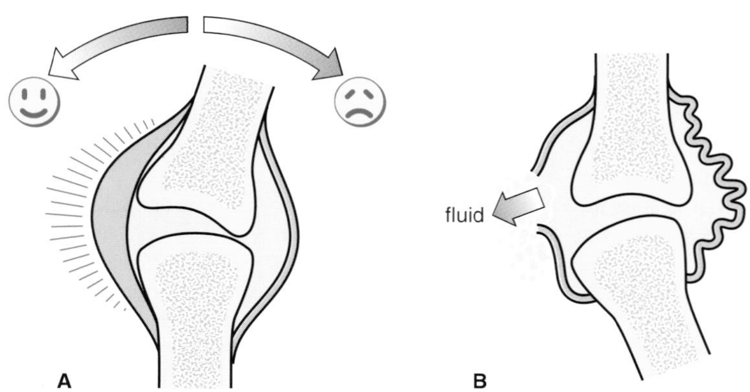

Fig. 8.6 A Sprain of capsule or ligament. B Rupture of capsule or ligament.

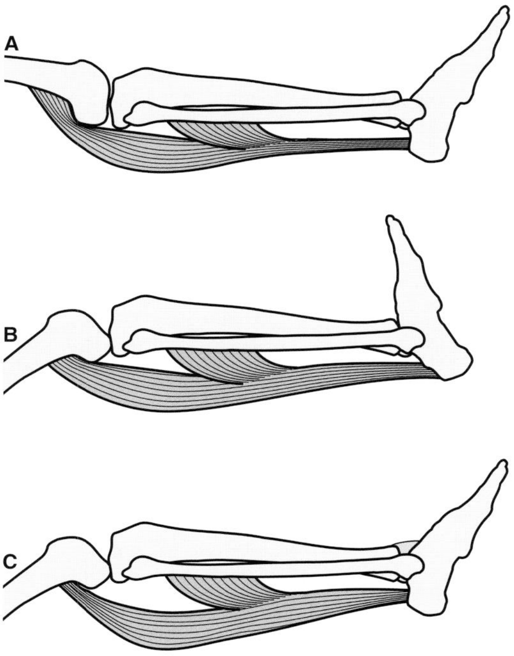

Fig. 8.7 Demonstrating that impairment of dorsiflexion at the ankle A. may be corrected by knee flexion if the cause is contraction of gastrocnemius muscle B. but will not correct if the pathology is in the ankle C.

action which stretches the damaged structure will elicit pain. Tendon rupture is associated with complete loss of active movement but a normal range of passive movement. Muscle or tendon pathology may also lead to joint contracture (Fig. 8.7).

THE GAIT

Abnormal gaits may be divided into two types – painful (antalgic) or painless.

Painful gait

In a moderately painful gait the patient spends as short a time as possible with the affected foot on the ground. This gives rise to a dot-dash pattern of rhythm, the dot representing the time spent on the painful limb. With more severe pain, the whole limb is held flexed and the foot is placed delicately on the ground for very short periods. The patient requires support to walk.

Painless gait

In a painless gait, the normal smooth rhythm is disturbed either because of a short limb, a deformed or stiff joint or weak muscles. The effect of muscle weakness will depend on the site and degree of muscle pathology. Unilateral abductor muscle weakness at the hip produces the Trendelenburg gait (p. 282). Bilateral weakness of gluteal muscles causes a waddling gait. If the gait is bizarre or seems greatly exaggerated in comparison with other objective findings, psychological causes should be considered. However, in adolescents disc problems may also present with a bizarre gait.

THE SPINE

Introduction

Although spinal examination can be subdivided into the examination of the movements of individual cervical, thoracic and lumbar segments, many spinal diseases are not confined to one segment and cause alteration in the posture or function of the whole spine. Spinal disease may occur in the absence of local symptoms and present with pain or neurological symptoms or signs in the trunk or limbs. The key to the accurate diagnosis of a spinal complaint lies in taking a careful history and eliciting signs and symptoms which help to distinguish mechanical or non-inflammatory from inflammatory spinal disease. Abnormalities of the normal spinal curves are common (see the Disorders box below).

DISORDERS
Causes of abnormal spinal curvature
Kyphosis (increased AP curvature) • Osteoporosis; infection; tumour
Scoliosis (lateral curvature) • Postural (correctable on flexion – not associated with vertebral rotation) • Inequality of limb length • Prolapsed intervertebral disc (Fig. 8.9, p. 269) • Inflammatory disorders
Kyphoscoliosis • Structural (uncorrected on flexion – associated with vertebral rotation) • Congenital (hemivertebra) • Acquired – idiopathic, neuromuscular, e.g. poliomyelitis
Lordosis • Reduced cervical – acute painful lesions • Increased cervical – ankylosing spondylitis • Reduced lumbar – ankylosing spondylitis, prolapsed intervertebral disc

HISTORY

Cervical spine

The commonest symptoms of a patient with neck pathology are pain and difficulty turning the head and neck. The pain may be localised to the head, neck, shoulder, arm, or interscapular region.

The patient may also report paraesthesiae in the arm due to nerve root irritation or, less commonly when the spinal cord is involved, symptoms of lower limb weakness, difficulty walking, loss of sensation and sphincter control. Disease of the upper cervical spine affecting the atlantoaxial joints produces pain radiating into the occiput in the distribution of the C2 nerve root. Disease of the middle and lower cervical spine tends to cause pain radiating into the upper border of the trapezius, interscapular region or into the arms, often associated with local tenderness. Irritation of the C6 and 7 nerve roots can give rise to widely referred pain in the interscapular region or into the radial fingers and thumb. Irritation of C8 can produce pain on the ulnar side of the forearm and into the ring and little fingers.

Thus in any patient with neck pain, and especially after trauma, careful enquiry into the distribution of pain and associated upper and lower limb neurological symptoms is essential. Neck pathology should also be considered in any patient complaining of diffuse pain in the arm (see Disorders box below), head, upper trunk or interscapular region, particularly if associated with sensory or other neurological disturbance.

DISORDERS
Causes of referred pain to the arm
• Cervical spine pathology
• Cervical rib
• Apical lung neoplasm (Pancoast lesion)
• Cardiac ischaemia
• Hiatus hernia

Thoracic spine

The presenting symptoms of pathology in the thoracic spine are usually localised spinal pain (see Disorders box) or pain radiating round the chest wall or, less frequently, symptoms of paraparesis including sensory loss, leg weakness, and loss of bladder or bowel control. Disc lesions are rare and may be accompanied by girdle pain radiating around the chest, mimicking cardiac or pleural disease. Pain arising from joints at the thoracolumbar junction can occur in ankylosing spondylitis and again may be confused with pulmonary, renal or cardiac problems. The patient with osteoporosis may complain of becoming progressively stooped (Dowager hump) with loss of height but without neurological features. Acute osteoporotic and malignant vertebral collapse are common causes of acute thoracic pain, and the latter is not infrequently associated with spinal cord compression.

With acute pain, infection should also be considered, especially when pain is associated with systemic upset or fever. When thoracic pain is poorly localised and no satisfactory explanation can be found, intrathoracic causes such as aortic aneurysm should also be considered.

DISORDERS
Causes of pain in the thoracic spine
Adolescents and young adults • Scheuermann's disease • Ankylosing spondylitis • Disc protrusion (rare)
Middle age and elderly • Degenerative change • Osteoporotic fracture
Any age • Tumour • Infection

Lumbar spine

Back pain is an almost ubiquitous experience and most adults will have experienced it by the time they are middle-aged. An important objective of the history is to distinguish those patients who have significant spinal pathology from those who do not. The important spinal conditions to be identified include acute disc protrusion, spinal stenosis, ankylosing spondylitis, osteoporotic fracture, infection, and tumours. Infection and tumours are likely to be associated with symptoms of ill health such as weight loss or fever. Abdominal and retroperitoneal pathology should also be considered. In the majority of patients, however, backache is either a manifestation of poor posture, or age-related degenerative changes in discs and facet joints (spondylosis), or a presenting symptom of psychosocial distress.

A common complaint is of low back pain after standing for too long, or sitting in a poor position. The symptoms tend to be worse as the day progresses and better after resting or on rising in the morning. This pattern is usually due to poor posture and related ligament stresses. Sometimes contributory factors such as inequality of leg length or psychosocial problems can be identified. In the latter case, there is often no clear pattern to the reported pain, and the possibility of mood disturbance should be considered.

In contrast, the insidious onset of backache and stiffness in a young adult suggests inflammatory disease such as ankylosing spondylitis. The symptoms are usually worse in the morning or after inactivity and ease with movement. Morning stiffness is more marked than in osteoarthritis, lasting 30–60 minutes. Often there are other clues to the diagnosis, such as involvement of peripheral joints, non-articular features such as iritis, or a family history of spondylarthritis.

Acute onset of low back pain, in a young adult, usually associated with bending or lifting, is the typical presentation of acute disc protrusion. Sudden movement, such as coughing, will exacerbate the pain. In addition, there may or may not be symptoms of compression of lumbar or sacral nerve roots (cauda equina syndrome). If sacral nerve roots are involved, there may be loss of sphincter control and perianal sensation. The acute episode may be superimposed on a background of preceding mild episodic backache due to disc degeneration. Acute back pain in the middle-aged, elderly or those with predisposing factors such as steroid therapy, may be due to osteoporotic fracture. The pain of this type of fracture is eased by lying, exacerbated by spinal flexion and is not associated with neurological symptoms.

An acute onset of severe progressive pain, especially if associated with systemic features such as malaise, weight loss or night sweats usually indicates pyogenic or tuberculous infection of the lumbar spine. The patient will report great difficulty in moving the spine. The infection may involve both the intervertebral discs and adjacent vertebrae, and at times may track into the sheath of the psoas muscle presenting as a painful flexed hip or as a swelling in the groin. In patients reporting unremitting spinal pain of recent onset, often with sleep disturbance, malignant disease involving a vertebral body should be considered. There may be other clues such as previous history of carcinoma, systemic symptoms or weight loss. Tumours rarely affect intervertebral discs.

Intermittent discomfort or pain in the lumbar spine occurring over a long period of time are the typical symptoms of degenerative disc disease. There is stiffness in the morning or after immobility. The pain and stiffness are relieved by gentle activity but recur with or after excessive activity. Over years or decades there is gradual loss of mobility of the lumbar spine, sometimes with spontaneous improvement in the pain as the facet joints become increasingly stiff.

Diffuse pain in the buttocks or thighs brought on by standing too long or walking is the presenting symptom of lumbosacral spinal stenosis, which can be difficult to distinguish from intermittent claudication (p. 108). Sometimes the pain is accompanied by tingling and numbness and can be difficult for the patient to describe. Typically the pain is relieved by rest or flexion of the spine. Stooping, or holding onto a supermarket trolley, may increase exercise tolerance. Narrowing of the spinal canal or neural exit foraminae, is usually caused by degenerative changes in the intervertebral discs and facet joints, and there is often a long preceding history of discomfort typical of degenerative joint disease.

KEY POINTS

- Establish the site and referral of pain and its response to rest, coughing, standing and activity.
- Establish the mode of onset and subsequent course.
- Enquire about neurological symptoms – especially those which may suggest spinal cord compression.

ANATOMY

Cervical spine

Nodding of the head occurs at the atlanto-occipital joint, rotational neck movements mainly at the atlantoaxial joint, whilst flexion, extension and lateral flexion occur mainly at the mid-cervical level.

The neural canal is almost filled by the cervical enlargement of the spinal cord and the emerging cervical roots pass through exit foraminae bounded by the facet joints posteriorly and the intervertebral discs and neurocentral joints anteriorly. The nerve roots, particularly in the lower cervical spine, may be compressed or irritated by lateral disc prolapse or osteophytes arising from the facet or neurocentral joints. A central disc prolapse may produce pressure on the cord itself.

Thoracic spine

This segment of the spinal column is the least mobile and maintains a kyphosis throughout life. Movement in the thoracic spine is mainly rotational and there is only a very small amount of flexion, extension and lateral flexion.

Lumbar spine

The lumbar spine has a smooth lordosis which may be lost in certain disorders such as ankylosing spondylitis and lumbar disc protrusion (Disorders box). The main surface markings are the spinous processes of L4/5 which are level with the pelvic brim and the 'dimples of Venus' which lie over the sacroiliac joints.

The principal movements are flexion, extension, lateral flexion and rotation. It is important to appreciate the normal range of spinal movements. Most patients will be able to bring the tips of their fingers at least to the level of the knees in forward flexion and lateral flexion. Extension is variable, but should be approximately 10–20 degrees. In flexion, the upper segments move first, followed by the lower segments to produce a smooth lumbar curve. Even with a completely rigid lumbar spine, if the hips are mobile, the patient still may be able to touch the toes.

In the adult, the spinal cord ends at the level of the second lumbar vertebra. Injury or lesions above this level may cause serious damage to the cord, which is permanent, and to the nerve roots, which may be temporary. Below the

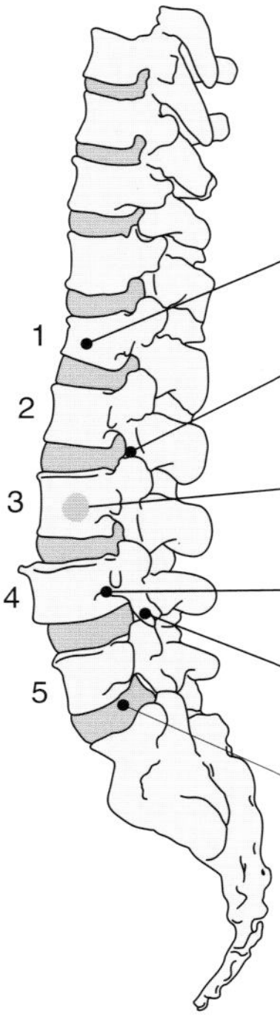

Fig. 8.8 Locomotor causes of back pain. Prolapsed invertebral disc occurs mostly frequently at the L4/L5 and L5/S1 levels.

level of L2, only the nerve roots can be damaged. Important locomotor causes of back pain are shown in Figure 8.8.

EXAMINATION OF THE SPINE

The examinations of the cervical, thoracic and lumbar spine are described separately, though in clinical practice the spine is often examined in its entirety.

Cervical spine

Examination sequence

- ☐ Note the posture of the neck and any abnormality, i.e. loss of lordosis, a torticollis (wry neck) or 'cock robin' deformity (see Disorders box).
- ☐ Palpate the bony contour. Note and localise the presence of tenderness in the spine, trapezius, interscapular and paraspinal muscles.
- ☐ Ask the patient to look right and left (80 degrees of rotation each way) and to tilt the head to the right and left (45 degrees of lateral flexion each way) and to flex (75 degrees) and extend (60 degrees) the neck. Note any asymmetry of movement.
- ☐ Gently perform passive movements if there is impairment of the active range.
- ☐ Perform a neurological examination of the upper and lower limbs, noting any sensory or motor abnormalities.

Common abnormal findings

- Local cervical tenderness may help to identify the site of pathology.
- Regional and paraspinal muscle tenderness, is commonly associated with neck pathology.
- Widespread muscle tenderness may be a feature of psychological distress.
- Loss of movement.
- Torticollis, associated with acute neck pain.
- Loss of cervical lordosis, associated with chronic neck pain.
- Loss of sensation in upper limb dermatomes, associated with nerve root irritation.

DISORDERS
Causes of abnormal neck posture
• Loss of lordosis or flexion deformity – acute lesions, rheumatoid arthritis
• Increased lordosis – ankylosing spondylitis
• Torticollis (wry neck) – sternomastoid contracture
• Lateral flexion (cock robin position) – erosion of lateral mass of atlas in RA

Thoracic spine

Examination sequence

- ☐ With the patient standing, inspect the posture from the front, back and side and note any deformity such as increased kyphosis (curvature in the AP plane) or scoliosis (curvature in the coronal plane).
- ☐ Examine the bony contour and define areas of tenderness.
- ☐ Where local tenderness is not detected, perform gentle percussion with a fist or tendon hammer.
- ☐ With the patient seated on the couch, observe the range of rotation from behind.
- ☐ Note whether spinal flexion does or does not correct any scoliosis which is present.
- ☐ Measure chest expansion which should usually be at least 5 cm.

Common abnormal findings

- Tenderness localised to the site of pathology.
- Kyphosis or kyphoscoliosis.

Lumbar spine

There are three important components to the examination of the lumbar spine. The first is to inspect for the presence of deformity (see Disorders box), the second is to assess the movements of the spine, and the third is to assess the effects of lumbar spinal pathology on the spinal cord or nerve roots.

DISORDERS
Some causes of abnormal lumbar posture
• Loss of lordosis – advanced age, ankylosing spondylitis, acute disc prolapse
• Scoliosis – acute disc prolapse (Fig. 8.9): – if lateral to nerve root, patient leans away from lesion – if medial to nerve root, patient leans towards lesion

Examination sequence

- ☐ With the patient standing, observe the posture from behind, checking that the spine is straight, and from the side checking that there is a normal lordosis.
- ☐ Observe the effect of flexion on any abnormal lateral curvature (scoliosis).
- ☐ Perform light percussion with the fist or tendon hammer. Note the presence of tenderness over the spinous processes and the paraspinal muscles.
- ☐ Whilst keeping the legs straight, ask the patient first to bend backwards, then forwards and then to each side. Note the range of movement in each direction and the contour formed by the spine.
- ☐ Carry out Schober's test where appropriate to quantify the range of lumbar spinal flexion (Fig. 8.10).

Schober's test

- ☐ Make a mark on the skin in the midline at the level of the dimples of Venus. Make two other marks, one 5 cm below and the other 10 cm above the first.
- ☐ Place a tape measure over the lumbar spine with the end (0 cm) at the lower mark and ask the patient to bend forwards.
- ☐ Record the movement of the upper skin mark with the tape measure. On flexion, the upper mark should normally move upwards by at least 5 cm.

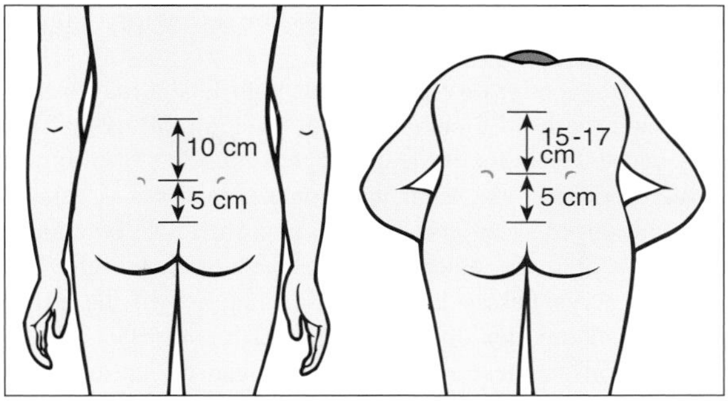

Fig. 8.10 Schober's test. Measuring forward flexion of spine.

Tests for nerve root compression

Prolapse of intervertebral discs occurs most frequently at the L4/5 or L5/S1 level, producing compression of the L5 and S1 nerve roots respectively. Tension can be applied to these nerve roots by flexing the hip with the knee straight – the so-called *straight leg raising test*. Normally, about 90 degrees of hip flexion should be possible but this varies considerably (70–120 degrees). When the root is stretched over a prolapsed disc, straight leg raising will be restricted

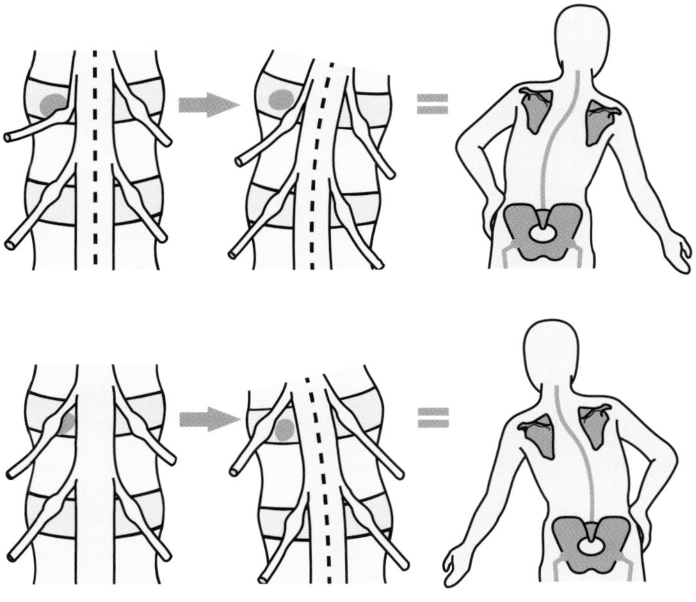

Fig. 8.9 Deviation of spine in prolapsed intervertebral disc.

and pain will usually be felt in the lumbar region, not just in the leg (Fig. 8.11B).

Less frequently, disc prolapse at high levels may occur, involving the L2, L3 or L4 roots of the femoral nerve. This may cause weakness of the quadriceps muscles, resulting in reduced power of extension at the knee, sometimes associated with a reduced knee jerk (L3/4). There may also be altered sensation over the anteromedial aspect of the thigh. The femoral nerve passes into the thigh anterior to the pubic ramus, and hip flexion or straight leg raising will relieve any tension on these roots. The roots can be stretched by extending the hip with the knee flexed (*femoral nerve stretch test*) (Fig. 8.12).

Additional tests are sometimes useful. The '*bowstring sign*' is another useful test and may be used to confirm nerve root irritation. If there is still doubt as to whether there is sciatic nerve root irritation, for example where malingering is suspected, other manoeuvres may be tried, such as the '*flip test*' (Fig. 8.13).

Examination sequence

Straight leg raising

- ☐ Examine the patient lying supine (Fig. 8.11A).
- ☐ With the knee flexed, check that passive hip flexion is normal.
- ☐ With the knee extended, raise the leg on the unaffected side by lifting the heel with one hand while preventing knee flexion with the other. Note the range of movement.
- ☐ Repeat this on the affected side, asking the patient to report as soon as it becomes painful and where the pain or paraesthesia is felt (Fig. 8.11B).
- ☐ When this limit is reached, gently dorsiflex the ankle, thereby applying further tension to the nerve root (*Bragaard test*) (Fig. 8.11C).

Bowstring sign

- ☐ Perform straight leg raising and at the limit flex the knee, reducing tension on the sciatic roots and hamstrings (Fig. 8.11D).
- ☐ Now further flex the hip.
- ☐ Gently extend the knee until the pain is reproduced once again (*Lasegue's sign*) (Fig. 8.11E).
- ☐ The posterior tibial nerve is now stretched like a bowstring across the popliteal fossa. Firm pressure is then applied with the thumb, first over the hamstring nearest the examiner, then over the nerve in the middle of the popliteal fossa and finally over the other hamstring tendon. Ask the patient which manoeuvre exacerbated the pain (Fig. 8.11F).
- ☐ The test is positive if the second manoeuvre is painful and if the resultant pain radiates from the knee to the back.

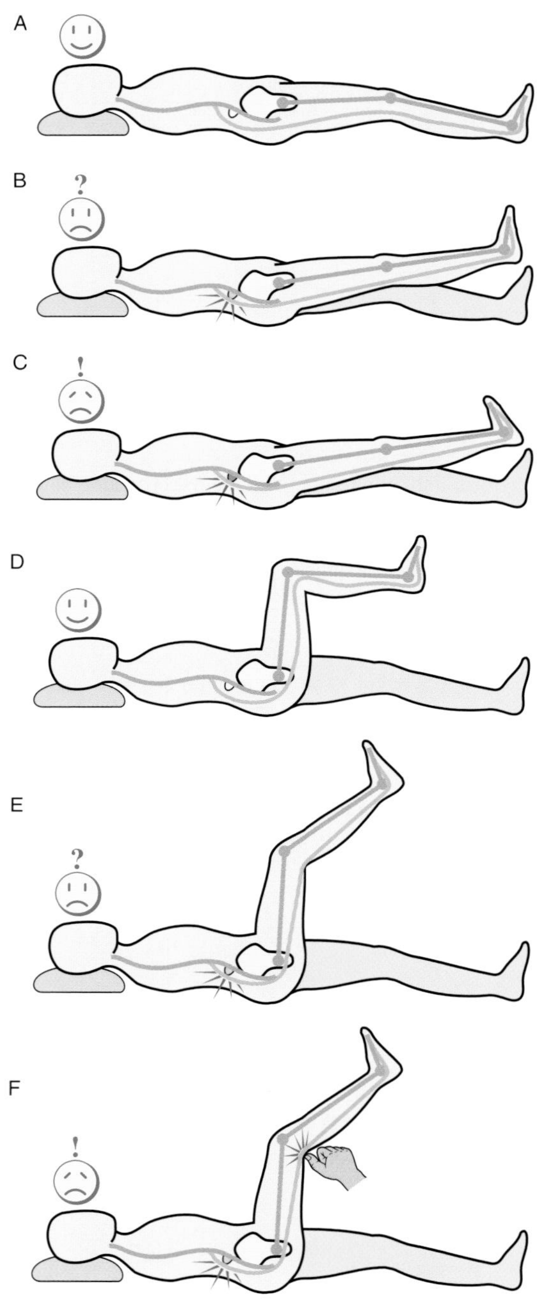

Fig. 8.11 Stretch tests – sciatic nerve roots. A Neutral; nerve roots slack. B Straight leg raising limited by tension of root over prolapsed disc. C Tension increased by dorsiflexion of foot (Bragaard test). D Root tension relieved by flexion at the knee. E With knee extension over prolapsed disc causing pain radiating to the back (Lasegue test). F Pressure over centre of popliteal fossa bears on posterior tibial nerve which is 'bowstringing' across the fossa causing pain locally and radiation into the back.

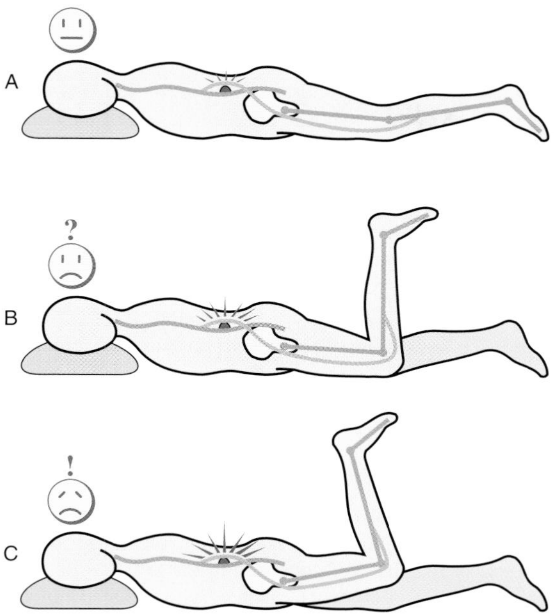

Fig. 8.12 Stretch test – femoral nerve. A Patient prone and free from pain because femoral roots are slack. B When femoral roots are tightened by flexion of the knee, pain may be felt in the back. C If still no pain, femoral roots are further stretched by extension of the hip.

Flip test

- ☐ Ask the patient to sit on the edge of the couch with the hips and knees flexed to 90 degrees and test the knee reflexes (Fig. 8.13A).
- ☐ Then, extend the knee, ostensibly to examine the ankle jerk.
- ☐ When there is root irritation, the patient will 'flip' backwards to relieve the sudden increase in tension on the nerve root (Fig. 8.13B).
- ☐ In the absence of significant nerve root irritation, the patient, distracted by attention to the ankle jerk test, may permit full extension of the knee, which is the equivalent of full 90 degrees straight leg raising (Fig. 8.13C).

Femoral nerve stretch test

- ☐ Ask the patient to lie prone or on the unaffected side if there is a painful flexion deformity of the hip.
- ☐ Flex the knee slowly, asking the patient to report onset of pain.
- ☐ If this fails to produce pain, in the thigh or back, gently extend the hip with the knee still flexed (Fig. 8.12).

Sacroiliac joints

There are situations where it is important to examine the sacroiliac joints, although the available clinical tests are not very reliable. Movements of these joints cannot usually be demonstrated clinically. During and immediately after pregnancy, laxity of the pelvis may occur causing instability in the pelvic girdle. This may allow a small amount of movement to be detected. This diagnosis is usually clear from the symptoms and the clinical context. Pain arising from the sacroiliac joints may radiate into the buttocks and

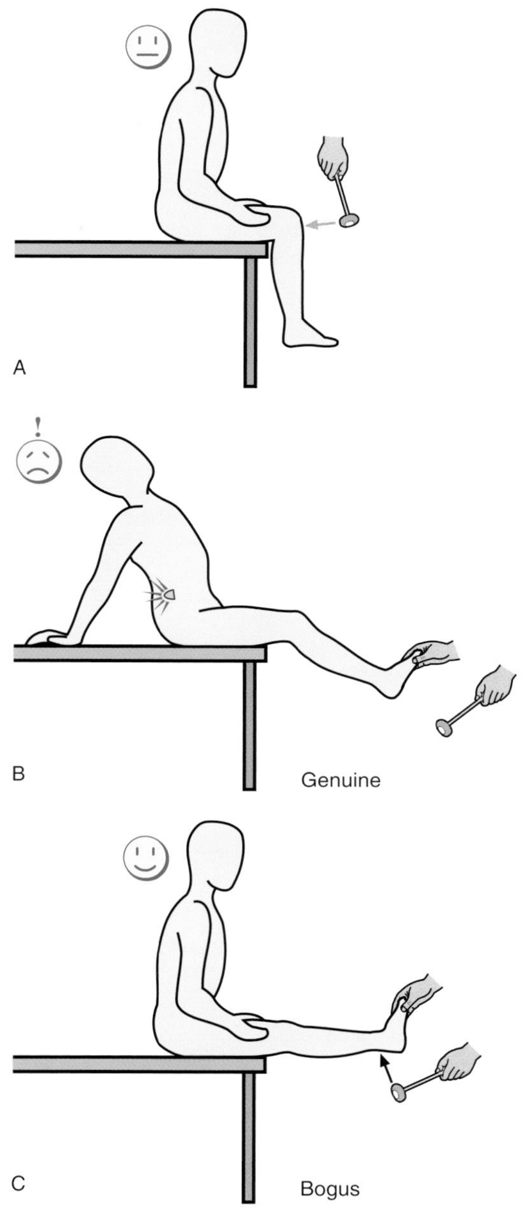

Fig. 8.13 Stretch test – sciatic nerve root. In the 'flip' test, when attention is diverted to the tendon reflexes the genuine patient will not permit full extension of the leg.

posterior thighs, but unlike sciatica, rarely extends below the knee. Local palpation over the sacroiliac joints is often unhelpful and may give rise to false positive and false negative results. Stressing the pelvis may produce buttock pain if these joints are inflamed.

Examination sequence

To stress the sacroiliac joints:

☐ Ask the patient to lie prone on a firm surface and apply firm pressure with the heel of the hand over the sacrum.

Or:

☐ With the patient supine, fully flex the hip and knee and, with firm pressure, adduct the thigh to stress the ipsilateral sacroiliac joint.

Common abnormal findings

- Restriction of spinal movement.
- Pain exacerbated by movement of the spine.
- Neurological signs associated with acute nerve root compression.

CASE HISTORY

A young man of 25 experienced intermittent lumbar backache after playing squash. After one of these episodes he developed acute lumbar backache while putting on his socks. The pain was extremely severe; he had difficulty moving and he had to crawl to the toilet. After 48 hours the pain spread into the posterolateral aspect of his right leg and across the dorsum of his foot and into his big toe. He had associated paraesthesia in this distribution. Coughing acutely exacerbated his discomfort. There was no systemic upset.

He could only get out of bed with assistance and stand with extreme difficulty. There was flattening of his lumbar lordosis. His pain was increased on attempted forward flexion and right lateral flexion of the spine. Straight leg raising on the right was reduced to 30 degrees. There was weakness of dorsiflexion of the big toe and depression of sensation across the dorsum of the foot and into the first interdigital cleft. The ankle jerk was intact. Rectal examination was normal. The history made infection or tumour unlikely and was highly suggestive of an acute prolapsed intervertebral disc. MRI scan confirmed the diagnosis.

Learning points

- The distribution of pain and the associated neurological signs indicate the level of the lesion (L4/5 disc).
- Abnormal sphincter tone and loss of perianal sensation suggest cauda equina compression which demands operative intervention.

KEY POINTS

- Note abnormalities of posture and distinguish between structural and postural scoliosis.
- Sites of spinal tenderness help to localise pathology.
- Assess range of movement and remember that even with a rigid spine a patient can touch the toes if the hips are mobile.
- Identify local or widespread muscle tenderness.
- Perianal sensory loss and sphincter tone should be assessed if sacral nerve root involvement is suspected.

THE LIMBS

The history and examination of the limb joints aims to distinguish between systemic conditions, which may cause pathology at several sites (e.g. rheumatoid arthritis), local conditions in which a single site is involved (e.g. tennis elbow) and conditions where limb symptoms are due to referred pain from disease of the spine or nerve roots. The distinction between inflammatory and non-inflammatory conditions is also made on the basis of the pattern of diurnal stiffness and pain, relation to activity and the presence of extra-articular features. It is also important to remember that pain arising in a joint may be referred and difficult for the patient to localise (Table 8.8).

UPPER LIMB: HISTORY

The presenting complaints arising from hands and wrists are usually stiffness, pain and loss of function. Pain and stiffness are usually well localised to the affected joints. In early inflammatory arthritis stiffness with reduced function may be the only symptoms, and pain may be minimal or absent. The complaint of local or diffuse swelling is common, but should always be confirmed on examination. The distribution of joint involvement is critical to diagnosis. If hand pain is diffuse or poorly localised by the patient, referred pain or a neurological problem such as carpal tunnel syndrome (Fig. 8.14) should be considered. This condition also frequently causes numbness and sleep disturbance. The patient may report hanging the arm down and shaking the hand to relieve the pain.

Pain due to pathology in the elbow joint is usually exacerbated by use and may be localised or referred to the forearm. The commonest problem is lateral epicondylitis or so-called 'tennis elbow'. Symptoms of pain in the upper outer arm or shoulder region with restriction of shoulder movements suggests pathology affecting one or more of the major structures of the shoulder girdle (i.e. glenohumeral, sternoclavicular or acromioclavicular joints, rotator cuff tendons or bone). Pain arising in the shoulder is felt over its anterior aspect or in the lateral aspect of the upper arm. The pain is exacerbated by lying on the shoulder and may cause sleep disturbance. Movements are likely to be both restricted and painful causing the patient to report difficulty putting on a jacket or reaching up to a shelf. Rotator cuff pathology tends to produce pain on elevating the arm. Pain which is

TABLE 8.8 Sites of somatic referral of limb joint pain

Shoulder	to	Lateral aspect of upper arm
Elbow	to	Forearm
Hip	to	Anterior thigh or knee or both

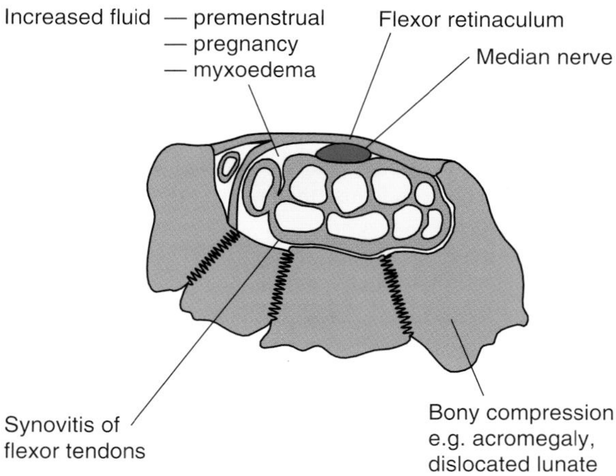

Fig. 8.14 Causes of median nerve compression.

difficult for the patient to localise, in the absence of shoulder restriction, is more likely to suggest referred pain from the neck or viscera.

A history of trauma is usually obvious and in young adults may be associated with dislocation of the shoulder. There is a tendency for this to be recurrent. Occasionally, dislocation may occur without an apparent history of trauma, such as after a nocturnal epileptic convulsion.

If the pattern of symptoms, e.g. diurnal variation, suggests an inflammatory disorder, a family history (Table 8.6) and symptoms of extra-articular features (Table 8.5) should be sought and close enquiry made about other joints (Table 8.2). The impact of upper limb symptoms on normal daily activities, i.e. extent of disability, should be documented (Table 8.9).

TABLE 8.9 Joints involved in performing daily activities

Pincer grip – for writing, turning key	Hand	Opposition of thumb to index
Gripping taps, handles, bottle tops	Hand, wrist	Grasp
Eating, cleaning teeth and face	Hand, elbow	Grasp, elbow flexion
Dressing, washing and grooming hair	Hand, elbow, shoulder	Pinch, grasp, elbow flexion Shoulder elevation/rotation
Cleaning perineum	Hand, wrist, elbow, shoulder	Grasp, wrist and elbow flexion Forearm supination Internal rotation shoulder

KEY POINTS

General

- Establish the site and distribution of pain and associated symptoms.
- Establish the daily pattern of symptoms.
- Enquire about extra-articular features and family history if a systemic inflammatory condition is suspected.
- Distinguish whether upper limb pain is due to local pathology or referred from the neck.
- Document functional difficulties.

Hand and wrist

- If pain is poorly localised, enquire about night pain and numbness in the hand.

Shoulder

- Remember that pain in the shoulder may be referred from the cervical spine, the root of the neck, pleura, diaphragm or peritoneum.

ANATOMY OF THE UPPER LIMB

The hand and wrist

The hand is a precision tool and a power tool. The flexor and extensor muscles of the forearm provide the powerhouse of the hand and wrist. However, without the use of intrinsic muscles of the hand, neither proper grip nor fine movements are possible. The interphalangeal joints allow only flexion and extension, with the metacarpophalangeal joints also allowing a little abduction and adduction when they are extended. The wrist provides flexion, extension, radial and ulnar deviation and circumduction.

The radial, ulnar and median nerves are all essential for normal hand function. The radial nerve innervates the wrist and finger extensors. The ulnar nerve innervates the adductor of the thumb and most of the interossei and lumbricals. The median nerve innervates the bulk of the flexor muscles in the forearm and the opponens and abductor muscles of the thumb.

The elbow

The joint is composed of two parts, the main joint between the humerus and ulna which allows flexion-extension and the superior radioulnar joint which allows supination-pronation.

The medial and lateral epicondyles, which are the respective common origins of the forearm flexor and extensor muscles, are superficial and easily palpated. With the tip of the olecranon the epicondyles form an equilateral triangle. The subcutaneous bursa overlying the olecranon is visible and palpable only when inflamed and swollen.

The shoulder

The lateral end of the clavicle and the acromion can be

easily identified allowing the location of the acromioclavicular joint above the glenohumeral joint. The tip of the coracoid process can be palpated, 1 inch below the clavicle under the anterior edge of the deltoid. The tendon of biceps can be palpated where it lies in the bicipital groove between the greater and lesser tubercles.

Movement of the shoulder is a complicated synthesis, with about 50% of movement occurring at the glenohumeral joint, about 50% as a result of the thoracoscapular mechanism and only a small amount at the acromioclavicular and sternoclavicular joints (see Fig. 8.18).

The rotator cuff comprises the conjoint tendons of supraspinatus, infraspinatus and teres minor. Infraspinatus and teres minor externally rotate the humerus. Supraspinatus stabilises the head of the humerus in the socket of the glenoid, which allows the deltoid muscle to abduct the arm. The rotator cuff (especially the supraspinatus tendon), the related subacromial bursa and the tendon of the long head of biceps, are the most common sites of pathology in the shoulder.

EXAMINATION OF THE UPPER LIMB

The hand and wrist

Examination of the hand consists of inspection, palpation and assessment of function. Since a full examination of function is lengthy, it is necessary to tailor the examination to the clinical history and the nature of the problem. For example, in a patient with lacerations of the digits, a thorough assessment of the integrity of the tendons, nerves and circulation is essential. In contrast, in a patient presenting with stiffness, pain and swelling of the hands the examination will be directed towards establishing the pattern of joint and tendon involvement (Table 8.2) and testing the principal hand functions, such as power grip and fine pinch.

Examination sequence

- ☐ Inspect the hands and wrists carefully (Table 8.10). Look specifically for skin and nail changes, muscle wasting, joint deformity and swelling of joints, tendon sheaths or surrounding tissue.
- ☐ Palpate the joints of the hands and wrists and periarticular soft tissues to elicit tenderness and to identify the bony or soft tissue nature of any swelling.
- ☐ Palpate the flexor tendon sheath, by placing the examining index finger across the volar aspect of the patient's fully extended fingers and then asking the patient to open and close the fingers, allowing crepitus to be detected.
- ☐ Palpate the flexor tendons from the sides to detect synovial swelling (the Savill pinch test).
- ☐ Palpate for local swellings of tendons, especially at the mouth of the fibrous flexor sheath. If a swelling on the tendon is felt, look for triggering of the finger (i.e. locking of the finger in flexion as the tendon nodule engages in the mouth of the fibrous sheath).
- ☐ Ask the patient to perform fine pinch (as if threading a needle).
- ☐ Note the grip strength by asking the patient to grasp two of the examiner's fingers. If the range of movements of the joints is not full, the patient may be unable to grip two or even three of the examiner's fingers.
- ☐ Note the range of wrist dorsiflexion (0–90 degrees).
- ☐ Note the range of wrist flexion (0–90 degrees).

Specific muscles and tendons

Undertake detailed testing of the individual muscles and tendons only if indicated.

- ☐ *Flexor digitorum profundus* (FDP) (flexes the distal interphalangeal joints). Ask the patient to flex the DIP joint (0–90 degrees) while holding the finger in extension at the PIP joint (Fig. 8.15A).
- ☐ *Flexor digitorum sublimis* (FDS) (flexes the PIP joints). It is necessary to eliminate the action of FDP which acts en masse. While holding the other fingers in full extension to block the action of FDP, ask the patient to flex the PIP joint in question (Fig. 8.15B).
- ☐ *Thenar muscle supplied by median nerve* (abduction 0–80 degrees). To test the action of abductor pollicis brevis, ask the patient to abduct the thumb vertically from the palm and to hold it against resistance. Test opposition by asking the patient to touch the terminal

TABLE 8.10 Examples of visible abnormalities of the hands associated with rheumatic disease

Abnormality	Appearance and consistency	Typical site	Associated rheumatic disease
Heberden's nodes	Small bony nodules	Dorsum of DIP joints	OA
Bouchard's nodes	Small bony nodules	Dorsum of PIP joints	OA
Rheumatoid nodules	Fleshy and firm	Extensor surface of knuckles	RA
Tophi	White subcutaneous	Juxta-articular	Gout
Calcific deposits	White subcutaneous	Finger pulp	SCL, DM
Dilated capillaries	(Use magnifying glass)	Nailfolds	SCL, DM, SLE

OA, osteoarthritis; RA, rheumatoid arthritis; SCL, scleroderma; DM, dermatomyositis; SLE systemic lupus erythematosus

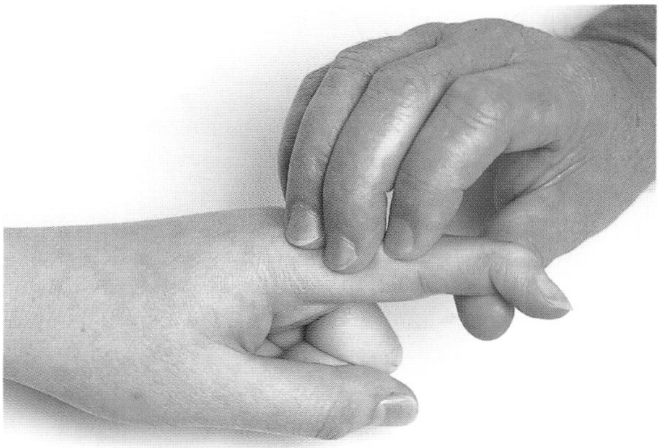

A

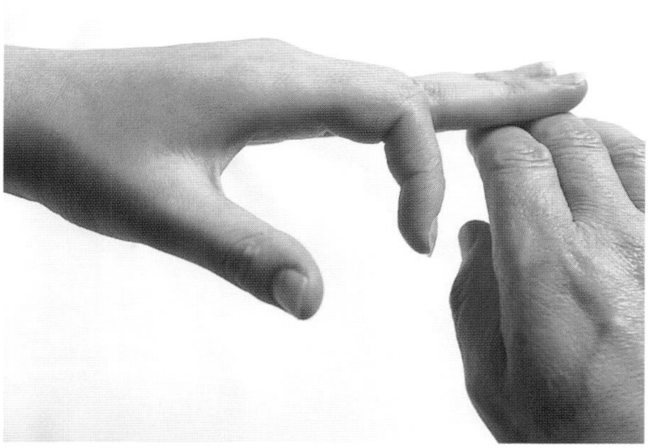

B

Fig. 8.15 A **Flexor digitorum profundus.** B **Flexor digitorum sublimis.**

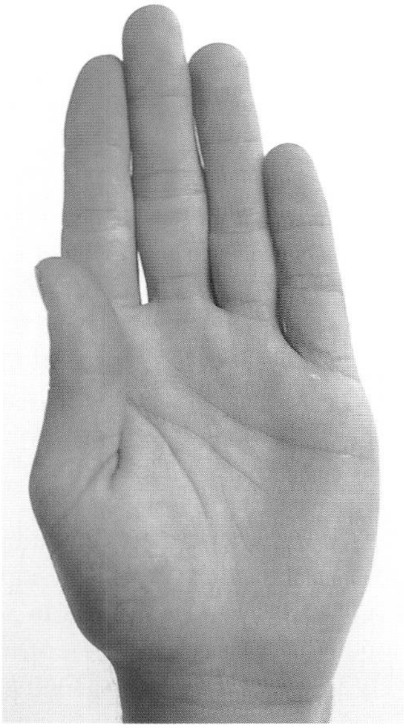

A

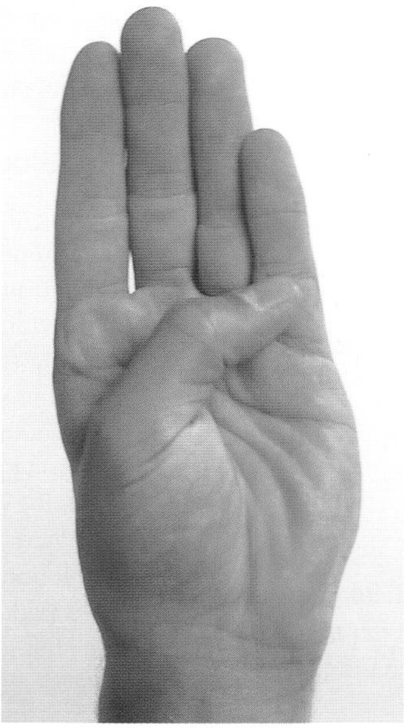

B

Fig. 8.16 A **Adduction and** B **opposition of the thumb.** Opposition involves rotation. It is commonly tested by asking the patient to touch the tip of the small finger with the thumb.

phalanx of the little finger with the thumb and to maintain this position against resistance (Fig. 8.16B).

- ☐ *Thenar muscle supplied by the ulnar nerve* (adduction of the thumb). Ask the patient to hold a card between the palm and the adducted thumb. If the adductor is weak, the thumb cannot be held straight and flexes at the MCP and IP joints (Froment's sign) (Fig. 8.17A).
- ☐ *Extensor pollicis longus* principally elevates the thumb (hitch-hiker's thumb). Ask the patient to place the palm on a flat surface and to lift the thumb like a hitch-hiker (Fig. 8.17B). The patient will only be able to do so if this tendon is intact.

Common abnormal findings

- Bony swelling and tenderness of DIP joints (Heberden's nodes), PIP joints (Bouchard's nodes) and first CMC joints owing to osteoarthritis.
- Soft tissue swelling and tenderness of joints and tendon sheaths owing to inflammatory arthritis.

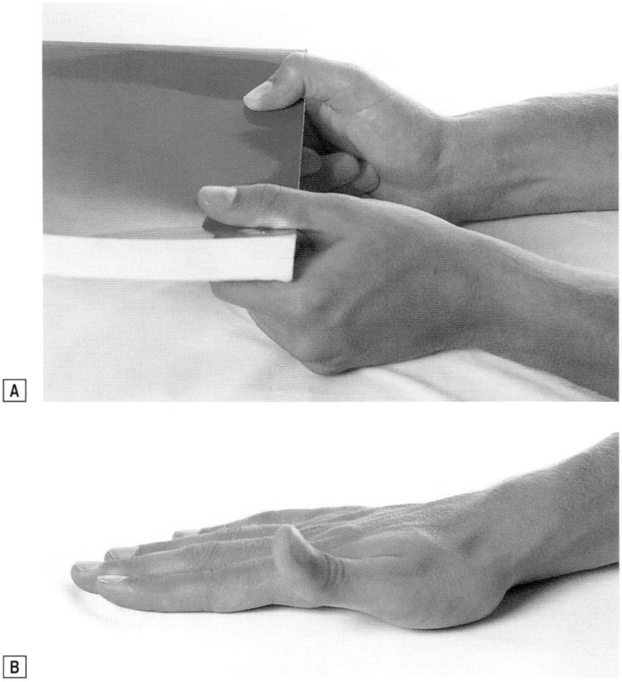

Fig. 8.17 A Thumb adductor showing weakness on the right side. B Intact extensor pollicis longus elevating the thumb off a flat surface.

- Trauma to tendons, joints and nerves. Division of tendons in the absence of joint disease results in loss of active movement but not passive movement.

The elbow

Examination sequence

☐ Inspect both elbows, noting any periarticular swelling; synovitis is most commonly observed over the posterolateral aspect of the joint between the lateral epicondyle and the olecranon.

☐ Palpate the elbow for bony contours, local tenderness, synovitis, nodules or bursae.

☐ Compare the range of active flexion and extension (0–150 degrees). Note the presence of flexion deformity or loss of range of flexion.

☐ Ask the patient to supinate (0–90 degrees) and pronate (0–90 degrees) the forearm. This is best performed with the elbows close to the patient's side and flexed to 90 degrees (failure to do this may give a misleading impression, since pronation can be simulated by abduction and internal rotation at the shoulder).

☐ To detect crepitus, palpate the elbow joint during flexion-extension and the head of the radius during supination-pronation.

☐ Test the integrity of the collateral ligaments with the arm fully extended.

Testing for epicondylitis

☐ Palpate for focal tenderness over the lateral and medial epicondyles at the site of the common extensor and common flexor origins.

☐ Ask the patient to grip tightly with the hand while the elbow is fully extended. If epicondylitis is present, the manoeuvre will elicit the patient's pain. The manoeuvre is usually less painful when the elbow is flexed.

Common abnormal findings

- Tenderness of epicondyles.
- Flexion deformity.
- Swelling of the olecranon bursa.
- Subcutaneous rheumatoid nodules.

Common disorders of the elbow

- Tennis elbow (lateral epicondylitis) or golfer's elbow (medial epicondylitis).
- Olecranon bursitis.

The shoulder

During the examination of the shoulder, it is necessary to determine which joint or structure is responsible for any limitation of movement. While examining for flexion and abduction, it is important to place a restraining hand on the scapula (or acromion). Once the limits of movement of the glenohumeral joint are reached, any movement of the scapula on the thorax is immediately detected. Loss of external rotation at the shoulder usually indicates glenohumeral joint pathology.

Where there is a rotator cuff syndrome, initiation of abduction will be painful if the supraspinatus tendon is inflamed. If the cuff is ruptured, the patient tends to shrug the shoulder when attempting to abduct. However, once the arm is abducted passively to about 45 degrees, the patient should then be able to continue active movement unaided from this position using deltoid. In the painful arc syndrome, the patient will usually experience pain in the mid arc of abduction or adduction (Fig. 8.19). Bicipital tendonitis can be identified by asking the patient to flex the elbow and to supinate the forearm against resistance, as both these manoeuvres should elicit pain.

Examination sequence

☐ Inspect and compare the shoulders from the front and the back. Note any muscle wasting, soft tissue swelling or difference in bony contour on the two sides.

☐ Note any tenderness or swelling over the anterior aspect and point of the shoulder, the acromioclavicular joint and sternoclavicular joint.

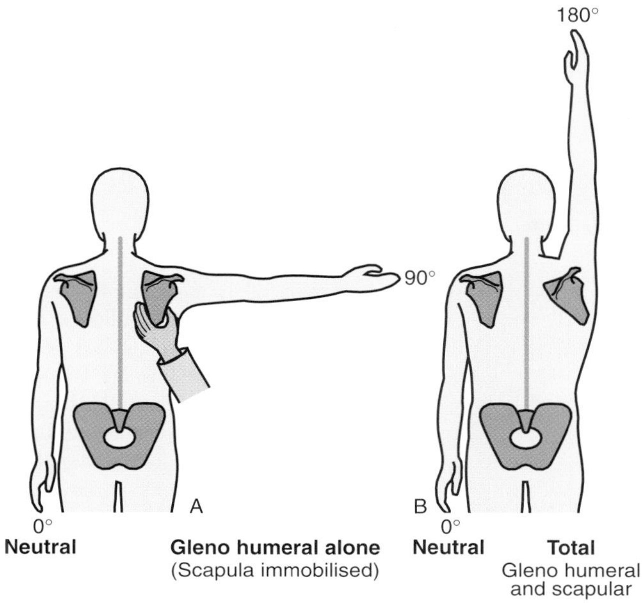

Fig. 8.18 Movements at the shoulder joint.

- ☐ Inspect the overall range of movement, noting whether movements are performed smoothly, symmetrically and without discomfort.
- ☐ Stand behind the patient and observe the overall range by asking the patient to place the hands at the base of the neck with elbows pointing sideways.
- ☐ Next, ask the patient to put the arms down and to reach behind the back to between the shoulder blades.
- ☐ Proceed with further examination only if pain, swelling or limitation of movement is present.

The glenohumeral joint

- ☐ Standing behind the patient, examine the range of external and internal rotation of each shoulder with the patient's arm by the side and the elbow flexed to 90 degrees.
- ☐ To examine the flexion and abduction, place a restraining hand on the acromion, or hold the blade of the scapula.
- ☐ Now ask the patient to flex the shoulder (normal range 90 degrees).
- ☐ Ask the patient to abduct the arm from the dependent position (normal range 90 degrees) until scapular movement is detected (Fig. 8.18A).
- ☐ If abduction cannot be initiated, the test for rotator cuff rupture should be performed.
- ☐ If the range of active abduction is restricted, test whether further passive abduction is possible. If impingement is present, this is painful. Impingement pain may also be elicited by rotating the arm while in the abducted position.
- ☐ If impingement pain is present, the tests for painful arc syndrome should be performed (see below).

The rotator cuff

- ☐ To elicit pain, ask the patient, with the arm by the side, to abduct the arm against resistance.
- ☐ If rupture is suspected, because abduction cannot be initiated, passively abduct the arm about 30–45 degrees from the patient's side. Ask the patient to attempt to continue active abduction (Fig. 8.19A).
- ☐ Test for a 'painful arc' by assisting the patient to raise the arm into full elevation and then asking the patient to lower the arm sideways (Fig. 8.19B).

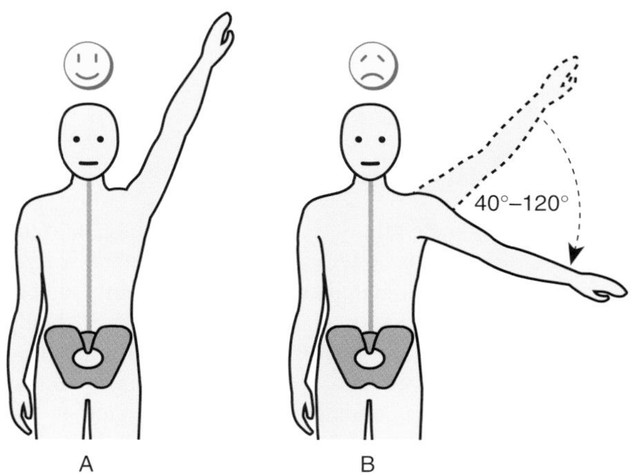

Fig. 8.19 Painful arc syndrome.

Testing for bicipital tendonitis

- ☐ To elicit tenderness palpate the tendon as it lies in the bicipital groove, on the anterior aspect of the shoulder.
- ☐ Ask the patient to flex the elbow against resistance.
- ☐ Ask the patient to supinate the forearm against resistance.

Common abnormal findings

- Wasting of the deltoid, in long-standing shoulder problems.
- Restriction of active movements.
- Tenderness over the insertion of the rotator cuff and the bicipital tendon owing to inflammatory and degenerative conditions affecting the rotator cuff.
- Impingement pain which is associated with rotator cuff pathology.

DISORDERS
Causes of shoulder girdle pain
• *Rotator cuff* – degeneration, tendon rupture, calcific tendonitis
• *Subacromial bursa* – calcific bursitis, polyarthritis
• *Capsule* – adhesive capsulitis
• *Head of humerus* – tumour deposit, osteonecrosis, fracture/dislocation
• *Joints*: – glenohumeral, sternoclavicular – synovitis, osteoarthritis, dislocation – acromioclavicular – osteoarthritis

KEY POINTS

- Note muscle wasting.
- Note which joints are painful. Localise tenderness or swelling and assess function.
- Note range of movement, joint stability and deformity.
- Check the integrity of individual tendons, muscles and nerves as appropriate.
- Assess the function of the hand (pinch and grip).

LOWER LIMB: HISTORY

If the pattern of symptoms (e.g. history of swelling, morning stiffness, response to activity and involvement of several joints) suggests an inflammatory disorder, a family history and symptoms of extra-articular features (Table 8.5) should be sought. If leg or foot pain is diffuse or poorly localised by the patient, referred pain, for example owing to lumbar nerve root pathology, should be considered. Pain in the knee is usually well localised while hip pain may be reported in the groin, anterior thigh or knee. The impact of lower limb symptoms on normal daily activities, i.e. the extent of disability, should be documented (Table 8.11).

TABLE 8.11 Activities of daily living involving the lower limb

- Walking, climbing stairs
- Dressing
- Rising and sitting
- Bathing
- Driving

The hip

With the exception of the congenitally dislocated hip, the major presenting symptom of hip disease is usually pain. Pain is usually felt in the groin, but may be reported in the thigh or knee or, less frequently, the buttock. The pain is usually worse on activity, and limits walking. There is often troublesome pain at night, which prevents sleep or awakens the patient when turning over during sleep. Some degree of stiffness is common and results in limitation of flexion which may be sufficient to prevent the patient putting on socks or shoes, or cutting the toenails. There may also be difficulty getting in and out of the bath or sitting on a low seat.

Fracture of the femoral neck is usually caused by a fall. In the presence of gross osteoporosis or tumour infiltration the nature of the injury may be quite trivial. If the fracture impacts, the patient may be able to get up and walk unaware that a fracture has occurred. Thus the ability to weight bear does not necessarily exclude a fracture of the hip. Violent injury, typically involving the front seat passenger in a car whose knee strikes the dashboard can cause the hip to dislocate posteriorly, resulting in agonising pain. The limb will be shortened and internally rotated.

The knee

In the absence of a history of trauma, the complaint of a relatively sudden onset of pain and swelling suggests diagnoses such as sepsis, crystal arthropathy (gout or pseudogout) or reactive arthritis (Fig. 8.20A). An insidious onset of chronic knee pain and swelling with stiffness, which is worse in the morning and after inactivity, is more typical of chronic monoarthritis. Enquiry about other joint symptoms, extra-articular features and family history will help with the diagnosis. A long history of painful knee, often with relatively little swelling, which is exacerbated by activity and causes progressive disability over months and years is more typical of degenerative disease. Night pain is an important feature of established degenerative disease. Pain in the knee which the patient has difficulty localising may be referred from the hip or, occasionally, the lumbar spine.

In the patient presenting after trauma, it is important to try to establish how the injury occurred and speed of onset of the swelling, since this information often assists in

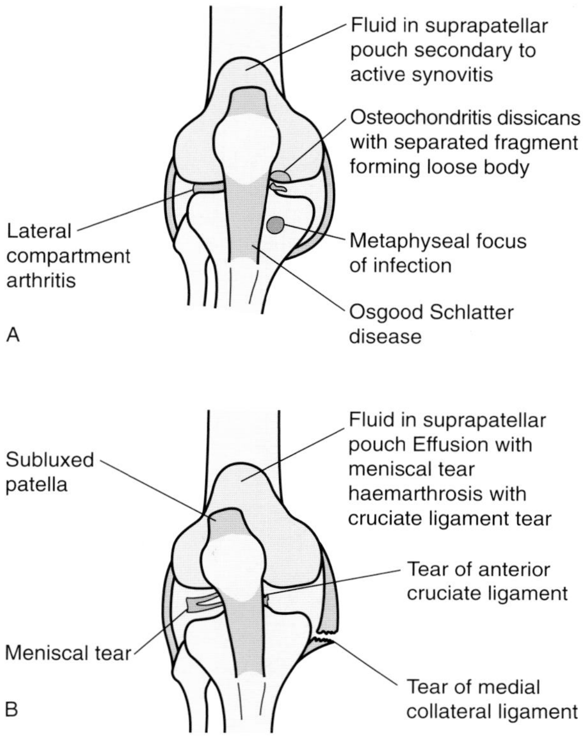

Fig. 8.20 A **Non-traumatic lesions about the knee.** B **Traumatic lesions about the knee.**

making the diagnosis (Fig. 8.20B). For example, rotation on a flexed knee, as when kicking a football is a typical cause of meniscal injury. The meniscus is avascular and when torn is associated with a slowly developing effusion. Abduction-adduction stresses across the knee, for example while skiing, are more likely to damage the collateral ligaments. Cruciate ligament injuries are also common and may be associated with a variety of mechanisms, such as hyperextension of the knee. Ligaments are vascular structures – thus after a tear of the collateral ligament there is bruising at the site of the injury, while after a cruciate ligament tear, a haemarthrosis rapidly develops. The patient should also be asked to try to identify the site of pain, which is usually localised to the site of injury or pathology.

Sometimes a knee effusion is associated with pain and swelling in the popliteal fossa. This is caused by synovial fluid passing through a one-way valvular system in the posterior capsule into the popliteal fossa producing a popliteal (Baker's) cyst. This may be asymptomatic but on occasions it can give rise to local pain. The history of a cyst, followed by an episode of acute pain in the calf, with a reduction in the size of the cyst is highly suggestive of a rupture of the cyst. This is sometimes misdiagnosed as a deep venous thrombosis.

The complaint of the knee 'giving way' is common. Such instability can occur as a result of inability to fully straighten the knee (locking), and this is often associated with a displaced segment of torn meniscus. Mobile loose bodies within the joint tend to produce intermittent locking when the knee suddenly gives way under the patient, and just as rapidly the obstruction frees and the knee returns to normal. A careful history may be required to distinguish between the complaint of locking and the sensation of stiffness and restriction felt in the degenerative knee, which is particularly noted by the patient after sitting.

The leg, ankle and foot

In adults, the clinical problems involving the ankle and foot can be divided into those presenting with or without a history of trauma.

History of trauma

'I twisted my ankle' is the typical history of the patient with an inversion injury. This can result in partial or complete tears of the lateral ligament complex, the latter often followed by a tendency to recurrent injury. The report of abrupt pain in the heel, typically occurring whilst the patient is playing tennis or squash, or even pushing a car, may be due to rupture of the Achilles tendon. Patients may think someone has kicked them. Patients on steroid therapy are prone to Achilles tendon rupture. After either penetrating or non-penetrating injury to the ankle, the tibialis posterior tendon may be damaged or ruptured. The patient reports local pain over the inner ankle and difficulty walking. If left untreated there may be rapid development of flat foot.

A history of pain in the forefoot localised to the second metatarsal, especially after an unusual degree of activity such as a lot of walking, suggests a stress fracture. The pain is usually relieved by rest and aggravated by weight bearing. The early diagnosis is made on the history and clinical findings, as X-rays may be normal for the first 10 days.

No history of trauma

Spontaneous forefoot pain, radiating into the contiguous sides of the third and fourth toes, and typically made worse when the patient wears tight shoes, suggests a plantar (Morton's) neuroma. Neuromata rarely affect other interdigital clefts.

Acute onset of pain and swelling, as in other joints, should prompt consideration of gout, infection and other acute inflammatory arthropathies. A history of insidious onset of pain in the foot, associated with stiffness or swelling, which is worse after inactivity and shows diurnal variation, may be due to rheumatoid arthritis or other inflammatory conditions. The forefoot is more commonly affected than the hindfoot. In more established cases, the metatarsal heads become prominent and the patient may report a sensation of walking on pebbles or broken glass.

The complaint of deformity of the great toe, either with or without pain on walking, is typical of hallux valgus. The pain is usually experienced over a soft tissue bunion overlying the exposed head of the first metatarsal, which can be associated with episodes of redness and swelling. Patients often have difficulty in obtaining suitable footwear. It is a very common problem and there is a family history of the disorder in two-thirds of patients. It is important to establish whether the toe is painful or not, because cosmetic treatment of deformity alone is not justified.

Pain under the heel on weight bearing, usually well localised to the medial tubercle of the calcaneum, may be due to plantar fasciitis. This may be a feature of seronegative spondyloarthropathies. Diffuse heel pain may also be a consequence of increased activity and poor footwear (e.g. jogger's or policeman's heel).

KEY POINTS

- Establish the site and distribution of pain and associated symptoms.
- Pain in the knee may be referred from the hip.
- The speed of onset of swelling after knee injury is of diagnostic help:
  - slow (6–24 hours) suggests avascular aetiology, e.g. meniscal tear
  - fast (within 1 hour) suggests vascular aetiology, e.g. cruciate ligament rupture.
- Increased hindfoot pain on uneven ground suggests subtalar joint pathology.
- Document functional difficulties; but remember that the ability to weight bear does not exclude an impacted fracture at the hip.

ANATOMY OF THE LOWER LIMB

The hip

As the hip is a ball and socket joint, flexion, extension, abduction, adduction, rotation and the combined movement of circumduction are all possible. The actual range changes through life, as does the posture of the joint. As age increases, the first movements to decrease are extension and internal rotation, followed by abduction. The femoral and obturator nerves supply sensory branches to the hip joint and knee joint, explaining the frequency of referred pain from the hip to the knee.

Hip abductor function may be deficient or absent following congenital or acquired dislocation of the hip, fracture of the neck of the femur, paralysis (as in poliomyelitis) or painful inhibition of function in arthritis. When the normal subject stands on one leg, the glutei contract, so that the opposite side of the pelvis is tilted up slightly; this mechanism allows the opposite leg to clear the ground while walking. If the glutei are deficient, the opposite side of the pelvis will tilt downwards and balance can only be maintained by leaning sideways to shift the centre of gravity over the affected hip (Trendelenburg's sign, Fig. 8.25). When walking, this causes the patient to dip or lurch towards the affected side. This can be corrected by the use of a stick in the opposite hand. With bilateral abductor impairment, the trunk leans from side to side, producing a characteristic rolling gait.

The knee

The main landmarks of the knee are illustrated in Figure 8.21. The patella and the tibial tubercle can be readily palpated

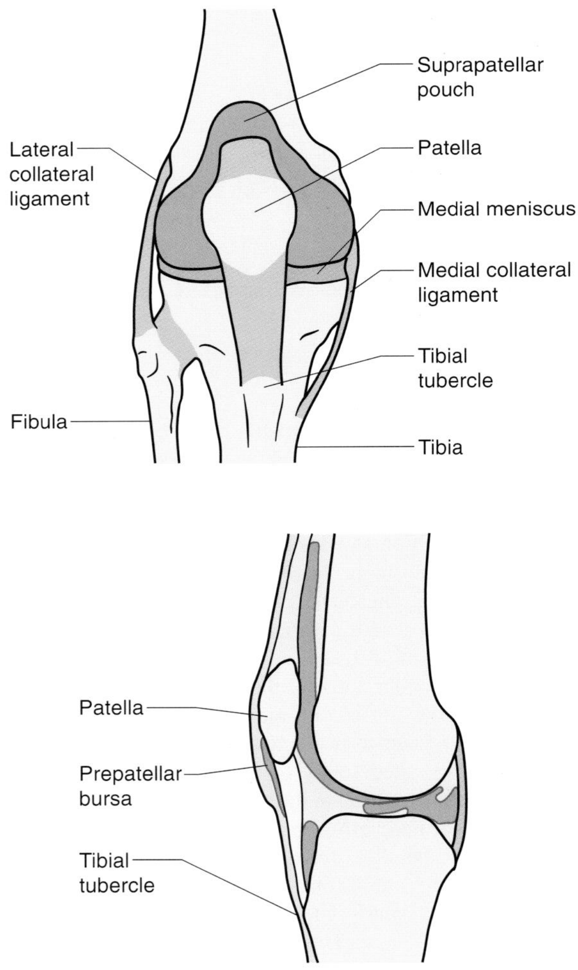

Fig. 8.21 Surface anatomy of the knee.

with the patellar tendon between these two structures. With the knee in flexion, the wide anterior joint line can be felt readily at the lateral and medial sides of the patellar tendon. The examiner can then palpate the femoral condyle above and the tibial plateau below, allowing the joint line to be defined and traced anteroposteriorly. Sites of tenderness can be related to the joint line.

The foot

For convenience, the foot may be divided into three regions: *the hindfoot* (talus and calcaneum), the *midtarsal region* (navicular, cuboid and cuneiforms) and *forefoot* (metatarsals and toes). For simplicity of description, the major movements are:

- ankle dorsiflexion and plantar flexion
- subtalar joint inversion and eversion
- midtarsal joint (talonavicular and calcaneocuboid joints) rotation (supination and pronation)
- forefoot (metatarsophalangeal joints) allow flexion and extension movements.

EXAMINATION OF THE LOWER LIMB

The hip

Examination sequence

Inspection – standing

☐ Observe the patient when standing and walking and note any abnormality of gait.

☐ Observe the patient from behind and look for scoliosis and pelvic tilting which may conceal a hip deformity or true shortening of one leg (Figs 8.22, 8.23, and 8.24). If pelvic tilt is present, examination of leg lengths is essential.

Test for stability of the hip – Trendelenburg's test

☐ Ask the patient to stand first on one leg and then the other.

☐ Observe any change in pelvic tilt on the non-weight-bearing side (Fig. 8.25).

Inspection – supine

☐ Inspect the patient supine, positioned so that the pelvic brim is at right angles to the spine.

☐ Inspect the posture of each leg and note any deformity, swelling or other signs of inflammation, muscle wasting, sinus formation or obvious asymmetry.

☐ Palpate for local tenderness over the front of the hip and over the greater trochanter.

☐ Measure leg lengths as follows:

- To measure 'apparent' shortening, place the legs parallel with the patient lying supine. Measure from a fixed point such as the xiphisternum or umbilicus to the tip of the medial malleolus on each side (Fig. 8.26).
- To measure 'true' shortening with the patient lying supine, place the normal limb in a comparable position of adduction or abduction to the abnormal limb. Measure from the anterior superior iliac spine to the medial malleolus (Fig. 8.27).

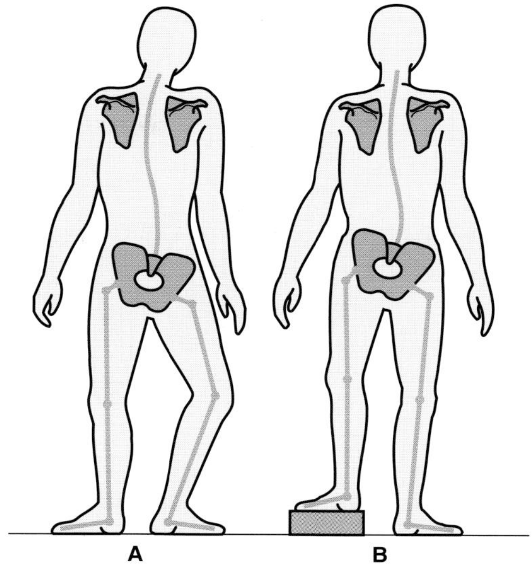

Fig. 8.22 [A] **Abduction deformity of the right hip.** [B] **A left shoe raise straightens the right leg but does not correct the pelvic tilt or the scoliosis.**

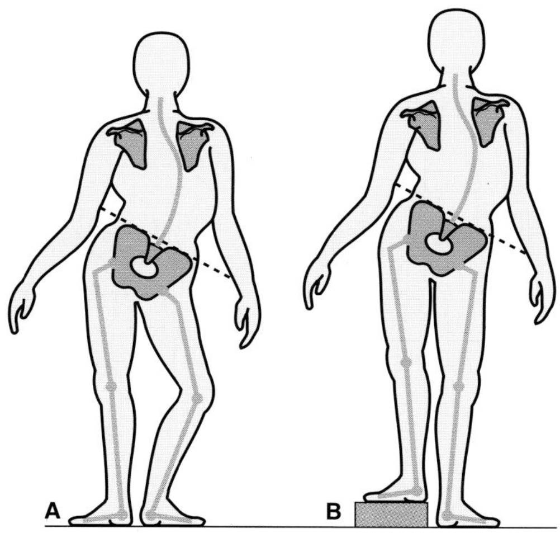

Fig. 8.23 [A] **Adduction deformity of the left hip.** [B] **A left shoe raise straightens the right leg without correcting the pelvic tilt or the scoliosis.**

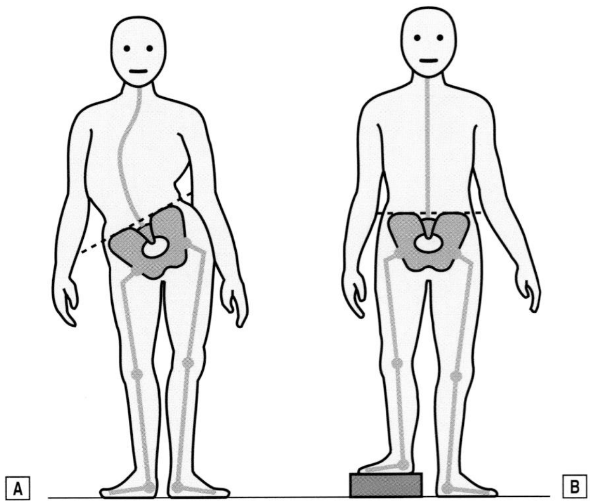

Fig. 8.24 Effect of true shortening of right leg on posture. A Causes pelvic tilt and scoliosis. B The pelvic tilt and scoliosis are fully corrected by providing a shoe raise.

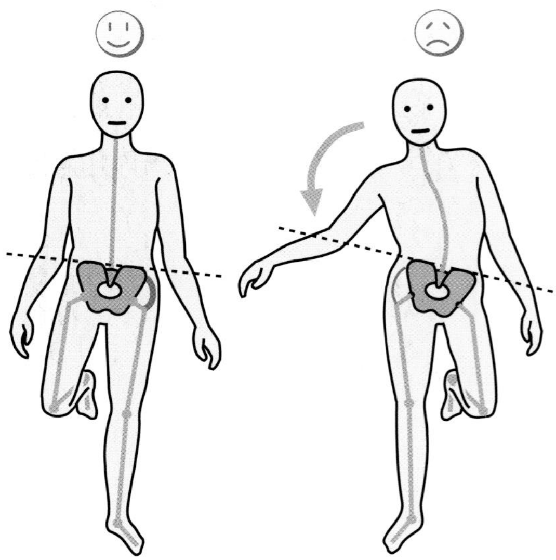

Fig. 8.25 Trendelenburg's sign. Powerful gluteal muscles maintain the position when standing on the left leg; weakness of the right gluteal muscles results in pelvic tilt when standing on the right leg.

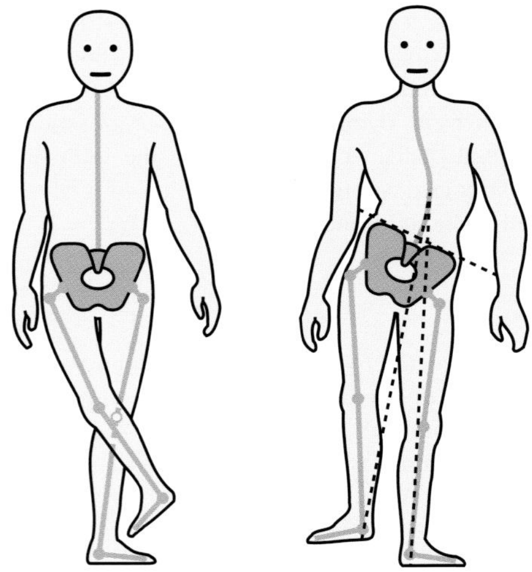

Fig. 8.26 Measurement for apparent shortening of the leg caused by adduction deformity of the right hip.

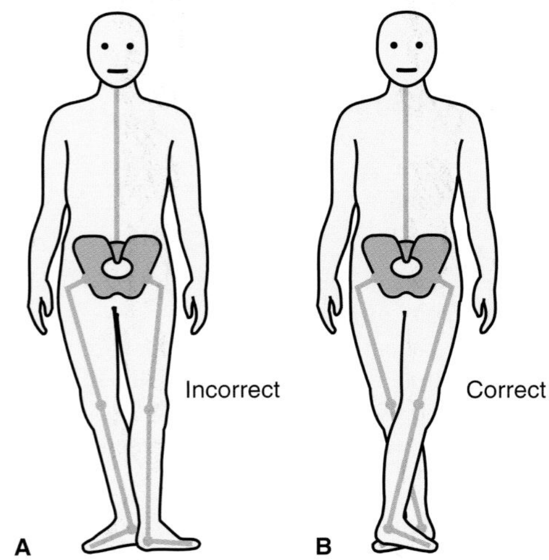

Fig. 8.27 Measurement for true shortening of the leg. The patient has an adduction deformity of the right limb. On placing the normal limb in the same position of adduction, the leg lengths are the same, excluding true shortening. A Incorrect because legs are not in a comparable position. B Correct because the legs are in a comparable position of adduction.

Movements

- ☐ Position the pelvis so that the pelvic brim is at right angles to the spine. (Any fixed adduction or abduction will usually be revealed immediately.)
- ☐ With one hand stabilising the iliac crest, use the other hand to flex each hip and note the range of flexion (0–120 degrees) (Fig. 8.28).
- ☐ Perform Thomas's test first on one side and then the other in order to unmask a flexion deformity of the hip concealed by the presence of a compensatory lumbar lordosis.
- ☐ Place one hand between the patient's lumbar spine and the examination couch.
- ☐ Flex the unaffected hip to its limit and continue to push to straighten the lumbar spine; as the lumbar lordosis is

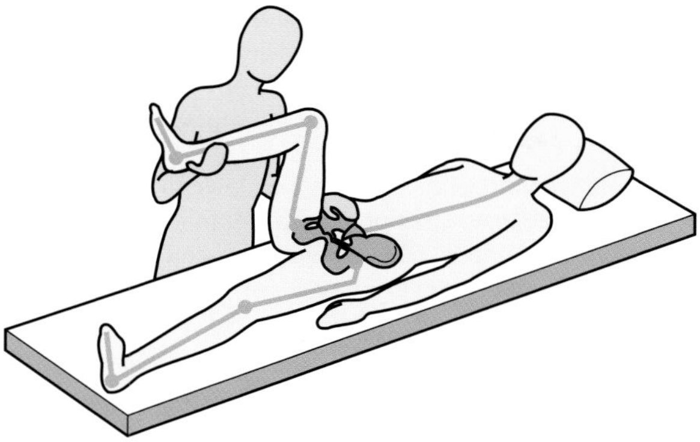

Fig. 8.28 Testing flexion of the hip.

obliterated, the examining hand is squashed between the patient's spine and the examination couch.

- ☐ The opposite leg, if abnormal, will rise off the table revealing the amount of flexion deformity present (Fig. 8.29B).
- ☐ Immobilise the pelvis by grasping the opposite iliac crest, then abduct (variable, minimum 45 degrees) (Fig. 8.30) and adduct (25 degrees) each hip, noting the range of movement. At each extreme the pelvis will be felt to tilt with the limb.
- ☐ To measure rotation with the hip flexed, flex the hip and knee to 90 degrees and use the tibia to assess the arc of rotation – internal rotation (30 degrees) and external rotation (45 degrees).

Or

- ☐ To measure with the hip extended, roll each leg on the couch and measure the range of rotation using the feet as indicators (90 degrees arc of movement).

Common abnormal findings

- Antalgic or Trendelenburg gait.
- Wasting of thigh muscles.
- Loss of flexion, rotation and abduction.
- Pain on passive rotation.
- Flexion and adduction contracture producing 'apparent' shortening of the limb.

The knee

The knee is particularly prone to injury because its stability through a full range of movement of 150 degrees is entirely dependent on the ligaments and muscles (Fig. 8.21).

A large effusion can often be easily seen on inspection as a 'horseshoe' swelling extending a hand's breadth above the patella. The presence of a moderately sized effusion can be confirmed by the '*patellar tap*'. Small effusions are best

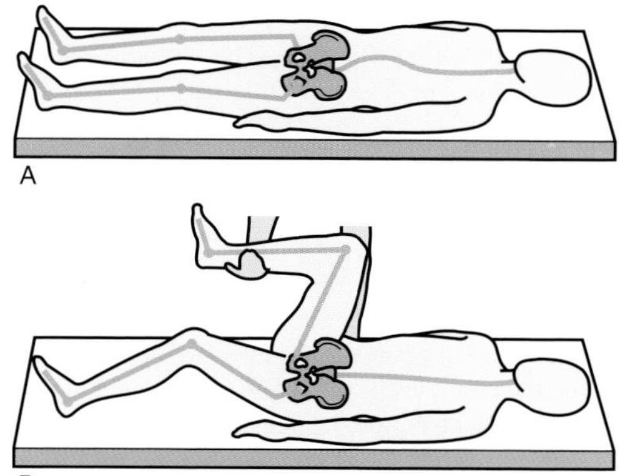

Fig. 8.29 Flexion deformity of the left hip. This may be concealed by lumbar lordosis [A] However, full flexion of the right hip reveals the flexion deformity on the left side [B] (Thomas's hip flexion test).

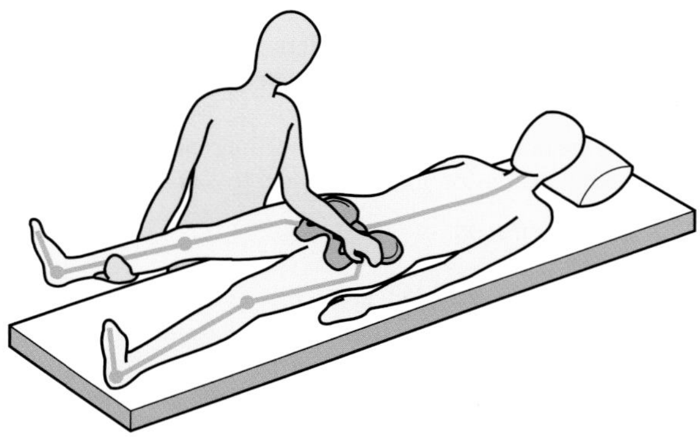

Fig. 8.30 Testing abduction of the hip.

DISORDERS

Limb length inequality due to hip pathology

Shortening
- True shortening – due to loss of bone or cartilage or femoral displacement:
  - Perthe's
  - Slipped femoral epiphysis
  - Avascular necrosis
  - Arthritis
  - Fracture/dislocation
  - Missed congenital dislocation of the hip
- Apparent shortening – due to adduction deformity giving rise to elevation of the pelvis on the side of the pathology
  - Arthritis

Lengthening
- Real lengthening:
  - Overgrowth, e.g. juvenile arthritis
- Apparent lengthening – due to abduction deformity causing downward tilt of the pelvis on the side of pathology:
  - Arthritis

detected using the '*massage test*'. There are various methods of performing this test. The method described is the chapter editor's preferred technique.

Examination sequence

- ☐ Note the patient's gait.
- ☐ With the patient standing, note the presence of genu valgum or genu varum.
- ☐ If genu valgum is present, measure the distance between the medial malleoli with the patient standing and knees just touching. In genu varum, measure the gap between the medial condyles of the femur with the feet together.
- ☐ With the patient supine, inspect the limb alignment and note any deformity, bony contour, loss of muscle bulk (especially quadriceps), erythema or swelling. A large effusion may be observed as a horseshoe swelling above the patella.
- ☐ If quadriceps wasting is present, record and compare muscle girth at a selected level above the patella (say 10 cm) in both thighs.
- ☐ With the knee flexed, palpate the joint line to elicit tenderness. Also note any tenderness above or below the joint line which may denote collateral ligament pathology.
- ☐ Note the presence of synovial swelling including any synovial distension in the popliteal fossa (Baker's cyst).

Testing for an effusion

'The patellar tap'

- ☐ With the knee extended, apply pressure with one hand to empty any fluid within the suprapatellar pouch into the retropatellar space. If there is sufficient fluid this will lift the patella off the underlying femoral condyle.
- ☐ With the fingers of the opposite hand, press down on the patella and fluctuation may be noticed. If this is repeated with a more brisk downward pressure on the patella, a tapping sensation may be felt as the patella hits the femur (Fig. 8.31). If the effusion is very tense the tap is difficult to elicit.

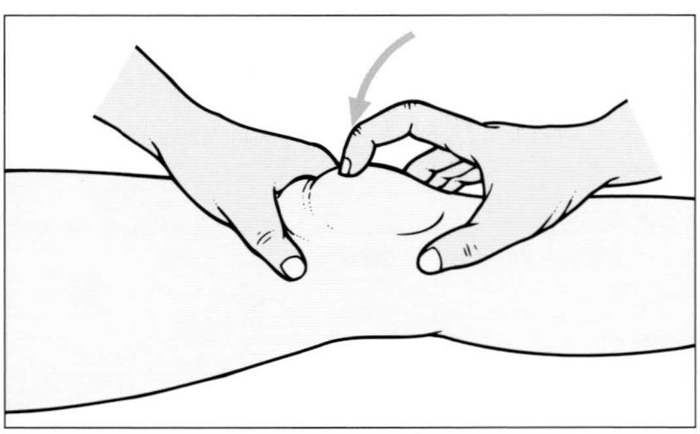

Fig. 8.31 Testing for an effusion by the patellar tap.

'The massage test' – to elicit a small effusion

- ☐ With the knee straight and the quadriceps relaxed, stroke any fluid on the medial side of the joint up and across into the lateral aspect of the suprapatellar pouch (Fig. 8.32A).
- ☐ Then, without delay, firmly stroke down the lateral side of the knee in an attempt to push any fluid back onto the medial side of the knee. If fluid is present, a fluid impulse will be seen to cause a transient bulge on the anteromedial side of the knee (Fig. 8.32B).

Movement

- ☐ With patient supine, note the presence of any flexion deformity of the knee. If the knee is flexed this may be due to pathology in knee, hip or both.
- ☐ Test whether full passive extension of the knee is possible, or whether it is a fixed incorrectable flexion deformity (contracture).
- ☐ Check for '*extensor lag*', which indicates quadriceps weakness. Ask the patient to lift the leg while attempting to keep the knee as straight as possible. If the patient cannot keep the knee fully extended, an '*extensor lag*' is present.
- ☐ Measure the range of active flexion using a goniometer (normal range 0–140 degrees). If there is a flexion deformity of say 15 degrees and the knee can be flexed to 110 degrees, the range of movement would be recorded as 15–110 degrees. At the limit of active flexion, check the range of passive flexion.
- ☐ When indicated, as in a suspected cartilage lesion, assess any minor limitation of full extension which may not be visible with the patient supine. Turn the patient into the prone position with the thigh supported on the

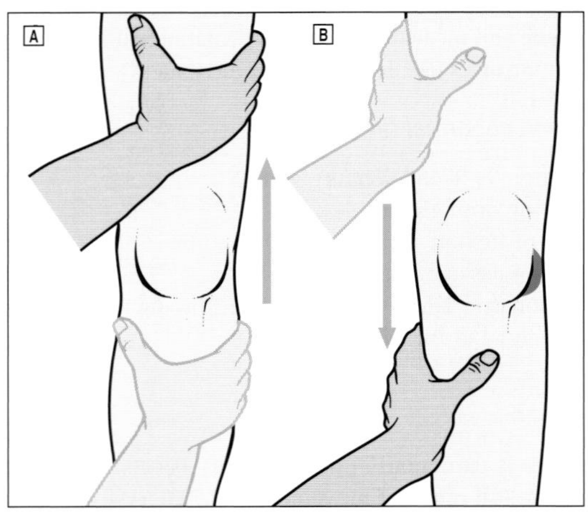

Fig. 8.32 Testing for an effusion in the right knee by the massage test. A Massage any fluid away from the medial side of the knee. B Apply firm downward pressure over the lateral side of the knee and observe for fluid displacement.

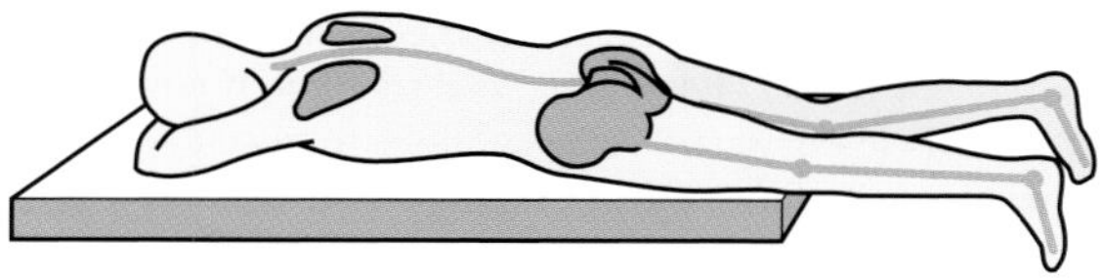

Fig. 8.33 Flexion contracture in presence of cartilage lesion.

bed and the lower leg projecting over the end of the examination couch. Observe the relative level of the heels. In the presence of a flexion deformity one heel will remain higher than the other (Fig. 8.33).

- ☐ When indicated, perform tests for instability, as described below.

Tests of the stability of the knee

Tests of knee stability are primarily of importance after injury. However, instability is also found in established arthritis with erosion of cartilage, because the collateral ligaments may become slack.

Testing the collateral ligaments

The collateral ligaments control mediolateral stability. With the knee fully extended, there is normally no abduction or adduction. If the ligament is lax, the knee opens when stressed. When this manoeuvre is performed on a strained ligament, no movement occurs, but pain is elicited over the damaged ligament. Remember that a small amount of movement is normally present when the knee is slightly flexed and 'unlocked'.

Examination sequence

- ☐ With the knee fully extended, hold the patient's ankle firmly between the examiner's elbow and side.
- ☐ Use both hands to attempt to abduct and adduct the tibia while keeping the knee straight (Fig. 8.34).

Or

- ☐ With the leg resting on the couch and one hand holding the ankle firmly, look for abnormal laxity by applying pressure with the other hand first over the medial and lateral aspects of the knee.

The cruciate ligaments

These ligaments are tested with the knee flexed to a right angle. In this position, there is normally a little anteroposterior glide of the tibia on the femur. Movement in excess of this is abnormal ('draw sign').

Examination sequence

- ☐ Place the knee in a flexed position and maintain the position by sitting gently against the patient's foot (Fig. 8.35).

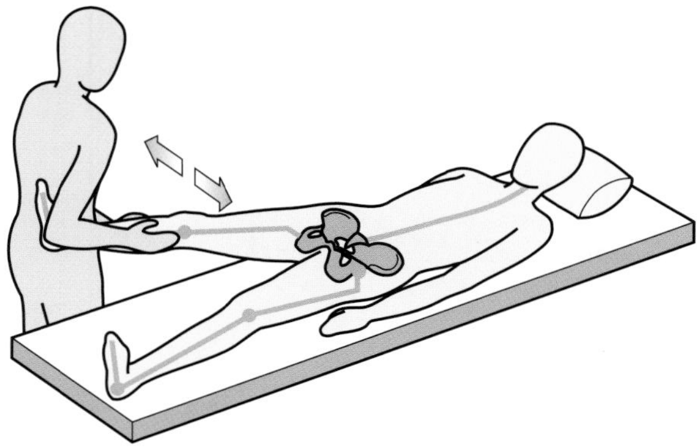

Fig. 8.34 Testing the collateral ligaments of the knee.

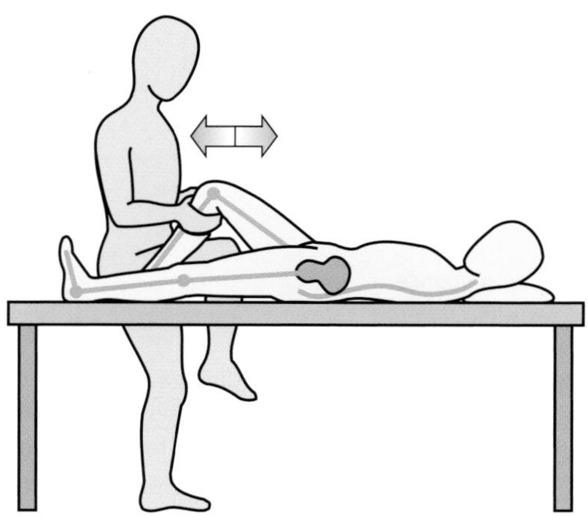

Fig. 8.35 Testing the cruciate ligaments of the knee.

- ☐ With both hands, first check that the hamstrings are relaxed, otherwise the test is invalid.
- ☐ Test the anterior cruciate ligament by grasping the tibia below and drawing it forward.
- ☐ Test the posterior cruciate ligament by pushing the tibia backwards.

Patellar instability

Recurrent subluxation of the patella may be associated with a small high-riding patella, genu valgum, joint hypermobility, trauma, or with wasting of the vastus medialis. If the patella has previously dislocated, the *'patellar apprehension test'* is usually positive.

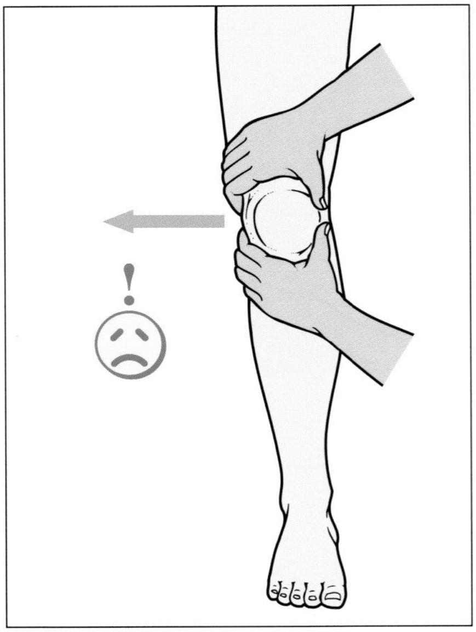

Fig. 8.36 Patellar apprehension test.

Examination sequence

- ☐ Perform the *patellar apprehension test* with the knee flexed to 30 degrees.
- ☐ Apply lateral pressure to the medial border of the patella. The patient demonstrates great apprehension in response to this manoeuvre and actively resists further flexion, fearing that the patellar may redislocate (Fig. 8.36).

Meniscal pathology

Meniscal tears are associated with a joint effusion and may cause 'locking'. Local tenderness is usually present at the site of pathology. An anterior beak tear, or bucket handle segment, may cause locking, but a tear of the posterior horn usually does not. The latter produces pain when the knee is in the flexed position.

Examination sequence

Testing for anterior horn lesions

- ☐ With the knee in the flexed position, palpate for tenderness in the anterior or middle third of the joint line.
- ☐ Next, determine whether there is a flexion contracture, if necessary by placing the patient in the prone position and looking for elevation of the heel (see Fig. 8.33).

Posterior horn lesions

- ☐ Grasp the patient's heel with the right hand and steady the knee with the left whilst palpating the joint line.
- ☐ Slowly extend the knee, repeat the manoeuvre with the tibia in external and then internal rotation. If positive, a clunk is felt or heard as the cartilage fragment is displaced and the patient experiences discomfort (McMurray's test).
- ☐ Ask the patient to go into a crouched position and waddle like a duck. The patient with a posterior horn lesion is unable to perform this manoeuvre.

Common abnormal findings

- Wasting of the quadriceps.
- Joint line tenderness at the site of intra-articular pathology.
- An effusion and synovial thickening.
- Flexion deformity.
- Pain on stretching a damaged ligament.
- Popliteal (Baker's) cysts in association with knee effusion.

CASE HISTORY

A 25-year-old man presents with a painful, acute swelling of his right knee. He had no other complaints. On detailed questioning, he mentioned that he played football weekly, but could not recall a specific history of trauma, previous joint problems or history of septic focus of the skin or throat. 2 weeks earlier, after eating out in a restaurant, he had loose bowels for 24 hours and felt unwell. He also admitted to a subsequent episode lasting a few days of urethral burning and discharge, most noticeable on passing urine for the first time each morning. He was married and had not had any casual sexual encounter.

On examination, the knee was held in about 30 degrees of flexion and although the patient was very unhappy to allow movement from this position, with care it could be flexed gently through 70 degrees. There was warm, boggy swelling of the knee, extending into the suprapatellar region. The joint was stable in all directions. He had mild tenderness, swelling and restriction of one ankle.

The history suggested a post-dysenteric arthritis and subsequent investigation confirmed that this was caused by enteric salmonella infection.

Learning points

- Although the lack of cellulitis and the retention of restricted knee movement are against a diagnosis of acute septic arthritis, this requires to be excluded by joint aspiration.
- Urethritis may be an inflammatory feature of reactive arthritis.
- The case illustrates the importance of taking a detailed history in patients presenting with locomotor symptoms.

The ankle and foot

Examination sequence

- ☐ Inspect the patient walking and note any abnormality of gait due to pain or deformity (Table 8.12).
- ☐ With the patient standing inspect the patient's feet and ankles and note the presence of:
  - hindfoot deformity (valgus or varus)
  - flattened (pes planus) or high (pes cavus) longitudinal arch
  - deformity of the toes (Figs 8.37, 8.38, 8.39 and 8.40).

CASE HISTORY

A 15-year-old girl was playing squash when she developed sudden acute pain in her knee and felt a tearing sensation as she fell. She was unable to continue with the game and the joint became swollen over the next few hours. The history of trauma suggested the possibility of damage to miniscus, ligaments or even bone.

Clinical examination revealed diffuse tenderness over the medial capsule, extending above and below the joint line but on stressing the collateral ligaments and cruciate ligaments the joint remained stable. She had a definite positive patellar apprehension test.

Learning points

- The case illustrates the diagnostic value of the patellar apprehension test.
- A medial capsular tear as a result of patellar dislocation should always be considered in the differential diagnosis of knee trauma, because sometimes the patella relocates so quickly that neither the patient nor the examining doctor may be aware of the problem.

TABLE 8.12 Abnormal gait due to ankle or foot pathology

Paralytic foot drop	High stepping and flapping
Fixed equinus deformity	High stepping and fixed
Talipes calcaneus	'Peg-leg' – lacking in spring
Hallux rigidus	Foot inverted and supinated
Stiff painful hindfoot and forefoot (e.g RA)	Slow, flat-footed and springless

- ☐ If there is pes planus, ask the patient to try to stand on the ball of the foot. If there is a mobile deformity, the longitudinal arch will be restored, but not if there is an underlying structural deformity to account for the flat foot (e.g. tarsal coalition).
- ☐ With the patient supine, note the condition of the nails and skin, and the presence of swelling or callosities.
- ☐ Palpate the hindfoot, mid-foot and forefoot to accurately localise any tenderness or swelling (see Disorders box below). Gently compress the forefoot to elicit tenderness.
- ☐ Note the active and passive range of movement of the ankle (normally dorsiflexion 10 degrees and plantar flexion 30 degrees).
- ☐ If ankle dorsiflexion is reduced, estimate the contribution of calf tightness as a possible cause by flexing the knee and re-examining the range of dorsiflexion (Fig. 8.7).
- ☐ To examine the subtalar and midtarsal joints, inspect the active and passive range of inversion and eversion of the heel (Fig. 8.41).
- ☐ Assess the composite range of movement of the subtalar and midtarsal joints. This is approximately 30 degrees of supination and 20 degrees of pronation.
- ☐ To examine the mid-foot joints only, immobilise the heel with one hand to block subtalar inversion and rotate the forefoot (Fig. 8.42).
- ☐ Carefully identify any restriction of movement in the individual toes.

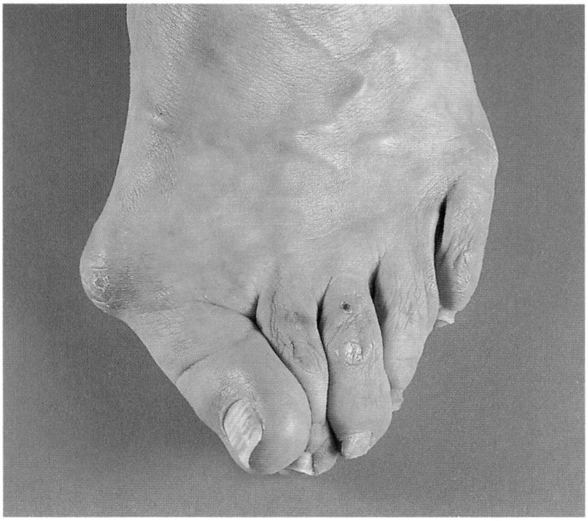

Fig. 8.37 Hallux valgus (left great toe).

Calf squeeze test to assess the integrity of the Achilles tendon

- ☐ Carefully palpate the Achilles tendon and gastrocnemius muscle and note the presence of tenderness, swelling or any defect in the tendon.
- ☐ With the patient prone or kneeling, gently but firmly squeeze the calf just distal to its maximum circumference. Note whether plantar flexion of the foot occurs. If it does not, the tendon is ruptured (Fig. 8.43).

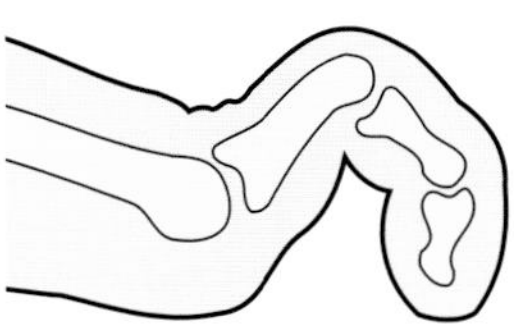

Fig. 8.38 Claw toe.

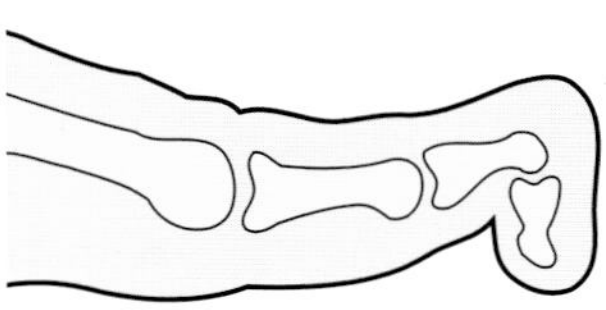

Fig. 8.39 Mallet toe.

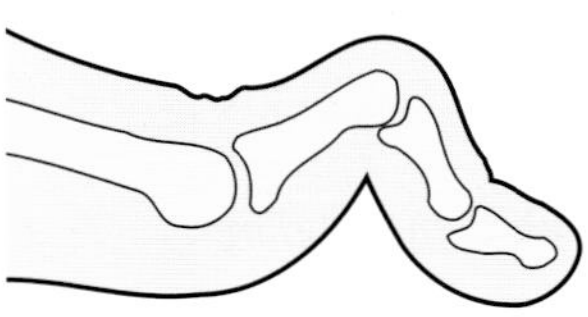

Fig. 8.40 Hammer toe.

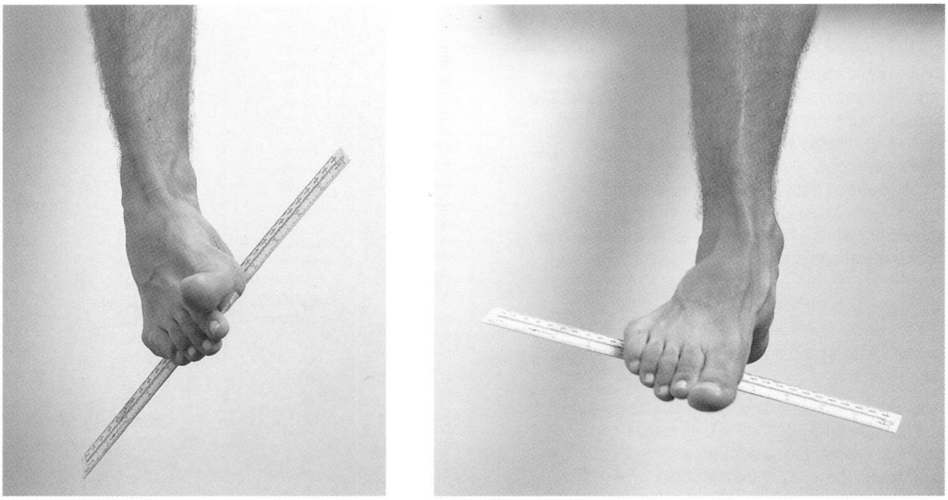

A B

Fig. 8.41 Examining the combined movements of the subtalar and midtarsal joints. A Supination (inversion). B Pronation (eversion).

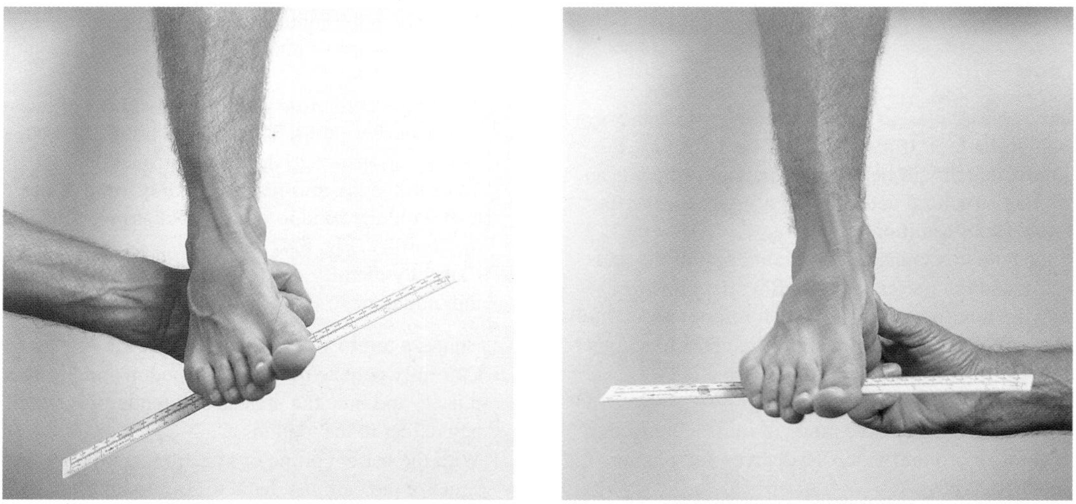

A B

Fig. 8.42 Examining movements of the midtarsal joints. Examiner holds the patient's heel to block subtalar movement. A The residual range of supination is due to midtarsal movement. B The residual range of prenation is due to midtarsal movement and is usually very limited.

Common abnormal findings

- Mobile flat foot (pes planus) and valgus hindfoot is common in all age groups.
- Hallux valgus deformity, with or without over-riding of the second toe in the middle-aged and elderly patient.
- Hammer or claw toe deformities in older patients.
- Heel pain (jogger's or policeman's heel) in middle-aged or older patients.

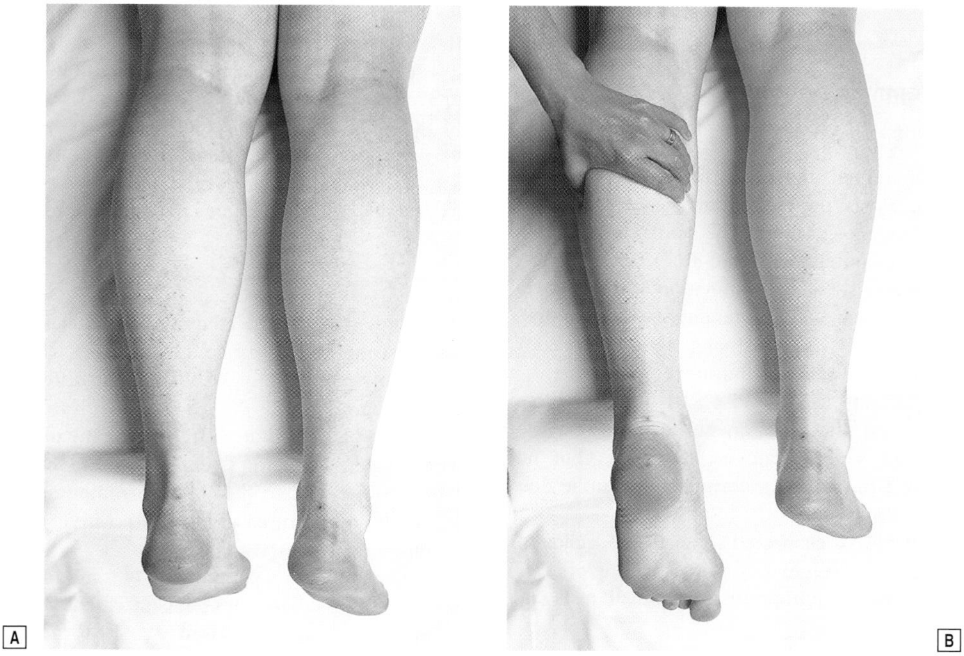

Fig. 8.43 The calf squeeze test for a ruptured Achilles tendon. A The control position. B Demonstrating an intact left Achilles tendon and plantar flexion of the foot.

DISORDERS
Site and pathology of pain in the heel and foot
The heel and hindfoot: ● Insertion of plantar fascia in calcaneum – plantar fasciitis ● Bone – calcaneal fracture; posterior bony prominence (pump heel) ● Ankle or subtalar joint – inflammatory or degenerative arthritis ● Tendon – tenosynovitis; partial or complete rupture of the Achilles tendon or posterior tibialis ● Retrocalcaneal bursa – bursitis
The forefoot: ● Bone – stress fracture of neck of second metatarsal ● MTP joints – synovitis ● Plantar nerve – Morton's neuroma ● Soft tissue contracture – clawing or hammer toe deformity

KEY POINTS

- Thomas's test is useful in unmasking flexion deformities of the hip.
- Any patient presenting with knee pain requires a careful examination of the hip.
- Always define the area of maximal tenderness.
- The patellar apprehension test may unmask an unstable kneecap.
- Assess function as well as joint movement.
- Examine the shoes for signs of abnormal wear.
- Deformity at one level may cause deformity at another.

CASE HISTORY

A 40-year-old taxi driver had no problems driving his taxi, but complained of increasing pain in the hindfoot, aggravated by walking over rough ground and causing sleep disturbance. On questioning, he explained that he had fallen from scaffolding 10 years previously, fracturing his heel and a thoracic vertebra. He had been unable to return to work as a roof tiler because of residual pain and stiffness in the hindfoot.

Clinically, he had a swollen hindfoot with tenderness over the sinus tarsi and the lateral border of the foot. There was no tenderness over the ankle joint line. He had a full range of flexion and extension at the ankle but no inversion of the subtalar joint and only minimal inversion of the midtarsal joint. X-ray examination confirmed the presence of a calcaneal deformity and osteoarthritis of the subtalar joint, almost certainly the result of arthritis secondary to previous calcaneal trauma.

Learning points

- This case illustrates the impact that impairment of a single joint may have on a specific occupation (roof tiler) but not on others (e.g. driving).

INVESTIGATION AND MANAGEMENT

Investigating common syndromes

The acute hot joint

In the absence of trauma, the main differential diagnosis lies between gout, sepsis, pseudogout and reactive arthritis. The most likely diagnosis should be apparent from the clinical history and examination (Table 8.13).

The single most useful test is examination of the synovial fluid aspirate for cell count and differential, presence of urate or pyrophosphate crystals on polarising light microscopy, or for infection by Gram stain and culture.

Acute-phase reactants (ESR and CRP) and full blood count may help with the assessment but they are not diagnostic. A raised serum urate is suggestive, but not diagnostic of gout. Conversely, a normal serum urate does not exclude gout.

If reactive arthritis is suspected, triggering organisms (chlamydia, salmonella, shigella, yersinia, campylobacter) should be sought using appropriate serological tests and direct culture.

X-rays of the joint may provide useful information, for example the presence of chondrocalcinosis (calcification of cartilage), in the menisci of the knee or the triangular ligament of the wrist, may be associated with pseudogout. Degenerative changes are a common and often coincidental finding, and should not deter careful search for other diagnoses.

Polyarthritis

The clinical history, a search for extra-articular features and careful identification of the joints involved should narrow the differential diagnosis, which may include seropositive or seronegative rheumatoid arthritis (RA), systemic lupus erythematosus (SLE), psoriatic arthritis, reactive arthritis and viral arthritis. Any investigations should be interpreted in the light of the clinical findings; none of the available tests is wholly reliable and none can be considered diagnostic.

X-rays of the hands, wrists and feet should be performed to identify whether there is periarticular osteoporosis or erosions. A normal blood count and ESR do not exclude polyarthritis, nor does a negative rheumatoid factor exclude RA. Conversely, the rheumatoid factor and antinuclear factor test respectively may each be positive in normal individuals as well as a wide variety of conditions other than RA and SLE. When the clinical picture suggests SLE or one of its variants, a number of other investigations, including tests for serum complement levels, antibodies against DNA and extractable nuclear antigens may be required.

TABLE 8.13 Differential diagnosis of acute hot joint

Gout	Risk factors (e.g. diuretics, alcohol), family history, male, typical joint – first MTP joint
Pseudogout	Older age, female, typical joint – knee or wrist
Sepsis	Fever, any age, any joint, risk factors (e.g. immunosuppression, drug abuse)
Reactive arthritis	Young adults, male or female, typical joints – knee, ankle or foot; bowel, ocular or urogenital symptoms

Back pain

A careful history and examination to establish the onset, site distribution of pain and any associated neurological symptoms is critical to establishing the differential diagnosis of back pain.

Imaging is widely used in the investigation of back pain. The choice of imaging is dependent on what information is being sought (Table 8.14). Plain radiographs give limited information and often give false positive or false negative results.

For example, in a patient with chronic low back pain and stiffness of an inflammatory character, ankylosing spondylitis should be considered. Here, the ESR may be raised or normal. Absence of the HLA-B27 tissue type makes the diagnosis unlikely but does not exclude it; furthermore, because about 12% of the general population carry this haplotype, its presence is not diagnostic of spondylitis. A plain X-ray of the pelvis may demonstrate sacroiliitis, and of the lumbar and thoracic spine may demonstrate 'squaring' of the vertebrae (the normal concave anterior and posterior surfaces of the vertebral body appear flattened owing to sub-ligamentous calcification forming deep to the longitudinal ligaments). As the disease progresses, frank ossification of the longitudinal ligaments becomes apparent.

COMMON PITFALLS AND HOW TO AVOID THEM

Osteomyelitis

- X-rays are normal for the first 10 days and do not exclude acute osteomyelitis. Bone pain and tenderness should be

TABLE 8.14 Choosing the imaging method in back pain

Suspected pathology	Imaging method
Degenerative change	None required
Sacroiliitis	Plain X-ray
Vertebral fracture	Plain X-ray, radionuclide scan, MRI
Spinal stenosis	CT scan, MRI
Disc prolapse	MRI or CT scan
Spinal cord compression	MRI scan
Tumour	MRI or radionuclide scan

considered to be due to osteomyelitis until proven otherwise because untreated acute osteomyelitis can become chronic within 48 hours, with all its possible attendant complications.

Urgent investigation, including blood cultures, and treatment is mandatory.

Septic arthritis

- Do not start antibiotics until the joint fluid has been aspirated for culture. Aspiration of the joint is essential to establish the precise diagnosis; otherwise identification of the organism may be impossible, prejudicing the outcome.

However, the patient should be started on antibiotics while awaiting the culture result.

Referred pain

- Hip or spinal pathology can present as a pain in the knee. If there are no supportive local clinical abnormalities in the knee joint, *think hip*, e.g. slipped upper femoral epiphysis in the adolescent.

Cauda equina lesions

- Acute disc lesions can produce cauda equina lesions, with effects on bowel and bladder function which may become permanent unless treated urgently. If there is impairment of sphincteric tone and perianal sensation, this represents a surgical emergency and urgent spinal decompression is required within 36–48 hours.

A significant cauda equina lesion can be excluded by carrying out a rectal examination.

Hip fractures

- Remember that a patient with an impacted fracture of the neck of the femur may walk away from the site of the accident. 50% of impacted fractures will subsequently displace and may create permanent problems of much greater magnitude.

Any pain in the hip exacerbated by rotation and associated with deformity requires investigation by X-ray examination.

Rupture of the Achilles tendon

- Complete rupture of the Achilles tendon can be easily missed. If diagnosis is delayed it may be extremely difficult to deal with surgically because of the separation of the ruptured tendon ends. The calf squeeze test is essential following any injury to the calf muscles.

Early synovitis

- Early synovitis may cause stiffness but little or no pain. Its detection allows prompt treatment in conditions such as rheumatoid arthritis and improves outcome. Careful examination is needed to identify joint swelling.

9 A system for case recording

N. R. COLLEDGE

INTRODUCTION

Previous chapters have illustrated the wealth of information that can be obtained from the history and physical examination. This information plays a key part in a patient's care so it is vital that it is recorded in a way that is concise and clear.

The purpose of the case record

The most important function of the case record is to allow information to be shared amongst the health professionals involved in a patient's care. Many hospitals now use multidisciplinary or unitary medical case records. The alternative is that each different profession documents information in its own 'specialist' notes. One patient can thus end up with separate sets of notes for nursing, physiotherapy, occupational therapy and social work as well as a medical case record, with much unnecessary duplication of information between them. The purpose of multidisciplinary notes is to avoid this duplication and to encourage a shared, holistic approach to care.

Within a case record, junior medical staff record their initial findings and plan of management. More senior medical staff may add comments regarding their own findings, and the proposed investigations and management. Records should be accurate, legible and clearly signed. This is especially so in specialities where doctors work a shift system. Should a patient present with a different problem in the future, it can be useful to compare the new findings with those found at the patient's earlier presentation. Other functions of the case record are shown in Table 9.1. It should be remembered that the case record is confidential and details must not be divulged to anyone who is not involved in the patient's care. The case record is a legal document which may be used in a court of law.

TABLE 9.1 Purpose of the case record

- Documentation of history and examination findings
- Sharing of information with medical colleagues and other health professionals
- Record of results of investigations
- Documentation of assessments by other health professionals, e.g. dietitians, therapists
- Record of decisions made regarding patient investigation and management
- Record of patient's progress
- Documentation of information and education provided to patient and patient's relatives
- Record of correspondence regarding patient's management

The patient's right of access

The Health Records Act of 1990 gives patients the right to see and receive a copy of their casenotes. It is unprofessional and potentially distressing to patients if judgemental or flippant comments are recorded. This should be borne in mind when details of a patient's behaviour, personality and relationships with other people are being described. Patients can be denied access to any part of their casenotes if it is considered that this would be likely to cause serious harm to their physical or mental health or damaging to any other individual. This may be important if a named third party, or somebody unnamed but who could be identified, has provided sensitive information, for example of sexual abuse. It is necessary to record such information on separate sheets of paper duly signed and dated by the clinician.

THE SYSTEM

The system for case recording is widely accepted, and indeed many hospital units now supply printed proformas as aides-mémoire. At first, case records can seem baffling because of the extent to which abbreviations are used. Because of pressure of time in clinical practice, these are acceptable but should not be overused. Those which are widely recognised have been included in the text. A particular feature is the use of the prefix '^{o}' to signify 'no', for example ^{o}tenderness, or ^{o}headache. Obscure acronyms should be avoided.

It is not necessary to record all the details of the history and examination in every patient. Some negative findings may be relevant but many can be safely omitted. It becomes easier to judge what does and does not need to be included with increasing experience. For instance, in a patient presenting with breathlessness, the negative details of the respiratory enquiry should be included while the negative responses to the gastrointestinal enquiry could be condensed to 'none' or 'nil'.

Drawings may be helpful, particularly of the abdomen (see Figs 5.9 and 5.10, p. 164) to illustrate the position of tenderness, masses or scars. They are also useful for recording the site and size of superficial injuries or ulcers. A sample case record is shown on the following pages with explanatory notes alongside each section in turn.

The history

Demographic details. The following should be recorded:

- Patient's name and address, date of birth and age
- Source of referral
- General practitioner's name and address
- Source of history, e.g. patient, relative, carer
- Date and time of examination.

03.08.99 MARY BROWN aged 76
14.00 — *32 Blackford Cresc.*
Edinburgh
DOB 17.09.22

Emergency admission to CCU via GP: — *Dr Wells*
History from patient — *High St.*
Edinburgh

Presenting complaint (PC). This is usually one or two words or a brief list as stated by the patient rather than in medical terminology, with the duration of each.

PC
Chest pain 2 hours
Breathless 1 hour
Dizziness 30 min

History of presenting complaint (HPC). This describes the onset and nature of each symptom and its course. The patient's account may have to be paraphrased or condensed. Details which are not relevant can be omitted, but if there is any doubt they should be included. Particularly important comments or descriptions should be included verbatim in inverted commas. Correct grammar is not necessary. It may be helpful to include other parts of the history if particularly relevant, such as the smoking history in patients with cardiac or respiratory presentations, or family history in those with disorders with a possible genetic trait such as hypercholesterolaemia or diabetes mellitus.

CCU – coronary care unit
GP – general practitioner
GTN – glyceryl trinitrate
SOB – shortness of breath

HPC
Severe pain 'like a band around chest' while watching TV which has now lasted 2 hours despite using GTN. Radiates to jaw and inner aspect of L arm.

Has gradually become breathless over last hour and dizzy in last 30 minutes.

First began 6 months ago: episode of lower retrosternal chest pain after walking about 1/2 mile uphill:

- *relieved by rest after 5 min*
- *no assoc. palpitations or SOB.*

Two further episodes over next 3 months.

3 months ago: increasing frequency of pain:

- *now brought on by walking 200 yards on the flat or climbing 1 flight of stairs*
- *worse after heavy meals*
- *other features of pain as before.*

2 months ago: visited GP who diagnosed angina. Prescribed GTN which gave effective relief.

1 week ago: 3 episodes of chest pain at rest, all immediately relieved by GTN.

Smokes 20/day since age of 19.

^{o}*blackouts,* ^{o}*pain in calves on exertion.*

Past medical history (PMH). By convention, this is tabulated in chronological order. It is useful to include important negatives, for example in a patient presenting with chest pain, it is useful to know of any previous myocardial infarction or angina or other risk factors for cardiovascular disease such as hypertension or diabetes mellitus. Jaundice is important because, if it is due to hepatitis B or C, the patient may present a risk to health workers.

COPD – chronic obstructive pulmonary disease
MI – myocardial infarction
DM – diabetes mellitus
J – jaundice
HBP – hypertension
RF – rheumatic fever
TB – tuberculosis

PMH

Tonsillectomy	*1952*	*Hospital X*
COPD	*Since 1990*	*General practitioner*
Perforated peptic ulcer	*1997*	*Hospital Y*

^{o}*MI,* ^{o}*DM,* ^{o}*J,* ^{o}*HBP,* ^{o}*Stroke,* ^{o}*RF,* ^{o}*TB.*

Drug history (DH). Drugs should also be tabulated. Any allergies, particularly to drugs, should also be included. If the patient has previously had an adverse drug reaction, this must be recorded prominently, for example on the front of the casenotes as well as within. It is also important to document details regarding some previously administered drugs, particularly corticosteroids.

NKA – no known allergies
Med – medication
QID – 4 times daily (TID – 3 times daily, BD – twice daily)

DH

	Dose	*Frequency*	*Duration*
Salbutamol inhaler	*2 puffs*	*QID*	*3 years*
Temazepam	*10 mg*	*at night*	*6 months*
Senokot (self-med.)	*2 tabs*	*2–3 times per week*	*10 years*
GTN	*1 tab*	*up to 10/day*	*2 months*

NKA.

Family history (FH). The causes of and ages at death of the patient's immediate family, i.e. parents, siblings and children, should be recorded. Other relevant details can be added below. The symbols used in the construction of a family tree or pedigree chart are shown in Figure 1.7, page 10.

FH

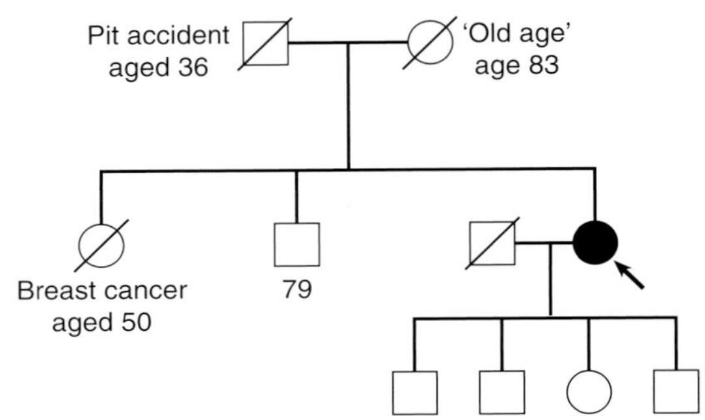

1 aunt died aged 57 of acute **MI**

Social history (SH). The following should be included. More or less detail will be required under each heading depending on the patient's circumstances (see Ch. 1, pp. 10–11):

- Occupation
- Marital status
  Sexual orientation and details of partners (only if appropriate)
- Living circumstances: type of housing and with whom
- Smoking, alcohol history and, when appropriate, illicit drug misuse
- Social support in the frail or disabled.

HH – home help

SH
Retired cleaner.
Widow for 3 years. Lives alone in sheltered housing.
Smoked 20/day from age of 19.
Teetotal.
HH once a week for cleaning and shopping. Daughter nearby visits regularly.

Systematic enquiry (SE). Positive responses to enquiry about the cardinal symptoms of those systems that do not feature in the presenting complaint should be documented. The full systematic enquiry is shown in Table 1.11 (p. 14) and is reproduced for convenience as Table 9.2.

CVS – cardiovascular system
RS – respiratory system
GIS – gastrointestinal system
GUS – genitourinary system
PMB – postmenopausal bleeding
NS – nervous system
LMS – locomotor system
ES – endocrine system

SE
CVS: See above.

RS: Long-standing cough most days with white sputum on rising in morning only. °haemoptysis.

Wheezy in cold weather.

GIS: Weight steady.

Nil else of note.

GUS: PARA 1+0. °PMB.

No urinary symptoms.

NS: Nil of note.

LMS: Occasional pain and stiffness in right knee on exertion for 5 years.

ES: Nil of note.

TABLE 9.2 Systemic inquiry: 'cardinal' symptoms

General health
General well-being
Sleep
Appetite
Weight change
Energy

Cardiovascular system
Ankle swelling
Palpitations
Breathlessness when lying flat (orthopnoea)
Attacks of nocturnal breathlessness (paroxysmal nocturnal dyspnoea)
Chest pain on exertion
Pain in legs on exertion

Respiratory system
Shortness of breath: exercise tolerance
Wheezing
Cough
Sputum production (colour, amount)
Chest pain related to respiration or coughing
Blood in sputum (haemoptysis)

Alimentary
Condition of mouth
Difficulty with swallowing (dysphagia)
Indigestion
Heartburn
Abdominal pain
Weight loss
Change in bowel habit
Colour of motion (e.g. pale, dark, black, fresh blood)

Urogenital
Pain on passing urine (dysuria)
Frequency of passing urine by day or night (nocturia)
Abnormal colour of urine (e.g. blood)
Number of sexual partners
Males
- If appropriate age, prostatic symptoms such as difficulty in starting to pass urine, poor stream, terminal dribbling
- If appropriate, mental attitude to sex (libido), morning erections, frequency of intercourse, ability to maintain erections, ejaculation, urethral discharge

Females
- If premenopausal, age of onset of periods (menarche), regularity of periods (e.g. 28-day cycle), length of period, blood loss (e.g. clots, flooding), date of last period, contraception if relevant, presence of vaginal discharge
- If post-menopausal, bleeding
- Stress and/or urge incontinence
- If appropriate, libido, pain during intercourse (dyspareunia)

Central nervous system
Headaches
Fits
Faints
Tingling (paraesthesiae)
Numbness
Muscle weakness
Hearing symptoms (e.g. deafness, tinnitus)
Excessive thirst
Sleep patterns

Visual
Appearance of eyes
Pain
Disturbance of vision

Locomotor
Joint pain or stiffness
Muscle pain or weakness

Endocrine
Heat intolerance
Cold intolerance
Change in sweating
Prominence of eyes
Swelling in neck

The examination

General (O/E):

- The patient's physical appearance, e.g. frail, drowsy, breathless
- The mental state, e.g. anxious, distressed, confused
- Whether clinically dehydrated
- Whether undernourished, cachectic or overweight and recorded weight and height
- Skin, e.g. cyanosis, pallor, jaundice and any specific lesions or rashes
- Breasts: normal or description of mass
- Hands: finger clubbing or other abnormality of skin or nails
- Lymph nodes: presence and site.

O/E

Anxious, frail, cachectic lady.
Weight 45 kg. Height 1.25 m.
2 cm craggy mass in upper, outer quadrant L breast. Fixed to underlying tissues.
Patient unaware of this.
1 cm node in apex of left axilla.
°pallor, °cyanosis, °jaundice, °clubbing.

Cardiovascular system (CVS). The following should be recorded:

- Pulse (P) rate, rhythm, character and volume
- Blood pressure (BP)
- Jugular venous pulse (JVP) height and character
- Presence or absence of ankle oedema
- Apex beat (AB) position, character, presence of thrills
- Heart sounds (HS), presence and description of added sounds and murmurs
- Peripheral pulses (PP)

  (Normal +, Reduced +/–, Absent –, Aneurysmal ++)
- Vascular bruits

  5ICS MCL – 5th intercostal space, midclavicular line
  ESM – ejection systolic murmur
  LLSE – lower left sternal edge

CVS

P90 reg, small volume, normal character. BP 140/80.
JVP + 3 cm, normal character. °oedema.
AB 5ICS MCL, °thrills.
HS I + II + 2/6, ESM at LLSE, °radiation.
°bruits.

PP:

	Radial	*Brachial*	*Carotid*	*Femoral*
R	+	+	+	+
L	+	+	+	+
	Popliteal	*Post. tibial*	*Dorsalis pedis*	
R	+/–	+/–	+/–	
L	+	+	+	

Respiratory system (RS):

- Any chest wall deformity
- Trachea central or deviated
- Signs of hyperinflation
- Expansion and its symmetry
- Percussion note (PN) and site of any abnormality
- Breath sounds (BS), any added sounds and site of abnormality
- Vocal resonance (VR) and site of abnormality.

RS

Trachea central. Reduced cricosternal distance and intercostal indrawing on inspiration.
Expansion reduced but symmetrical.
PN resonant.
BS vesicular and quiet.
VR normal and symmetrical.

Abdominal system (AS):

- Mouth: any abnormality
- Abdomen:
  - any scars and their site
  - altered shape, e.g. distended, scaphoid
  - hernial orifices
  - any tenderness and guarding
  - any masses including their size, site and character
  - any enlargement of the liver, kidneys or spleen (often shortened to LKKS)
  - presence of ascites
  - bowel sounds (BS)

AS

Normal oral mucosa.
Upper midline scar.
Hernial orifices intact.
°tenderness or guarding.
°masses.
°LKKS or ascites.
BS normal.
PR not performed.
PV not performed.

- Rectal examination (PR): if not performed, record as such
- In women: vaginal examination (PV); only perform if relevant
- In men: external genitalia.

Nervous system (NS). The following should be noted:

- In older patients, record the abbreviated mental test (AMT) score (Ch. 1, p. 19)
- Speech abnormality
- Cranial nerves: record abnormalities only
- Fundoscopic abnormalities
- In those with impaired consciousness, head injury or where raised intracranial pressure is a possibility, record the Glasgow Coma Score (GCS).

The rest of the examination can be tabulated. The presence or absence of, for example, tremor, gait abnormality, fasciculation, dyspraxia, two-point discrimination, stereoagnosis, or sensory neglect should be recorded when relevant, but not routinely.

PERLA – pupils equal and reactive to light and accommodation
NAD – no abnormality detected
UL – upper limb
LL – lower limb
K – knee
A – ankle
B – biceps
T – triceps
S – supinator
Pl – plantar (flexor – ↓; extensor – ↑)
n – normal
+++ increased, ++ normal, + diminished, – absent

NS

AMT 9.
Cranial nerves II–XII: PERLA, NAD.
Ophthalmoscopy: °lens opacities, fundi poorly visualised; NAD.
Speech normal.

	Right		*Left*	
	UL	*LL*	*UL*	*LL*
Power	*5*	*5*	*5*	*5*
Tone	*n*	*n*	*n*	*n*
Light touch	*n*	*n*	*n*	*n*
Position	*n*	*n*	*n*	*n*
Coordination	*n*	*n*	*n*	*n*

Reflexes	*K*	*A*	*B*	*T*	*S*	*Pl*
R	++	+	++	+	+	↓
L	++	+	++	+	+	↓

Locomotor system (LMS):

- Deformities of the bones or joints in the limbs or spine
- Limitations of range of movement (ROM) in any joint.

LMS

Heberden's nodes on 2nd and 3rd fingers bilaterally.
Full ROM in all joints.
Crepitus in right knee. No other bony abnormality.

Clinical diagnosis or impression

- Record your conclusions from the history and examination and the most likely diagnoses in order of probability.
- In patients with multiple pathology, it is useful to construct a problem list so that the key issues can be grasped at once.

Impression

Active problems:

1. *Chest pain suggestive of unstable angina or acute myocardial infarction (MI)*
2. *Left breast lump and axillary node suspicious of neoplasia*
3. *Smoker.*

Inactive problems:

1. *Stable COPD*
2. *Perforated duodenal ulcer 1992*
3. *Possible osteoarthritis of right knee.*

Plan

- List the investigations required. When a result is already available, for example of an electrocardiograph, record it.
- Record any immediate management instigated.
- If uncertain about an investigation or treatment, precede with a '?' and discuss with a more senior member of staff.

Plan

ECG performed on admission shows sinus rhythm and deep ST depression in leads II, III and aVF.

Serial cardiac enzymes
Repeat ECG in 4 hours
Chest X-ray
Full blood count
Urea and electrolytes, glucose, cholesterol and triglycerides

Oxygen and cardiac monitor
Aspirin (already given)
Nitrate infusion
Enoxaparin
Diltiazem (beta-blocker contraindicated owing to COPD)
Advice to stop smoking

When stable:

1. *review anti-anginal management*
2. *referral for mammography and fine needle aspiration of breast lump*
3. *spirometry and assessment of inhaler technique.*

Information given

Document briefly what you have told the patient and any other family member. It is also important to document any diagnosis that you have not discussed.

Signature. A case record must always be signed, with the signatory's name printed below along with his or her status, e.g. Final year medical student, House Officer, Consultant.

Information given

Patient and daughter informed that chest pain is either an MI or a severe attack of angina. Treatment explained. Daughter warned of difficulty in predicting outcome.

NB. Breast lump not mentioned at this stage until further discussion with senior staff.

A. Doctor
A. DOCTOR
(House Officer)

Progress notes

All important information should be documented. This will vary depending upon the clinical situation. It should include:

- changes in the patient's symptoms
- the examination findings in the relevant system(s)
- results of new investigations
- the clinical impression of the patient's progress
- the plan for the patient's further management, particularly changes in drug treatments
- information or education given to the patient or the patient's relatives
- in patients undergoing rehabilitation, functional progress reported by nurses and therapists.

Entries should be made if the patient's condition changes unexpectedly, but it is also necessary to document day-to-day progress. The frequency of entries will depend on the speed with which the situation is changing. In an intensive therapy setting this may be several times a day, while in

3.8.99
1800

Ward Round – Dr Consultant

No further chest pain.

O/E
P70, BP 100/70.
JVP not elevated, °oedema.
HS I + II and ESM as above.

Chest clear.

Breast lump noted.

ECG at 4 hours – resolution of inferior ST changes.

CK: (1) 60
(2) 100.

Impression
Probable unstable angina – now settling.
Await final CK.

less acute settings, daily or even alternate daily notes may be more appropriate. All entries must be signed and dated.

CONCLUSION

Well-kept casenotes are vital for efficient and effective patient care. Mastering the skill of 'writing up' a case history can seem a daunting prospect at first, but with practice it becomes a routine part of everyday clinical practice.

Plan

Continue enoxaparin until pain-free for 48 hours.
Wean off IV nitrate from 0900 tomorrow.
For echocardiography in view of murmur.
Spirometry and assessment of inhaler technique.

Consultant to discuss finding of breast lump with patient and daughter.

A. Doctor
A. DOCTOR
(House Officer)

Index

A

B

C

T